THERAPY FOR NEUROLOGIC DISORDERS

THERAPY FOR NEUROLOGIC DISORDERS

Edited by

WIGBERT C. WIEDERHOLT, M.D.

Department of Neurosciences
School of Medicine
University of California, San Diego
La Jolla, California

1807 1982
175 YEARS OF PUBLISHING

A WILEY MEDICAL PUBLICATION

JOHN WILEY & SONS

New York • Chichester • Brisbane • Toronto • Singapore

Cover design by Wanda Lubelska

Library of Congress Cataloging in Publication Data

Main entry under title:

Therapy for neurologic disorders.

(A Wiley medical publication)
Includes index.
1. Nervous system—Diseases—Treatment.
I. Wiederholt, Wigbert C. II. Series.
RC349.8.T76 616.8′046 81-14768

ISBN 0-471-09508-7 AACR2

Printed in the United States of America

10 9 8 7 6 5 4 3 2 1

Contributors

J. Bruni, M.D., F.R.C.P.(C)
Postdoctoral Fellow in Neurophysiology and Neuropharmacology, Neurology Service
University of Florida College of Medicine
Veterans Administration Hospital
Gainesville, Florida

John P. Conomy, M.D.
Associate Clinical Professor
Department of Neurology
Case Western Reserve University Medical School
Chairman, Department of Neurology
Cleveland Clinic Foundation
Cleveland, Ohio

Marinos C. Dalakas, M.D.
Senior Staff Fellow
National Institute of Neurological Communicative Diseases and Strokes
National Institutes of Health
Bethesda, Maryland

W. King Engel, M.D.
Professor
Department of Neurology
Director, Center for Neuromuscular Diseases
University of Southern California School of Medicine
Los Angeles, California

Claudia M. Greco, M.D.
Assistant Professor of Pathology
University of California Medical Center, San Diego
San Diego, California

Charles Jablecki, M.D.
Assistant Professor
Department of Neurosciences
University of California Medical Center, San Diego
San Diego, California

Kenneth P. Johnson, M.D.
Professor and Chairman
Department of Neurology
University of Maryland School of Medicine
Baltimore, Maryland

Herbert R. Karp, M.D.
Professor and Chairman
Department of Neurology
Emory University School of Medicine
Atlanta, Georgia

Ronald M. Kobayashi, M.D.
Associate Clinical Professor
Department of Neurosciences
University of California, San Diego School of Medicine
La Jolla, California
Neurologist, Neurology Medical Clinic
Donald N. Sharp Community Hospital
San Diego, California

Lawrence F. Marshall, M.D.
Associate Professor
Department of Surgery
Chief, Neurosurgical Service
University of California Medical Center, San Diego
San Diego, California

George W. Paulson, M.D.
Clinical Professor
Department of Neurology
Ohio State University
School of Medicine
Program Director of Neurology
Riverside Methodist Hospital
Columbus, Ohio

Robert I. Roelofs, M.D.
Associate Professor
Department of Neurology
University of Minnesota
School of Medicine
Minneapolis, Minnesota

William A. Sibley, M.D.
Professor and Head
Department of Neurology
University of Arizona
Tucson, Arizona

Robert G. Siekert, M.D.
Professor
Department of Neurology
Mayo Medical School
Consultant in Neurology
Mayo Clinic
Rochester, Minnesota

B. J. Wilder, M.D.
Professor
Department of Neurology and
Neurosciences
University of Florida College of
Medicine
Chief, Neurology Service
Veterans Administration Medical Center
Gainesville, Florida

Dewey K. Ziegler, M.D.
Professor and Chairman
Department of Neurology
University of Kansas College
of Health Sciences
Kansas City, Kansas

Preface

Neurology is sometimes perceived as a medical specialty of astute diagnosticians who have little else to offer. During the last 25 years, however, exciting developments have taken place that are beginning to change this image. While advances have been too slow for those of us who have dedicated our professional lives to the care of patients with neurological disorders, therapeutic interventions—specific and nonspecific—that exist today could only be dreamed of several decades ago. Even though no specific treatment is available for some major neurological disorders, the judicious use of supportive therapies, including antibiotics, has had a significant impact on longevity and the quality of the lives of patients with chronic neurological disorders.

This book brings together the expertise of individuals who are recognized as leaders and innovators in their respective fields. The main focus is, of course, on therapy, and an attempt has been made to limit discussion of nontherapeutic modalities to those having a direct bearing on standard therapies and those that may lead to the development of new forms of treatment in the future. The book does include some treatment methods that are still experimental and some that are not accepted by the neurological community at large. Time will tell whether or not some of these treatments are dead-end roads or will open up exciting new vistas. Regardless, the widespread interest and enthusiasm in treating neurological disorders will directly or indirectly benefit our patients.

No attempt has been made to be all-inclusive. Regrettably, but unavoidably, when this book reaches its readers, some therapies may already be outdated. Fortunately, this also implies that the field is moving forward with great vigor and hope for the future.

W.C.W.

Acknowledgments

I am grateful to all contributors for lending their expertise to this book, for the efforts that went into their chapters, and for their patience while this endeavor came to fruition.

I would like to acknowledge Dr. Morton Rubinstein who, several years ago, provided the initiative and stimulus to begin work on this book.

The staff of John Wiley & Sons, Inc., have been most helpful; their assistance is greatly appreciated. Ms. Alice Macnow, in particular, is thanked for her effort.

A special thanks to my secretary, Mrs. Jean O. Robinson, whose patience, endurance, and good humor kept everything going.

W.C.W.

Contents

THERAPY FOR
NEUROLOGIC DISORDERS

1
Treatment of Certain Metabolic Encephalopathies

John P. Conomy

The metabolic encephalopathies comprise a heterogeneous and often ill-defined group of illnesses in which disturbances of brain function arise as a result of some illness outside the central nervous system (CNS). Metabolic encephalopathies disturb both the organization and function of the brain. All of these disorders are potentially reversible to a reasonably complete degree. Treatment of the metabolic encephalopathies is directed toward correction of the underlying condition as well as toward special measures designed to protect the nervous system from the deficiency of necessary substrates, the effects of toxins, and the residua of increased intracranial pressure when it exists.

Neurological literature, including publications of contemporary vintage, frequently suggests that distinctions exist between metabolic and structural disease of the brain, but in the final analysis that distinction may be highly artificial. It has been said that the metabolic encephalopathies lead first to a disturbance in functioning of the machinery of the nervous system, and then to the destruction of the machinery itself. The end results of metabolic CNS destruction are frequently visible with the microscope and occasionally to the naked eye. Many metabolic encephalopathies have clear and well-established structural counterparts. The characteristic gliosis of encephalopathy associated with liver failure is an example of such a counterpart. It is true that the pathologic basis of metabolic encephalopathies tends to be most apparent at the microscopic level, but striking gross pathologic changes in metabolic encephalopathies occasionally are encountered. The pseudolaminar necrosis and cavitary softening seen in anoxic encephalopathy are examples of gross pathologic change.

In a general way, the pathologic changes in metabolic encephalopathies tend to involve the entire brain. At times regional pathologic preponderance and selective zones of injury are observed. Selective and symmetric regions of injury are common in encephalopathies associated with nutritional deficiency, as exemplified by Wernike–Korsakoff disease. Encephalopathies associated with substrate deficiencies or failure of internal organs have less of a tendency to produce symmetric pathologic changes or to obey precise anatomic boundaries. The metabolic encephalopathies tend to affect neuronal structures (brain cortex, subcortical nuclei) more than they do white matter, although the latter may not be spared entirely. Demyelination of white matter, for instance, is a consequence of anoxic encephalopathy in individuals with long survival or in delayed-onset anoxic encephalopathy (1). In most metabolic encephalopathies, however, the clinical findings are far more impressive than are the pathologic changes. In some encephalopathies that are fatal, such as certain instances of chronic dialysis dementia, the macroscopic and microscopic appearance of brain may be virtually normal.

The etiologic approach to the metabolic encephalopathies assumes that either an endogenous or exogenous toxin or the lack of some essential metabolic substance produces brain disease. This is clearly the case in hypoglycemic and hypoxic encephalopathies, but it is less clearly proven in certain of the more chronic encephalopathies, such as some that are associated with long-standing renal or hepatic insufficiency. In these illnesses, the possible participation of viral, biochemical, or other injurious factors is not completely known. This chapter does not attempt to review, classify, and describe comprehensively the treatment of all the metabolic encephalopathies. To do so would require one or perhaps several textbooks, since virtually all categories of organ failure, intoxication, poisoning, or systemic disease affect the nervous system. This chapter will review the encephalopathies that are common and whose treatment has undergone change in the last decade as a result of advances in either pharmacology or technology. The chapter also will discuss selected forms of encephalopathy that confront the practicing neurologist but that generally are not covered in standard sources.

CLINICAL FINDINGS IN METABOLIC ENCEPHALOPATHIES

The clinical picture in the metabolic encephalopathies is dominated by certain common findings. These include defects in consciousness, intellectual function, and motor activity, with the frequent imposition of seizures. In general, focal neurologic abnormalities are not common in the metabolic encephalopathies (a few exceptions are mentioned below). The predominant focal findings in a patient with depressed consciousness should lead the examiner to the consideration of some other illness of the nervous system, such as tumor, hemorrhage, infarction, or demyelinating disease. Sensory and visual field disturbances are rare in metabolic brain disorders.

Defects in Consciousness and Intellectual Function

The general pattern of defects in the realm of the so-called higher cortical function in metabolic encephalopathies usually begins with distraction and slowness of thought. Defects in memory and concentration are usually evident next and ordinarily occur before the expression of psychotic thinking, delirium, and hallucinations. Depressed consciousness, stupor, and, finally, coma complete the natural progression of metabolic encephalopathies.

Abnormalities of Motor Function

Generalized muscle weakness without focal features is common to all the metabolic encephalopathies. Weakness frequently is limiting, and the patient loses voluntary mobility, at least in moderately advanced encephalopathies. Ataxia is not uncommon and occasionally is clearly of cerebellar type. Its presence, however, usually does not explain the motor limitations of most patients with metabolic brain disturbances. Muscle tone is variably affected, with hypotonia characteristic of most cases. Marked increases in muscle tone, however, occur in some instances of acute cerebral anoxia, uremia, and hepatic failure. Patients with metabolic encephalopathy associated with hepatic failure may show syndromes of spasticity or rigidity. Patients with liver coma rarely display decerebrate or decorticate postures. These postures resolve with successful treatment of the encephalopathic state. Isolated, random, and multifocal muscle twitching is common in metabolic encephalopathies and is frequently seen in particular in encephalopathies associated with renal failure and hyperosmolar states.

Seizures and Other Involuntary Movements

Any type of seizure, with the exception of true petit mal epilepsy, may be encountered in the metabolic encephalopathies. Nonfocal, generalized, grand mal seizures are most frequent and occasionally precede disorders of consciousness and intellectual function. They may constitute the initial clinical expression of metabolic brain illness. Most seizures that occur in metabolic encephalopathies, however, tend to do so later in the course of the disease, particularly in the setting of depressed consciousness. Myoclonic seizures, either as single, isolated jerks with consciousness preserved or as massive, repetitive episodes in an unconscious patient, are the next most common type of seizure found in metabolic brain disorders; in addition, they are the most resistant to treatment. Myoclonic fits occur commonly in anoxic and uremic encephalopathies. Although focal seizures are not common in metabolic encephalopathies, many cases of hyperosmolar nonketotic hyperglycemic encephalopathy and occasional instances of lead encephalopathy provide clear exceptions to this observation.

Involuntary movements other than seizures are common in metabolic encephalopathies and occur in general in patients with abnormalities of mental state. Asterixis refers to a flapping tremor of the outstretched limbs. It is common in encephalopathy associated with liver failure but is not pathognomonic of that disease. First described in liver disease in 1949 by Adams and Foley (2), asterixis has been documented since in individuals with chronic renal disease, pulmonary insufficiency, gastrointestinal disturbances, and a variety of drug intoxications (3). While asterixis is commonly elicited in the outstretched hands and arms, it may at times be widespread (see section on hepatic encephalopathy). Chorea, dystonia, and athetosis comprise other abnormal involuntary movements associated with internal organ failure. These movements tend to occur in long-standing and advanced instances of disease.

TREATMENT OF METABOLIC ENCEPHALOPATHIES

Treatment of the metabolic encephalopathies frequently is complex, always supportive, and, in general, is aimed at correction of the underlying condition either by removal of some systemic toxin or by administration of the depleted systemic substrate. Treatment is directed less frequently at the nervous system itself; if it is, it usually aims at reduction of elevated intracranial pressure (as in Reye's syndrome), the treatment of seizures (as in uremic encephalopathy), or at prevention of deficiencies of brain substrate or cofactor (e.g., administration of glucose in hypoglycemic encephalopathy, administration of thiamine in parenteral hyperalimentation). The "toxin" that causes brain impairment in the common encephalopathies related to organ failure, such as those associated with liver and kidney disease, is unknown. Ammonia and various amines compete for the dubious honor in the case of liver disease (see below). Some nitrogenous waste or, perhaps, the hydrogen ion itself may be the culprit in the case of kidney failure. Treatment of these conditions and the others discussed in this section is virtually never aimed at the correction of a single factor alone, but rather at the simultaneous or sequential correction of a number of abnormalities that characterize the patient's clinical state. Improvement and restoration of brain function generally occurs as a by-product of the correction of multiple systemic abnormalities. Uremic encephalopathy is a clear example of this general pattern; the patient with uremia is victimized not only by an increased nitrogen load, but also by acidosis of body fluids, hypocalcemia, vascular hypertension, fluid overload, frequent hyponatremia, and a host of other metabolic disturbances. Restoration of more normal brain function depends on treatment of all of these imbalances.

It is characteristic of patients with metabolic encephalopathy, particularly encephalopathy caused by organ failure or severe electrolyte disturbances (e.g., syndrome of inappropriate antidiuretic hormone secretion) that improvement of certain laboratory parameters (e.g., restoration of electrolyte balance) precedes the clinical improvement of brain function. Several hours, sometimes days, may pass before the patient appears to be as well clinically as they do according to laboratory reports. Exceptions to expected improvement must be made for individuals in whom substantial cerebral anoxia accompanies metabolic encephalopathy, since improvement in these patients is a function of the duration of the insult. Anoxic anoxia, severe hypoglycemia, and iatrogenic Wernicke–Korsakoff disease are clear examples of metabolic encephalopathies that remain severe or become permanent or fatal in spite of eventual correction of the metabolic disorder. Why patient improvement so frequently lags behind correction of metabolic abnormalities in many of the ultimately correctable metabolic encephalopathies is unclear. However, nearly all such conditions are associated with significant and frequently prolonged depression of cerebral respiration and blood flow; the encephalopathies of hepatic and renal disease are clear examples. The neurologist must advise his or her colleagues of this lag in patients whose improvement has not kept pace with documented correction of the underlying disease or abnormal metabolic state. Much of the treatment of metabolic encephalopathies has become highly technologized. The frequent use of life-support systems (e.g., dialysis, controlled ventilation, prolonged parenteral alimentation, hemoperfusion, continuous intravascular and intracranial monitoring) is increasing, and these methods constitute major additions to the "new neurology".

HEPATIC ENCEPHALOPATHY

In his writings Hippocrates described abnormalities of mental state that culminated in coma in jaundiced patients (4). Bright in 1836 (5) and Frerichs in 1860 (6) gave clear and complete accounts of rapidly developing coma in patients with obvious fulminant liver disease. While jaundice need not be present for a diagnosis of hepatic coma, that state accompanies liver disease of any cause and is encountered most frequently in patients with Laennec's cirrhosis and in those with viral, toxic, or drug-induced hepatic necrosis. Hepatic coma usually develops fairly rapidly and may be precipitated by excessive gastrointestinal protein load, gastrointestinal bleeding, intercurrent infection, hypokalemia, or the use of certain drugs, such as thiazide diuretics. Individuals with long-standing, slowly progressive liver disease or portal-systemic shunts may develop chronic forms of hepatic encephalopathy in which dementia and movement disorders similar to those encountered in Wilson's disease are seen. Patients with chronic portal-systemic encephalopathy occasionally may develop spinal cord disease that produces spastic diplegia (7).

At the outset of cerebral symptoms, patients with hepatic coma most commonly first show evidence of distraction, excitement or apathy, memory impairment, and disorganization of personal activity. Their complaints, however, may include generalized weakness, muscle aches, vague headache, and a variety of other minor woes. This prodromal phase is often associated with mild hypothermia. The prodrome may be very brief or, depending on the extent of liver damage and the cause, may last for days. Delirium, hallucinations, and seizures are not frequent prodromal symptoms in hepatic coma, although any of them may occur. Their presence, however, should suggest some additional illness, such as drug or alcohol withdrawal, brain injury, or infection. Asterixis develops and parallels the progressive confusion of hepatic encephalopathy. The movement disorder ordinarily can be detected in the tongue and feet whenever it is present in the hands. The actual flapping motion of asterixis has been shown to be associated with electromyographic silence in muscle (8). This silence, in turn, is thought to be due to inhibitory influences on alpha motor neurons which originate in these brain cells as by-products of metabolic disturbance. On rare occasions, asterixis is so widespread that it approaches true myoclonus in its effects and may impair walking. Asterixis also may be present unilaterally in an otherwise unimpaired limb, although this rarely occurs. In my experience, this finding should lead to a search for a structural lesion that involves the contralateral hemisphere. Ericson et al. have reported unilateral asterixis with stenosis of the contralateral carotid in a patient with renal failure (9). Asterixis does not occur in paralyzed limbs.

As hepatic encephalopathy develops, confusion worsens and gives way to stupor then to coma. Coma is marked ordinarily by a lack of focal signs except for variably and occasionally unilaterally abnormal plantar reactions. Hepatic coma may develop with dramatic suddenness in some patients and, in a few, it may coexist with focal neurologic findings. Conomy and Swash (10) have described the sudden appearance of decorticate and decerebrate postures in a group of patients with hepatic coma. The postural abnormalities cleared with treatment of the encephalopathy. These individuals resemble patients with brain-stem infarctions or hemorrhages in the appearance of postural abnormality; however, cranial-nerve, caloric, and oculocephalic examinations do not suggest structural disease of the brain stem tegmentum, or tectum.

As hepatic encephalopathy worsens and tends toward coma, respiratory hyperventilation becomes prominent. The pattern of respiration is rapid, deep, and regular, clearly resembling that seen in central pontine hyperventilation. As a consequence of uninhibited respiratory drive, patients in hepatic coma are generally alkalotic as a result of pulmonary loss of carbon dioxide. Fetor hepaticus, an indescribable pulmonary stench, characterizes hepatic coma and has been shown to be caused by the accumulation of dimethylsulfide and, to a lesser extent, methane thiol in the exhaled breath (11).

Etiology of Hepatic Coma

The central role of abnormal nitrogen metabolism, particularly that involving ammonia, has been explored for more than 100 years. It is far from clear, however, that excessive amounts of ammonia alone is the cause of hepatic encephalopathy or hepatic coma. In cases of hepatic encephalopathy in which hepatocellular failure is prominent, hyperammonemia is accompanied by faulty production of glucose, impaired hepatic glycolysis and gluconeogenesis, impaired operation of the Krebs–Henseleit urea cycle, and reduced clearance of toxic substances other than ammonia resulting from bacterial action upon proteins and amino acids in the gut. In instances of hepatic encephalopathy associated with portocaval bypass, both hyperammonemia and impaired clearance of toxic factors originating in the gut are present. Thus, it is not clear that increased levels of ammonia alone are responsible for hepatic coma. Short-chain fatty acids also have been shown to be increased in the blood and cerebrospinal fluid (CSF) of patients with hepatic encephalopathy produced by any of various causes (12). Infusion of these fatty acids has been shown to cause reversible coma in laboratory animals. The etiologic factors related to the genesis of hepatic coma have been reviewed recently by Fisher and Baldessarini (13) and by Schenker et al. (14).

Laboratory Abnormalities in Hepatic Encephalopathy

Abnormalities of liver function usually are present in hepatic coma, but their severity is not necessarily correlated with the severity of the encephalopathy or with the presence or absence of coma. In some patients with portocaval bypass, results of routine tests of liver function may be normal, yet the patient may have severe encephalopathy (10). Although patients with hepatic encephalopathy generally have some degree of hyperammonemia, the hyperammonemia does not bear a clear relation to the severity of the brain disturbance.

Most patients with fully developed hepatic coma are hyponatremic, hypokalemic and alkalotic and show depression of blood urea nitrogen (BUN). Acidosis, although it appears in very few patients, may be caused by production of lactic acid. Cerebral blood flow is reduced in hepatic coma, probably as a function of alkalosis and depression of $PaCO_2$, and the cerebral metabolic rate of oxygen also is reduced. Hypoglycemia and concomitant renal failure are not uncommon findings; the latter is marked by rising levels of BUN, creatinine, and serum potassium associated with declining urinary output.

The CSF usually is normal in all respects but may be tinged yellow from the presence of bilirubin if the victim is moderately jaundiced. It should not be assumed, however, that even slight CSF xanthochromia is due to bilirubin since individuals with liver disease are also frequently autoanticoagulated and may have intracranial hemorrhagic conditions. Computed tomographic brain scanning is a safe and useful diagnostic aid in this setting for determining whether there is intracranial hemorrhage. While modest elevation of CSF protein may occur for unknown reasons in fewer than 10% of patients with hepatic coma, even modest elevations usually indicate a serious underlying disease, such as cryptococcal meningitis (15).

The Electroencephalogram in Hepatic Encephalopathy

The electroencephalogram (EEG) is generally conceded to be a sensitive but nonspecific test both for hepatic encephalopathy and for monitoring its course. In the early 1950s, Adams and Foley (16) described characteristic changes in the EEG of patients with encephalopathy. As the encephalopathy worsens, minor EEG abnormalities give way to paroxysmal slowing, evident first frontally and then centrally. As coma deepens, high-voltage, bilaterally synchronous activity described as mountainous and monotonous predominates the entire record, including the recorded regions of the posterior brain. Silverman (17) described pseudo–petit mal and other pseudoparoxysmal EEG records in patients with hepatic encephalopathy. In my experience, pseudo–petit mal records are uncommon and occur only in the early stages of hepatic stupor. Other pseudoparoxysmal records are more common. EEG changes reverse with successful treatment and worsen with clinical deterioration. For this reason, the EEG can be a fairly sensitive monitoring device in the course of treatment of hepatic encephalopathy.

Acquired Chronic Hepatocerebral Degeneration

In 1965, Victor et al. (18) described 27 patients who developed chronic encephalopathy associated with acquired (non-Wilsonian) liver disease. These individuals displayed various but ordinarily severe combinations of dementia, dysarthria, ataxia, pyramidal-tract signs, and involuntary movements of the choreoathetoid variety. Both their clinical pictures and the pathologic changes, including the appearance of Opalski cells, in the brain resembled those seen in Wilson's disease. Persons with acquired chronic hepatocerebral degeneration clearly lack the family history of liver or brain disease, Kayser–Fleischer rings, and characteristic abnormalities of copper metabolism diagnostic of Wilson's disease (19). It subsequently has become clear that persons with any type of long-standing liver disease, including postnecrotic and biliary cirrhosis, can develop a persistent and progressive syndrome in which dementia and movement disorders are the most prominent features. Such cases also suggest that the neurologic disorder in Wilson's disease may be more a by-product of the hepatic abnormality in that condition that a direct result of cerebral copper intoxication. Both reduction of protein load in the gut and colonic exclusion have been attempted as treatment in patients with acquired chronic hepatic encephalopathy. Prognosis is poor in these patients, however. A few improve, particularly if they are treated in the early stages of the illness and if they are capable of some functional hepatic regeneration and recovery. Patients with advanced disease usually remain disabled by a combination of dementia and movement disorder.

Treatment of Hepatic Encephalopathy

Hepatic encephalopathy is preventable if the susceptible patient is identified before symptoms appear and if dietary management, gut sterilization, or other therapeutic measures tailored to the individual are carried out. Offending drugs must be avoided, and intercurrent illness that may precipitate encephalopathy must be prevented or treated promptly. While hepatic coma is potentially reversible, mortality in fully developed episodes is 60% or higher. Mortality depends on the degree and duration of the encephalopathy, the age of the patient, the nature of the underlying liver disease, and the extent and types of intercurrent illnesses (20,21). The appearance of encephalopathy of any degree in a patient with well-compensated liver failure and without apparent cause (e.g., infection, drugs) should always suggest occult gastrointestinal bleeding from esophageal varices, gastric or duodenal ulcer, or intestinal tract tumor. In patients who lack an obvious cause, the initial step in neurologic assessment is a rectal examination with testing of the stool for the presence of blood.

General principles of treatment in hepatic encephalopathy consist of the reduction of gastrointestinal protein load (including blood), correction of fluid and electrolyte abnormalities, avoidance of potentially injurious drugs and substances, and use of therapies that diminish the intestinal production of ammonia or enhance its elimination from the body. The use of pharmacologic agents to correct the hypothesized alteration of brain neurotransmitters has attained some popularity recently. Heroic measures, such as cross-circulation and liver transplantation, are employed infrequently and usually are reserved for acute, severe instances of liver disease in previously healthy individuals with advanced and fulminating encephalopathy. Current treatment modalities are summarized below and are outlined in Table 1.

Reduction of Gastrointestinal Protein Load

Reduction of protein load in the gut is achieved by temporary restriction of dietary protein and removal of blood from the stomach or colon by appropriate means (i.e., colonic lavage, endoscopic aspiration). Correction of bleeding varices

Table 1. Treatment of Hepatic Encephalopathy

PROPHYLACTIC TREATMENT
Reduction of dietary protein load
Avoidance of injurious drugs
Tranquilizers, thiazides, narcotics, short-acting barbiturates, glutethimide, and others
Reduction of total nitrogen burden
Diet, gut sterilization with antibiotics, lactulose, judicious blood transfusion, surgical colonic exclusion
Avoidance of injurious procedures
Rapid diuresis, removal of large amounts of ascites by paracentesis
ACTIVE TREATMENT
Pharmacologic
Electrolyte correction
Administration of glutamic and other amino acids
Acetohydroxamic acid
Vitamins
Corticosteroids
Colonization of bowel with *Lactobacillus*
Technologic
Gastrointestinal lavage
Colonic bypass
Exchange transfusion
Hypothermia
Dialysis
Hemoperfusion
Cross-circulation

and other sources of blood loss is performed by various types of intestinal intubation, lavage, and tamponade. Dietary protein should be restricted to 20–40 g/day in persons with mild encephalopathy. Patients with moderate or more severe encephalopathies and who are able to eat should receive protein-free diets.

Reduction of Gastrointestinal Ammonia Production

Most ammonia in the body is produced by bacteria in the gut, particularly in the colon. Use of enemas to remove colonic contents is followed by either gastric or colonic instillation of neomycin sulfate (4–6 g/day for stuporous or comatose patients, followed by 2 g/day in divided doses if the antibiotic is to be used after resolution of severe encephalopathy). Neomycin, as well as other antibiotics, reduces the production of ammonia by coliform bacteria. If neither oral nor rectal neomycin can be used for any reason, treatment with parenteral tetracycline is suggested, with the caveat that high doses of tetracyclines can be hepatotoxic. Colonization of the gut with *Lactobacillus,* an organism that does not produce ammonia, has been tried but has proved to be impractical.

Correction of Fluid and Electrolyte Abnormalities

The frequent association of hypokalemia and hyponatremia with hepatic encephalopathy has been pointed out. These deficiencies should be judiciously corrected. Hypomagnesemia is not uncommon and must be treated as well. Hypophosphatemia of moderate degree is common, and profound hypophosphatemia is rare in hepatic encephalopathy (see section on hypophosphatemic coma). The alkalosis that frequently occurs in patients with hepatic coma usually resolves with correction of the hypokalemia and resolution of the hyperventilatory state. Concomitant renal failure (hepatorenal syndrome) is a constant hazard and requires monitoring of urine output and BUN, creatinine, serum potassium, and serum calcium levels. Glycolysis and gluconeogenesis are impaired in patients with hepatic encephalopathy, and sufficient calories must be provided to offset these disorders. This can be accomplished safely over the short term by administration of parenteral glucose.

Avoidance of Injurious Drugs, Substances, and Procedures

A number of drugs, substances, and procedures are known either to precipitate or worsen hepatic encephalopathy. It is best to avoid tranquilizers, thiazide diuretics, narcotics, short-acting barbiturates, paraldehyde, and certain hypnotics (glutethimide and chloral hydrate). The hepatic hazards of large doses of tetracycline have been pointed out already. Rapid diuresis by any means, including rapid removal of large volumes of ascitic fluid, can result in significant hypovolemia, which is a precipitating cause of hepatic encephalopathy. The hazards of blood transfusion and nosocomial sepsis related to procedures such as dialysis or use of steroid drugs are well known.

The measures listed above constitute the major aspects of treatment of hepatic encephalopathy. A number of other new, adjunctive, or less clearly beneficial treatments also may be directed toward patients with brain dysfunction secondary to hepatic disease.

Lactulose Therapy

Lactulose (β-1,4-galactosidofructose) is a synthetic disaccharide that is derived from lactose. It is neither degraded nor absorbed to any appreciable extent in the upper gastrointestinal tract of humans but is acted on by bacterial fermentation in the colon, in which lactic and acetic acids are produced. These acids lower the pH of the colonic contents, which, in turn, promotes the egress of ammonia from the blood to the colonic lumen (22). Lactulose also is a cathartic that is comparable to sorbitol and may reduce ammonia levels partially through enematic action (23). In the course of facilitating loss of colonic ammonia, lactulose produces flatulence, abdominal distention, nausea, vomiting, and a tendency toward diarrhea. Individual daily doses must be balanced against these side effects. Lactulose has been used successfully in treatment of chronic hepatic encephalopathy and in prevention of recurrent, episodic encephalopathy associated with liver failure in susceptible persons. The use of lactulose may permit liberalization of protein intake in some patients prone to encephalopathy; thus, its use may improve their nutritional status as well. Lactulose is available as a syrup that contains both galactose, lactose, and other sugars in addition to lactulose. Administration usually consists of an oral dose of 20–30 g/day (30–45 ml of syrup). Double the amount may be given the first day or two of treatment if rapid action is desired and if the patient can tolerate the gastrointestinal side effects.

L-Dopa Therapy

In the early 1970s, investigators working independently in England, France, and the United States reported beneficial effects of L-dopa on the course of severe hepatic encephalopathy (24–26). Selected patients with severe degrees of coma were shown to become increasingly alert and to respond with purposeful motor activity after treatment with L-dopa. Treatment consists of administration of large amounts of L-dopa (up to 5 g/day) via a nasogastric tube. The alerting effect of L-dopa in liver coma is thought to be fairly specific, since the infusion of norepinephrine and epinephrine did not have a similar effect (24).

The theoretic basis for the use of L-dopa in patients with hepatic encephalopathy originates in the fact that the drug increases systemic levels of certain biogenic amines, such as β-phenylethanolamine and octopamine. These substances may act as false neurotransmitters in the brain and thus contribute to the evolution of coma. Their deleterious action allegedly is subverted by excess brain dopamine that originates as L-dopa. Most series of patients with hepatic encephalopathy who received L-dopa and who experienced success have been small in size, uncontrolled, and included patients who received a number of other therapies shortly before or simultaneously with L-dopa. Furthermore, many patients with liver coma do not respond to L-dopa. At present there is no general agreement about the use of this drug in the treatment of encephalopathy associated with liver failure. Bromocriptine, a dopamine-receptor agonist with prolonged action, has recently been reported to be beneficial in the treatment of chronic hepatic encephalopathy when the agent is combined with restriction of dietary protein (27).

Drugs That Limit Ammonia Production or Increase Ammonia Removal

Certain amino acids and amino-acid derivatives that are capable of removing ammonia from the circulation have been used in the treatment of hepatic encephalopathy. Glutamic acid, arginine, and protamine are examples of such substances. All of them have enjoyed periods of popularity, but it is not clear that they are effective in treatment. Acetohydroxamic acid, an inhibitor of bacterial urease in the gastrointestinal tract, is a drug that recently has been used in an attempt to limit ammonia production in the gut (28). Since intestinal hydrolysis of urea by ureases of bacterial origin is a major biologic source of ammonia, theoretically the substance may be useful. The use of this drug in treatment, however, along with immunization-induced inhibition of urease, is not yet clearly established. Exchange resins that release potassium are used occasionally in therapy, but they carry a risk of hyperkalemia because, in general, these resins exchange potassium for ammonia in the gut. Serum potassium must be monitored frequently during the course of therapy with these drugs.

Recolonization of the Colon

Recolonization of the bowel with *Lactobacillus,* which, unlike coliform bacteria, do not produce ammonia, also has been attempted in the treatment of hepatic encephalopathy. Lactobacilli are fed to patients, and with a sufficient bacterial load, the organisms competitively colonize the large bowel. This theoretically attractive therapy has not yet achieved firm standing in the therapeutic armamentarium.

Use of Vitamins

Both pyridoxine and lipoic (thiotic) acid have been suggested as remedies for hepatic encephalopathy, but neither has been shown to be particularly effective (29). Thiamine should be administered to patients with hepatic encephalopathy because that condition is associated frequently with chronic alcoholism or malnutrition. The likelihood of dealing with a vitamin-deficient patient in the course of treatment of hepatic encephalopathy is great. It is probable that the administration of replacement doses of multivitamins ultimately will be of some benefit to these patients.

Use of Adrenal Steroids for Hepatic Coma

The use of corticosteroids is clearly beneficial in patients with chronic active hepatitis, particularly in females with nonalcoholic cirrhosis (30) and in cases of idiosyncratic, drug-induced liver damage, whether it occurs as an isolated illness or accompanies the Stevens–Johnson syndrome. Although initial, encouraging reports of the therapeutic effects of steroids in clearly developed hepatic encephalopathy (31) have not been confirmed by subsequent experience, their use in treatment of this illness is fairly widespread, and their dubious benefit must be weighed against the potential side effects.

Colonic Bypass Procedures

Colectomy and intestinal bypass procedures have been used in the treatment of acute and chronic hepatic encephalopathy. Both techniques prevent the colon from maintaining a cesspool connection with the systemic circulation with respect to ammonia (32). Surgical procedures of this type, however, are associated with significant morbidity and mortality because they must be performed in patients who are very ill. In both rerouting procedures, the terminal ileum remains capable of being colonized with coliform bacteria. The recolonized segment then can act as a new nidus for the formation of ammonia and nitrogenous waste.

Heroic and Experimental Procedures for Hepatic Coma

A number of procedures have been developed during the last 15 years that are heroic, experimental, or both in relation to the treatment of hepatic encephalopathy and hepatic coma. These methods are applied most frequently to patients with subacute, progressive, severe encephalopathies that develop in the course of massive hepatic necrosis that is viral, toxic, or drug induced. They have been employed less frequently for hepatic coma resulting from chronic liver disease.

Exchange transfusion in hepatic encephalopathy is carried out with heparinized, fresh, whole blood. The procedure has been shown to be beneficial in some instances of transfusion hepatitis, infectious hepatitis, and drug-related hepatic necrosis, but it does not appear to be beneficial in halothane-induced acute liver atrophy (33). Even after successful exchange transfusion, some patients do not improve; if they do improve, they may subsequently succumb to some complication of the liver disease.

Hypothermic total-body perfusion, hemodialysis, peritoneal dialysis, plasmapheresis, hemoperfusion, and liver transplantation are other heroic measures that are employed rarely but that occasionally have benefit in patients with fulminant liver necrosis and severe encephalopathy. Cross-circulation of the patient's blood with that of other humans or of baboons, or perfusion of the patient's blood through a liver removed from a cow, pig, or other animal or through artificial organs also has been attempted with varying results. Clinical trials of dialytic procedures, cell–plasma separation, and plasma perfusion are now under way in a number of institutions that treat patients with chronic hepatic encephalopathy. As the safety and reliability of the new technology increases, it is likely that such methods will in the future be removed from the category of heroic procedures.

Among the new techniques that are gaining some acceptance is hemoperfusion. In hemoperfusion, solutes are extracted from blood through their adherence to charcoal (charcoal hemoperfusion); or to some other sorbent in an extracorporeal system. A number of synthetic sorbents have been developed for differential solute affinity. Early trials with hemoperfusion were fraught with difficulties produced by cell damage and trapping of formed blood elements in the perfusion device or by failure or embolization of the sorbent. Technical advances that vary the size of the sorbent particulate, or that use coatings and filtration devices have overcome these difficulties, and the techniques of hemoperfusion are now seeing more widespread use in the treatment of encephalopathies associated with hepatic failure, uremia, and exogenous poisoning (34,35).

REYE'S SYNDROME (REYE–JOHNSON SYNDROME)

A severe and frequently fatal encephalopathy that occurs in childhood and is associated with fatty degeneration of the viscera was described in 1963 by Reye et al. (36) in Australia. At the same time that this report appeared, Johnson et al. (37) in the United States described a similar illness. The cause of the syndrome is unknown. Mortality is high in spite of increasingly technologically oriented supportive treatment, such as hemodialysis and monitoring of intracranial pressure. Reye's syndrome represents generalized pathologic dysfunction of the heart, lungs, pancreas, skeletal muscle, brain, liver, and kidneys.

The disease usually afflicts children between the ages of 6 months and late teens (average 6–10 years). Nearly every case occurs within one week after the onset of varicella, influenza, or some other banal infection, usually of a respiratory type. Vomiting is the rule during the day or two before the first symptoms of encephalopathy appear. Anorexia, apathy, and listlessness are early markers of the disease, and lethargy, immobility, agitated delirium, confusion, and slurred speech follow. Coma with elevated intracranial pressure, decerebrate or decorticate posture, and hyperventilation may supervene. Profound coma, loss of brain-stem reflexes, and flaccid paralysis are the cardinal signs before death. An increased incidence of Reye's syndrome followed an epidemic of influenza B in the United States in the winter of 1973–1974 (38). A number of other viruses have been implicated in the disorder, but their etiologic relation to Reye's syndrome has not been proved. These include type 1 vaccinelike poliovirus (39), herpesvirus, myxovirus-paramyxovirus-like organisms (40), and picornavirus (41).

Pathology

Light microscopy of tissue in Reye's syndrome discloses infiltration of fatty droplets without an inflammatory reaction. Electron microscopic studies of hepatic mitochondria in Reye's syndrome reveal characteristic abnormalities that include swelling, decreased matrix density, and loss of dense bodies. The formation of fatty droplets represents collections of triglycerides in the hepatic cells. The mitochondrial abnormalities in the liver are reversible in patients who survive the illness (42).

Reye's syndrome is not the only encephalopathy of childhood that produces stupor, coma, and hepatic pathology. Acute liver disease with encephalopathy that does not involve other organ systems can occur in childhood and can be confused with Reye's syndrome (43). The confusion between Reye's syndrome and diseases similar to it can be resolved with liver biopsy, which, if it must be performed, should be done within the first two days of the clinically symptomatic phase of the disease (44). Liver biopsy can be performed safely in children with Reye's syndrome within 24 hours after administration of vitamin K to correct abnormal prothrombin time.

Brain pathology in Reye's syndrome consists of damage to glial cells, myelin, and neurons (45). Astrocytes show swelling of both the cell bodies and their processes, and pyknosis occurs in the neurons. Blisterlike vesicles arise from myelin sheaths throughout the brain. Electron microscopy shows damage to the mitochondria of neurons not unlike that seen in the liver. These findings occur in association with increased brain weight resulting from edema and with gross evidence of cerebral herniation in patients dying of the disease.

Laboratory Findings

Laboratory findings in Reye's syndrome consist of hypoglycemia, hypoxemia, vascular hypertension, and elevated intracranial pressure. Lethargy and stupor occur early in the disease, and coma evolves rapidly. Huttenlocher (46) has developed a system of staging the severity of Reye's syndrome on the basis of levels of consciousness and other neurologic findings. The cause of coma cannot be attributed directly to liver failure, since liver failure is only one aspect of the illness. It is known, however, that the hepatic lesion of Reye's syndrome limits the production of ornithine transcarbamylase and carbamyl phosphate synthetase (47). In addition to the viral and biochemical abnormalities of Reye's syndrome, an aflatoxin (a toxic metabolite of *Aspergillus flavus*) has been identified in the liver of a 15-year-old patient dying of the disease (48). As with hepatic coma, levels of short-chain fatty acids have been shown to be elevated in the blood of patients with Reye's syndrome (49).

Treatment

Treatment of Reye's syndrome (Table 2) is based on early recognition of the clinical condition, strong supportive care, and constant monitoring of vital functions, including intracranial pressure. Respiratory intubation and monitoring of blood gases are essential in comatose persons. Patients with Reye's syndrome generally are alkalotic, and precautions must be taken not to raise the P_{CO_2} while

Table 2. Modalities of Treatment in Reye's Syndrome

EEG monitoring
Intravascular monitoring
Plasma volume
Venous pressure
P_{CO_2}, P_{O_2} (blood)
Ventilatory control
Regulation of P_{CO_2}
Pharmacologic reduction of intracranial pressure
Mannitol
Dexamethasone
Urea
Parenteral correction of hypoglycemia and electrolyte abnormalities
Exchange transfusion
Dialysis
Hemodialysis
Peritoneal dialysis

the intracranial pressure is elevated. Elevation of the P_{CO_2} would increase intracranial pressure as a consequence of expansion of the vascular compartment of the intracranial contents. Ventilatory control must be achieved, and it is necessary at times to induce paralysis of respiration pharmacologically in an effort to maintain such control. Intracranial pressure is usually controlled with osmotic diuretics, particularly mannitol. Urea and dexamethasone also have been employed to reduce brain swelling. Intracranial pressure can be monitored with either a subarachnoid (Richmond) screw or an intraventricular cannula connected to a pressure transducer. Monitoring of all other vital functions must also be maintained. Constant attention must be given to serum concentrations of potassium, phosphorus, and calcium and to the development of azotemia. Serum osmolality and urine output also must be monitored carefully.

Exchange transfusion and peritoneal dialysis have been used in the treatment of Reye's syndrome with variable effectiveness (50). Exchange transfusion has been shown to lower elevated intracranial pressure (51).

In spite of immense treatment efforts, Reye's syndrome remains a highly fatal illness. DeVivo and colleagues (52) have shown that early treatment and vigorous supportive care lead to increased rates of survival, even when exchange transfusion and peritoneal dialysis are not performed. Mortality was 86% in Reye's original report of 1963. A decade later, in the 1973–1974 epidemic, mortality in 349 cases was 41% (53).

ENCEPHALOPATHY ASSOCIATED WITH RENAL DISEASE

There are few other areas of modern medicine in which advances in treatment and technology have been employed as rapidly and with such obvious benefit as they have in the treatment of renal disease. Individuals with acute or chronic kidney failure now enjoy better-quality survival and, with the use of various forms of dialysis and renal transplantation, long periods of freedom from disease. At times, frank and outright cure of kidney failure is possible. New treatment methods, however, have given rise to new varieties of neurologic disease, and this fact is particularly obvious in the area of chronic renal failure. The neurologic aspects of renal disease have been reviewed comprehensively by Raskin and Fishman (54) and by Tyler (55).

The forms of nervous system illness that we will consider in the setting of renal disease include uremic encephalopathy, dialysis dysequilibrium syndrome, dialysis dementia, and Wernicke–Korsakoff disease. Treatment of these conditions is summarized in Table 3. The last three illnesses on the list arise, not from renal disease per se, but from some aspect of its treatment. They are far more common as complications of therapy for chronic rather than acute renal failure. In the setting of renal disease, as in the setting of any other organ failure, it is prudent to exclude other varieties of brain illnesses from the differential diagnosis of encephalopathy. In renal disease, these other illnesses include brain tumors, CNS lymphomas, fungal and parasitic infections of the brain, and rare instances of central pontine myelinolysis. Brain tumors occur more frequently in persons who have undergone renal transplantation, and the incidence of sarcomas of brain among recipients of transplanted kidneys is much greater than in a control population. CNS lymphomas, as with lymphomas in other systems and organs, are more common in these patients as well. Chronic immunosuppression is thought to play a role in the genesis of brain sarcomas and of systemic and nervous system lymphomas. Systemic toxoplasmosis, cryptococcosis, and cytomegalovirus infections are common in immunosuppressed individuals with renal disease.

Uremic Encephalopathy

As with most encephalopathies associated with organ failure, there is no characteristic course of illness and no outstanding or pathognomonic sign or symptom that distinguishes uremic encephalopathy from that associated with a variety of other organ failures, intoxications, or poisonings. Uremic encephalopathy is characterized by fluctuating and progressively severe clinical signs, which usually include slurred speech, mental confusion, and slowness of thought. Disorientation, ataxia, and weakness frequently accompanied by asterixis and muscle twitching appear early in the course of the disease. Myoclonus, while common in uremic encephalopathy, appears later. Confusion and mental sluggishness give way to stupor and then to flaccid coma. Delusions and hallucinations are not uncommon as uremic encephalopathy progresses. The uremic encephalopathic state, however, is not associated with papilledema. When papilledema appears in uremia, some preexisting intracranial disease, such as subdural hemorrhage, brain tumor, or hypertensive encephalopathy, must be considered. Tremulousness is extremely common in uremic encephalopathy, and the distal tremor resembles that seen in hyperthyroid states. Aside from myalgic twitching, asterixis, and myoclonus, other movement disorders rarely occur in uremic encephalopathy. Chorea and hemiballism, however, have been reported. Tetany sometimes occurs in chronic renal failure and ordinarily is seen in patients with hyperphosphatemia. Tetany coexists paradoxically with acidosis and is common in patients with asterixis and myoclonus.

Table 3. Encephalopathies That Occur in the Course of Renal Disease

Type of Encephalopathy	*Treatment Measures*
Uremic encephalopathy	Protein restriction, correction of acidosis, fluid restriction, correction of hyponatremia, hypocalcemia, hyperkalemia, hyperphosphatemia, treatment of vascular hypertension, prevention of vitamin deficiency including Wernicke-Korsakoff disease, prevention of viral hepatitis, treatment of seizures, dialysis, hemoperfusion, renal transplantation
Dialysis dementia	Anticonvulsants, tranquilizers, chelators, physostigmine, intensified dialysis (?) (all treatment generally ineffective)
Dialysis dysequilibrium syndrome	Fluid restriction, sedation, anticonvulsants, electrolyte correction
Treatment-related Wernicke-Korsakoff syndrome	Thiamine, multivitamins
Hyperosmolar hyperglycemic nonketotic encephalopathy	(See Table 9)

Paratonia, grasp reflexes, and a large range of nonlocalizing signs also occur in uremic encephalopathy. Plum and Posner (56) have reported hemiparesis in this condition as well. Decerebrate and decorticate postures have been reported in uremic encephalopathy, but, in my experience, these occur far less frequently in this disease than they do in advanced states of hepatic coma. Convulsions, usually of a major type, are a late and frequently preterminal event in uremic encephalopathy. These usually are generalized in their clinical appearance and by EEG criteria, but focal convulsions of unexplained cause occasionally occur. At times, seizures are precipitated by administration of penicillin, which, since it is not excreted by the failing kidney, acts as an epileptogenic substance (57).

The EEG of patients with uremic encephalopathy shows stages of change similar to those seen in hepatic coma. As the encephalopathy becomes more severe, background slowing progresses; the degree of slowing is correlated generally with the severity of the encephalopathy. Focal or generalized epileptic activity may be encountered.

Treatment of Seizures in Uremia

The treatment of seizures in uremic encephalopathy calls for an understanding of the pharmacology of anticonvulsant drugs in the setting of renal failure. The chronic uremic state is associated with low levels of plasma phenytoin and a short phenytoin half-life at ordinary doses on standard treatment regimens (58). Phenobarbital can be used in chronic renal failure but must be used with caution because of its obligate renal excretion.

Phenytoin can be used to control convulsions in uremic encephalopathy. It must be understood, however, that metabolism of phenytoin is enhanced in uremia, that its half-life is shortened, and that albumin binding is diminished.

The mean half-life of phenytoin in a uremic stale has been shown to be 8.1 hours, roughly one-third of its ordinary half-life. Blood levels of phenytoin in uremic patients remain lower than they do in healthy persons, regardless of the mode of administration (59,60). The plasma level of diphenylhydantoin at any dose is monitored best when blood levels are determined by the enzymatic-immunologic method, which measures both free and plasma-bound phenytoin. The drug should be administered three times a day rather than once a day because of the alterations in half-life. Administration of phenobarbital also should be monitored by determinations of plasma levels. Phenobarbital has been shown to be a safe and effective anticonvulsant when given at a total dose of 90–180 mg/day in patients with chronic renal failure (61). Status epilepticus is not common in patients with uremic encephalopathy. If it does occur, however, it should be managed with parenteral administration of either diazepam or diphenylhydantoin. It is important to obey precisely the guidelines that have been suggested for the treatment of status epilepticus in nonuremic patients (62). Although lidocaine has been suggested as an anticonvulsant agent for intravenous (IV) use in uremic encephalopathy, the drug has never enjoyed widespread use or popularity. In spite of theoretic advantages of its use (i.e., its metabolism is relatively unaffected by the uremic state), it seems to offer no advantages over more conventional drugs.

Meningeal Signs and CSF Findings in Uremia

Neck stiffness is a well-known physical sign and is seen in up to one-third of patients with uremic encephalopathy (63). Up to one-half of these patients have a mononuclear pleocytosis in the CSF. Chamber counts usually reveal only a few cells, but several hundred mononuclear cells per cubic centimeter occasionally are found within the sterile CSF of comatose patients. Fifty percent or more patients with uremic encephalopathy have a modest increase in CSF protein, but values greater than 100 mg/dl should not be attributed to uremic encephalopathy per se but should suggest tumor, chronic infection, subdural hemorrhage, or some other structural cause of protein elevation. CSF urea is increased in uremic encephalopathy, since urea is a small and easily diffusible molecule.

Brain Pathology in Uremia

In contrast to the clinical richness and immense variation of the uremic encephalopathic state, the nervous system pathology in patients dying of acute or chronic renal encephalopathy shows little brain alteration. A mild or moderate generalized gliosis involves the brain cortex. During life, utilization of cerebral oxygen is diminished and there is a diminution in adenosine triphosphatase (ATP) activity in the brain. The state of uremic encephalopathy is associated with elevated levels of calcium in the brain and with cerebral accumulation of various organic acids. In patients dying of uremic encephalopathy, the major neuropathology is due to intercurrent disease, particularly hypertension. Brain infarcts and areas of intracerebral hemorrhage are frequently encountered and are associated with hypertension and with the bleeding disorders seen in chronic uremia. Uremic encephalopathy alone does not cause brain edema, and the condition is not associated with an increase in intracranial pressure.

Treatment of Uremic Encephalopathy

The treatment of encephalopathy associated with acute renal failure (e.g., acute renal tubular necrosis attributable to any of various causes) is accomplished ideally by supportive care in conjunction with dialytic therapy. In acute renal failure, dietary protein should be restricted to 40–60 g/day, and occasionally less than this amount can be tolerated. The dietary intake of potassium and sodium should be strictly limited because of the cardiotoxicity and fluid retention associated with an inability to excrete these electrolytes. At times, control of hyperkalemia involves the use of exchange resins, which also require constant monitoring of serum and urine electrolytes. Fluids should be restricted to no more than 500 cc/day more than the estimated losses in urine and via the gastrointestinal tract. Vitamin supplementation, particularly with thiamine and pyridoxine, should be ensured. If acidosis supervenes, administration of bicarbonate becomes necessary; however, attention must be given to an accompanying sodium overload if sodium bicarbonate is used. Hyponatremia that occurs in the course of acute renal failure is usually dilutional in origin and is treated by restriction of fluid intake rather than by administration of additional sodium. Hyperphosphatemia, which at times is associated with hypocalcemia, can be managed by administration of phosphate-binding gels, such as those containing aluminum hydroxide. The use of such gels has been implicated in the etiology of chronic dialysis encephalopathy (see below).

Chronic or recurrent encephalopathy associated with renal failure is managed by a combination of supportive measures, dialysis, and renal transplantation. Pruritus, anorexia, nausea, constipation, and diarrhea are common in chronic renal failure. They respond unpredictably and unsatisfactorily to a variety of drugs. At times these symptoms respond better to dietary management with diets containing 40 g or less of dietary protein per day. One such diet, the Giovannetti diet, consists of protein-free cereals with protein supplementation by milk and eggs. It has been suggested that such an unpalatable diet not be employed until the glomerular filtration rate (GFR) falls below 10 ml/min.

If hypertension is not the cause of chronic renal failure, it becomes a supervening issue with respect to treatment in about 80% of patients with chronic renal disease. Hypertension is aggravated by sodium and water retention. Methyldopa and propranolol are commonly used to control blood pressure associated with chronic renal failure. Thiazide diuretics tend to be less satisfactory as therapeutic agents, since they are not useful when the GFR falls below 15 ml/min. It has been suggested recently that furosemide in a daily oral dose of 40 mg may be useful in the treatment of hypertension under these circumstances (64). The appearance of edema may signal the nephrotic syndrome in patients with chronic renal failure. The syndrome can be diagnosed by the appearance of increasing excretion of urinary protein and by the development of progressive hyperlipidemia. Cardiac failure, as evidenced in chronic renal failure by pulmonary edema, usually is associated with volume overload and responds poorly to cardiac glycosides. These drugs must be used with caution in patients with chronic renal failure because renal excretion is impaired in these individuals. In general, patients with chronic renal failure require about one-third of the average maintenance dose of cardiac glycosides that patients not afflicted with chronic and severe kidney disease require. Pericarditis, pericardial effusions, and pericardial tamponade comprise other hazards to the heart in chronic renal failure. Cardiac tamponade in particular is a hazard in early portions of dialysis programs. Pericarditis in chronic renal failure may go on to produce restrictive and constrictive heart failure because of replacement of both pericardial effusions and exudates with fibrous tissue if the fluids are not removed.

Most patients with chronic renal failure are anemic as a result of either the suppression of erythropoietin activity or the imposition of hemolytic anemias, or both. Patients with polycystic kidney disease are an exception to this rule, since most of them have adequate levels of hemoglobin throughout the course of their disease and dialysis. Patients with chronic renal failure also are at risk from bleeding. Their platelet count usually is normal or slightly reduced, but the aggregating ability of the platelets is reduced considerably. Catabolism of fibrinogen is enhanced, and a syndrome of disseminated intravascular coagulation can result under these circumstances (65). Symptomatic proximal myopathy occasionally accompanies osteomalacia and renal osteodystrophy. Infections, however, remain the most serious and common problem in management of chronic renal failure. Bacterial and fungal infections remain the leading causes of mortality in patients with chronic renal failure. Viral hepatitis (hepatitis B) in particular is a hazard in patients undergoing chronic hemodialysis, but rates of infection (up to 50%) can be minimized by hepatitis B screening programs and by administration of hepatitis B immunoglobulin. Accelerated atherosclerosis, peripheral neuropathy, and ascites further complicate the clinical course of patients with chronic uremia. Those on chronic dialysis programs are further susceptible to acute or subacute intoxication with trace substances (nickel, zinc, aluminum, fluoride) derived from dialytic solutions and to spallation (the embolization of plastic materials and plasticizers from tubing and machinery used in treatment). Manis and Friedman (35) have reviewed the current medical treatment of irreversible uremia.

Dialysis Dysequilibrium Syndrome

The dialysis dysequilibrium syndrome designates a wide and not entirely predictable constellation of neurologic symptoms that occur during or after hemodialysis or peritoneal dialysis. The syndrome has been the subject of reviews by Wakim (66) and Arieff et al. (67). The symptoms of dialysis dysequilibrium syndrome usually consist of headache, nausea, cramps, stupor, and generalized convulsions. The syndrome has occurred, at least in minor form, in up to 10% of patients undergoing dialysis of any sort. Unlike uremic encephalopathy, dialysis dysequilibrium syndrome is accompanied by increased intracranial pressure. The syndrome is more common when dialysis is performed rapidly or during the early phases of a blood dialysis program. Although the syndrome occurs frequently during the process of dialysis, it may not be evident for up to 24 hours after completion of dialysis. Papilledema occurs in this condition but only rarely.

The cause of the dialysis dysequilibrium syndrome is believed to be a pathologic shift of water into the substance of the brain. There is evidence to suggest that the rapid reduction of plasma urea in the course of dialysis is accompanied by a less rapid reduction in brain urea. This situation creates an osmotic gradient from blood to brain, causing water to shift into the brain in an attempt to create osmotic equilibrium. This process is known as the *reverse urea effect.* Several other theories have been suggested, all with some degree of scientific substantiation, to explain the events that occur in the dialysis dysequilibrium syndrome. *Idiogenic osmoles* are low-molecular-weight substances that are present in the brain of uremic animals. These substances also may create osmotic gradients and lead to the imbibition of brain water, resulting in symptoms of dysequilibrium. The role of idiogenic osmoles in humans with this condition is unclear. Lowering of the CSF pH in the course of hemodialysis by the efflux of accumulated organic acids also has been suggested as an etiologic event in the dialysis dysequilibrium syndrome. Alteration of the relationship between brain and serum sodium in the course of dialysis is yet another suggested cause. Overhydration from excessive water loading and abnormalities in the ratio of serum potassium to serum calcium also have been implicated in the etiology of this condition.

The treatment of the dysequilibrium syndrome consists of reduction of water overload, correction of electrolyte imbalances, symptomatic treatment of seizures, and mild sedation with benzodiazepines should agitation and delirium accompany the condition. Phenothiazine drugs also may be given, if necessary, since their degradation is performed by the liver rather than by the kidney. In moderate or severe renal failure, maintenance doses of phenothiazines may be required no more than every 12–24 hours. Cerra et al. (68) and Hagstam et al. (69) have suggested that the use of mannitol or albumin during dialysis lessens the frequency and severity of the dialysis dysequilibrium syndrome. Bennett et al. (70) have provided a guide to the use of pharmacologic agents in the setting of dialysis.

Subdural hemorrhage that occurs in the absence of known trauma is easily confused with the dialysis equilibrium syndrome. This is particularly common in people with chronic renal failure, and its presence should always be excluded in the person who appears with agitation, delirium, and obtundation, with or without focal neurologic signs. The source of subdural hemorrhage in patients with chronic renal failure is related to the tendency toward bleeding and to the platelet abnormalities of chronic uremia. Computed tomography should be performed to exclude the presence of subdural hemorrhage in the course of dialysis (Fig. 1).

Progressive Dialysis Encephalopathy (Chronic Dialysis Dementia, Dementia Dialytica)

This unique condition was first reported in 1972 by Alfrey and colleagues (71). The current clinical understanding of this condition and suggestions for its treatment have been reviewed by Lederman and Henry (72). This syndrome occurs as a consequence of renal failure of any type and is more frequent in patients undergoing chronic hemodialysis than in those treated by other

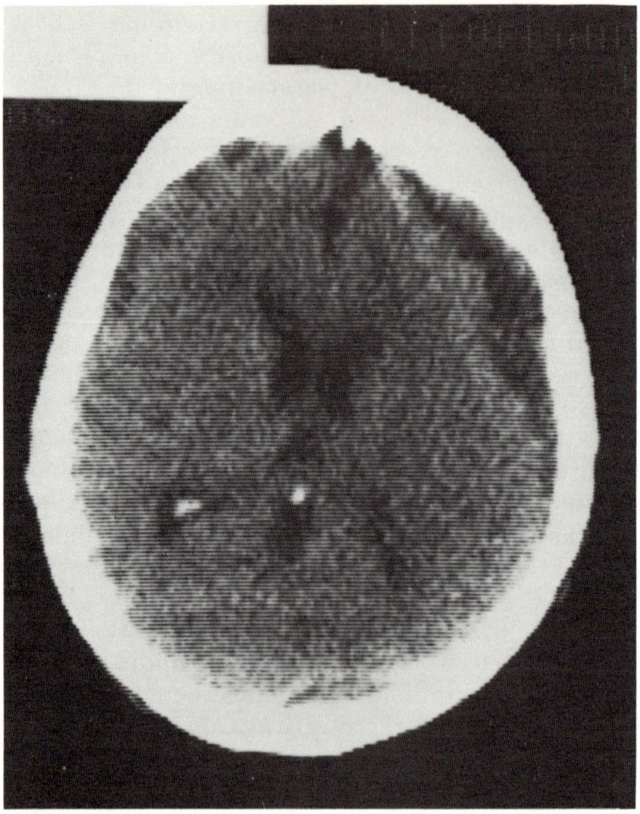

Figure 1. This computed tomographic brain scan was obtained in a woman undergoing dialysis for chronic renal failure. She had thrombocytopenia and recent worsening of her azotemia. Her neurologic course was marked by the development of stupor without focal signs. The computed tomogram shows bilateral subdural hemorrhages that mimicked metabolic encephalopathy.

methods. The duration of illness varies, ranging from one month to three years, with an average duration of six months before death. The most common clinical presentations are the appearance of progressive dementia, accompanied by psychosis with delusions and hallucinations, in the setting of agitated behavior. Stuttering, stammering, dysarthric speech, myoclonus, and multifocal and generalized seizures complete the clinical picture. While speech is dysarthric, language is further impaired. Dysphasic and dyspractic elements of language have been clearly identified in this condition (73). The EEG of patients with progressive dialysis encephalopathy is characterized by slowing, with the frequent appearance of shifting, nonfocal, paroxysmal bursts of high voltage, sometimes associated with polyspike activity.

The cause of progressive dialysis encephalopathy is unknown. Abnormalities in metabolism of trace metals have been suggested, including disturbances in brain concentrations of tin, rubidium, and aluminum. The role of aluminum has received particular attention because excesses of this element are known to act as a neuronal toxin. It has been suggested that excess brain aluminum may be derived from the large quantities of aluminum hydroxide gels used to treat patients with chronic renal failure in an effort to control their hyperphosphatemia (74). Dialysate baths may provide an additional source of aluminum and other trace metals that ultimately may be deposited in the brain. A variety of other causes of this usually fatal illness have been suggested and include slow viral infection, intoxication from organic acids, dopamine deficiency, and phosphate deficiency. The clinical course of dialysis dementia is one of an eventual and usually rapid death. Stabilization of the syndrome and spontaneous remission after a period of worsening have been reported, but such instances are rare.

The treatment of the dialysis dementia syndrome consists of alleviating the symptoms, and the results are unpredictable and imperfect. Dialysis may either improve the syndrome temporarily or worsen it. It is known to subside temporarily after renal transplantation but has appeared de novo after renal transplantation has been performed. Increasingly frequent dialysis treatments and the administration of physostigmine, rubidium, dimercaprol, penicillamine, vitamins, corticosteroids and anticonvulsants seem to have little predictable beneficial effect on the condition. Parenteral administration of diazepam may control myoclonus and seizures temporarily (75), but my experience and that of my colleagues suggest that administration of this drug results in variable and, at best, temporary benefit. Myoclonic seizures in patients with this disorder at times are produced by voluntary muscle activity, such as attempts to speak. Characteristic or outstanding pathologic changes in the brain have not been reported in patients dying of progressive dialysis encephalopathy. The residual effects of chronic hypertension and chronic uremic states predominate, but, as in most brain complications of chronic renal failure, the pathology is decidedly bland in contrast to the clinical state.

Wernicke–Korsakoff Encephalopathy in Renal Disease

Wernicke–Korsakoff disease with typical clinical and pathologic findings has been reported in both children and adults undergoing chronic dialysis (76,77). Patients who are afflicted by this condition in general are those who have not received supplemental thiamine in the course of their treatment. Why some patients develop this condition in the course of dialysis is not known. Evidently consistent fluctuations in blood levels of thiamine do not occur during the course of hemodialysis. Of six patients studied by Lasker et al. (78), only one exhibited a significant reduction in plasma levels of thiamine; the same patient had a 40% reduction in plasma levels of thiamine in the course of hemodialysis. It seems prudent, however, to anticipate this preventable neurologic catastrophe and to be certain that patients undergoing dialysis are treated with therapeutic amounts of thiamine before and during the course of their treatment. Oral administration of 50 mg thiamine hydrochloride per day in this setting is recommended.

PANCREATIC ENCEPHALOPATHY

Pancreatic encephalopathy arises in the course of episodes of acute pancreatitis in association with acute chronic or relapsing pancreatic disease. In general, abdominal pain and a multitude of other systemic signs precede symptoms of brain illness. Systemic signs include hypovolemic and cardiogenic shock, hypocalcemic tetany, elevation of serum levels of pancreatic enzymes, and hyperlipidemia. When hemorrhage occurs, ductal obstruction or severe pancreatic edema or inflammation involve the region of the head of the pancreas. Levels of hepatic enzymes and bilirubin also may be elevated as a result of obstruction and retrograde inflammatory changes in the bile ducts. The onset of the brain illness usually is abrupt and frequently is accompanied by focal or generalized seizures and obtundation. Focal signs of hemispheric disease, such as aphasia and hemiparesis, are not uncommon. Prolonged coma, frequently accompanied by decerebrate and decorticate postures, also may be seen in this rare complication of acute pancreatic disease. CSF pressure may be elevated, and mononuclear pleocytosis of modest degree (10–50 cells) may be encountered. It should be noted, however, that fatal instances of pancreatic encephalopathy have been recorded in which the CSF was entirely normal (79). Cerebral angiograms may display vascular shifts consistent with the mass effects of random, acute hemispheric lesions. In such cases, the lesions are felt to be due to the lytic effects of liberated pancreatic enzymes, including lipases and proteinases, on brain tissue. Although the pathology of this disorder has been the subject of several studies, the pathogenesis of brain illness in acute pancreatitis is unclear. The brain lesions generally are demyelinative in nature, and the demyelination has been attributed to a number of causes, including anoxia and direct lipolytic attack.

Systemic hypoxia sometimes occurs concomitant with acute pancreatitis. Hypoxia may result from both hypovolemia and cardiogenic factors, but systemic fat embolism probably plays a role as well. Demyelination in such a setting may be attributed to the effects of prolonged hypoxia on the brain. Johnson and Tong (80) have described fat embolism in the brain arteries of patients dying of pancreatic encephalopathy and associated demyelinative lesions; however, this is not a common finding. Sherins and Verity (79) have described central pontine myelinolysis associated with acute hemorrhagic pancreatitis in a person who also was a chronic alcoholic and who had brain lesions of the corpus callosum and suggesting Marchiafava–Bignami disease. The individual they reported also experienced delirium tremens and had a clinical course marked by hyperglycemia and hypernatremia. Sharf and Bental (81) have reported a clinical instance that they believe represents focal brain autodigestion caused by liberated pancreatic enzymes. Postmortem examination of similar cases has been offered by Vogel (82).

Treatment of Acute Pancreatic Encephalopathy

Most recorded instances of acute pancreatic encephalopathy are fatal, but recovery after severe and prolonged multifocal illness also has been reported (81). Treatment of this disease is directed toward the basic underlying condition and to the control of seizures and elevated intracranial pressure. Relief of pain in patients with pancreatitis should be achieved with meperidine, since it is far less likely to constrict the sphincter of Oddi that is morphine or other narcotics. Thus, the risk of further parenchymal damage to the pancreas by retention of pancreatic secretions is lessened. Shock resulting from retroperitoneal blood loss can frequently be severe. Evidence of such blood loss may not appear for several days and then announce itself in the form of a bruising discoloration about the costal margins and flanks (Grey–Turner sign) or about the region of the umbilicus (Cullen's sign). Shock is treated best by administration of blood or plasma substitutes. Pancreatic secretion can be inhibited with use of a variety of synthetic anticholinergic drugs. Efforts have been made to counteract the activity of liberated enzymes by administration of antienzymes (81). Hypokalemia and hypocalcemia are treated with appropriate electrolyte replacement. Hyperglycemia and hyperosmolality are distinct hazards in this condition and may contribute to the occasional instances of central pontine myelinolysis encountered in the setting of acute pancreatitis. Antibiotics should be administered to prevent peritonitis. Surgical intervention usually is not required but may be necessary in difficult cases in which laparotomy is necessary to establish the diagnosis.

NEUROLOGIC ASPECTS OF HEAT-INDUCED ILLNESS

The states of illness discussed thus far have had in common the failure of some vital organ that leads to progressive dysfunction of the brain. Thus, they are metabolic encephalopathies in the traditional and established sense. Heat-induced illness differs from these conditions in that the etiologic agent of the illness is a form of physical energy (thermal energy) and the target organ in the disease production is the brain itself rather than a supporting organ. A similarity between heat-induced illness and metabolic encephalopathy becomes apparent, however, if we consider the brain as a system of mutually supportive structures and regions in which the metabolic failure of one constituent induces functional failure of other constituents and, finally, of the whole system. In this way we can infer, from both clinical and experimental observation, that the symptoms of heat-induced illness are induced by dysfunction of the nervous system, and that the lethal aspects of heat stroke itself, although multisystemic in expression, are based on the metabolic failure of the hypothalamus and the consequent collapse of the autonomic nervous system.

Maintenance of body temperature requires that heat production be balanced with heat loss. Heat gain is largely the result of metabolic processes and solar radiation, and, at high environmental temperatures, heat gain is also accomplished through conduction and convection through the skin. In a hot environment, heat loss is accomplished by evaporation of water from both sensible and insensible sources in the body. Conduction and convection contribute further to the body's conservation of thermal energy and produce heat loss when evaporation is limited by high environmental humidity.

Heat balance in humans ultimately is a function of the hypothalamus. The final common thermal pathway involves the autonomic nervous system. Anderson and Haymaker (83), Myers (84), and Myers and Yaksh (85) have reviewed the physical, biochemical, and hypothalamic aspects of heat regulation in humans and animals. Heat loss with respect to brain mechanisms, seems to be triggered by activation of temperature-dependent neurons in the rostral hypothalamus. Stimulation of this cell group leads to the release of noradrenalin from terminals in the caudolateral hypothalamus, producing panting and cutaneous vasodilatation. Heat gain is mediated by a serotonin pathway that converges on the posterior hypothalamus. Activation of this pathway leads to inhibition of the noradrenergic pathway for heat loss. Activation of the serotonergic pathway also leads to complex neuroendocrine responses, such as inhibition of vasopressin release, peripheral vasoconstriction, shivering, elevation of arterial blood pressure, increased production of thyrotropin-releasing hormone production, and thyroxine release.

The major clinical aspects of heat-induced illness have been reviewed by Gottschalk and Thomas (86) and by Shibolet et al. (87). A great deal of nosologic confusion exists with regard to heat-induced illness in humans, and the following classification is taken from classifications offered by Haymaker and Anderson (83) and by Leithead et al. (88). Table 4 outlines the major nosologic categories of heat-induced illnesses, their prominent clinical manifestations, and principles of clinical treatment.

Heat Cramps

Heat cramps are painful contractions of the voluntary muscles. Patients who experience such cramps usually have exercised in a hot environment and have lost excessive amounts of water and sodium in the form of sweat. Heat cramps

Table 4. Classification and Treatment of Heat-Induced Illness

Category of Illness	*Prominent Symptoms and Signs*	*Major Treatment Modalities*
Heat cramps	Painful cramps in voluntary muscles, normal or slightly elevated body temperature	Prescribe rest, replace fluids
Heat exhaustion	Headache, nausea, vomiting, drenching sweat; syncope, possible cramps; normal, subnormal, or slightly elevated body temperature	Prescribe rest, replace fluids and electrolytes
Borderline heat-induced hyperpyrexia	Headache, nausea, vomiting, anhydrosis, shock, body temperature of 103–106°F	Lower body temperature, replace fluids and electrolytes, treat shock
Heat stroke	Stupor or coma, shock, anhydrosis, ± volume loss, cardiac dysrhythmias, possible DIC,[a] hyperkalemia, renal failure, acidosis, adrenal failure, body temperature of 106–109°F	Replace fluids and/or blood, treat shock and cardiac abnormalities, achieve base replacement of steroids, administer exchange resins, possibly give dialysis, lower body temperature

[a]Disseminated intravascular coagulation.

ordinarily are associated with nausea and frequently are prodromal symptoms of the more serious conditions of heat stroke and heat exhaustion. Heat cramps are treated by rest and replacement of both salt and water. Loss of these constituents in this situation is not isotonic; water is relatively more depleted than electrolytes, and water replacement is of paramount importance.

Heat Exhaustion

Mild heat exhaustion results from more extensive losses of salt and water than those associated with heat cramps. The clinical picture includes exercise-induced collapse and syncope. Severe heat exhaustion is accompanied by headache, nausea, vomiting, severe sweating, and a shocklike state. Loss of water and salt are more severe in the latter form. Body temperature in heat exhaustion can be normal, subnormal, or elevated, but patients with this condition generally are wet from the loss of sweat. This becomes an important physical sign in the differentiation of this condition from heat stroke. It should be noted, however, that certain people can lose large volumes of sweat in environments that produce rapid evaporation, so that they may be both volume depleted *and* dry. Football players who practice on hot, windy days and who suffer heat exhaustion are examples of such individuals. With failure of the autonomic system, including failure to sweat, heat exhaustion blends into heat stroke.

Borderline Heat-Induced Hyperpyrexia

Borderline heat-induced hyperpyrexia may follow heat exhaustion and includes all the symptoms and signs related to the latter. In borderline heat-induced hyperpyrexia, the body temperature is elevated to between 40 and 41°C (103 and 106°F). Loss of sweating occurs. The condition is also termed *anhydrotic heat exhaustion.* In contrast to persons with heat stroke, those with borderline heat-induced hyperpyrexia are conscious and coherent. Treatment consists of lowering body temperature, and correcting shock and hypovolemia, and replacing electrolytes.

Heat Stroke

As its name implies, heat stroke frequently arises with dramatic suddenness. It also may represent the end stage of the other heat-induced conditions discussed earlier. It tends to victimize nonacclimatized individuals and frequently is a phenomenon of the first heat wave of summer. It is disproportionately a disease of the old and infirm and particularly affects victims of heart disease, alcoholism, or malnutrition. The poor are likely to be victimized because they lack access to air conditioners. Military recruits, bakers, merchant marines stationed in the tropics and others who exercise excessively in the heat also are at increased risk. Persons taking anticholinergic drugs, including drugs used as tranquilizers or in the treatment of Parkinson's disease, are at particular risk. Although collapse is sudden, there may be premonitory symptoms of confusion, vague aches and pains, nausea, and similar nonspecific complaints.

Persons with heat stroke generally present in a coma, with hot, dry skin and a body temperature of 42–43°C (106–109°F). Seizures are a frequent finding, and tachycardia and vascular shock are part of the clinical picture. Dehydration is seldom severe in true heat stroke, a fact that has ramifications in treatment. Frequent complications of heat stroke include myoglobulinuria, acidosis, and the multiorgan effects of disseminated intravascular coagulation.

Treatment

The basic aims of treatment of heat stroke consist of the lowering of body temperature, preservation of fluid and electrolyte balance, support of the circulatory system, and minimization of tissue injury. Management also frequently consists of treatment of severe acidosis and of cardiac and renal failure.

Except for persons whose heat stroke is associated with prodromal loss of salt and water, victims may not have marked volume depletion. Care must be taken, therefore, not to induce volume overload in these individuals. Monitoring of central venous pressure usually is mandatory under these circumstances. Hypernatremia, if it occurs, usually is mild, and severe hyponatremia is not common. Patients with heat stroke may be severely hyperkalemic to the point of cardiac and renal toxicity because of the breakdown of red blood cells. Myoglobulinuria and rhabdomyolysis aggravate hyperkalemia further and lead to renal impairment. The disseminated intravascular coagulation associated with heat stroke has ramifications in all organ systems. Evidence of thrombotic and hemorrhagic disease are widespread and can be found literally in every part of the body.

Patients with heat stroke should be given oxygen to correct the associated hypoxia and acidosis. Base deficits must be calculated and replacement carried out with sodium bicarbonate. Seizures can be treated with parenteral diazepam or, if they become recurrent, with diphenylhydantoin under appropriate monitoring. If cardiac failure supervenes in heat stroke, it usually is characterized by high-output failure and should be treated by digitalization. Hemorrhage, intravascular thrombosis, and hypofibrinogenemia can be treated with heparin. In some severe instances, administration of ϵ-aminocaproic acid (6 g IV initially, followed by 0.5 g IV every hour) is necessary to control fibrinolysis. Replacement of whole blood and blood products (platelets, plasma) also may be instituted, if clinically warranted. Corticosteroids may be beneficial for treatment of both shock and disseminated intravascular coagulation, but their role in salvage is dubious. Corticosteroids certainly are indicated in the clinical course of heat stroke if hemorrhagic adrenal failure is suspected. It must be cautioned that the use of corticosteroids may aggravate hypofibrinogenemia.

The most important aspect of treatment is lowering of the body temperature. This can be accomplished with application of cold packs, placing the patient in ice, or sponging the patient with icy solutions. Shivering and vasoconstriction may be reduced by massage and by administration of either diazepam or small doses of chlorpromazine. Systemic hypotension must be treated as any other condition of cardiovascular shock.

Heat stroke has been associated with a mortality as high as 50% in some series. Severe residua of heat stroke, particularly brain dysfunction, occur in a large percentage of survivors (89). The pathologic changes that occur in the brain superficially resemble those seen in anoxic encephalopathy. This fact is not surprising, since at 43°C, the temperature at which heat stroke generally occurs, neurons become incapable of critical levels of nucleotide metabolism and glucose transport (90). Furthermore, it has been shown in primates that, at the critical temperature of 43°C, cerebral blood flow becomes impaired and major EEG deterioration occurs (91). Heat stroke thus represents a metabolic encephalopathy that is evidenced first by hypothalamic failure, next by metabolic failure of large numbers of brain neurons, and finally, and often fatally, by the wreckage of the metabolic machinery of the cells involved.

ENCEPHALOPATHIES THAT OCCUR DURING PROLONGED PARENTERAL ALIMENTATION

Wernicke–Korsakoff Disease

Wernicke–Korsakoff disease is associated characteristically with chronic alcohol abuse and neglect of nutrition. Its occasional appearance in the setting of chronic renal disease and dialysis has been discussed already. Persons who require prolonged parenteral therapy, particularly IV hyperalimentation, now comprise another source of morbidity and mortality from Wernicke–Korsakoff disease. Even though a patient may not have a history of alcoholism, dietary neglect is substantiated clearly in such individuals, particularly with regard to the lack of thiamine. The occurrence of Wernicke–Korsakoff disease in the setting of parenteral hyperalimentation constitutes a completely preventable illness and provides the clinician with the opportunity to provide gratifying treatment of a severe and occasionally fatal brain illness. Neurologists in particular should not fail to recall that one of Wernicke's original three patients was not an alcoholic, but was a 20-year-old woman who suffered from chronic vomiting caused by pyloric stenosis resulting from the ingestion of sulfuric acid during a suicide attempt (92). In certain hospital settings, prolonged parenteral alimentation has replaced alcoholism as the most frequent context for the precipitation of Wernicke–Korsakoff disease.

The clinical picture in patients who develop Wernicke–Korsakoff disease during prolonged IV feeding is the same as that seen in patients whose dietary habits have been ruined by alcoholism. Irritability, somnolence, and moodiness give way to extraocular muscle palsies, nystagmus, ataxia, and amnestic mental changes. In the ordinary patient who receives prolonged parenteral hyperalimentation, the clue commonly provided by a history of alcoholism is missing, and a dietary history that substantiates thiamine deficiency may emerge only on review of complicated and extensive nutritional records. Wernicke–Korsakoff disease also should be considered in patients who display this clinical picture and who, for reasons of prolonged starvation or intestinal bypass surgery, have neglected proper nutrition in the treatment of obesity (93). In the alcoholic patient, in the patient undergoing prolonged IV alimentation, and in the intentionally or therapeutically starved patient dying of this syndrome, the pathology is similar and absolutely characteristic of that associated with classic Wernicke–Korsakoff disease (94). In Wernicke–Korsakoff disease associated with prolonged IV therapy, the diagnosis frequently is not made until postmortem examination. Publications by Nadel and Burger (95) and Kramer and

Goodwin (96) have called attention to the setting of IV hyperalimentation as a cause of Wernicke–Korsakoff disease; increased awareness from these and other reports and better recognition of situations that give rise to this illness should lead to higher rates of recovery for these unfortunate patients.

Blass and Gibson (97) have identified a partial defect in thiamine metabolism in alcoholic patients who acquire Wernicke–Korsakoff syndrome. They showed transketolase activity in the fibroblasts of alcoholic patients with Wernicke–Korsakoff disease to be less than that in similarly matched alcoholic controls without the illness. This suggests a genetic susceptibility to Wernicke–Korsakoff disease that is unmasked only under circumstances of dietary failure. Whether this situation also pertains to persons who acquire Wernicke–Korsakoff disease in other settings is not known at present.

Wernicke–Korsakoff disease that occurs in the setting of prolonged IV alimentation should be treated as it would be in any other setting. Generous amounts of thiamine (400 mg/day) should be administered parenterally. This may seem like an astronomic amount of this vitamin-cofactor, but the dose is well tolerated, does no harm, and, on the contrary, is known to do a great deal of good.

Hypophosphatemic Encephalopathy

Hypophosphatemia as a cause of severe encephalopathy has been identified more frequently in recent years as a result of the use of multichannel blood autoanalyzers. Encephalopathy, at times evolving into coma, occurs with severe hypophosphatemia and generally is seen when serum phosphate in susceptible individuals falls to levels of less than 1 mg/dl. Severe hypophosphatemia occurs in a variety of circumstances, including ethanol withdrawal, hypothermia, diabetic ketoacidosis, overuse of phosphate-binding antacids, recovery from burns, and prolonged respiratory alkalosis (98). Prolonged IV hyperalimentation has provided another cause of profound hypophosphatemia (99,100), with resultant tendencies toward severe metabolic encephalopathy. Hypophosphatemia in this setting appears to be a response to the sudden infusion of a large carbohydrate load.

The clinical expression of hypophosphatemic encephalopathy varies. Many patients appear to tolerate moderate and prolonged reductions in serum phosphate with few or no symptoms. In some patients with profound hypophosphatemia, progressive obtundation with or without accompanying delirium leads to coma. In others, the progression of encephalopathy is accompanied by a variety of multifocal and nonfocal signs, including shifting abnormalities in muscle tone and seizures. Some patients with hypophosphatemia demonstrate generalized muscle weakness and complain of distal paresthesias (101). The EEG in hypophosphatemic encephalopathy is characterized by generalized shifting and nonspecific slowing and by the occasional appearance of seizure discharges. Through the courtesy of Dr. Michael Devereaux (Department of Neurology, Mt. Sinai Hospital of Cleveland, Ohio) and Dr. Roland Philip (Head, Department of Surgery, Kaiser Foundation, Cleveland), I have learned of one instance of hypophosphatemic coma in which the EEG was characterized by prolonged and sustained electrocerebral silence. The patient was not hypothermic but had been treated with prolonged IV hyperalimentation. She experienced multifocal seizures but went on to recover slowly after parenteral administration of phosphate.

Hypophosphatemic encephalopathy usually occurs in persons with other underlying causes of stupor, coma, or other expressions of metabolic brain illness. It rarely exists with purity, but it should not be excluded as a cause of metabolic brain illness. Treatment of hypophosphatemic encephalopathy consists of the parenteral administration of phosphate. This can be accomplished in adults by the administration of 10 mg of potassium acid phosphate per hour IV, with serial determinations of serum electrolytes during the course of administration. As with most other metabolic encephalopathies, clinical recovery lags far behind laboratory confirmation of metabolic correction. It is not uncommon for clinical recovery to occur over the course of two or three days after the levels of serum phosphate have been corrected (102).

Hyperglycemic Hyperosmolar Nonketotic Encephalopathy

Hyperglycemic hyperosmolar nonketotic encephalopathy is an infrequent complication of parenteral alimentation. Large carbohydrate loads precipitate the condition, and known and latent diabetics are at special risk. The condition has a large number of possible etiologies and is discussed fully in a subsequent section.

HYPERTENSIVE ENCEPHALOPATHY

Hypertensive encephalopathy refers to a clinical syndrome of global disturbance of brain function associated with greatly elevated systemic blood pressure. Its mechanisms are not completely known, and a variety of theories have been advanced to explain its pathogenesis (103–106). These include disordered regulation of the brain vasculature, reflex vasospasm, and pressure-induced injury to vascular walls. Whenever hypertensive encephalopathy occurs, it does so in a patient with underlying hypertensive disease in whom elevations of blood pressure have recently reached the so-called malignant range (i.e., diastolic elevations of greater than 120 mm Hg). In eclamptic women, the symptoms of hypertensive encephalopathy can occur with blood pressures in the vicinity of 160/100 mm Hg; however, in actuality, most patients with hypertensive encephalopathy have blood pressures in the vicinity of 250/150 mm Hg. It must be recalled that nearly all hypertensive encephalopathy is preventable by adequate treatment of hypertension. The neurologist should be aware of hypertensive encephalopathy as a special hazard to quadriplegic patients through mechanisms of autonomic dysreflexia (107). Fujishima and colleagues (108) have published experimental evidence to suggest that the vasculopathy of hypertensive encephalopathy results from excesses of circulating renin in circumstances of renal vascular–related hypertension.

Clinical Picture

The clinical picture of hypertensive encephalopathy has been reviewed by Gifford and Westbrook (109). Hypertensive encephalopathy is associated with hypertension from any cause and can occur at any age. It is most common in essential hypertension, in hypertension secondary to renal or renal vascular illnesses, and in hypertension associated with pregnancy. It is rare in hypertension caused by primary aldosteronism or by coarctation of the aorta. In some patients, the inciting cause is not a rise in blood pressure. Other persons who develop hypertensive encephalopathy usually are found to have known hypertension and for some reason have experienced a hiatus in their antihypertensive drug therapy.

Headache is the cardinal feature of hypertensive encephalopathy. It develops gradually, usually gaining momentum from 24–72 hours before the time an individual seeks medical attention. Headache is generalized and constant. Confusion, somnolence, and irritability occur in many patients and follow the onset of headache by several hours at least. Visual blurring and vomiting are not uncommon. Generalized seizures are not as frequent a finding. Focal brain deficits are even less common, but episodic cortical blindness, diplopia, focal convulsions, and other migratory focal neurologic complaints may be encountered occasionally. In most cases, neurologic examination discloses ischemic retinal hypertensive changes, with marked arterial narrowing as the most common ocular finding. Retinal exudates, hemorrhages, and papilledema are encountered less commonly, but they are by no means rare. CSF pressure usually is increased but may be normal, even in patients with advanced encephalopathy and in the face of incontrovertible elevation of the optic-nerve heads. CSF pressure bears no constant relation to the presence or absence of papilledema. Retinal vascular changes produce the funduscopic abnormality in this setting. The protein and cellular content of the CSF generally are normal, but alterations may follow the appearance of structural brain lesions. Modest elevations in CSF protein and red or white blood cell counts may be found subsequently. Azotemia and moderate degrees of renal failure are common in hypertensive encephalopathy, and uremia usually worsens with advancing degrees of brain disturbance.

The differential diagnosis of hypertensive encephalopathy includes all aspects of vascular ruin that may befall the brain of hypertensive individuals. The term *hypertensive encephalopathy* itself has given rise to some confusion, since it has been used in the past to designate brain infarctions and hemorrhages that occur in hypertensive patients. Fortunately, the confusion that has resulted from the imprecise application of the diagnostic term seems to be waning. The presence of infarctive, hemorrhagic, or traumatic structural lesions can be excluded by computed axial tomography and by observation of the clinical course. The EEG is abnormal in hypertensive encephalopathy but is in no way diagnostic. Random slowing, which at times is pseudorhythmic, and occasional epileptiform discharges can be found on the EEG. Uremic encephalopathy represents the point of greatest contention in the differential diagnosis of hypertensive encephalopathy. Although the analogies and similarities between the two conditions are many, one fundamental distinction remains: patients with hypertensive encephalopathy improve, usually markedly, with treatment of their blood pressure *alone,* even if they remain azotemic or become increasingly so. Patients with uremic encephalopathy do not respond in this fashion.

The pathologic changes in hypertensive encephalopathy have been emphasized by Chester et al. (110). The characteristic lesions consist of fibrinoid necrosis of arterioles and thrombosis of small arterioles and capillaries within the nervous system. These changes are not confined to the brain or spinal cord, but also involve the eyes, kidneys, and other organs. Lesions of the nervous system occur predominantly in the brain stem, basal ganglia, and, to a somewhat lesser degree, the cerebral hemispheres and spinal cord. Vascular lesions are associated with microinfarcts and petechial hemorrhages. The appearance of cerebral edema is inconstant, since it is prominent in some patients and is not found in others (103,108). Hypertensive encephalopathy and uremic encephalopathy may coexist clinically and pathologically in the same patient.

Pharmacologic Treatment

Hypertensive encephalopathy is a true neurologic emergency. Suspicion of its diagnosis on the basis of history, signs, and symptoms is sufficient reason to institute prompt treatment, preferably within the confines of an intensive care unit and with cardiac monitoring. There is no room for inordinate delay in the treatment of this disease.

Drug treatment of hypertensive encephalopathy in adults has been reviewed by Vidt and Gifford (112) and in children, by Fleischmann (113). Efficacious drugs that are available for parenteral use can be divided into two categories: those that act as direct vasodilators, and those whose action is exerted through modification of CNS mechanisms (neurotransmitter blocking agents). Table 5 gives a summary of drugs used in hypertensive encephalopathy. In most instances of hypertensive encephalopathy, parenteral vasodilators are the drugs of choice. Irrespective of the pharmacologic agent used, extreme vigilance in monitoring blood pressure is critical in the treatment of hypertensive emergencies, since the danger of converting a hypertensive crisis to a hypotensive catastrophe is ever present.

Direct Vasodilator Agents

Diazoxide should be administered to adults IV in a 50- or 100-mg rapid bolus, and its effects should be monitored frequently over the subsequent five to 15 minutes. Rapid injection is essential, since protein binding occurs quickly and abolishes the vasodilator effect of the drug. In extreme situations, a bolus of 300 mg may be administered as the initial dose. The clinical effects of diazoxide are noted usually within the first 10 minutes after injection. In children, doses of 3–5 mg/kg are administered as a rapid bolus and repeated in 15 to 20 minutes, if necessary. The effect of a large bolus of diazoxide may be effective for up to 12 hours. The drug has the advantages of seldom producing serious hypotension, and it does not induce somnolence, the presence of which may interfere with assessment of the patient's neurologic state. Diazoxide must be used with caution in patients with cerebral or coronary vascular insufficiency. The drug is known to induce hyperglycemia in some individuals; thus, levels of blood sugar must be monitored closely if sustained treatment with diazoxide is necessary.

The parenteral use of *hydralazine* should be reserved for management of hypertensive encephalopathy that complicates glomerulonephritis or eclampsia. The drug can be infused IV at a rate of 0.5–1 mg/min. Blood pressure should be monitored constantly during infusion. The effects of parenteral hydralazine are

Table 5. Treatment of Hypertensive Encephalopathy

Type of Drug	*Method of Administration*
Direct Vasodilator Agents	
Diazoxide	3–5 mg/kg in children; 50–100 mg IV bolus in adults. Repeated at 5–15 minute intervals.
Hydralazine	0.5–1 mg/min IV in adults; 0.15–0.2 mg/kg/min IV in children. Continue at IV rate to control constantly monitored blood pressure.
Sodium nitroprusside	Prepare light-protected solution of 50–100 mg/L; deliver IV at rate of 1–10 μg/min to control constantly monitored blood pressure. Check levels of serum thiocyanate.
Neurotransmitter Blocking Agents	
Trimethephan	Prepare solution of 10 ml trimethephan (50 mg/ml) in 500 cc 5% dextrose in water. Deliver at rate of 4–100 drops/min (average, 60 drops, or 3–4 mg/min) to control strictly monitored blood pressure.
Reserpine	Give 0.5–1 mg IM in adults, followed by 2–5 mg every 3–4 hours. Drug has erratic effect, long duration of action.
Methyldopate ester	Give 100–500 mg IV in adults. Repeat at 4- to 6-hour intervals or longer. Occasionally larger initial doses are used. Drug has slow onset and long duration of action.
Phentolamine	Give 5 mg phentolamine mesylate IV in adults, 1 mg IV in children. Repeat as needed. Drug has rapid onset of action and short duration of effect.

noted usually within 10 minutes of administration. Hydralazine shares with diazoxide the advantages of not producing serious hypotension or sedation. The use of hydralazine, however, is contraindicated in patients with coronary artery insufficiency, since the drug increases cardiac work by increasing stroke volume and heart rate. Hydralazine can be given to children in doses of 0.15 mg/kg intramuscularly (IM) or 0.2 mg/kg IV.

Sodium nitroprusside is prepared in solutions of either 50–100 mg/L of 5% dextrose in water. Infusion should be started at a rate of 1 μg/min. Infusion rates faster than 10 μg/min are rarely required in either children or adults. The clinician must establish the least effective parenteral dose rate by monitoring patient response. It is essential to use freshly prepared solutions of sodium nitroprusside, and, because the drug deteriorates in the presence of light, the IV bottle should be wrapped in foil or some other opaque substance for protection. Once prepared, a solution of sodium nitroprusside should not be kept for more than four hours. If more nitroprusside is needed, a new solution must be made. The onset of clinical action of sodium nitroprusside is immediate, as is the cessation of action. Cessation of administration leads to a prompt rise in blood pressure; the use of the drug, therefore, requires constant monitoring of blood pressure during slow IV infusion. Levels of sodium thiocyanate should be monitored in patients who are receiving sodium nitroprusside, and the drug should be discontinued if thiocyanate levels exceed 10 mg/dl. Thiocyanate intoxication is a special hazard in patients with renal failure, and some of these individuals who experience a hypertensive emergency may require dialysis combined with nitroprusside administration. Nitroprusside is an extremely effective drug in the treatment of hypertensive encephalopathy and can be used when other drugs have failed. Constant observation by trained personnel is necessary during its use.

Neurotransmitter Blocking Agents

Trimethaphan and similar neurotransmitter blocking drugs cause inhibition of both the sympathetic and parasympathetic nervous systems. This class of agents have been used far less frequently in recent years than in the past because of the advent of more effective and somewhat safer direct vasodilator drugs. The neurotransmitter blocking agents, exemplified by trimethaphan, exert their hypotensive effects in primarily orthostatic fashion. Thus, larger doses are required to lower blood pressure in a reclining patient than in a patient standing upright. The inhibition of parasympathetic nerves associated with the use of such drugs leads to ileus and urinary retention, which may further complicate the treatment of hypertensive encephalopathy, or at least demand discontinuation of the agent. Ganglion-blocking agents should not be used in the management of hypertensive encephalopathy associated with prepartum eclampsia because these agents can produce ileus and respiratory embarrassment to the fetus.

Administration of trimethaphan is begun by the preparation of a solution containing 500 mg trimethaphan (one 10-ml ampule) in 500 cc of 5% dextrose in water. In adults, infusion should begin at a rate of 60 drops (3–4 mg) per minute, and blood pressure should be monitored constantly. Maintenance rates vary from four to 100 drops per minute. If serious hypotension occurs that threatens cerebral, cardiac, or renal perfusion, it is necessary to administer IV phenylephrine, methphentermine, or norepinephrine.

Reserpine and *methyldopate ester* also have been used in the management of hypertensive encephalopathy. However, these drugs share the disadvantages of slow onset of action and sedative effects. Reserpine is one of more than 20 rauwolfia alkaloids and is derived from *Rauwolfia serpentina,* a plant indigenous to the Indian subcontinent. The drug's pharmacologic actions are complex and produce mental depression, antipsychotic effects, enhanced gastric secretion, vascular congestion of mucosal surfaces, and lowering of convulsant thresholds, in addition to its effects on vascular hypotension. Reserpine acts by depleting tissue stores of catecholamines and by blocking membrane reuptake of catechols that are released from presynaptic terminals. Reserpine is no longer frequently used in the treatment of hypertensive emergencies. It is given by IM administration, and its absorption and onset of action are erratic. It may aggravate seizures in eclamptic women, and its tendency to produce mucosal congestion may result in respiratory distress in the newborn. If reserpine is used, it should be given in an initial IM dose of 0.5–1 mg in adults, followed by 2–5 mg every three to four hours to maintain acceptable blood pressure. Like methyldopate ester, reserpine may be useful in clinical situations in which control of blood pressure is desired for hours rather than for minutes. Unlike the direct vasodilators, the effects of reserpine and similar drugs are long lasting.

Methyldopa (methyldopate ester) inhibits the formation of dopa and thus of norepinephrine by inhibiting production of dopa-decarboxylase. Methyldopa also inhibits the formation of serotonin from 5-hydroxytryptophan. The drug's antihypertensive action, however, may result from ganglionic blocking activity not directly related to inhibitory effects of these enzymes. Methyldopate ester is administered IV in initial doses of 100–500 mg, with repetition and variation of the dose at four- to six-hour intervals (occasionally at 10–16-hour intervals), depending on response of the blood pressure. In some instances of hypertensive encephalopathy, initial doses of 1,000–3,000 mg have been given, but this method has not gained wide acceptance because of the associated risk of long-lasting hypotension. Once blood pressure is controlled with methyldopate ester, further medication may not be required for 24–60 hours. If serious hypotension occurs while a patient is being treated with methyldopate ester, blood pressure may be raised by administration of phenylephrine or norepinephrine, since adrenergic receptors are not blocked by methyldopa.

Phentolamine, a drug that blocks alpha-adrenergic receptors, is specifically indicated for the management of hypertensive crises caused by high levels of circulating catecholamines. Administration of phentolamine is indicated specifically for hypertensive crises associated with pheochromocytoma or sudden catecholamine release precipitated by simultaneous ingestion of monamine oxidase inhibitors and tyramine-containing food, or in patients whose long-term treatment with clonidine has been withdrawn abruptly. Phentolamine is also used to control hypertension, tachycardia, and other systemic effects of noradrenalin overflow in the course of surgery for correction of pheochromocytoma. In the treatment of noradrenergic hypertensive crises, phentolamine mesylate should be given IV in doses of 5 mg in adults (1 mg in children) and repeated as needed to control blood pressure.

New Drugs

Two new drugs that have shown promise in the treatment of hypertensive encephalopathy are *clonidine* and *nifedipine.* Clonidine acts on the CNS by direct stimulation of alpha-adrenergic receptors; this, in turn, leads to diminution of sympathetic nerve tone and to reduced reactivity of vascular smooth muscle. Niarchos (114) has reported reasonably good results with the clinical use of clonidine. In his study, the drug was shown to have a much slower onset of action than vasodilators, but its parenteral use was free from serious side effects, such as catastrophic hypotension. *Nifedipine* is a vasodilator which inhibits calcium flux during excitation-contraction of vascular muscles, including the heart. Guazzi and colleagues (115) have suggested that the drug is safe and effective in hypertensive crises. Nifedipine has the particular advantage of oral or sublingual administration, and its onset of action is rapid when given by these routes. It also increases cardiac output in cases where myocardial failure complicates hypertensive encephalopathy. The general effectiveness of clonidine and nifedipine in hypertensive encephalopathy, however, await the results of further clinical trials.

SYNDROME OF INAPPROPRIATE ANTIDIURETIC HORMONE SECRETION (SCHWARTZ–BARTTER SYNDROME)

The syndrome of inappropriate antidiuretic hormone secretion (SIADH) occurs in a wide variety of clinical settings, such as malignancies, trauma, hemorrhage, endocrinopathies, pulmonary disorders, and drug-related disorders (Table 6). Every setting in which SIADH occurs is associated with hypotonic plasma and hyponatremia due to the aberrant or otherwise inappropriately sustained secretion of antidiuretic hormone (ADH). In these situations, decreasing plasma osmolality fails to turn off the production of ADH by the hypothalamus or other cellular sources of the substance. Secretion of ADH promotes resorption of water from the renal distal convoluted tubule and the collecting tubule. ADH is bound to carrier proteins called neurophysins, of which there are at least three distinct types (116). This binding occurs at the cell membrane of ADH-producing pituitary cells and is found also in some nonendocrine ADH-producing tumors, such as oat-cell carcinoma of the lung (117). Neurophysins may have some peripheral action on the transport of water and sodium, and the possibility that neurophysins along with ADH are responsible for the pathogenesis of SIADH is unsettled. Bartter has summarized the symptoms that occur in SIADH as water overload leading to water intoxication (118). Its laboratory hallmarks are hyponatremia and hypo-osmolality of plasma and other body fluids that occur simultaneously with hyperosmolar urine in a patient who is not hypovolemic or dehydrated. Normal renal and adrenal function permit laboratory diagnosis more readily than does abnormal function, but it is clear that SIADH may occur in the setting of either normal or abnormal function.

The clinical symptoms of SIADH are a function of both the absolute level and the rate of decline of plasma sodium and of the fall in osmolality of body fluids. Individuals who develop SIADH slowly and to only a mild or moderate degree, (e.g., those with certain nonendocrine tumors) may be asymptomatic and have serum sodium values of between 120 and 130 mEq/L. Such patients, however, are at risk if they are subjected to large fluid loads because they will develop water intoxication. Patients with mild or chronic SIADH from any cause may exhibit symptoms of anorexia, lassitude, confusion, muscle aches, and lack of concentration. Such patients can be treated with water restriction, a therapy that is frequently greeted with little compliance and that is difficult to maintain outside of controlled settings such as hospitals. Both oral lithium carbonate and demeclocycline, a tetracycline antibiotic, have been employed in the treatment of SIADH, and both permit more liberal water intake. These drugs act to produce nephrogenic diabetes insipidus by toxic action on the renal tubule. Lithium carbonate is administered to adults in doses of between 600 and 900 mg/day to maintain levels of serum lithium of 1–1.2 mEq/L. Demeclocycline is given in doses ranging from 600–1,200 mg/day (1,315 mg/kg/day). Of the two drugs, demeclocycline is believed to have the advantages of lesser toxicity, better patient tolerance, and the capability to produce a potentially more reversible form of renal tubular dysfunction than lithium (119,120).

Patients with severe or rapidly developing SIADH may become agitated and violent, experience generalized or multifocal seizures, and lapse into coma.

Table 6. Causes of SIADH (modified from Bartter)

Endogenous Production of Hypothalamic ADH
CNS disorders
Meningitis
Stroke
Brain injury (postoperative states, severe concussion, chronic subdural hemorrhage)
Brain abscess
Acute viral encephalitis
Subarachnoid hemorrhage
Hypothalamic lesions in acute intermittent porphyria
Intracranial tumor
Peripheral Nervous System Disorders
Guillain–Barré syndrome
Hemorrhage
Pulmonary Disorders
Pneumonia
Tuberculosis
Fungal pulmonary diseases
Endocrinopathies
Addison's disease
Myxedema
Hypopituitarism
Idiopathic SIADH
Other Disorders
Cardiac failure
Hepatic cirrhosis
Syndrome of normotensive juxtaglomerular hyperplasia with hyperkalemia and alkalosis (Bartter's syndrome)
SIADH in patients with mechanical ventilatory assistance
Aberrant ADH production
Lung carcinoma
Carcinoma of the gut
Pancreatic cancers
Carcinoma of the ureter
Hodgkin's disease
Drugs
Vasopressin
Oxytocin
Vincristine
Chlorpropramide
Thiazides
Atromid-S
Tegretol
Nicotine
Cyclophosphamide

SOURCE: Bartter FC: The syndrome of inappropriate secretion of antidiuretic hormone (SIADH). DM, November 1973, pp. 1–47.

Stretch reflexes vary and may be either hyperactive or lost; similar variations are to be expected in posture, plantar responses, and a variety of other neurologic functions. Periodic Cheyne–Stokes respirations and central hyperpnea may be seen. In profound hyperosmolar coma, body temperature falls to subnormal levels.

Individuals with severe and life-threatening SIADH can be treated with a combination of furosemide and hypertonic saline (121). Furosemide can be given in a dose of 1 mg/kg IV at the outset, and samples of urine sodium should be evaluated hourly. Urinary losses of sodium should be replaced with 3% sodium chloride administered IV every hour. Intermediate degrees of SIADH resulting from transient causes (e.g., trauma) that produce symptoms but are not life threatening can be treated in hospitalized patients simply by water restriction and general supportive measures. Intravenous infusion of sodium may not be necessary in these patients, and thus it is possible to avoid the obligate risks entailed by expansion of plasma volume.

Neurologists should be aware that patients who require mechanical ventilatory assistance may develop SIADH. Such individuals include those with myasthenia gravis, high lesions of the spinal cord, and Guillain–Barré syndrome. The following is an example of such a patient.

CASE STUDY: SIADH IN A PATIENT REQUIRING MECHANICAL VENTILATION

A 49-year-old woman underwent removal of a large schwannoma at the level of C2 and subsequently developed adhesive arachnoiditis. She entered the Cleveland Clinic Foundation five years after her original surgery because she was experiencing progressive respiratory impairment characterized by mechanical weakness of the chest wall and diaphragm, hypercapnia, and hypoxia. At entry her serum sodium level was normal. She refused tracheostomy but accepted treatment with a negative-pressure chest curaisse device. Her respiratory function improved, but five days later she became delirious and then comatose. Levels of arterial blood pH and blood gases were normal, but her serum sodium level was 107 mEq/L. Serum osmolality was 214 mOsm/L and urine osmolality was 329 mOsm/L. In spite of treatment with furosemide and IV hypertonic sodium chloride, the patient died during an episode of seizures (J.P. Conomy, J.M. Polensky, unpublished data).

Table 7. Treatment of SIADH

Severe, Life-Threatening SIADH
Furosemide, 1 mg/kg IV
Hypertonic saline (3%): amounts to be based on renal loss[a]
Fluid restriction
Supportive care
Moderate SIADH
Fluid restriction
Supportive care
Chronic or Mild SIADH
Fluid restriction
Avoidance of water intoxication
Lithium carbonate, 600–900 mg/day orally in adults[a]
Demeclocycline, 13–15 mg/kg/day orally in adults[a]

[a]See text for full description of administration.

In this setting it is likely that a combination of prolonged recumbency, high levels of arterial P_{CO_2}, and ineffective cardiac atrial filling led to overproduction of ADH, since all of these factors are known to increase ADH levels. Table 7 provides a summary of treatment measures for SIADH according to severity of the clinical state.

HYPERGLYCEMIC HYPEROSMOLAR NONKETOTIC ENCEPHALOPATHY (SYNDROME OF HYPEROSMOLAR COMA)

The syndrome of hyperglycemic hyperosmolar nonketotic encephalopathy is important because patients who develop this condition are commonly under the active care of a physician and frequently are hospitalized. Coma usually evolves rapidly and is typically associated with focal or generalized seizures, epilepsia partialis continua, or multifocal fits. Symptoms and signs of hyperglycemic hyperosmolar nonketotic encephalopathy are related to hyperosmolarity of the extracellular fluid predominantly caused by increased amounts of glucose, which occasionally approach astronomical levels (600–3,000 mg/100 ml). The syndrome is superimposed on a background of insulin deficiency, corticosteroid administration, severe burns, pancreatitis, pancreatic carcinoma, dialysis, parenteral hyperalimentation, hypothermia, extensive surgical procedures, pathologic gorging of carbohydrates, and severe infections. All these conditions have in common diminished utilization of glucose, due to diminished insulin reserve (juvenile diabetes mellitus), large parenteral or alimentary intake of carbohydrates (resulting from gorging or hyperalimentation), increased gluconeogenesis (resulting from corticosteroid administration), diminished peripheral utilization of glucose (resulting from hypothermia or burns), or failure of the kidneys to excrete glucose (renal failure).

The clinical picture in hyperglycemic hyperosmolar nonketotic encephalopathy is produced by a combination of brain dysfunction and hypovolemia. In addition to stupor, convulsions, and coma, symptoms of shock frequently occur. In many patients, polyuria, thirst, confusion, and delirium may follow the fully developed syndrome by a day or two (122). Laboratory findings in patients with hyperosmolar coma consist of extreme serum hypo-osmolarity, extreme hyperglycemia, hypovolemia, and normal or moderately elevated levels of serum ketones, sodium, potassium, and free fatty acids. BUN is characteristically elevated. Systemic acidosis may be present and is due to lactic acidemia.

Hyperglycemic hyperosmolar nonketotic encephalopathy occurs most frequently in patients with known juvenile- or adult-onset diabetes. For this reason, the condition must be distinguished from diabetic ketoacidosis. Seizures, while uncommon in diabetic ketoacidosis, are a clinical hallmark of hyperglycemic hyperosmolar nonketotic encephalopathy. Serum osmolality, BUN, and serum levels of glucose and sodium are higher in hyperglycemic hyperosmolar nonketotic encephalopathy than in diabetic ketoacidosis. However, patients with diabetic ketoacidosis exhibit high degrees of ketonemia and ketonuria accompanied by great elevations in plasma free fatty acids, whereas patients with hyperglycemic hyperosmolar nonketotic encephalopathy have much lower levels of these moieties. Individuals with diabetic ketoacidosis usually require large amounts of insulin to correct their abnormalities, whereas patients with hyperglycemic hyperosmolar nonketotic encephalopathy require less insulin. While dehydration is common to both states, it generally is more severe in hyperglycemic hyperosmolar nonketotic encephalopathy.

Therapy for this hyperosmolar state is aimed at reduction of hyperglycemia and correction of hypervolemia. Feig and McCurdy (123) have recommended the following treatment plan: Once the syndrome is identified, patients should be started on a regimen of isotonic saline. When adequate blood pressure and urine output are ensured, isotonic fluids, such as half-normal saline, should also be started. Five units of regular insulin should be given at the outset, followed by five units every two hours until glucose values fall to acceptable levels (250 mg/100 ml or less). Since patients with hyperglycemic hyperosmolar nonketotic encephalopathy are frequently potassium depleted, potassium chloride or potassium phosphate should be added to the IV fluids in patients who are not hyperkalemic or significantly acidotic. Serum levels of potassium should be monitored frequently.

The extent of dehydration and hypovolemia is frequently very severe in many patients with hyperglycemic hyperosmolar nonketotic encephalopathy. Such patients may require as much as 6–8 L of fluids to correct their deficit, with up to half the amount required in the first 8–12 hours of therapy. Patients with hyperglycemic hyperosmolar nonketotic encephalopathy are not insulin resistant, and most of them need only 50 units, and almost never more than 350 units, of insulin to correct their difficulties.

Diphenylhydantoin should be used cautiously to treat seizures in hyperglycemic hyperosmolar nonketotic encephalopathy, since the drug impairs in-

Table 8. Diagnosis of Hyperglycemic Hyperosmolar Nonketotic Encephalopathy

Clinical Circumstances
Diabetes mellitus
Pancreatic disease
Burns
Renal failure
Parenteral hyperalimentation
Clinical Findings
Polyuria
Thirst
Focal or generalized seizures
Coma
Shock
Laboratory Findings
Serum hyperosmolarity
Extreme hyperglycemia
Little or no ketoacidosis
Hypovolemia
Increased BUN
Normal or increased levels of serum sodium

Table 9. Treatment of Hyperglycemic Hyperosmolar Nonketotic Encephalopathy

Give isotonic NaCl until adequate blood pressure is established and urine flow is ensured.
Give hypotonic NaCl thereafter to correct hypovolemia.
Give parenteral potassium unless hyperkalemia or significant acidosis is present.
Give insulin in *relatively small amounts:* 5 units regular insulin IM every 2 hours.
Start 5% dextrose in water or 5% dextrose in normal saline when blood sugar is in 250–300 mg/100 ml range.

sulin release, a feature that is basic to the etiology of the clinical syndrome in the first place (124). Goldberg and Sandbar (125) have implicated use of diphenylhydantoin in the precipitation of hyperglycemic hyperosmolar nonketotic encephalopathy. Additional drugs that may be shown to impair insulin release or carbohydrate tolerance and thus should be avoided in this condition include thiazides, chlorpromazine, and nalidixic acid. Patients with hyperglycemic hyperosmolar nonketotic encephalopathy who remain hypotensive and oliguric in spite of volume replacement have a gloomy prognosis, with mortality as high as 75%. Tables 8 and 9, respectively, summarize the diagnosis and treatment of hyperglycemic hyperosmolar nonketotic encephalopathy.

BRIEF REVIEW OF LEAD POISONING (SATURNISM)

Lead encephalopathy in its characteristically severe and fully developed form occurs in up to 14% of cases of lead poisoning in adults (126) and in a much higher proportion of infants and children. In a review from Australia, Freeman (127) has estimated that up to 90% of infants and children with chronic severe lead poisoning develop clearly recognizable encephalopathy. Lead encephalopathy in its classic form is characterized by a history of environmental exposure to lead. The clinical and laboratory signs consist of pallor, irritability, epigastric pain, vomiting, basophilic stippling of red blood cells, anemia, and, occasionally evidence of nephropathy. Lead lines may be seen at the gingival margins or at the mucocutaneous junction of the rectum. The urine contains increased levels of lead or can be shown to do so by a challenge with a chelating agent. Urine levels of Δ-aminolevulinic acid and coproporphyrins may be increased. The neurologic picture in classic lead encephalopathy consists of confusion; delirium; severe, sustained, and unusually focal or generalized seizures that are unusually refractory to treatment; coma; increased intracranial pressure associated with moderate elevation in CSF protein; and mononuclear CSF pleocytosis (10–50 cells). Infants may show enlarged head circumference resulting from brain swelling, and both children and adults may exhibit papilledema.

Treatment of lead encephalopathy consists of measures to reduce intracranial pressure (administration of mannitol or urea); administration of pharmacologic agents to prevent further absorption of lead from sources that may be remaining in the intestinal tract (2,3-dimercaptopropranol, BAL, 3–5 mg/kg IM every four hours for four to five days); and administration of agents that remove lead from sources in tissue (BAL and calcium edetate, calcium disodium versenate, 50 mg/kg/day parenterally, or 50–75 mg/kg/day orally in children and adults). Oral calcium edetate should be avoided in patients who are likely to have lead in their gastrointestinal tract, since, although calcium edetate is a chelator, it promotes absorption of lead through the alimentary tract. Hyperthermia, dehydration, and electrolyte imbalances may accompany lead encephalopathy and must be treated specifically. Chisholm (128) and Menkes (129) have published protocols for the treatment of lead encephalopathy.

In an interesting and worthwhile publication, Guinee (130) has reviewed the historic and epidemiologic features of lead poisoning. Frank and clearly identifiable encephalopathy of the type described above is no longer as common as it once was because of both increased recognition of the syndrome and such public health and safety measures as reduction of lead in paints and toys. Most persons with identifiable lead encephalopathy have blood levels of lead greater than 100 μg/ml. As Lin-Fu has pointed out, a lead level that is not associated with overt clinical evidence of lead toxicity is not necessarily normal (131). Although persons with elevated lead levels in tissue may not be symptomatic in the classic sense, they may not be free of detectable neurologic or systemic disease. Precisely what levels of lead in blood and tissue are acceptable is open to debate; however, a cutoff point in blood of 40 μg/100 ml is now generally agreed on as this arbitrary and historically unstable value. Blood levels of lead ranging from 20–100 mg/100 ml have held the honor transiently in the past. What does seem to be emerging from a large number of careful studies in the past 20 years is the notion that the lower the blood and tissue levels of lead, the better.

Epidemiologic studies of children over the past two decades have established that certain populations are at special risk of lead poisoning. These include economically disadvantaged urban children, and children living in the environs of lead mines, smelters, and processing plants. All children who live in urban environments generally have higher blood levels of lead than do children who live in rural environments. This difference probably is attributable to greater exposure of the former group to industrial and vehicular effluents. In addition, some adults who do not work in lead-related industries have been shown to have high levels of lead in their blood. People in this category include residents of traffic-congested center cities, traffic policemen, persons who work in firearms testing centers, and workers on highways and in traffic tunnels. Blood levels of lead in these groups are two to three times higher than those found in controls of similar age and sex (132).

There is mounting evidence that lead exposure in children may be associated with brain deficits that are far more subtle than those seen in fully developed, classic lead encephalopathy (131,133). Developmental and neuropsychological studies evaluating motor and mental achievement and learning abilities strongly suggest that children with undue but not clearly toxic tissue burdens of lead are neurologically impaired as compared with controls. Aspects of brain function that have been best studied are measures of intelligence quotient and classroom behavior. These suggest that lead exposure produces deficits in these areas at levels below those that produce symptoms severe enough to be diagnosed clinically as lead encephalopathy. Less quantifiable disorders that may be expressions of subclinical encephalopathy in children or adults, such as withdrawal, anxiety, lack of affection, temper tantrums, inattention, and hyperkinesis, are studied less readily but certainly cannot be excluded as manifestations of a brain disorder that falls short of evolving into confusion, stupor, seizures, and coma. Furthermore, it is not clear that chronic lead exposure or lead poisoning in childhood may not lead to serious health impairment in adult life. Studies from Australia suggest that childhood lead poisoning leads to chronic nephritis, gout, and mental impairment in adulthood (134); these inferences, however, are not yet solidly established. It is clear that lead fragments retained in the body can lead to episodes of frank and fully developed lead encephalopathy more than two decades later. Some rare forms of motor neuron disease that clearly resemble amyotrophic lateral sclerosis have been associated with chronic lead exposure and high tissue levels of the element (135,136).

Social and technological advances and changes in public health practices have worked to change the pattern of dispersion of lead encephalopathy, and recent advances in both detection and understanding have suggested that this disorder may exist in a form less obvious than severe, subacute brain illness. Problems of pica and industrial exposure have not been solved, however, and recreational exposure to lead still occurs through the use of certain drinking vessels and sniffing of gasoline. Very recent series of adults with lead poisoning demonstrate that lead encephalopathy continues to be a hazard for moonshiners and their customers (137), as well as for persons who retain lead bullets in their bodies, particularly if lead fragments manage to find their way to synovial cavities (138).

ACKNOWLEDGMENT

I wish to thank Jeannette Conomy, B.S.N., and Karen Barnes, Ph.D., for their suggestions regarding the manuscript, and Susan Cummins, Diane Crouse and Linda Sands for their skillful help. The Reinberger Foundation, whose support has provided the opportunity for many of the observations reflected in this presentation, is gratefully acknowledged.

REFERENCES

1. Plum F, Posner J, Hain RF: Delayed neurological deterioration after anoxia. Arch Intern Med 110:56–63, 1962.
2. Adams RD, Foley JM: Neurological changes in more common types of severe liver disease. Trans Am Neurol Assoc 74:217, 1949.
3. Tyler HR, Leavitt S: Asterixis. J Chronic Dis 18:409–411, 1965.
4. Hippocrates: On regimen in acute diseases. In *The Genuine Works of Hippocrates,* vol. 2. Translated by FD Adams. New York, William Wood, 1929, p. 270.
5. Bright R: Observations of jaundice. Guys Hosp Rep 1:604–637, 1836.
6. Frerichs FT: *A Clinical Treatise on Diseases of the Liver.* Translated by C. Murchison. London, New Sydenham Society, 1860.
7. Gautier G, Wildi E: L'encephalo-myelopathie porto-systemique. Rev Neurol 131:319–338, 1975.
8. Leavitt S, Tyler HR: Studies in asterixis. Arch Neurol 10:360–368, 1964.
9. Ericson J, Warren SE, Gribik M, et al: Unilateral asterixis in a dialysis patient. JAMA 240:671, 1978.

10. Conomy JP, Swash M: Reversible decerebrate and decorticate postures in hepatic coma. N Engl J Med 278:876–879, 1968.
11. Chen S, Ziev L, Mahadevan V: Mercaptans and dimethylsulfide in the breath of patients with cirrhosis of the liver. J Lab Clin Med 75:628–635, 1970.
12. Walker CO, McCandless DW, McGarry JD, et al: Cerebral energy metabolism in short chain fatty acid–induced coma. J Lab Clin Med 76:569–583, 1970.
13. Fisher JE, Baldessarini RJ: Pathogenesis and therapy of hepatic coma. Prog Liver Dis 5:363–397, 1976.
14. Schenker S, Breen KJ, Hoyumpa AM: Hepatic encephalopathy: current status. Gastroenterology 66:121–151, 1974.
15. Dillon D, Schenker S: Cerebrospinal fluid protein concentration in hepatic coma. JAMA 221:507, 1972.
16. Adams RD, Foley JM: The neurological disorder associated with liver disease. Res Publ Assoc Res Nerv Ment Dis 32:198–237, 1953.
17. Silverman D: Some observations on the EEG in hepatic coma. J Electroenceph Clin Neurophys 14:53–59, 1962.
18. Victor M, Adams RD, Cole M: The acquired (non-Wilsonian) type of chronic hepatocerebral degeneration. Medicine (Baltimore) 44:345–396, 1965.
19. Goldstein NP, Owen CA: Introduction to Symposium on copper metabolism and Wilson's disease. Mayo Clin Proc 49:363–367, 1974.
20. Trey C, Lipworth L, Davidson CS: Parameters influencing survival in the first 318 patients reported to the fulminant hepatic failure surveillance study. Gastroenterology 58:306, 1970.
21. Plum F, Caronna JJ: Can one predict the outcome of medical coma? Ciba Foundation Symposium 34:121–136, 1975.
22. Elkington SG, Floch MH, Conn HO: Lactulose in the treatment of chronic portal-systemic encephalopathy. N Engl J Med 281:408–412, 1969.
23. Kosman ME: Lactulose (Cephulac) in portosystemic encephalopathy. JAMA 236:2444–2445, 1976.
24. Parkes JD, Sharpstone P, Williams R: Levodopa in hepatic coma. Lancet 2:1341–1343, 1970.
25. Fisher JE, Baldessarini RJ, Wurtman RJ: False neurotransmitters in hepatic failure. Lancet 2:75–81, 1971.
26. Sarragin A, Emerit J, Oliver L, et al: Traitment du coma hepatique par L-dopa. Presse Med 79:2226–2227, 1971.
27. Morgan MY, Jakobovitz A, Elithorn A, et al: Successful use of bromocriptine in the treatment of a patient with chronic portasystemic encephalopathy. N Engl J Med 296:793–794, 1977.
28. Summershill WHJ, Thorsell F, Femkerg J, et al: Effect of urease inhibition in hyperammonemia clinical and experimental studies with acetohydroxamic acid. Gastroenterology 54:20–26, 1968.
29. Davidson CS: Hepatic coma. In *Gastroenterology*. Edited by HL Backus. Philadelphia, WB Saunders, 1976, pp. 435–450.
30. Juhl E, Winkel P, Tygstrup N: Sex ascites and alcoholism in survival of patients with cirrhosis. N Engl J Med 291:271–274, 1974.
31. Katz R, Velasco M, Klinger J, et al: Corticosteroids in the treatment of acute hepatitis in coma. Gastroenterology 42:258–266, 1962.
32. The colon: cesspool or nutrient factory? (editorial) N Engl J Med 267:891–892, 1962.
33. Burnell JM, Dawborn JK, Epstein RB, et al: Acute hepatic coma treated by cross-circulation or exchange transfusion. N Engl J Med 276:936–944, 1967.
34. Nose Y, Malchesky PS, Castino F, et al: Improved hemoperfusion systems for renal-hepatic support. Kidney Int 10(Suppl 7):S244–S247, 1976.
35. Manis T, Freidman A: Dialytic therapy for irreversible uremia (Part II). N Engl J Med 301:1321–1328, 1979.
36. Reye RDK, Morgan J, Baral J: Encephalopathy and fatty degeneration of the viscera: a disease entity in childhood. Lancet 2:749–752, 1963.

37. Johnson GM, Scurletis TD, Carroll NB: A study of 16 fatal cases of encephalitis-like disease in North Carolina children. NC Med J 24:464–473, 1963.

38. Corey L, Reuloen R: Reye's syndrome 1974: an epidemiologic approach. In: *Reye's Syndrome.* Edited by JD Pollack. New York, Grune and Stratton, 1975.

39. Brunberg JA, Bell WE: Reye's syndrome: an association with type-1 vaccine-like poliovirus. Arch Neurol 30:304–306, 1974.

40. Tang TT, Siegesmund KA, Sedmak GV, et al: Reye's syndrome: a correlated electron-microscopic, viral and biochemical observation. JAMA 232:1339–1346, 1975.

41. Alvira MM, Mendoza M: Reye's syndrome: a viral myopathy? N Engl J Med 292:1297, 1975.

42. Partin JC, Schubert WK, Partin JS: Mitochondrial ultrastructure in Reye's syndrome (encephalopathy and fatty degeneration of the viscera). N Engl J Med 285:1339–1344, 1971.

43. Gall DG, Cutz E, McClung HJ, et al: Acute liver disease and encephalopathy mimicking Reye syndrome. Pediatrics 87:869–874, 1975.

44. Bobo RC, Schubert WK, Partin JC, et al: Reye's syndrome: treatment by exchange transfusion with special reference to the 1974 epidemic in Cincinnati, Ohio. Pediatrics 87:881–886, 1975.

45. Partin JC, Partin JS, Schubert WK, et al: Brain ultrastructure in Reye's syndrome. J Neuropathol Exp Neurol 34:425–444, 1975.

46. Huttenlocher PR: Reye's syndrome: relation of outcome to therapy. J Pediatr 80:845–850, 1972.

47. Snodgrass PJ, DeLong R: Urea cycle enzyme deficiencies and increased nitrogen load producing hyperammonemia in Reye's syndrome. N Engl J Med 294:855–860, 1976.

48. Carballo E, Ellefson RD, Gomez MR: An aflatoxin in the liver of a patient with Reye–Johnson syndrome. Mayo Clin Proc 51:48–50, 1976.

49. Trauner DA, Nyhan WL, Sweetman L: Short chain organic acidemia and Reye's syndrome. Neurology 25:296–298, 1975.

50. Samaha RJ, Blau E, Berardelli JL: Reye's syndrome: clinical diagnosis and treatment with peritoneal dialysis. Pediatrics 53:336–340, 1974.

51. Berman W, Pizzi F, Schut L, et al: The effects of exchange transfusion in intracranial pressure in Reye's syndrome. J Pediatr 87:887–891, 1975.

52. DeVivo D, Keating JP, Haymond MW: Reye's syndrome: results of intensive supportive care. J Pediatr 87:875–880, 1975.

53. Morbid Mortal Weekly Rep 23:115, 1974.

54. Raskin NH, Fishman RA: Neurologic disorders in renal failure (2 parts). N Engl J Med 294:143–148, 204–210, 1976.

55. Tyler HR: Neurologic disorders in renal failure. Am J Med 44:734–746, 1968.

56. Plum F, Posner JB: *The Diagnosis of Stupor and Coma.* Philadelphia, FA Davis, 1972, p. 184.

57. Oldstone MBA, Nelson E: Central nervous system manifestations of penicillin toxicity in man. Neurology 16:693–700, 1966.

58. Conomy JP: Long-term use of the major anticonvulsant drugs. Am Fam Physician 18:107–116, 1978.

59. Letteri JM, Mellk H, Louis S, et al: Diphenylhydantoin metabolism in uremia. N Engl J Med 285:648–652, 1971.

60. Kutt H, and McDowell F: Management of epilepsy with diphenylhydantoin sodium: dosage regulation for problem patients. JAMA 203:969–972, 1968.

61. Merrell JP, Hamper CL: *Uremia Progress in Pathophysiology and Treatment.* New York, Grune and Stratton, 1971.

62. Conomy JP, and McNamara JO: Emergency management of the patient with seizures. Postgrad Mcd 55:59 74, 1974.

63. Madonick MJ, Berke K, Schiffer I: Pleocytosis and meningeal signs in uremia: report of 62 cases. Arch Neurol Psychiatr 64:431–436, 1950.

64. Bank N, Lief P, and Piczon O: Use of diuretics in the treatment of hypertension secondary to renal disease. Arch Intern Med 138:1524–1529, 1978.

65. Wardle EN: Fibrinogen catabolism studies in patients with renal disease. Q J Med 42:205–219, 1973.

66. Wakim KG: The pathophysiology of the dialysis dysequilibrium syndrome. Mayo Clin Proc 44:406–429, 1969.

67. Arieff AI, Massry G, Barrientos A, et al: Brain water and electrolyte metabolism in uremia: effects of slow and rapid hemodialysis. Kidney Int 4:177–187, 1973.

68. Cerra FB, Anthone R, Anthone S: Colloid osmotic pressure fluctuations and the disequilibrium syndrome during dialysis. Nephron 13:245–252, 1974.

69. Hagstam KE, Lindergard B, Tibbling G: Mannitol infusion in regular haemodialysis treatment for chronic renal insufficiency. Scand J Urol Nephrol 3:257–263, 1969.

70. Bennett WM, Singer I, Coggins CJ: A guide to drug therapy in renal failure. JAMA 230:1544–1553, 1974.

71. Alfrey AC, Mishel JM, Burks J, et al: Syndrome of dysproxia and multifocal seizures associated with chronic hemodialysis. Trans Am Soc Artif Intern Organs 18:257–261, 1972.

72. Lederman RJ, Henry CE: Progressive dialysis dementia. Ann Neurol 4:199–204, 1978.

73. Rosenbeck JC, McNiel MR, Lemme ML, et al: Speech and language findings in a chronic hemodialysis patient. J Speech Hear Disord 40:245–251, 1975.

74. Alfrey AC, LeGendre GR, Kaehny WD: The dialysis encephalopathy syndrome: possible aluminum intoxication. N Engl J Med 294:184–188, 1976.

75. Nadal AM, Wilson WP: Dialysis encephalopathy: a possible seizure disorder. Neurology 26:1130-1134, 1976.

76. Faris AA: Wernicke's encephalopathy in uremia. Neurology 22:1293–1297, 1972.

77. Lopez RI, Collins GK: Wernicke's encephalopathy: a complication of chronic hemodialysis. Arch Neurol 18:248–259, 1968.

78. Lasker N, Harvey A, Baker H: Vitamin levels in hemodialysis and intermittent peritoneal dialysis. Trans Am Soc Artif Intern Organs 9:51–56, 1963.

79. Sherins RJ, Verity A: Central pontine myelinolysis associated with acute hemorrhagic pancreatitis. J Neurol Neurosurg Psychiatr 31:583–588, 1968.

80. Johnson DA, Tong NT: Pancreatic encephalopathy. South Med J 70:165–167, 1977.

81. Sharf B, Bental E: Pancreatic encephalopathy. J Neurol Neurosurg Psychiatr 34:357–361, 1971.

82. Vogel FS: Cerebral demyelination and focal visceral lesions in a case of acute hemorrhagic pancreatitis with a consideration of the possible role of circulating enzymes in the causation of the lesions. Arch Pathol 53:355–362, 1951.

83. Haymaker W, Anderson E: Disorders of the hypothalamus and pituitary gland. In: *Clinical Neurology.* Edited by AB Baker and LH Baker. New York, Harper and Row, 1976.

84. Myers RD: Temperature regulation: neurochemical systems in the hypothalamus. Edited by W Haymaker, E Anderson, and WHJ Nauta. Springfield, IL, Charles C Thomas, 1969.

85. Myers RD, Yaksh TL: Control of body temperature in the unanesthetized monkey by cholinergic and aminergic systems in the hypothalamus. J Physiol 202:483–500, 1969.

86. Gottschalk PG, Thomas JE: Heat stroke. Mayo Clin Proc 41:470–482, 1966.

87. Shibolet S, Coll R, Gilat T, et al: Heatstroke: its clinical picture and mechanism in 36 cases. Q J Med 6:525–548, 1967.

88. Leithead CS, Guthrie J, DeLaPlace S, et al: Incidence, aetiology and prevention of heat illness on ships in the Persian Gulf. Lancet 2:109–115, 1958.

89. Salem SN: Neurologic complications of heat stroke in Kuwait. Ann Trop Med Parasitol 60:1784–1788, 1966.

90. Nemoto EM, Frankel HM: Cerebral oxygenation and metabolism during progressive hyperthermia. Am J Physiol 219:1784–1788, 1970.

91. Meyer JS, Honda J: Cerebral blood flow and metabolism during experimental hyperthermia. Minn Med 50:37–44, 1967.

92. Wernicke C: *Lehrbuch der Gehirnkronkheiten fuer Aerzte und Studierinde.* Kassel, Theodor Fisher. 1881, pp. 229–242.

93. Drenick EJ, Joven CB, Swenseid ME: Occurrence of acute Wernicke's encephalopathy during prolonged starvation for the treatment of obesity. N Engl J Med 274:937–939, 1966.

94. Victor M, Adams RD, Collins GH: *The Wernicke–Korsakoff Syndrome.* In *Contemporary Neurology Series.* Edited by F Plum and FH McDowell. Philadelphia, FA Davis, 1971.

95. Nadel AM, Burger PC: Wernicke encephalopathy following prolonged intravenous therapy. JAMA 235:2403–2405, 1976.

96. Kramer J, Goodwin JA: Wernicke's encephalopathy: complication of intravenous hyperalimentation. JAMA 238:2176–2177, 1977.

97. Blass JT, Gibson GE: Abnormality of a thiamine-requiring enzyme in patients with Wernicke–Korsakoff syndrome. N Engl J Med 297:1367–1370, 1977.

98. Knochel JP: Hypophosphatemia. Clin Nephrol 7:131–137, 1977.

99. Havill JH, Rothwell PRG, Chin L: Hypophosphatemia and paresthesias during parenteral nutrition. NZ Med J 83:403, 1976.

100. Lichtman MA: Hypoalimentation during hyperalimentation. N Engl J Med 290:1432, 1974.

101. Silvas SE, Paragas PD: Paresthesias, weakness, seizures, and hypophosphatemia in patients receiving hyperalimentation. Gastroenterology 62:513, 1972.

102. Lee JL, Sibbald WJ, Holliday RL, et al: Hypophosphatemia associated with coma. Can Med Assoc J 119:143–145, 1977.

103. Byrom FB: The pathogenesis of hypertensive encephalopathy and its relation to the malignant phase of hypertensio-experimental evidence from the hypertensive rat. Lancet 2:201–211, 1954.

104. Lassen NA, Aganoli A: The upper limit of autoregulation of cerebral blood flow on the pathogenesis of hypertensive encephalopathy. Scand Clin Lab Invest 30:113–116, 1972.

105. Skinhoj E: The sympathetic nervous system and the regulation of cerebral blood flow in man. Stroke 3:711–716, 1972.

106. Dinsdale HB: Hypertension in the blood brain barrier. In: *Advances in Neurology.* Edited by J Cervos-Navarros. New York, Raven Press, 1978, pp. 341–346.

107. Naftchi N, Demmeny M, Lowman E, et al: Hypertensive crises in quadriplegic patients. Circulation 57:336–341, 1978.

108. Fujishima M, Onoyama K, Oniki H, et al: Effects of acute hypertension on brain metabolism in normotensive, renal vascular hypertensive, and spontaneously hypertensive rats. Stroke 9:349–353, 1978.

109. Gifford RW, Westbrook E: Hypertensive encephalopathy: mechanisms, clinical features, and treatment. Prog Cardiovasc Dis 17:115–124, 1975.

110. Chester E, Agamanolis DP, Banker BQ, et al: Hypertensive encephalopathy: a clinical pathologic study of 20 cases. Neurology 28:928–939, 1978.

111. Adams RD: Vascular diseases of the brain. Annu Rev Med 4:213–252, 1964.

112. Vidt D, Gifford RW: Management of hypertensive emergencies. Cleve Clin Q 45:299–306, 1978.

113. Fleischmann LE: Management of hypertensive crises in children. Pediatr Ann 6:410–414, 1977.

114. Niarchos AP: Evaluation of intravenous clonidine in hypertensive emergencies. J Clin Pharmacol 18:220–228, 1978.

115. Guazzi M, Olivari MT, Polese A, et al: Nifedipine, a new antihypertensive with rapid action. Clin Pharmacol Ther 22:528–532, 1977.

116. Martin JB, Reichlin S, Brown G: Neural regulation of water and salt metabolism: physiologic function and diseases. In: *Clinical Neuroendocrinology. Contemporary Neurology Series,* vol. 14. Edited by F Plum and FH McDowell. Philadelphia, FA Davis, 1977, pp. 63–92.

117. Hamilton BPM, Upton GV, Amatruda TT: Evidence for the presence of neurophysin in tumors producing the syndrome of inappropriate antidiuresis. J Clin Endocrinol Metabl 35:764, 1972.

118. Bartter FC: The syndrome of inappropriate secretion of antidiuretic hormone (SIADH). DM November 1973, pp. 1–47.

119. Forrest JN, Cox M, Hong C, et al: Superiority of demeclocycline over lithium in the treatment of chronic syndrome of inappropriate secretion of antidiuretic hormone. N Engl J Med 298:173–177, 1978.

120. De Troyer A: Demeclocycline: treatment for syndrome of inappropriate antidiuretic hormone secretion. JAMA 237:2723–2726, 1977.

121. Hantman D, Rossier B, Zohlman R, et al: Rapid correction of hyponatremia in the syndrome of inappropriate secretion of antidiuretic hormone. Ann Intern Med 78:870–875, 1973.

122. Tyler FH: Hyperosmolar coma. Am J Med 45:485–487, 1968.

123. Feig PU, McCurdy DK: The hypertonic state. N Engl J Med 297:1444–1454, 1977.

124. Malherbe C, Burill KC, Levin S, et al: Effects of diphenylhydantoin on insulin secretion in man. N Engl J Med 286:339–342, 1972.

125. Goldberg EM, Sanbar SS: Hyperglycemic, non-ketotic coma following administration of Dilantin (diphenylhydantoin). Diabetes 18:101–106, 1969.

126. Cantarow A, Trumper M: *Lead Poisoning.* Baltimore, Williams and Wilkins, 1944.

127. Freeman R: Chronic lead poisoning in children: a review of 90 children diagnosed in Sydney, 1948–1967. 2. Clinical features and investigations. Med J Aust 1:648, 1970.

128. Chisholm JJ: Management of increased lead absorption and lead poisoning in children. N Engl J Med 289:1016–1018, 1973.

129. Menkes JH: *Textbook of Child Neurology.* Philadelphia, Lea and Febiger, 1974, p. 342.

130. Guinee VF: Lead poisoning. Am J Med 52:283–288, 1972.

131. Lin-Fu JS: Undue absorption of lead among children: a new look at an old problem. N Engl J Med 286:702–710, 1972.

132. U.S. Department of Health, Education, and Welfare: *Survey of Lead in the Atmosphere of Three Urban Communities.* Publication No. 999-AP-12, Washington, D.C., U.S. Government Printing Office, January 1965.

133. Neadleman HL, Gunnoe C, Leviton A, et al: Deficits and classroom performance of children with elevated dentine levels. N Engl J Med 300:689–695, 1979.

134. Henderson DA: A follow-up of cases of plumbism in children. *Aust Ann Med* 3:219–223, 1954.

135. Boothby JA, DeJesus PV, Rowland LP: Reversible forms of motor neuron disease. Arch Neurol 31:18–23, 1974.

136. Pethaw A, Sawatzky A, Hallier CR, et al: Lead content of neuromuscular tissue in amyotrophic lateral sclerosis. Br J Ind Med 31:275–287, 1974.

137. Whitfield CL, Ch'ien LT, Whitehead JD: Lead encephalopathy in adults. Am J Med 52:289–298, 1972.

138. Dillman RO, Crumb CK, Lidsky MJ: Lead poisoning from a gunshot wound. Am J Med 66:509–513, 1979.

2
Treatment of Neuromuscular Diseases

W. King Engel
Marinos Dalakas

DEFINITION

A number of neuromuscular diseases can be treated either symptomatically or semietiologically/pathogenically. *Neuromuscular diseases* are disorders of the motor unit. The *motor unit* consists of one *lower motor neuron* (LMN) and the few hundred *muscle fibers* innervated by it. Diseases caused by an abnormality of the LMN are generally termed *neuropathies;* those not caused by an LMN disorder are called *myopathies.* In some instances, the diagnosis of myopathy is made by exclusion. *Junctional disorders* are ones in which the defect is at a *neuromuscular junction* (NMJ), on either the LMN side of the muscle-fiber side, or both. This chapter is concerned with myopathies and disorders of the NMJ (basic biology of the motor unit, LMN, NMJ, and muscle are reviewed elsewhere [1–8]). The chapter reflects our approach to treating neuromuscular disorders. Approaches of other investigators are described in other volumes (3,5,9–12).

TYPES OF TREATMENT

Under the broad heading of treatment we includ the following: (*1*) treatment per se (including pharmacologic, roentgenographic, and physical alterations of plasma or cells). Treatment can be etiologic, pathogenic, or symptomatic in nature; (*2*) respiratory assistance; (*3*) prevention, such as genetic counseling; (*4*) physical medicine, such as manipulations, training, or bracing; (*5*) surgical correction; (*6*) nursing care; (*7*) interpersonal relations, such as that between doctor and patient or nurse and patient, or group discussions; and (*8*) habilitation and rehabilitation, both vocational and nonvocational.

Treatment per se is discussed in the section on each disease. Some side effects of drugs are given, but for a full listing one must consult package inserts, *The*

Physician's Desk Reference (a commercial compendium of package inserts of many drugs; it does not include all effective uses of the drugs listed), texts of pharmacology and therapeutics, and other sources. Doses and schedules given here are suggestions based on our experience and should be modified if clinical judgment so indicates.

In order to evaluate the benefit of a particular treatment or the progression of disease, we developed a simple bedside system and for 20 years have found it valuable. For each patient we identify and record a few simple tasks (such as having the patient raise each leg off the bed, elevate both hands above ear level when seated, comb their hair, shave, arise from a specific chair with arms crossed on the chest) that the patient cannot quite accomplish, as well as tasks that he or she can barely do. If the condition improves, the can't-quites become just-barelys or better; if the condition worsens, the opposite occurs.

Respiratory assistance is described in the section on myasthenia gravis. It is also especially applicable to the relapsing neuropathies (e.g., dysimmune, porphyric), infrequently applicable to dysimmune dermatomyopathy/polymyopathy, and, after due consideration, may be applicable to certain patients in whom the chance of recovery is very slight (e.g., those with amyotrophic lateral sclerosis [11] or progressive hereditary myopathy, such as acid maltase deficiency).

Use of genetic counseling for prevention of neurologic disease must be based on accurate diagnosis of the patient, as established by relevant diagnostic parameters as discussed here and elsewhere (1–8,10,11). Such parameters include clinical examination; histochemistry of muscle biopsy sample; clinical electrophysiology of muscles and nerves; laboratory examination of blood, spinal fluid, and urine; metabolic loading and imbalancing tests; x-ray films and isotope scans; and, in some instances, a short therapeutic trial as a diagnostic test. Counseling also must be based on a study of probable and possible carriers and on knowledge of genetic patterns that the disease or syndrome has expressed previously.

Physical medicine, of which we are strong enthusiasts, has potential benefits for all patients with neuromuscular disease. Many patients receive major benefit from such therapy, regardless of whether specific treatment of the disease is available.

Surgical correction should be accomplished with the simplest procedure that will achieve the *functional* goal (as opposed to a cosmetic goal) but also with an understanding of the expected course of the disease, the possible worsening effect of prolonged bed rest or other immobilization, and, in regard to scoliosis, worsening of respiratory capacity to the point of lifelong insufficiency (we are aware of the deaths of two scoliosis patients that probably resulted from such a sequence). Corrections of the limbs and spine are discussed elsewhere (13–16). Surgery to correct ptosis of the eyelid should not be rushed into and should virtually never be done in patients with a treatable disease such as myasthenia gravis. Lid crutches help many such patients. One surgical failure that occurs in these cases is overcorrection, which results in exposure keratopathy, which, in turn, can lead to the emergence of corneal perforation. A silastic suspension can also be considered (17). The dysphagia of oculopharyngeal dystrophy sometimes responds well to cricopharyngeal myotomy (18).

Nursing care can be an important, and sometimes critical, aspect of treatment (see section on myasthenia gravis) in the care of patients with neuromuscular disease (11,19).

Interpersonal relations play an important role in the management of patients with neuromuscular disease. Such relations include explanations to the patient by the physician regarding medical matters and by the nurse on nursing matters. In some circumstances, group discussions among patients and among relatives who have similar problems can be valuable. Severe disabling fear or anxiety expressed as neuromuscular impairment can be termed *hysteria*, but this state is more common in milder degrees. Sometimes anxiety is the only factor to cause symptoms of weakness, but often it is superimposed on a definite but mild neuromuscular disease that becomes obscurred by the anxiety. The fear or anxiety often can be managed by the nonpsychiatric physician through careful inquiry into anxiety-provoking factors, such as fear of the diagnosis or interpersonal relations in the patient's family or work situation. Whether or not those factors can be resolved perfectly, the patient whose anxiety expresses itself as neuromuscular impairment often can be helped by the physician's encouragement to increase gradually activity in a closely supervised setting that will allow "face saving for the subconscious."

Habilitation and rehabilitation must be considered in every patient who is handicapped with neuromuscular disease. Measures include keeping the disabled patient on the job (either out of the home or at home) at long as possible, fitting the patient to a new job that they can do, ensuring physical access to the job and to necessities (e.g., restrooms), and enhancing the awareness of family, friends, employers, and the public to needs of the disabled patient.

DISORDERS OF THE NEUROMUSCULAR JUNCTION (NMJ)

Myasthenia Gravis

Clinical Features and Diagnosis

Myasthenia gravis (MG) is a dysimmune disease that causes weakness resulting from defective transmission at the NMJ. The major clinical finding is rapid muscle fatigability, which affects most severely the musculature innervated by the cranial nerves and the musculature of the trunk and proximal limbs, although the weakness often affects all muscles to some degree. Diagnostic features include the pattern of involvement, rapid fatigability with recovery after a few minutes' rest, clinical response to anticholinesterases (e.g., edrophonium, neostigmine, pyridostigmine), marked worsening with administration of d-tubocurarine (curare),* decrement on repetitive electric stimulation at low fre-

*A systemic curare test, which occasionally is necessary in difficult patients consists of intravenous (IV) administration of doses (0.0020625 mg d-tubocurarine per kg body weight) that are each 1/80 of the curarizing dose. The curare is given from a 5-ml syringe containing 8/80 of the curarizing dose (0.0165 mg/kg) in a total volume of 4 ml (i.e., 0.5 ml per dose) each minute until weakness occurs, or to a maximum of eight doses (20). Our guidelines for the results are as follows: positive is weakness at 5/80 or less, negative is no weakness at 8/80, and uncertain is weakness at 6/80–8/80. Weakness induced by the d-tubocurarine is reversed by IV administration of edrophonium, 2–10 mg. The test

quencies (2–5 Hz) or pathologic jitter (21) that are repaired by anticholinesterase, and serum IgG antibody against nicotinic acetylcholine receptor (nAChR) (22,23). (The IV lactate test, presumably based on its worsening of MG by lowering of plasma Ca^{2+}, is another possible diagnostic procedure [24] but is not widely used.)

The pathogenesis of typical MG involves an abnormal circulating IgG (22,23) directed against the nAChR at the muscular, and probably to some extent at the neuronal, portion of the NMJ (25,26). The antibody damages and simplifies nAChR-containing junctional membranes (27–30), probably by antigenic modulation and perhaps to some degree by antibody-dependent complement-mediated focal lysis, resulting in net loss of nAChR (23,27,28). Anti-AChR antibodies can be identified by morphologic methods in 68% (25,26) and by radioimmunoassay (RIA) in 87% of MG patients (patients with negative results by RIA are usually mildly affected or in remission) (22,23). Higher titers are in general more frequently associated with patients who have detectable thymoma than with nonthymoma patients less than 40 years old. Although no clear relations exist between antibody titer and severity of disease in a group of MG patients, it does often parallel the course in a given patient (22,23).

The anti-nAChR antibody in patients with early MG is IgM, which then converts to IgG (31). This sequence of events suggests a response to a recent immunologic challenge, and it is known that the thymus is required for such conversion. Different antibodies against nAChR can exist in the same patient (23,32–34). Probably not all of these antibodies are pathogenic, and possibly not all the pathogenic ones are measured in the RIA (35); thus, the antibody response in MG is usually polyclonal (33). The RIA does not measure the antibody that is directed against the ACh recognition site of nAChR because it is blocked by the effects of ^{125}I-α-bungarotoxin in the assay (36). The pathogenic IgG probably is directed preferably against extrajunctional nAChR, some of which also is present at the junction, rather than against purely junctional nAChR (37). There do exist patients with MG and monoclonal gammopathy (38,39); in some, the pathogenic antibody was not thought to be the IgG-kappa spike. Anti-nAChR antibody in cerebrospinal fluid (CSF) is detectable in most MG patients and is said to be synthesized "locally" (31); anti-nAChR antibody had been suggested earlier as the cause of brisk reflexes typical of MG patients. The antibody causes these reflexes by blocking the AChR of the inhibitory Renshaw cells (which inhibit the inhibitors) (W.K. Engel, unpublished observations). An anti-nAChR antibody of children with MG that affects T cells may be important pathogenically (as may be a non-IgG humoral factor, possibly of thymic origin) (40). (The antimuscle/antithymus–epithelial cell antibody (41–43], which cross-reacts with the I-band sarcoplasmic reticulum [44], may be either the same as anti-nAChR or produced concomitantly with nAChR [45].

Mechanisms of initiating the dysimmune state may differ among MG patients. Some seem to exhibit genetic susceptibility, as reflected by histocompatibility

---

should be done in the presence of an anesthesiologist or anesthetist who can intubate and ventilate the patient if respiratory insufficiency develops. (We are intuitively skeptical of the scientific standardization of the forearm-regional curare test because the test requires that curare be diffused retrograde into the veins, contrary to valvular traffic, into the muscle of an ischemic limb.)

leukocyle antigen (HLA) tissue typing of MG patients with variables of different age of onset and presence or absence of thymoma (32,46–48). In animal model systems, certain genes control glycoproteins of cell surfaces, cellular interactions of responses, and production of antibodies (49); there is also genetic influence or susceptibility to experimental allergic myasthenia gravis (EAMG) (50). The cause of production of the abnormal IgG in MG is still speculative (51–54). MG patients also may exhibit dysimmune manifestations that are related to other tissues (46,55–59).

The thymus seems to play a central role in the pathogenesis of MG. Of adult MG patients including most young adults, 72% have hyperplasia as evidenced by lymphoid germinal centers, 10% have thymoma (defined as proliferated thymic epithelial cells and occurring generally in patients aged 40 or older), and 18% (usually older patients) have atrophy (60) but not absence (61). In young adults, thymectomy is especially therapeutic. However, we feel that thymectomy is somewhat beneficial at any age (61), suggesting that thymic abnormality plays a role at all ages (61). The reason for the beneficial effects of thymectomy is still not certain. Human thymic epithelial cells contain nAChR (53) and thymosin (54) (they do not contain myofibrils, however, and thus are not "myoid" [51–63]). These substances are present in the hyperplastic thymus, in the thymomatous thymus (about 30% of patients with thymoma have MG [64]), and even in the "atrophic" thymus of middle-aged and older MG patients (53,54,61). Although their possible role as an antigenic site containing a "foreigned molecule" (i.e., one related to infestation by a virus, mycoplasma, or other organism, or to an environmental toxin) has been raised (51–53), this hypothesis remains unconfirmed. It has been suggested that thymosin from thymic epithelial cells (54) or perhaps another thymic non-IgG factor (40,65) may play a facilitative role. (Conversely, an inhibitor of thymic hormone activity has been found in the serum of patients with lymphoblastic leukemia [66].) A few immunologic studies have been made of thymic lymphocytes in patients with MG (67); however, no enzymatic studies, which are becoming important in the study of lymphoid malignancies (68) have yet been conducted. Abnormalities of T-lymphocytes that affect the control of IgG production may be relevant to the study of the thymus, and some studies have been made in MG (67). In MG (as well as in dysimmune dermatomyopathy/polymyopathy), perhaps a double-infection mechanism coupled with genetic susceptibility, such as occurs with malaria and Epstein-Barr virus to impair T-lymphocyte control and result in Burkitt lymphoma (69), should be considered. MG patients and their relatives have an increased frequency of other dysimmune diseases and of certain HLA determinants, suggesting a genetic predisposition to dysimmune disease (23,32,46,48,70). MG may be of slightly different pathogenesis in different age groups; onset that occurs between the ages of 20 and 40, affects women predominantly (female-to-male ratio of 2:1), while onset that occurs between the ages of 50 and 70 affects males primarily (23).

Spontaneous remission in MG occurs infrequently during the first year after onset and are quite uncommon thereafter. MG is a highly treatable disease but can be life threatening when it affects the respiratory or swallowing muscles (the latter can result in aspiration of food).

Transient neonatal myasthenia occurs in approximately 12% of the offspring of mothers who have MG (putatively, an amniotic factor, possibly alpha fetoprotein, may be protective and may account partially for this low percentage [71]). It is a myasthenic weakness that begins at the time of birth and lasts a few days to a few weeks (average, 18 days) (72). Presumably, it is caused by placental transmission of the toxic IgG from the mother (47). Clinical improvement correlates with a decrease in titers of anti-AChR antibody (half-life, 10 days) (73), although correlations are not perfect. After the disease passes at this time in life it never recurs.

Congenital or *infantile MG* is a chronic disorder that begins in infancy or early childhood. It has a prolonged course and is relatively unresponsive to thymectomy or treatment with anticholinesterase or prednisone, Occasionally patients do respond (W.K. Engel, unpublished observations) (40), however, making a trial of medical treatment and thymectomy worthy of consideration. Anti-AChR antibodies typically are not present (75). Congenital MG sometimes is hereditary; the hereditary form may not be dysimmune and, therefore, would not be expected to respond to antidysimmune therapy.

Ocular MG, by definition, affects the eyes only. However, ocular involvement usually is the harbinger of more generalized involvement, especially in patients younger than 50 years. In older patients (older than 50), MG can remain confined to the eye muscles for a long or indefinite period. In these patients, any measurable anti-nAChR antibody is usually present in low titer (22,23).

Drug-induced myasthenia can result from use of D-penicillamine (which is used to treat rheumatoid arthritis and hepatolenticular degeneration) in both numans and experimental animals (76). The disease resembles spontaneous MG clinically, electrophysiologically, and in its response to pharmacologic therapy. It is accompanied by thymic hyperplasia (76) and by anti-nAChR antibodies that decrease to normal values after the causative drug is withdrawn (32,78–80).

Experimental allergic myasthenia gravis (EAMG) (23,81–83) can be induced in animals, according to genetic susceptibility (50), by repeated injection of the antigen nAChR from the electricity-producing organ (a kind of specialized muscle) of electric fish or electric eel. The disorder involves a pathologic IgG that is directed against the nAChR. The disease can be treated with anticholinesterases (81), prednisone, or azathioprine (35). Monoclonal anti-nAChR IgG (mIgG) produced by hybridomas can also induce an MG state in animals that responds to treatment with anticholinesterases (84).

Management

An experienced team approach is invaluable in handling the complex therapeutic program often required for MG. Treatment can involve (*a*) "whipping" the NMJ with anticholinesterase or, much less effectively, with guanidine or geramine diacetate [85,86] or (*b*) attacking the underlying dysimmune phenomenon by removing IgG through plasmapheresis, removing B-lymphocyte "IgG factories" and T-lymphocytes by lymphocytopheresis, impairing or destroying B and/or T lymphocytes chemically (with prednisone, azathioprine, cyclophosphamide, methotrexate, or other drugs), immunologically (with antilymphocyte globulin or antithymic lymphocyte globulin or by irradiation of thymus, spleen, or total body), or removing the thymus surgically. Antidysimmune therapy in MG, used empirically years before discovery of the pathologic

IgG, aims to eliminate the provocative antigen (if it is in the thymus), eliminate possibly facilitative nonlymphocytic cells (e.g., thymic epithelial cells), and either eliminate pathologic lymphocytes or suppress them until the provocative antigen abates or a state of immune tolerance to the antigen develops.

Pathogenically, MG probably is a monophasic disease, but certainly the phase can last a long time, usually many years (in contrast to the shorter phase of a few years in childhood dysimmune dermatomyopathy), necessitating antidysimmune treatment for many years.

Anticholinesterases. Anticholinesterases prolong the presence of ACh at the NMJ, presumably compensating for the reduced amount of nAChR. In comparing the effects of MG to those of curare poisoning, Denny-Brown (D. Denny-Brown, personal communication) noted that the antidote physostigmine was the first popular treatment of MG and was astonishingly effective (87). Other anticholinesterases, such as pyridostigmine, neostigmine, and the short-acting diagnostic agent edrophonium, are now preferred. Although the usual diagnostic dose of edrophonium is said to be 10 mg given IV, we prefer to give 2 mg IV as the first dose; if there is no beneficial or untoward effect after 60 seconds, we give the remaining 8 mg. Atropine sulfate should be on hand, and 0.4–0.6 mg should be given IV immediately if severe side effects occur. This dose may be repeated, if necessary. Some physicians prefer to give the atropine first routinely, since the drug blocks the muscarinic side effects of the anticholinesterases. When it is difficult to interpret the response or to identify a placebo reaction, the edrophonium test should be confirmed with use of a control in the form of either saline or a drug that is known to have an effect (e.g., nicotinic acid, 50 mg IV, causes a vasodilatory flush). Rare patients have been known to collapse momentarily with the edrophonium test (W.K. Engel, unpublished observations) (51), presumably as a result of syncope caused by vagal bradycardia or standstill. Administration of a predose of atropine should obviate this reaction. In patients taking anticholinesterases, the physician also may use atropine before intubation or enema, procedures that could provoke vagal slowing. Caution should be used in giving edrophonium to patients with cardiac dysrhythmia or bronchial asthma. We also keep an Ambu ventilating bag and mouth airways on hand during testing with edrophonium. In an infant or young child, intramuscular (IM) neostigmine, 0.1–0.5 mg, with atropine is sometimes preferable for the diagnostic test because its action begins after the acute crying associated with injection has subsided and persists longer than edrophonium.

Oral anticholinesterase is preferred for treatment of MG. The dose equivalences are as follows: pyridostigmine bromide, 60 mg orally or 2 mg IM or very slowly IV; neostigmine bromide, 15 mg orally, or neostigmine methosulfate, 0.5 mg IM, subcutaneously, or very slowly IV. Pyridostigmine "timespan" tablets, 180 mg, are used in some stable myasthenic patients for sustained release during sleep. However, the tablets can be difficult to regulate because they are absorbed erratically. We do not use them in unstable myasthenic patients. The initial dose can be 30 mg (one-half tablet) pyridostigmine (the most commonly used therapeutic anticholinesterase) t.i.d. or q.i.d. (onset of effects occurs in 10–20 minutes, peak action occurs in one to two hours, action ceases in three to four hours; action of parenteral dose ceases somewhat sooner). The dosage can be increased gradually, as required, to 60–120 mg or, cautiously, to 180 mg, and can be given as frequently as every four hours while the patient is awake (less is needed during sleep). In severe cases, if the physician is supervising the patient's program carefully, the dosage can be given every three hours. It is important that there be an increase in the patient's strength after the initial dose and then a decrease before the next dose. Since both overdosage and underdosage with anticholinesterases can result in weakness, the doses must be given sufficiently far apart so that the increase and decrease in strength can be observed (this is especially important in the initial management or during unstable periods). If the changes in strength do not occur, the possibility of overdosage must be considered more strongly.

Common side effects of anticholinesterases include increased weakness in MG, abdominal cramps, diarrhea, salivation, sweating, and urinary urgency and frequency (sometimes erroneously prompting the patient to consult a urologist). Fasciculations occur less frequently in MG patients than in others, perhaps because the anti-nAChR antibody (51) blocks the presynaptic nAChR (25,88). Increased vagal tone of the heart and bronchioles is a theoretical concern. All the side effects are muscarinic except the weakness and fasciculations, which are nicotinic. We almost never give maintenance atropine (or similar drugs) to block the muscarinic side effects because these reactions are important warning signals of anticholinesterase overdosage, and we certainly never give the atropine to a newly treated or unstable patients.

Crisis in MG refers to a situation in which the patient recently has become severely weak, usually with difficulty in breathing, and does not respond to anticholinesterases or other treatment. It often is revealed that the patient has received increasing dosages of anticholinesterase and has exhibited a diminishing response. A precipitating event of the crisis could be intercurrent infection, aspiration, postpartum state, or a drug mentioned below. Other precipitating events may not be evident. The crisis can be either *myasthenic*, caused by worsening of the disease plus a relative unresponsiveness to anticholinesterase therapy, or, less commonly, *cholinergic*, caused by anticholinesterase toxicity. Differentiation between the two types is sometimes difficult. The first approach is to review the treatment pattern and response of the preceding 24–48 hours and the preceding week or two. Some physicians advocate IV administration of edrophonium to decide whether the patient is underdosed or overdosed. This approach, however, is fraught with danger because of the following considerations (51). (*1*) An edrophonium test in the crisis or precrisis setting should be performed only if respiratory vital capacity is to be monitored, since respiratory impairment is the one muscle weakness that can be life threatening. (*2*) In the myasthenic patient, some muscles can be overdosed at the same time that others can be underdosed. If, after administering edrophonium, the physician sees the patient's eyes open wider and is not measuring vital capacity, the vital capacity might actually be decreasing from overdosage. On the basis of the ocular response, it might seem logical to increase the dose of anticholinesterase; however, such a move would worsen respiratory function and could precipitate respiratory failure or, if not managed in time, death. (*3*) If edrophonium is given while the action of a pyridostigmine dose is decreasing rather than peaking, the patient may exhibit a false-positive response to the edrophonium. This might lead the physician to increase the pyridostigmine dose, which, in turn, could cause greater cholinergic overdosage at the peak of the drug action (along with possible respiratory failure and copious orotracheobronchial secretions). (*4*) Edrophonium can have a measurable action that is longer than the expected 10 minutes (e.g., 60–150 minutes [89]). Thus, the effects of frequent doses of edrophonium can be cumulative by themselves and with those of pyridostigmine. Our general rule is that, if the patient is in a serious crisis and we are uncertain whether he or she is overdosed or underdosed, we withhold all anticholinesterase medication and have respiratory assistance at hand. If the patient weakens first or remains unchanged, he or she probably was either underdosed with anticholinesterase or partly refractory; if the patient initially becomes stronger, he or she probably was overdosed. If the patient has borderline respiratory failure and cannot be improved otherwise, it is often beneficial, for uncertain reasons, to stop all anticholinesterase medication for several days while the patient is ventilated artificially by a respirator (this procedure is becoming less necessary with the availability of emergency plasmapheresis/lymphocytopheresis). Withholding anticholinesterases also reduces anticholinesterase-induced excess secretions and gastrointestinal hyperactivity and often results in the return of anticholinesterase sensitivity. Thus, overdosage with the anticholinesterases used in MG is treated passively by awaiting catabolism/excretion. (Oximes, such as pyridine aldoxine methiodine, are not used in MG as they are in cases of poisoning from long-acting organophosphorus anticholinesterases, such as malathion and parathion.)

Active aspects of treating a crisis include respiratory management, emergency plasmapheresis/lymphocytopheresis, and treatment of collateral predisposing factors and complications (e.g., pulmonary infections, obstructions, edema). These measures should be carried out by an experienced team, often in an intensive care setting. With this approach, mortality in our experience has been zero. A combination of prednisone and azathioprine can be started if a major infection is not present. After several days, when the patient is stabilized, anticholinesterases can be either resumed cautiously at half the precrisis dosage or continued to be withheld; we prefer to withhold, if possible.

In animals, neostigmine can produce abnormalities of LMN endings at the junctions (90); it is not known whether such toxicity with anticholinesterases occurs clinically, but it does not seem to be a common problem.

In some patients there has been a question of poor intestinal absorption of pyridostigmine (pills occasionally are recovered intact in the feces). Blood levels of the drug have been studied with gas chromatography (91). Because assays of blood levels are not generally available, virtually all MG patients must be managed empirically. Even when such assays are available, the measurement might not be very helpful because, as mentioned previously, some muscles can be overdosed while others are underdosed (51). Furthermore, even if blood levels of pyridostigmine are to be adequate, in an unresponsive patient the anticholinesterase dosage should be either increased empirically in order to detect possible peripheral resistance or lowered it to detect unusual sensitivity to intoxication.

Other Whips. Not widely used but of some benefit to occasional MG patients is guanidine, ephedrine, KCl. If benefit is going to appear, it should do so during the day the drug is given at its optimal dosage. Germine diacetate, a stabilizer of postsynaptic and presynaptic plasmalemma, has showed promise but is no longer available (85,86).

Adrenocorticosteroids and adrenocorticotropic hormone (ACTH). At a time when prednisone (which is converted in the liver to prednisolone) was generally described as being contraindicated in patients with MG (92,93), *high-single-dose alternate-day prednisone* (HSDAD-Pred) was introduced as the pharmacologic method of choice for treatment of the disease (94,95). This approach was based on the facts that MG was considered a dysimmune disease, that HSDAD-Pred was being used for other dysimmune neuromuscular diseases (96,97), and that a 10-day course of ACTH at 100 units IV per day had been used previously as a standard but only temporarily beneficial measure (98–100). Our program now is to treat the MG patient with 100 mg HSDAD-Pred for a long period (19,51). The entire dosage and program are arbitrary and empiric—there is no exact method for predetermination.

Initially we treat the average adult for three to four weeks with a single dose of 100 mg prednisone per day and then taper to an alternate-day program by gradually reducing the off-day dose. Tapering extends over 10 weeks by dropping the off-day dose by 10 mg per week (or faster if necessitated by side effects, but with the greater attendant risk of breakthrough of disease). The last reduction (i.e., to zero on the off-day) is accomplished gradually by reducing the number of milligrams to 10, 5, 2.5 and finally to zero in weekly decrements. On the first totally off-day the patient is observed for symptoms of hypoadrenalism; with gradual reduction, these symptoms seldom occur, and when they do they are mild. (Some patients require a continued small dose of prednisone, 5–15 mg, on the off-day to control their symptoms.) Reduction of HSDAD-Pred must be done very gradually, by decrements of 5 mg not more often than about every three to four weeks, assuming that the prednisone therapy is having a beneficial effect and side effects are minor. (Prednisone given as a therapeutic trial in a disease and found ineffective is reduced swiftly, especially if side effects occur.) With dosages of less than 30 mg, reductions are made in 2.5-mg decrements to a dose of 15 mg q.o.d. and then continued by 1-mg decrements to not less than 10 or 5 mg. In our experience, the last dose should be maintained indefinitely.

Another method of beginning prednisone in patients with MG is with a schedule of incremental doses (101) as a program of single daily doses program (102). The approach can be used when there is concern either about the side effects of prednisone (e.g., in a patient who previously has had a gastrointestinal ulcer or who has hypertension or diabetes mellitus and in whom an alternative, noncorticosteroid drug such as azathioprine or cyclophosphamide is contraindicated) or about a possible adverse action of the prednisone alone or with an anticholinesterase. The program can begin with a single dose of 15–30 mg per day and increase by 5–10 mg every one to four days.

Prednisone can benefit 80% or more of MG patients (12,19,51,94,103–105) and at any age and most especially in older men (19). Although its use has been criticized on grounds that a randomized control study has not yet been conducted (12), we do not consider this to be a significant objection. Certainly there are other ways to establish efficacy of a treatment, as we did in our original studies. In them, the patient served as his or her own control and demonstrated (*1*) a progressively declining course or a long plateau that did not respond to any other treatment before prednisone was started, followed by a response that always occurred within a few days or weeks and with no other change in therapy (there was no improvement when anticholinesterases were stopped several days before prednisone therapy was begun); (*2*) a distinct cycle of improving and worsening that was related to on-day versus off-day administration of prednisone, especially early in the course of treatment; (*3*) worsening when prednisone was tapered too quickly (discovered in retrospect); and (*4*) resumption of response when the prednisone dose was increased (19,94,95). Our avoidance of anticholinesterase drugs in these studies permitted clear attribution of benefit to the prednisone. We still believe that, in order to minimize problems of anticholinesterase overdosage, dosages of anticholinesterases should be reduced as much as possible or eliminated without endangering or crippling the patient, before prednisone therapy is begun. If the patient is already assisted by a respirator, elimination of the drug can be done safely and will also obviate the risk of anticholinesterase induced secretions. With therapeutic levels of prednisone, most patients show sustained improvement in a few days to a few weeks. If a response is not obtained, we continue therapy for at least three months, and preferably six months. If the patient improves considerably, tapering from 100-mg to zero on the alternate-day schedule is begun cautiously after about one to six months.

An obligatory aspect of our prednisone regimen is a collateral program designed to prevent or diminish some of the drug's side effects (19,96,97). The program consists of (*1*) antacids between meals (e.g., aluminum hydroxide [Amphogel], which can constipate; combined magnesium and aluminum hydroxides [Maalox], which can loosen stools; a combination or alteration of both; or a magaldrate [Riopan], which is very slightly lower in sodium) and/or frequent between-meal and bedtime feedings of milk or other bland food; (*2*) a diet low in sodium (2 g/day) and carbohydrates and high in protein; and (*3*) 80–120 mEq/day of oral liquid potassium as KCl in divided doses (K-Lyte, which contains $KHCO_3$, should not be used because the bicarbonate can accelerate renal potassium loss).

Side effects of prednisone include atrophy of type II muscle fiber (52,106–109), which can exacerbate weakness produced by the disease; hyperglucosemia; glucosuria; hypertension; sodium retention; potassium loss; gastrointestinal ulceration and bleeding; rounding, hirsutism, and redness of the face; cushingoid body habitus; acneiform rash; osteoporosis (osteopenia) and vertebral collapse; aseptic necrosis of the femoral or humeral head; cataracts; glaucoma; psychoses; and possibly decreased resistance to infection. We have not seen gastrointestinal ulceration or bleeding in patients treated on our program and adequately on the collateral program (thus, we do not use prophylactic cimetidine). The various acute and subacute side effects are much fewer with the HSDAD-Pred program, and even with the single-daily-dose program, than with the divided-daily-dose program, even when the single-daily-dose program results in the same or somewhat higher total dosage per 48 hours. For example, we have not observed gastrointestinal problems, psychosis, or susceptibility to infection with our program. However, prolonged treatment does allow long-term side effects to appear. These include osteoporosis and avascular necrosis of bones. Osteoporosis is particularly apt to occur in menopausal and postmenopausal women and is less common in other patients. This effect may be related to glucocorticoid receptors of bone cells and to the intermodulation among glucocorticoids, other hormones, and vitamin D (110). Although in children corticosteroids tend to retard growth in stature, this effect is considerably reduced by HSDAD-Pred therapy (111,112). Decreased birth weight of full-term infants born to mothers who take 10 mg corticosteroids per day was reported recently (113) but remains to be confirmed.

Whether there is truly an adverse interaction between prednisone and anticholinesterases, as was originally thought (114) is not known; it is not a major clinical problem. Definite, however, is the occurrence in occasional patients of *ingravescent overdosage* with anticholinesterase if the drug is continued at moderate or high dosage after the addition of prednisone. This reaction occurs as the patient improves as a result of the prednisone. The weakness that patients can develop from anticholinesterase overdosage can mimic myasthenic weakness. The suspected overdosage can be analyzed by reducing the anticholinesterase cautiously and looking for improvement. Cholinergic side effects (described earlier) strongly suggest anticholinesterase overdosage; however, sometimes overdosage occurs either without these symptoms or without the patient's recognition of them. (Noncholinergic diarrhea can result from antacids made with magnesium and aluminum hydroxides.) Patients sometimes take atropine (inadvisedly) to conceal the muscarinic side effects, thereby forgetting them. We are reluctant to use atropine in MG patients to conceal anticholinesterase side effects, and we never use it when the patient is first taking the drugs becasue it prevents him or her from learning the important side effects and warning signals of overdose. (In an occasional patient, the physician may try to achieve more optimal anticholinesterase dosage by masking the muscarinic side effects with oral belladonna tincture, 0.3–0.5 ml, or with atropine, about 0.3–0.5 mg, three to four times a day.) Whether there is a true worsening of MG when the patient begins prednisone (i.e., aside from that caused by anticholinesterase overdosage) is controversial. Some investigators claim that such worsening occurs in 80% of patients (105), but we have not seen it, perhaps because we keep the anticholinesterase dosage as low as possible. Because of this potential worsening, MG patients should begin prednisone therapy only under very close supervision, in a hospital, if possible.

The exact site and mode of benefit from prednisone in dysimmune diseases is not certain (115). Prednisone probably affects lymphocytes (and perhaps macrophages) in the thymus, lymph nodes, gut, spleen, bone marrow, and circulation (whether it also affects abnormal thymic epithelial cells has not been investigated [51].) Certainly the thymus is not the only site of prednisone action, because patients who have not responded to thymectomy can benefit, often remarkably, from long-term HSDAD-Pred therapy or daily doses of prednisone (94,96). The drug diminishes numbers and functions (116) of circulating T and B lymphocytes markedly (T lymphocytes are affected more than B lymphocytes). The effect is maximal at about eight hours after a single dose and ceases by 24 hours (116). The therapy may simply put lymphocytes out of circulation temporarily rather than lyse them (117,118). Because this measurably brief action is in contrast to the cumulative benefit of the continued HSDAD-Pred program, prolonged prednisone therapy might be having a more enduring but unmeasured effect on at least a certain subpopulation of lymphocytes. Since prednisone (or polyinosine-cytosine poly-l-lysine [Poly ICLC] [119]) can have a beneficial effect within hours, it is likely to interfere with an adverse metabolic action of lymphocyte products at the NMJ (or, in dysimmune neuropathy, at the Schwann cell or axon [120]). In humans, glucocorticoid blocks both the proliferative response of T and B lymphocytes to antigenic stimulation and synthesis of lymphokines probably in the following way: The cytoplasmic glucocortocoid receptor of the lymphocyte complexed with the glucocorticoid enters the nucleus and binds to a nuclear receptor. This results in synthesis of messenger ribonucleic acid (RNA) and then, in the cytoplasm, of synthesis of a protein capable of inhibiting transport of glucose and amino acids across the plasmalemma. The resulting fuel restriction in the lymphocyte blocks its ability to synthesize additional RNA and protein that are required for proliferation (121). Antiinflammatory glucocorticoids also inhibit prostaglandin biosynthesis by preventing release of arachidonic acid from phospholipids through macrocortin, an intracellular polypeptide that acts as a second messenger and whose synthesis depends on de novo biosynthesis of RNA and protein (122). Among the nonneoplastic lymphocytes, only activated ("stimulated") lymphocytes contain abundant glucocorticoid receptors and thus are inhibitable by corticosteroids (123). These few "blastic" cells presumably are the aberrantly "turned on" lymphocytes that must be inhibited in order to treat dysimmune diseases. (This situation may be related to the clinical benefit that is sustained by low-dose [5–15 mg q.o.d.] prednisone, and to a lag of three to four months in recurrence of symptoms with cessation of the low-dose corticosteroid [51].)

Another biological factor that may be pertinent to glucocorticoid therapy is the relative affinity of corticosteroids for the corticosteroid-binding globulin in plasma, as compared with the intracellular cytoplasmic receptor (123). (Glucocorticoids have other effects on lymphocytes that do not act via glucocorticoid receptors [123].) EAMG can be prevented experimentally by optimal treatment with glucocorticoids (or azathioprine) (35,124). Alternate-day prednisone does not affect cutaneous delayed hypersensitivity (CDH) or increase susceptibility to infection (118). Corticosteroids can affect humoral immune mechanisms in humans by lowering total serum levels of both IgG and circulating antibodies by inhibiting synthesis of immunoglobulins (125). In MG, anti-nAChR antibodies are decreased during corticosteroid therapy (126–128). Prednisone is also an anti-inflammatory agent and decreases polymorphs, monocytes, and fluid accumulation in inflammatory foci.

It is curious that clinically the dose of prednisone can be gradually tapered to a very low level, such as 10 or 5 mg HSDAD, and still maintain a therapeutic effect. However, if that dose is stopped and MG reappears (which it nearly always does in one to four months), the disease often canot be brought under control until the dose is reinstituted at very high levels, such as 100 mg HSDAD or even daily

(19,51).* For this reason, it has been our practice to recommend that patients in remission continue to take 5–15 mg prednisone (or another immunosuppressant, such as azathioprine) for a prolonged period.

If weakness increases during the tapering of prednisone, it is not necessary to raise the dose of prednisone immediately if the increase is slight. It is better to keep the dose at the same level for a few weeks, because often the disease can be brought back under control. The prednisone dose should be increased only if the worsening is significant. When weakness worsens to such a degree, increasing the dosage to the last previous step usually is not effective. For example, if weakness appears after the alternate-day dose is decreased from 70 to 65 mg, significant weakness usually is not corrected by raising the dosage to 70 mg; rather, it requires raising the dosage to 80–85 mg and sometimes to 100 mg. If such an elevation is needed, the prednisone must be reduced very gradually as the disease is brought under control.

Patients who fail to respond to 100 mg prednisone sometimes benefit from doses as high as 150 or even 200 mg, either HSDAD or daily for some time (W.K. Engel, unpublished observations) (19,51,94,96,102). The risk of side effects is correspondingly increased, although some patients have no more side effects at very high doses than others do at 100 mg, perhaps because the drug is metabolized differently at different dosages. (Desirable for the future would be [*1*] a method of testing a patient with a single dose to learn the individualized optimal pharmacologically effective dose, and [2] a corticosteroid with a higher ratio of benefits to side effects. Also, in treating some forms of cancer, patients receive doses of 1 g prednisone per day for seven to 10 days. Such an approach might be considered in resistant cases of MG, although risks of side effects would be increased.)

Azathioprine, Cyclophosphamide, and Methotrexate. These other long-term immunosuppressants affect various cell-mediated and humoral immune responses. Of them, *azathioprine*, which is converted in the liver to the hypoxanthine analogue 6-mercaptopurine, interferes with metabolism of inosinic acid and synthesis of purine. These responses result in numerous cellular effects. It is our drug of choice and the one we have used, with or without prednisone, for many years in the treatment of dysimmune neuromuscular diseases. We use it (*1*) whenever prednisone alone is not beneficial, (*2*) if prednisone is relatively contraindicated, and (*3*) for the past few years in a starting combination with HSDAD-Pred. Azathioprine can inhibit synthesis of immunoglobulins in humans (133), decrease anti-nAChR titers in MG patients (31,134), and suppress EAMG (35). The dose of azathioprine that we give begins at 3 mg/kg body weight per day, in a single dose. It takes about seven to 14 days to manifest its laboratory effect (e.g., leukopenia, other evidence of bone marrow suppression) and one to 12 weeks to manifest its clinical effect. Clinical benefit may occur without reduction of white blood cells (WBCs), but in the absence of clinical response the dosage can be increased gradually to titrate reduction in WBCs. Care must be taken that the polymorph count does not fall below 1,500–2,000 mm^3 in the

*In our opinion, it is unlikely that the known action of prednisone at the NMJ (24,128–132) can account for these phenomena.

steady state (remembering that a decrease in the lymphocyte count is desired) or that the numbers of platelets and erythrocytes do not fall too low. (In chemotherapy for multiple myeloma, polymorph counts are, under careful observation, dropped in pulses to less than 500 mm^3 [135].) Accordingly, doses of azathioprine (and other cytotoxic agents) must be monitored closely and adjusted for maintenance in a therapeutic but safe range.

A side effect of azathioprine that we have recognized as rather common is fever (W.K. Engel, unpublished observations) (51). Fever can appear one to three weeks or several months after beginning azathioprine; if the patient is also on a HSDAD-Pred program, the fever occcurs only during the prednisone off-day. The first step in assessing the fever is to take chest films and blood cultures to determine whether pneumonitis, tuberculosis, or bacteremia are the causative factors. Although infection must be considered and sought, it is important to stop the azathioprine. Fever resulting from azathioprine regresses over the next one to three days. After an afebrile period of about a week, the azathioprine can be reintroduced cautiously. During reinstatement of the drug, the patient should be watched carefully for reappearance of the fever; this is a worthwhile measure because, if the patient's fever was caused by an intercurrent viral (or other) infection, the azathioprine need not have been stopped.

The other, more usual side effects of azathioprine are suppression of bone marrow production in regard to granulocyte, erythrocyte, and platelet series, and hepatocellular damage (with elevation of levels of serum transaminases, 5-nucleotidase, and alkaline phosphatase but not of creatine phosphokinase). Less frequent side effects are alopecia, pancreatitis (noted in patients with regional enteritis [136]), gonadal involvement, and possibly delayed risk of neoplasia (137). Opportunistic infections have not been a problem at the doses we have used. Because of potential clinical teratogenicity (still a controversial point), it may be that azathioprine (and the other cytotoxic drugs) should be withdrawn in both men and women several months before conception and avoided during pregnancy. (Because allopurinol impairs the catabolism of azathioprine, either the two drugs should not be used concurrently or the dose of azathioprine should be reduced to about 25% of the original dose.)

Azathioprine can be effective in 80% or more of MG patients. However, some investigators find that efficacy may not be evident for many months to years (138–140). The long delay in these studies may have been related to their using a dosage that was less than effective (139,141) (i.e., less than 3 mg/kg). Some of the most startling improvements we observed in patients with dysimmune diseases occurred in those who followed unplanned "overdosing" (according to total leukocyte counts) with azathioprine or cyclophosphamide (W.K. Engel, unpublished observations). By pressing the dosage to the highest level tolerable, benefit can appear within one to 12 weeks.

If the patient is being treated with both prednisone and azathioprine, we prefer to reduce the prednisone gradually and maintain the azathioprine dosage, because the side effects of long-term prednisone seem to be more significant than those of long-term azathioprine.

Cyclophosphamide, an alkylating agent (142) that substitutes chemical groups of nucleic acids and proteins and cross-links DNA, is our alternative drug of choice in this group. The starting single daily dose is 1–2 mg/kg/day, as in other dysimmune diseases (143,144). The drug also has a delay of seven to 14 days before laboratory manifestations of improvement and a delay of one to 12 weeks before clinical effects are evident. The doses can be increased cautiously, again to titrate reduction of the polymorph count to not less than 1,500–2,000 in the steady state. Common side effects of cyclophosphamide include suppression of bone marrow production and hemorrhagic cystitis. Alopecia, gonadal dysfunction, possibly delayed neoplasia (e.g., leukemia, lymphoma, bladder cancer) (145), and possibly bladder and pulmonary fibrosis also may occur. Some researchers believe that there is virtually no risk in using cyclophosphamide if the total WBC count is maintained at not less than 3,000 (118) (i.e., if the neutrophil count remains greater than 1,500). Bone marrow function must be monitored throughout treatment. The clinical benefit is said to be correlated with chronic lymphocytopenia rather than with functional impairment of surviving lymphocytes (118) (although this conclusion may not have taken into account the most relevant functions). Cyclophosphamide preferentially kills rapidly dividing lymphocytes; however, it also can affect resting cells, and it first preferentially reduces B cells (118). Cyclophosphamide can decrease elevated levels of serum immunoglobulin; suppress antibody response and cutaneous delayed hypersensitivity (CDH) to a new antigen while it essentially spares preestablished CDH; decrease blastic responses to specific antigenic stimulation; and leave responses to mitogens unchanged (118).

Methotrexate, an antagonist of folate metabolism, can be considered a possible third choice. It can be given IV or IM once a week, or orally if it can be regulated satisfactorily. A low starting dose can be increased gradually according to the patient's tolerance, and it can be titrated upward, but not to reduce counts of polymorphs, platelets, or erythrocytes excessively or to produce other side effects. Although we, like others (146), have used IV methotrexate successfully in some patients with dysimmune neuromuscular diseases who cannot take azathioprine or cyclophosphamide, we have had difficulties with side effects of overdosage, particularly in the form of oral and intestinal ulcers. Diarrhea, suppression of bone narrow production, and liver damage also can occur. (Higher-dose methotrexate combined with rescue of folinic acid [leukovorin] (147) has not yet been attempted as an approach to treatment of neuromuscular diseases.)

Other immunomodulators that have not received a trial in MG include polyinosine-cytosine poly-l-lysine (Poly ICLC), ostensibly an interferon inducer but actually a potent lymphocytopenic agent (119); interferon; chlorambucil (an akylating agent) (148); melphalan (an akylating agent); and cyclosporin A (lymphoma induced by Epstein-Barr virus [149] and other toxicities [150] may be a problem). Danazol, which can suppress pituitary output of follicle-stimulating hormone and luteinizing hormone, has been effective in treatment of a lupus erythematosus–like aspect of hereditary angioneurotic edema, possibly by virtue of the drug's androgenic properties (151), and might be considered for use in other dysimmune diseases. However, it can cause myopathy in susceptible persons (W.K. Engel, S. Hosea, M. Frank, unpublished observations).

Plasmapheresis (Plasma Exchange). Plasmapheresis grew out of the concept of thoracic-duct drainage and knowledge of the circulating pathogenic IgG. Approximately 4 L of the patient's plasma is removed and is replaced with either human serum albumin or an artificial plasma, or a combination of both (the replacement fluids are expensive). Plasmapheresis is often remarkably beneficial in crisis situations (23,127,152); it can result in increased strength, so that the patient can avoid using a respirator or, if already assisted by one, can stop using it (in this respect, plasmapheresis can also be used prethymectomy). The procedure can be performed every day or every other day for three to five times, and then one to three times a week for three to four weeks. The patient may improve in the first 24 hours, or after a few days. All types of MG patients can benefit from plasmapheresis except some with chronic congenital MG. Benefit is achieved by a washing out of the toxic circulating IgG; however, a washing out of excess anticholinesterase medication could also be a factor. Furthermore, plasmapheresis can reduce plasma levels of cholinesterase to 38%, which conceivably could play a role in prolonging the action of not only exogenous succinylcholine (153) but perhaps also of junctional ACh. Plasmapheresis also might wash out a putative pathogenic thymic hormone (40,54,66), some other detrimental substance, or immune complexes (doubtful) (154).

It is doubtful, both theoretically (W.K. Engel, unpublished observations) and empirically (32,155) that plasmapheresis has a long-term effect. Only if the procedure is done repeatedly can it have a sustained cumulative benefit. In order to maintain the clinical benefit, plasmapheresis must be used in conjunction with immunosuppressive agents, such as a prednisone-azathioprine combination, to stop production of pathologic IgG (32,127). When such a combination is used over a long period, however, it becomes doubtful whether plasmapheresis adds benefit to the effects of two drugs that already are known to be beneficial (W.K. Engel, unpublished observations) (32,51,139–141,156). Furthermore, plasmapheresis diminishes levels of circulating normal IgG more effectively than anti-nAChR, whereas glucocorticoids and azathioprine increase these levels (31). In our experience, periodic maintenance plasmapheresis can soon lead to venous thrombosis, and loss of vascular access. For repeated plasmapheresis (which we try in other conditions but not in MG), we prefer to establish an arteriovenous fistula in the forearm rather than install a plastic shunt.

Potential side effects of plasmapheresis are detailed elsewhere (152,157). Investigators have not noted a problem of decreased levels of circulating therapeutic drugs in MG patients who are treated with plasmapheresis. There is not always a good correlation between the beneficial response to plasmapheresis and the reduction or the absolute level of the anti-nAChR IgG antibody, although the titer usually does decrease (22,32,157,158). In plasmapheresis of MG and other dysimmune patients, we routinely perform concurrent *lymphocytopheresis* with the same machine to remove putatively offending B and T lymphocytes along with their offensive products.

Thoracic duct drainage was successful as an acute therapy of myasthenic patients in crisis (139). The process removed both serum IgG and lymphocytes. Although removal of these elements may have contributed to the improvement, weakness returned acutely after reinfusion of the IgG (but not of the lymphocytes) (139). Complications of thoracic-duct drainage include stenosis or fistula of the duct. The procedure is not generally used for treatment of MG. Lymphocytes are removed more safely by lymphocytopheresis during plasmapheresis.

Antithymocyte Globulin (ATG) and Antilymphocyte Globulin (ALG) Serum (IgG fraction). ATG and ALG can have a very potent antilymphocyte effect. After a single program of treatment, the circulating lymphocyte count can remain low for months to several years. The treatment must be considered with caution. While theoretically it can be of benefit in MG (one study reports clinical benefit from ALG [159]), it is not generally used in MG. ATG has been used recently in some transplantation procedures and dysimmune diseases; its side effects are significant.

Radiation Therapy. Irradiation of the thymus has been carried out in some centers (160) but not with universal appeal, apparently because of its inconsistent results. For the past few years we have been giving 6,000 rad to the anterior mediastinum after thymectomy in patients with histologically diagnosed thymoma and have had excellent results in four cases (although the effects lasted only about 10 months in one patient, who then responded to HSDAD-Pred plus azathioprine). We recently have introduced *splenic irradiation* as a new approach to the treatment of MG. Three of five patients with chronic MG that was resistant to thymectomy responded well to prednisone and azathioprine after receiving 1,000 rad to the spleen (100 rad/day for 10 days) in each of two to three courses (161). We chose splenic irradiation because lymphocytes are the most sensitive of the circulating cells to radiation and they occur in large numbers in the spleen. In fact, we have suggested that the benefit of mediastinal or thymic and post-thymectomy irradiation relates to damage to lymphocytes (circulating cells and those in nodes and bone marrow) rather than to damage to thymic epithelial cells (161).

Total body irradiation (150 rad given over five weeks) has been very successful in one otherwise unresponsive patient with virtually end-stage polymyositis (162) and is being tested in MG patients; the first such patient is now showing distinct improvement (W.K. Engel, A. Lichter, M.C. Dalakas, unpublished observations).

Thymectomy. Thymectomy is an established treatment of MG and benefits 75% or more patients (12,61,163). With thymectomy, the benefit can appear in a few weeks to a few years (164). Thymectomy is most effective in young adults (whose hyperplastic thymus contains active lymphoid germinal centers) and is somewhat more effective in patients who have had the disease for fewer than five years. However, we (61) and other workers (165) have found it beneficial in all age groups and in both sexes, although it has been least so for patients with chronic infantile or early juvenile-onset MG. We feel that the thymus is an important aspect of the pathogenesis of the disease and should be removed. Even in older patients with MG, whose thymus usually is described as "involuted" (if it is not thymomatous), we always find nodules of cells, lymphocytes, and epithelial cells (the last occur both in Hassell's corpuscles and scattered; all of these contain thymosin [54,61]), throughout the anterior mediastinal fat and sometimes in the pericardium. It should be recalled how few cells in the hypothalamus and pituitary can affect total body function profoundly; therefore, even the few small nests of abnormal lymphocytes in the thymus could, in fact, be programming an abnormality, perhaps in conjunction with the observed thymic epithelial cells that contain nAChR (53) and thymosin (54). All thymomas should be excised, whether or not the patient has MG. Thymomas can be detected best, albeit inperfectly, by computed tomography.

In all age groups, except when another aspect of the patient's condition presents a contraindication, early thymectomy is favored (19,61,164). We perform thymectomy whenever anticholinesterases alone do not provide excellent control and before we start corticosteroid therapy, in an attempt to obviate the need for corticosteroids. Exceptions to this policy include older, generally fragile patients who do not have a radiologically detectable mediastinal mass that suggests thymoma and especially if their MG is mainly ocular. Such patients usually respond very well to corticosteroid therapy (19,166). A decrease in titers of anti-nAChR antibody after thymectomy is a disputed effect but does tend to occur (23,32,167,168). Thymoma, defined solely as proliferation of thymic epithelial cells (169), occurs in 10% of adults with MG. Of these, 72% occur in patients aged 40 and older (62). In contrast to patients in other series (170), our MG patients who underwent thymectomy (plus mediastinal irradiation, 6,000 rad) are all doing very well; some of them are taking prednisone with or without azathioprine.

We do not like the suprasternal (transcervical) surgical route for thymectomy because with it even experienced thoracic surgeons can find it impossible to remove all of the identified thymic tissue, especially the bottom half of one or both lobes. Since we presume that it is important to remove thymic tissue as completely as possible, our surgical colleague, C.L. McIntosh, prefers a transsternal approach, with an inverted Y-shaped sternal incision from the center of the manubrium to the third intercostal space on each side. Hyperextension of the patient's thoracic region then allows excellent visibility for removing all evidence of thymic tissue (which occasionally can also be strung along the mediastinum and pericardium and even extend upward into the neck) or, in older patients, for cleaning out all the fatty tissue in the anterior mediastinum.

Rethymectomy sometimes is necessary, especially after a previous transcervical operation, and can lead to improvement if a residual or recurrent thymus is found and removed (61). Of patients with thymoma, 30% develop MG a year or more after thymectomy (171). We performed rethymectomy in one such patient with medically uncontrolled MG; the patient achieved nearly complete remission and later gave birth to a healthy child after 20 years of apparent infertility (W.K. Engel, C.L. McIntosh, unpublished observations). We have experienced zero mortality in 85 transsternal thymectomies (61,172), as also was found at Columbia (172). Morbidity is related mainly to pain for a few days. The pain can reduce vital capacity by 1–2 L for the first few days; it can be controlled well with small IV doses of morphine which actually increase respiratory function. Bleeding, pneumothorax, and infection are to be watched for. After thymectomy, tracheal extubation should be done only when ventilatory function is adequate. The anesthesiologist and the neurologist should agree on the time of extubation, taking into account not only the current vital capacity, but also two additional factors: (*1*) the fatigue component of MG, and (*2*) the commonly observed transient increase of muscle function in MG for a few to 24 hours after thymectomy (possibly resulting from stress-released endogenous corticoids) (W.K. Engel, unpublished observations). The chest tube usually is removed after 24 hours. There is no evident long-range harmful effect of thymectomy (W.K. Engel, unpublished observations) (165,170,173–180).

Management of corticosteroids and anticholinesterases during thymectomy is as follows. (*1*) Oral corticosteroids are replaced by hydrocortisone, 100 mg IV every six hours, until the patient can resume oral medication. (*2*) Anticholinesterase medication preferably is omitted the day of surgery in order to reduce bronchial secretions. If withdrawal of the drug is not possible, it can be given orally as usual on the morning of surgery (depending partly on how early the surgery will be) (alternatively, some physicians prefer to give slightly less than corresponding oral amount IM (e.g., oral to IM pyridostigmine, 30:1; oral to IM neostigmine, 15:0.5) with atropine. Postoperatively, anticholinesterase medication should be withheld until weakness occurs, at which time the drug should be replaced initially at half the preoperative dose. Pyridostigmine or neostigmine administered IM is given until the patient can take oral medication. On the evening of surgery, patients who have not been receiving corticoids sometimes experience a transient increase in strength, possibly resulting from stress-released endogenous corticoids. This usually is followed by weakening the next day, and decisions regarding management should not be influenced by this transient phenomenon.

Anti-idiotype Antibodies (Conjectural Treatment). The anti-nAChR IgG that is responsible for weakness in MG is, within the horde of antibodies in a given patient, probably molecularly unique in amino-acid sequences (181), especially in its variable N-terminal F_{ab} region. Thus, the pathogenic nAChR can be isolated (through affinity binding to nAChR columns and used to make highly specific monoclonal antibody against its unique molecular aspects only (in other dysimmune diseases, a technique for obtaining the human monoclonal pathologic antibody [182] may be useful). When the fabricated antibody is administered to the patient, it theoretically could destroy both the circulating pathogenic IgG and the clone of the B lymphocytes producing it, assuming that that IgG suffuses their surface (183) (i.e., anti-missile missiles and anti-missile-launcher missiles). A variation of this is to label the antibody (or a miniature antibody, i.e., a smaller molecule with the same antibodylike specificity) with a very small amount of a deadly radioisotope or chemotherapeutic drug that would kill the target B lymphocytes only at close range.

Induction of Immune Tolerance (Conjectural Treatment). An ideal treatment of MG (and other dysimmune diseases) would be induction of lasting tolerance to the provocative antigen(s) without adverse affects on the patient. A start toward this has been made in EAMG by immunization of animals with denatured nAChR (35,166).

Respiratory Care. Every patient with MG (and every patient with neuromuscular disease) should have vital capacity measured at the first examination. Measurement should be repeated at every outpatient visit or every day (or more frequently, if indicated) during hospitalization (19). We use a Wright respirometer for this purpose. If there is a question that an MG patient (or, presumably, any patient) needs the help of a respirator, the mechanical assistance should be used. In an average-sized adult, a vital capacity of less than 1 L (i.e., less than 25% of the predicted value) suggests impending respiratory failure. Although the bedside measurement is the best single test, measurements of altered arterial P_{CO_2}

and Po_2 also can be used as warnings, especially measurements of retained CO_2 (19). Other signs of respiratory insufficiency include anxiety, depression, loss of ability to speak for more than a few seconds, dysphonia, headache, and hypertension. A decrease in vital capacity can be caused by a mucous plug in a bronchus or bronchiole or by the onset of pulmonary infection, as well as by muscle weakness. These conditions should be sought.

Acute respiratory failure can be managed temporarily with a hand-operated Ambu ventilating bag and a mouth airway. These devices should always be readily accessible during examination of a myasthenic patient who could develop respiratory failure, and they should be kept on hand wherever the patient goes as long as the concern is present. In a hospital setting, respiratory failure can be managed acutely by transnasal or transoral insertion of a cuffed endotracheal tube that is connected to the respirator (such as a Bennett MA-1). A soft-cuffed endotracheal tube can easily be left in place for one week and with caution for two or three weeks. Suction of the tracheobronchial tree is somewhat less effective through an endotracheal tube than through a tracheostomy tube (W.K. Engel, unpublished observations) (184). Sterile technique should be used for suction through either an endotracheal or a tracheostomy tube. If respiratory assistance will be needed for more than two to three weeks, elective tracheostomy should be performed under brief general anesthesia. We prefer a Portex soft-cuffed tracheostomy tube because patients tolerate it better. Size 27–33 is preferable; suction becomes difficult with tubes smaller than this.

Intubation with a cuffed tube also can be used to protect the airway, namely, if impaired swallowing results in aspiration, obstruction of bronchioles, and pneumonitis.

When we give patients mechanical respiration, we stop all anticholinesterases for at least a few days (and usually longer) to determine the status of the MG, to reduce the often copious orotracheobronchial secretions the drugs produce, and to avoid complicating interpretation of the effects of other treatments. We also try to avoid giving atropine because it can produce thickened sticky secretions that are difficult to remove by suction.

A myasthenic patient (or a patient with relapsing dysimmune neuropathy) does not become "habituated" to the respirator as might a patient with chronic lung disease. For this reason, as MG patients become stronger, they do not need to be weaned from the respirator. Instead, they are removed from the respirator for increasing periods of time during the day (within their limits of respiratory comfort), starting with a few minutes every hour, to test respiratory strength. When patients are first removed from the respirator, they must be under constant observation by trained medical personnel who can replace the connection to the respirator instantly if necessary. During the period of transition, patients should sleep with the respirator connected to ensure constant respiration throughout the night. Other aspects of care for patients with respiratory weakness include suction of secretions (by sterile technique if the patient is intubated), chest clapping, and, in some situations, postural drainage and intermittent positive pressure three to four times per day to expand the lungs. Further details on nursing are described elsewhere (11,19). In general, we are slow to take out the tracheostomy tube. Before a tracheostomy tube is removed, the cuff should be deflated and the tube plugged for a varying number of days or weeks to be certain that the patient can breathe and swallow safely without assistance.

For mild chronic respiratory insufficiency, a Thompson portable respirator can be very satisfactory. It utilizes an air-bladder positive-pressure pneumobelt attached like a girale about the abdomen to provide rhythmic external pressure.

Nutrition. Nutrition is important to MG patients. If they cannot swallow, a nasogastric tube should be inserted (the red rubber type is preferred [19]). Because MG is nearly always treatable, we have not yet had to perform esophagostomy (which we prefer to gastrostomy in untreatable diseases [185]). Patients who have problems with choking or aspiration usually avoid these problems by avoiding food; however, this approach results in malnutrition. When the first signs of choking appear, a nasogastric tube and/or a cuffed tracheostomy or cuffed endotracheal tube (swallowing can be difficult with the cuff inflated) must be placed. A diet containing 1,500–2,000 calories and 2 g sodium should be given in divided feedings. Patients in the recovery phase sometimes become too bold in trying to eat, which can lead to aspiration and possibly death. Moreover, swallowing sometimes is the last important function to return as the patient improves. When recovering patients eat without an inflated cuffed tube, they must proceed carefully, and sometimes excruciatingly slowly, from water to clear liquids, full liquids, purées, soft solids, and, finally, regular food.

Nursing Care. Attuned, experienced nursing is very important in management of the MG patient and in early recognition of potentially life-threatening situations, such as decreased vital capacity, blood in secretions from a well-established tracheostomy tube or in residua from the nasogastric tube, and alterations in responsiveness and behavior (11,19). In addition, nursing can provide range-of-motion exercises to prevent contractures, oversee active exercise, participate in very early mobilization to a chair (even while the patient is using a respirator), help support the patient psychologically, provide intellectual stimulation and understanding communication, and help convince the patient of the treatability of MG. Our nursing approach is detailed carefully elsewhere (19).

Myasthenic Hazards

Detrimental Drugs. Certain drugs are detrimental to patients with MG. Several antibiotics (especially the aminoglycosides "mycins"), including gentamicin, neomycin, dihydrostreptomycin, streptomycin, amikacin, sisomicin, kanamycin, tobramycin, kanendomycin, dibekacin, viomycin, colistin, polymyxin A and B, bacitracin, and possibly tetracyclines (although the last have been used without harm) (186–188) can reduce the amount of ACh that is released presynaptically at the NMJ. The effects of this resemble the defect caused by the production of excess Mg^{2+} (189,190) (they also may have a lesser, curarelike postsynaptic effect [190]). When this effect occurs, calcium is the most effective agent for improving neuromuscular transmission; anticholinesterases are said to be less effective. Temporary intubation and ventilation may be required until the effect of the antibiotic dissipates. Antibiotics that appear to be safe include ampicillin, erythromycin, and often the tetracyclines. Quinine can worsen the condition of the myasthenic patient, apparently by increasing the excitability threshold of the muscle fiber; quinine is present in tonic water (e.g., in gin and tonic). Antiarrhythmic drugs, such as quinidine, phenytoin, procainamide, and propranolol (and perhaps other β-adrenergic blockers) might worsen MG and should be used with caution; however, certainly some have been used without harm in MG patients (160). It is possible that chlorpromazine has worsened MG in some cases (191). Succinylcholine does not have a prolonged effect in myasthenic patients as it does in patients with deficiency of plasma cholinesterase. Similarly, myasthenic patients do not have a greatly prolonged response to d-tubocurarine; however, they do have an increased sensitivity to it, which is the basis of the diagnostic test described earlier (20).

Other Factors. Intercurrent infection (including inoculation, vaccination, and allergic episodes) can worsen MG, perhaps by general acceleration of production of antibodies and precipitate a crisis. Some females with MG have increased weakness just before the onset of their menstrual period and for the first day or two of it; however, suppression of ovulation by birth control pills has not offered consistent benefit in these patients. Emotional stress also can worsen the myasthenic state and precipitate a crisis. Heat (e.g., hot showers, sunlight) can weaken myasthenic patients temporarily. The increased physical burden of pregnancy, labor, and the sleep-deprived care required by a newborn can weaken a myasthenic woman. (There may also be an immunologic explanation for postpartum weakness: sudden loss of soluble factors produced by the hypertrophied suppressor T-lymphocyte system of the normal fetus [192] that may have benefited the patient transiently during pregnancy.) Hyperthyroidism also can worsen MG (193) as can hypothyroidism (58).

Summary of Our Therapeutic Program for Adults with MG

1. Patients with minimal disease who are controlled *satisfactorily* with small or medium doses of pyridostigmine, our drug of choice, do not need additional treatment. Satisfactory means that the patient can do daily activities to his or her satisfaction. For example, diplopia unacceptable to a neurosurgeon is tolerable to other patients.
2. Patients controlled unsatisfactorily (according to the criterion in 1), regardless of age, and those who are suspected of having thymoma, should undergo thymectomy unless there are contraindications (e.g., cardiac, renal, thromboembolic, or other accompanying problems, or general fragility of old age).
3. Patients not controlled according to the criteria in 1 and 2 or those who are not controlled by the criterion in 1 but who do not undergo thymectomy are given prednisone plus azathioprine as long-term treatment.
4. Patients who do not respond to the treatment in 3 can be given a trial of prednisone plus cyclophosphamide or prednisone plus methotrexate.

4a. The recently introduced total body irradiation may, with more experience, prove to be preferable to the treatment in 4 and perhaps even to that in 3.

5. Plasmapheresis is reserved for short-term use in acute (crisis) and subacute (precrisis) situations.

Management of Neonatal Myasthenia.

The most important aspect of managing the infant with transient neonatal myasthenia is anticipation. Every child of a myasthenic mother should be considered potentially to have this disorder, which appears in the first three days of life and often at birth. Edrophonium is a short-acting diagnostic agent; the dose for infants is about 0.5 mg IV or 1–2 mg IM (responses to IM administration are delayed two to 10 minutes). i.m. Pyridostigmine, 0.05–0.15 mg/kg body weight IM, or neostigmine methylsulfate, 0.1 mg IM, are longer-acting diagnostic and therapeutic measures. The infant should be watched for muscarinic side effects, and it may be necessary to give about 0.007–0.01 mg/kg atropine subcutaneously or IM, perhaps before the anticholinesterase. In addition, a respirator should be available. Feeding through a nasogastric tube also may be necessary. The weakness of neonatal myasthenia lasts a few days to a few weeks (average, 18 days) but can persist for up to two to three months (194). During this time, it is important to guard against pulmonary or other complications. Treatment with oral anticholinesterase medication also can be given according to the oral:IM ratios outlined earlier. Dosages can be decreased as the infant's condition improves. (All anticholinesterase dosages specified in this section are according to the package inserts as detailed in the 1980 edition of the *Physician's Desk Reference.*) The fact that plasmapheresis has virtually cured one infant (195) supports the pathogenic role of transplacental transfer of toxic maternal IgG (with or without other soluble factors).

Non-MG Junctional Defect that Responds to Corticosteroids

A new clinicopathologic disease that presumably affects the NMJ was manifested in a seven-year-old boy who, at age 14 months, developed nonfamilial, generalized weakness of the limbs and trunk that began proximally and spread distally. The condition progressed to severe disability at age 18 months and remained at that level (196). Eyes, face, jaw, and tongue were not involved, and there was no fluctuation or clinical atrophy. At age seven, studies revealed mild atrophy of type II muscle fiber only, brief duration, small amplitude action potential (BSAP) pattern on electromyogram (EMG), normal motor-nerve conduction velocity, a 15% decrement (borderline) at 5 Hz that decreased to 7% with administration of edrophonium. Neostigmine caused moderate clinical improvement for a few days; this was followed by worsening, and guanidine gave no benefit. However, prednisone, 1.5 mg/kg/day in a single dose, which then was tapered to every other day, has given dramatic, sustained benefit for three years. The disease has been shown repeatedly to be responsive to prednisone by the fact that it worsens when the dose is lowered and subsides again when the dose is restored (196). Plasma nAChR antibodies and carnitine values were not abnormal. A 14-year-old boy with similar findings has had a similarly gratifying response to prednisone (W.K. Engel, unpublished observations). The reason that a prednisone-responsive functional defect was suspected in these patients was the lack of correlation between striking muscle weakness and minimal histochemical changes seen in the muscle biopsy specimen. Recognition of this disorder is important because it is an example of the treatable limb-girdle syndrome.

Facilitating Myasthenic Syndrome

Facilitating myasthenic syndrome (FMS) (197–199) usually occurs in persons of middle and advanced age. Patients show weakness of the proximal muscles of the limbs and trunk but little or no involvement of cranial nerve musculature. Dryness of the mouth and reduced tendon reflexes often occur. FMS usually is associated with a remote neoplasm, especially a bronchogenic one, and the neuromuscular syndrome can be manifest before the tumor is identified. However, FMS is not associated with neoplasm (197,199,200) in 20–30% of patients. The diagnosis can sometimes be made clinically by noting whether strength increases (e.g., in the deltoid muscle, biceps brachialis, or wrist extensors) as the patient pushes repeatedly against resistance. On the EMG, the amplitude of the first potential is low (normal in MG), and there is marked facilitation at high-frequency (10–50 Hz) stimulation. At low-frequency stimulation (2–5 Hz) there is no change in facilitation and there even may be a mild decrease. FMS is thought to involve defective release of ACh from the presynaptic nerve terminal, possibly expressed as too few quanta of ACh. The mechanism of the remote neoplastic effect is not known, although a "Sparafucile" effect resulting from an abnormal molecule produced by the tumor has been proposed (51) (see discussion of adult dysimmune polymyopathy with neoplasia). In fact, such an abnormal molecule may have been demonstrated in vitro with a tumor extract from one patient (201), but plasmapheresis has not been beneficial (202).

Treatment of FMS is with guanidine, which enhances the release of ACh from the presynaptic terminal (198). The dosage is increased over one to two weeks from 10 mg/kg/day to a maximum of about 30 mg/kg/day. Side effects of guanidine include paresthesias of the mouth and extremities, nausea, vomiting, dizziness, and, rarely, suppression of bone marrow production and liver toxicity. Calcium also enhances release of junctional ACh, but its benefit in FMS remains conjectural. One patient with nonneoplastic FMS was benefited by and dependent upon prednisone (199). Although the effect of prednisone in other FMS patients is not well established, the drug could be tried cautiously. Associated neoplasms should be sought and treated.

Acetylcholinesterase Deficiency at the NMJ

A new junctional syndrome has been described recently (203). It is characterized by generalized weakness that increases with exertion, easy fatigability, hyporeflexia, and clinical refractoriness to anticholinesterase drugs and to guanidine. The EMG showed decremental muscle response to all frequencies of stimulation, repetitive muscle response to single stimulation of nerve, marked decrease in the morphologic size of motor-nerve terminals, normal postsynaptic nAChR, and absence of acetylcholinesterase (16 S) at the NMJ. Anti-nAChR antibodies were not detected (208). Prednisone improved the clinical symptoms slightly but did not change the transmission defect that was evident on the EMG (203).

Possible Defect of the ACh-Induced Ion Channel

Another recently identified junctional syndrome is familial and is characterized by slowly progressive proximal and distal muscle weakness and wasting in the cranium, trunk, and limbs starting in infancy or early adulthood; lack of response to edrophonium; absence of nAChR antibodies; repetitive muscle-action potentials from one nerve stimulus; decrement on the EMG at 2–3 Hz; abnormal jitter and blocking; markedly prolonged duration of MEPPs and EPPs that is worsened by neostigmine; decreased MEPP amplitude; paucity of type II muscle fiber; tubular aggregates and vacuoles in muscle fibers near the NMJ; morphologically decreased nerve-terminal area with increased density of synaptic vesicles; and shortened postsynaptic membranes with focal degeneration associated with loss of nAChR (204). The postulated cause is a prolonged open time of ACh-induced ion channels secondary to degeneration of junctional folds. There is no known treatment for this condition.

Botulism

Botulism usually occurs, within 12–36 hours, from consumption of improperly canned foods or foods that contain botulinum toxin that is produced in the container by the anaerobic bacterium *Clostridium butulinum* (205). Wound botulism is also known to occur (205). Botulinum toxin (206,207) impairs the release of ACh by blocking the ability of Ca^{2+} moving intracellularly to trigger exocytotic release of ACh from the presynaptic motor axonal terminal at the NMJ. Limbs, respiration, and musculature of the cranial nerves are affected. As in FMS, the EMG initially is facilitative, can show BSAPs (205) and later may show features of denervation. The effects of *C. botulinum* can be treated clinically with guanidine (205); however, because the illness usually is severe, maximum doses of 30, or possibly up to 50 mg/kg/day orally should be given immediately. Ca^{2+} is less effective. (Although the pharmacologic effects of *C. botulinum* can be counteracted by venom from the black widow spider, this technique is not yet used clinically.) Clinical improvement with guanidine is most notable in ocular muscles and less so in other areas, including respiratory muscles (208). The most important aspect of management is respiratory assistance. Antitoxin also can be used and has been reported to be beneficial if given early in the course of the illness (209). However, a 21% rate of adverse reactions to antitoxin of equine origin has been reported (210,211). *Wound botulism* requires additional attention to the wound. *Infantile botulism* is a newly recognized phenomenon, the alleged toxin being produced in the intestine by ingested *C. botulinum* organisms or spores (212,213). The disease is believed to affect infants aged 3–26 weeks and is characterized by generalized weakness, difficulties in feeding, hypotonia, respiratory insufficiency, and constipation. Infantile botulism is suggested as a cause of "floppy baby" and as a possible cause of sudden infant death syndrome (213–215). It can be treated with respiratory assistance and general supportive measures and appears to be self-limited. Antibiotics against the clostridial organism and parenteral antitoxin can be used but are of uncertain benefit (214). The use of guanidine in infantile botulism has not been reported but can be considered.

Other Toxins that Affect the NMJ (216,217)

Clinically, these other toxins are rarely encountered, but it is important to be aware of them. Treatment in these cases usually is supportive, with respiratory aid if necessary. (*1*) *Presynaptic toxins.* Black widow spider venom (α-latrotoxin) can cause spasms, presumably by its action of increasing influx of Ca^{2+} into motor-nerve terminals, leading to dispersion, fusion, and exocytosis of ACh-containing vesicles (218). Butulinum toxin, β-bungarotoxin, notexin, and crotoxin impair ACh release. Hemicholinium, notexin, and taipoxin block uptake of choline. (*2*) *Postsynaptic toxins.* α-bungarotoxin, α-cobratoxin, d-tubocurarine, MG IgG, and erabutoxin B block the postsynaptic nAChR and presumably also bind to the small amount of nAChR that is also found on the presynaptic axon terminal (23,24). Histrionicotoxin, amantadine, and atropine bind to and can inhibit the ion-conductance modulator of nAChR (minimally in the case of the last two). Relatively short-acting therapeutic anticholinesterases and long-acting ones (e.g., diisopropylfluorophosphate, malathion, parathion) bind to and inhibit the action of acetylcholinesterase. (*3*) *Toxins that affect ion channels.* These toxins can affect the general function of nerve- and muscle cell plasmalemma. The Na^+ channel is blocked by tetrodotoxin and saxitoxin and is kept open by veratrine (to which geramine diacetate is related), batrachotoxin, aconitine, grayanotoxin, crotamine, scorpion toxin, and sea anemone toxin. (*4*) *Myonecrotic toxins.* Myonecrotic toxins cause necrosis of muscle fiber and include phospholipase A_2, toxins of elapids (which need Ca^{2+} to lyse muscle cells), diisopropylfluorophosphate (causes damage especially at the junctional region), and notexin. (*5*) *Other.* Ciguatera intoxication (caused by consumption of tropical fish that have ingested a toxin ultimately from a phytoplankton dinoflagellate) affects the NMJ and/or terminal axons by an unknown mechanism (219).

Tick Paralysis

An ascending motor paralysis that results in respiratory paralysis and death can be caused by the excretion of a toxin from a female tick. The toxin blocks nerve transmission in the tertinal portion of the motor nerves (205). Treatment consists of complete removal of the tick, which can be hiding in head or pubic hair, the ear, or the vulva (220).

Plasma (Nonspecific) Cholinesterase Deficiency

Plasma cholinesterase deficiency is an autosomal recessive hereditary disorder (221,222) that is symptomless until the homozygous patient is given succinyl choline as a muscle relaxant during surgery (i.e., the disorder predisposes the patient to succinylcholine intoxication). The patient then remains paralyzed for several hours to one to two days. The paralysis is caused by failure of the plasma enzyme to hydrolyze the succinylcholine. Treatment consists of management of respiratory failure as long as necessary and of warning the patient and his or her other physicians of the danger posed by succinylcholine. The risk may also apply to other members of the patient's family, and they should be tested for this deficiency by analysis of plasma cholinesterase. This can be done easily by an electrophoretic-histochemical procedure (223) or by direct quantitative assay (224). d-Tubocurarine can be used as a muscle relaxant in future surgery.

DISORDERS OF MUSCLE

Dysimmune Dermatomyopathy and Dysimmune Polymyopathy

It is possible to debate the precise definitions of dermatomyositis and polymyositis. However, in order to obviate ruminative arguments (225), we drop the somewhat misleading suffix "itis" (although certainly not denying that "itis" occurs in biopsy specimens of a number of patients in this category, more often in adults than in children) and introduce the term *dysimmune* to delineate one general category that is based on presumed pathogenesis. Because dysimmune dermatomyopathy (DDM) and dysimmune polymyopathy (DPM) have in common pathologic features, pathogenesis (by definition dysimmune, of which there are several components, in somewhat different expressions in different patients), and treatment (antidysimmune), we will consider them together as the *DDM/DPM complex.* Childhood DDM seems to be a distinct entity, and whether or not DPM occurs in childhood has not been established. In adults there also occurs typical DDM, as well as DPM that seems to be virtually the same as typical DDM but without skin lesions. In cases of putative adult DPM that are difficult to diagnose, a trial with antidysimmune therapy sometimes can be diagnostic (the only known exception is the response of patients with carnitine deficiency to prednisone [226–229]). If uncertainty still exists, the label "27-YOOC" (muscle disease of unknown type, continuous weakness) can be applied to emphasize the uncertainty (230). In DDM/DPM, inflammation in the biopsy specimen is not a diagnostic sine qua non (108,231). Virtually all DDM/DPM patients respond to prednisone or some other antidysimmune treatment to some degree or some length of time. Whether or not the improvement is sustained determines the outcome. Lack of sustained response in some patients emphasizes the need for better antidysimmune programs. The outcome of treatment in various centers is a function partly of how vigorously and carefully antidysimmune treatment is applied (i.e., how assiduously benefit is sought by pushing the treatment to the margin of safety. and how carefully side effects are avoided by fine tuning the therapeutic program). Nondysimmune inflammatory and infectious myopathies will also be reviewed in this section.

Childhood DDM/DPM.

Childhood DDM/DPM begins at any age of childhood, although it is very uncommon in children younger than two years. Usually it is gradual in onset but sometimes is fulminant. Muscle weakness is much greater proximally in the limbs and trunk. Swallowing sometimes is affected. There is often weakness of the flexor muscles of the neck, but other cranial nerve musculature typically is spared. The skin rash consists of redness of the face (somewhat accentuated in a butterfly distribution on the cheeks, bridge of the nose, and under the lower eyelids), eyelids, elbows, upper chest, and knees; and sometimes a diffuse mottling of the extremities. The rash is a mottled or diffuse red, often with a bluish hue and often associated with dilated capillaries in the rash area. Typically there is redness, ulceration, or scarring over the knuckles of the hands and fingers and dilated capillary loops at the base of the fingernails. Facial edema may be present. The gastrointestinal tract sometimes is involved, with ulcerations and bleeding that in most patients are not necessarily attributable to corticosteroids because these signs occur in untreated patients as well (232). However, ulcerations and bleeding also can be drug induced in patients treated with high daily divided doses of corticosteroids without adjunct antacids or between-meal feedings.

Childhood DDM/DPM is usually a self-limited disorder, although in some patients the disease lingers for decades. Although spontaneous arrest and improvement of childhood DDM/DPM can occur early, the disease generally progresses for several (approximately three to 10) years, after which time its activity seems to stop spontaneously (with or without residual), never to return. If it is not treated it can lead to death resulting from aspiration pneumonitis, respiratory insufficiency, or gastrointestinal bleeding. The serum mucle enzymes (creatine phosphokinase [CPK], glutamic oxaloacetic transaminase, glutamic pyruvic transaminase, lactic dehydrogenase, aldolase) are often elevated. That these enzymes come from muscle rather than the liver can be determined by the elevation of CPK and by lack of elevation of alkaline phosphatase, 5-nucleotidase, or other indicators of liver function. In some patients with childhood DDM/DPM, serum muscle enzymes are not elevated, even in the presence of significant and progressive untreated muscle weakness. The sedimentation rate is often elevated. In childhood DDM/DPM, the EMG shows a BSAP pattern (55,233), sometimes with fibrillations.

The muscle biopsy specimen usually is diagnostic. It shows active muscle involvement with necrosis and phagocytosis of fibers, "regen-degen" fibers (highlighted by the alkaline-phosphatase reaction) (W.K. Engel, unpublished observations) (231,234), some of which are multivacuolated fibers (106–108). Any macrophages that are present are highlighted by their pronounced staining by nonspecific esterase and acid-phosphatase reactions (W.K. Engel, unpublished observations). In spite of the suffix "itis," the biopsy specimen often does not show a dysimmune inflammation of lymphocytic infiltration around fibers and/or blood vessels; accordingly, inflammation is not a histologic criterion for diagnosis (W.K. Engel, unpublished observations) (108). (One must not perform biopsy on a muscle site that has recently been punctured by a needle [e.g., for EMG or therapeutic injections] because the specimen may show needle-induced myopathy/myositis [235,236].)

A characteristic abnormality of blood vessels in childhood DDM/DPM is thickening, particularly of small venules and arterioles. The thickening is associated with deposition of immunoglobulins and complement and is found in most patients with childhood DDM/DPM (and in a smaller percentage of adults) (237). The thickening is also associated with accumulation in the vessels of types I and III collagen and procollagen and of fibronectin (238). Such vessels usually do not show lymphocytic infiltration.

Two features that confirm placement of childhood DDM/DPM in the category of collagen vascular disease (which includes lupus erythematosus, in which the biopsy specimen usually is abnormal and indistinguishable from that of childhood DDM [W.K. Engel, unpublished observations] [108]) are the perifascicular smallness of the muscle fibers and the positive reaction of connective tissue with alkaline phosphatase (2,108,231). The architecture of the small fibers in the perifascicular region is abnormal. They have an overall looser (watery-looking) structure, one or several small vacuoles, darker staining with oxidative enzyme, large, round nuclei, and sometimes other regen-degen features (106,108,239). Endomysial and perimysial connective tissue is proliferated in association with accumulation of types I and III collagen and of fibronectin (which are not disease specific, since the same accumulations occur in Duchenne muscular dystrophy [238]). The streaks of staining with alkaline phosphatase in perimysial and endomysial connective tissue are not seen in healthy human muscle (the only normal positive reaction with alkaline phosphatase occurs in small arterioles [234]). The streaks are disproportionately strong in DDM/DPM patients and probably reflect more rapid fibroblastic proliferation (they are occasionally present, but to a much lesser degree, in Duchenne muscular dystrophy if there is a large amount of active necrosis; the only other condition in which the streaks are prominent is in the active proliferating phase of myositis ossificans [W.K. Engel, unpublished observations]).

Two additional features of the muscle biopsy specimen that are highly suggestive of DDM/DPM are calcium in perimysial and endomysial connective tissue and thickening of small blood vessels. Excess calcium can be seen in any muscle fiber that shows major or minor damage. In DDM/DPM much more calcium is deposited in regions of connective tissue than is seen in other non-dysimmune myopathies (e.g., Duchenne muscular dystrophy) (231). The calcium deposition probably is related to fibroblastic responses and to the presence of excessive alkaline phosphatase and inflammatory cells (if they occur) (231). The skin biopsy specimen in DDM/DPM can show lymphocytic infiltration, often around blood vessels, increased amounts of alkaline phosphatase, and increased calcium deposits in the connective tissue (W.K. Engel, unpublished observations) (231).

The details of the pathogenesis of childhood DDM/DPM are not known. In general, however, the disease is considered to be a dysimmune process. Pathogenesis may consist of a direct attack on muscle by immunoglobulins and/or lymphocytes, but this is uncertain. A major component probably is ischemia caused by blockage of small vessels by immunoglobulins (with or without the Ig complex), deposition, and collagen proliferation (perhaps secondary to the Ig deposition) within their walls (237,238). The possible role of viruses in DDM/DPM is uncertain. Although virus particles have been reported to occur in muscle (241–243), living organisms have not been isolated and transmission of disease has not been observed. DPM that seems to appear after viral infection (244), immunization (245,246), administration of penicillamine (247) or procainamide (accompanied by immunologic evidence of lupus erythematosus [248]), and severe sunburn [W.K. Engel, unpublished observations] has been noted in occasional cases, and the common mechanism could be dysimmune. The acute transient myositis seen in children, which is often related to influenza virus (244,249, 250), may be an important model of a very brief, self-limited type of DDM/DPM or of an initial viral-myositis phase of DDM/DPM. If so, it raises the question of whether to institute early and/or prolonged antiviral treatment in DDM/DPM (see comments on viral infection and lymphocytes under *Myasthenia Gravis*). (From a biochemical standpoint, a scleroderma-like illness is reported to have developed during therapy with 1-5-hydroxytryptophan and carbidopa (250).)

Treatment. Treatment of childhood DDM/DPM is designed to stop manifestations of the disease before they become crippling or fatal. Whether antidysimmune treatment hastens the eventual limitation (possibly self-limitation) of the disease is not known; nevertheless, therapy certainly allows the patient to survive in good condition until the time of limitation. Treatment of the basic disease consists of the antidysimmune approach, as outlined in the section on MG. Although we previously have started with prednisone alone (1.25–1.5 mg/kg in a single daily dose for two to four weeks, then tapered to HSDAD), we now sometimes start with prednisone plus azathioprine (or, if the patient cannot tolerate this, prednisone plus cyclophosphamide), as in MG. Some physicians have used methotrexate, but we find it inconvenient and difficult to manage. In a young, growing patient, certain side effects deserve additional consideration. Corticosteroids can impair growth, but this effect generally is only slight to moderate with HDAD-Pred therapy. When the DDM/DPM is severe or life threatening, a reduction in the patient's eventual stature is acceptable. Furthermore, azathioprine and cyclophosphamide may affect gonadal function.

The method of beginning and reducing the dosage of prednisone and other drugs is the same as in MG (although the initial worsening seen in MG does not occur). In DDM/DPM, dosage is determined primarily according to muscle strength. Concurrently, the serum muscle enzymes, if elevated, are used as an indication of continued leakage of muscle fibers. However, an increase in serum muscle enzymes is considered to be only a possible harbinger of exacerbation. Accordingly, a slight increase in serum muscle enzymes that appears in association with decreasing dosage does not necessitate an immediate increment in dosage, even if there is slight increase in weakness (as long as there is not a major increase in weakness). Rather, the dosage should be kept the same; this often is followed in a few weeks by a return of serum muscle enzymes and of strength to the previous level and further improvement. After four to eight weeks of stabilization, the medication can cautiously be reduced further. If, on keeping the dosage at the same level, the weakness increases or its persistence is of concern, the dosage must be increased. As in MG, we prefer to stop the prednisone before stopping the azathioprine or the cyclophosphamide. If treatment is to be prolonged, a small amount of the drug can be given; in childhood DDM/DPM, medication can be withdrawn sooner than in MG or adult-onset DDM/DPM (e.g., after two to four years of stability and virtual clinical normality). In mild cases of DDM/DPM, some physicians prefer to withhold treatment and await spontaneous remission; this issue is unsettled, since both treatment and lack of treatment carry known and unknown risks.

In a DDM/DPM patient who shows increasing muscle weakness along with signs of prednisone toxicity, the question arises as to whether the weakness is caused by prednisone-induced atrophy of type II muscle fiber or by worsening of disease. The two pathogenic phenomena can coexist, and many patients on an effective program of prolonged HSDAD-Pred can exhibit slight atrophy of type II muscle fiber. Even patients who are not receiving treatment can have moderate to prominent atrophy of type II fiber as a result of the basic DDM/DPM (or MG), especially when contractures cause immobilization and/or disuse of a muscle. Nevertheless, we try to determine the major cause of weakness in the following ways: (*1*) review the past one to two months in regard to muscle strength and mobility, serum muscle enzymes and other clinical evidence of disease activity, and evidence of drug side effects (all these in relation to any changes in medication that had been made); (*2*) decide whether the progress of the disease or prednisone toxicity is the more likely cause; (*3*) arbitrarily choose to raise or lower the prednisone dosage accordingly; (*4*) await an answer, which will be evident in about one to eight weeks. Although a repeat muscle biopsy can be performed to determine remaining disease activity, this often is not helpful in determining the cause of increased weakness. In fact, it can be misleading because histochemical evidence of disease activity can exist even though prednisone toxicity is causing the increased muscle weakness (W.K. Engel, unpublished observations).

Because childhood DDM/DPM usually is a limited (possibly self-limited) monophasic disease that does not recur once it is completely inactive, the drugs can be withdrawn after clinical stability is achieved and after a few years of dosage at a very low maintenance level.

Plasmapheresis (127,152) would seem to be a logical approach to treatment if pathologic antibodies or immunoglobulin complexes, circulated in DDM/DPM; we would add lymphocytopheresis to any plasmapheresis that is done. The use of plasmapheresis in DDM/DPM has not been studied fully although there are anecdotal reports of patients who improved with this therapy. As in MG, it is important to distinguish between the effects of plasmapheresis and those of drugs taken concurrently. Because the delayed side effects of total body irradiation (described in the section on adult DDM/DPM) remain somewhat uncertain, it seems best not to apply this modality to children yet, except possibly in extreme situations. Administration of ALG or ATG also would be a logical approach that has not been studied in DDM/DPM. Penicillamine, which occasionally can induce dysimmune disease (e.g., MG), can reduce circulating immune complexes and immunoglobulins in primary biliary cirrhosis (253) but has not been used in childhood DDM/DPM.

Vascular occlusion is considered a pathogenic factor in childhood DDM/DPM (106–108,232,237). Accordingly, vasodilation and/or anticoagulation (achieved with a variety of agents, including aspirin and antithrombotic agents such as dipyridamole and other phosphodiesterase inhibitors that potentiate endogenous prostacycline [254]), and/or thrombolytic agents (e.g., urokinase, streptokinase [255]) would seem logical considerations for therapy; however, none of these substances have been studied carefully. Danazol may increases clearing of immune complexes, and it is known to improve a lupuslike aspect of hereditary angioneurotic edema (151). Thus, we suggest that danazol could be considered for use in childhood DDM, although it also can cause myopathy (151).

Calcium deposition in connective tissue of muscle, subcutaneous, and cutaneous regions occurs in most children and adults with DDM/DPM, as evidenced histochemically and by clinical scanning with ^{99m}Tc-diphosphonate (231,256), and larger deposits can be demonstrated by x-ray or ultrasound. In some children the calcification can be massive and can cause severe crippling, pain, and skin breakdown and infection. Radiologically, the larger calcium deposits have a flocculent appearance. When widespread, the deposition is called *calcinosis universaliss*; it is a complication of childhood DDM/DPM and not a distinct disease. When calcinosis increases we consider it a sign of smoldering disease activity and an indication for antidysimmune treatment (51,231). Treatment of the calcium deposition with ethylenediaminetetraacetic acid, EGTA, and diphosphonate has been unsatisfactory (252). Aluminum hydroxide was reported to be beneficial in one case (257) but has not come into general use. We have documented remarkable clinical and radiologic improvement and virtually complete regression of calcium deposits in some children (and also some adults) with DDM/DPM when the basic disease was successfully treated with prednisone plus azathioprine (W.K. Engel, unpublished observations). The mechanism of the metastatic calcium deposition is not known. We have postulated (51,231,258) that the excess alkaline phosphatase found in the connective tissue of DDM/DPM muscle, subcutaneous tissue, and skin splits phosphate from various organic phosphate compounds (e.g., adenosine triphosphate, adenosine diphosphate, adenosine 5′-monophosphate, and other nucleotides), and that the phosphate combines with the ubiquitous calcium of extracellular fluid to produce deposits of calcium phosphate, probably as apatite crystals. (Whether local increase of γ-carboxyglutamic acid (259) has a pathogenic role is uncertain.)

Contractures often are a major problem in childhood DDM/DPM. They can be prevented or progressively lessened through medical therapy that consists of persistent passive stretching with the aid of an experienced physical therapist. With training, the patient's family can learn the procedures (108).

While the patient is responding to medical treatment, *active exercise* (but not beyond the point of fatigue) also is important for rebuilding muscle fibers by stimulating protein anabolism.

Adult DDM/DPM

The clinical and pathologic features of the adult DDM/DPM complex resemble those of childhood DDM/DPM. Although some investigators believe that patients with muscle involvement alone (DPM) differ from those with muscle involvement plus skin involvement (DDM), we do not subscribe to such a distinction (with the exception of patients with vacuolar myopathy); hence our use of the term *DDM/DPM complex.* In adults, DDM is less common than DPM but, in our experience, is neither more severe nor less responsive to treatment than DPM. Arthralgias are common in adult DDM/DPM but myalgias are not (W.K. Engel, unpublished observations). The pathology of adult DDM/DPM can be like that of the childhood form, or it can show rather evenly scattered (nonperifascicular) necrotic/phagocytosed fibers and regen-degen fibers; more commonly (but not always) there are perivascular lymphocytic and macrophagic inflammatory-cell responses. Although not all cases of DDM or DPM are of exactly the same etiology or pathogenic mechanism, we consider them all to be dysimmune; thus, because of our incomplete knowledge at present, any possible differences in the syndromes do not indicate different treatments. Mechanisms of killer T lymphocytes and rhabdomyocytoxic immunoglobulins have been sought (260–264), but studies have not demonstrated a consistent pathogenic mechanism. DPM/DDM may occur alone or in the course of collagen-vascular disease, especially with systemic lupus erythrematosus, rheumatoid arthritis, Sjögren's syndrome, major vasculitides (including polyarteritis and necrotizing vasculitis [W.K. Engel, unpublished observations] [265]), and sometimes with progressive systemic sclerosis (scleroderma). Some features of DDM/DPM may reflect disorders that are not muscle related or skin related, such as arthralgias, Reynaud's phenomenon, or abnormalities of circulating immunoglobulins (e.g., antinuclear antibodies, rheumatoid factor). There may be increased sedimentation rate, and cardiac arrhythmias, conduction abnormalities, increased left-ventricular function during systole, and mitral-valve prolapse associated with cardiomyopathy also may occur (266,267) and should be treated if significant. Occasionally a patient with DDM/DPM has a parent or sibling with DDM/DPM or another dysimmune disease (e.g., lupus erythematosus, MG, multiple sclerosis) (W.K. Engel, unpublished observations). Muscle involvement that occurs in other collagen-vascular diseases is indistinguishable histochemically from that in DDM/DPM (W.K. Engel, unpublished observations) (108).

Treatment. Treatment of adult DDM/DPM is the same as for the childhood form. Some adult DDM/DPM patients obtain remarkable benefit from corticosteroids with or without azathioprine (or cyclophosphamide or methotrexate), and some do not. Patients also may have good muscle response and poor skin response. We now prefer to start with prednisone plus azathioprine and eventually (after very gradual tapering) withdraw the prednisone first. If the disease is well controlled but worsens then with a reduction in dosage, the condition may or may not respond again (i.e., now that it has become very difficult to control). Overall, the response of adult-onset DDM/DPM is less satisfactory than that of childhood DDM/DPM, although with treatment some adults achieve remarkable and prolonged remission. Our experience has led us to recommend that adult DDM/DPM patients in remission continue to take 5–15 mg single-dose alternate-day prednisone (or another immunosuppressant) for a prolonged period (as we also recommend for MG) (this is not an unequivocally established plan). Calcinosis of tissue can occur in the adult form of DDM/DPM but not with the massive deposits that can occur in the childhood form. This feature also can respond to treatment of the basic disease (256). Dysimmune diseases associated with neoplasia probably affect lymphocytes or thymic epithelial cells or both. Peptides produced by neoplastic and/or fetal cells have been reported (268), some of which also affect lymphocytes (192) or thymic epithelial cells (66). Such effects could conceivably be irreversible even after removal of the neoplasm. In patients with DDM/DPM associated with scleroderma, both muscle and skin usually respond poorly.

The use of total body irradiation in adult DDM/DPM is derived from our use of splenic irradiation in MG (161); both approaches were developed because lymphocytes are considered to be the most sensitive of circulating cells to x-irradiation. Our experience to date with this technique in DDM/DPM has been with one 40-year-old woman who had DPM for five years and had become refractory to prednisone, intolerant to azathioprine, and responsive to but then intoxicated by methotrexate and cyclophosphamide. Inadequate vascular access prevented plasmapheresis or lymphocytopheresis. She was totally paralyzed proximally and nearly so distally (unable to hold a pencil), unable to swallow her secretions, had a vital capacity of 0.6 L. She needed the aid of a nasogastric tube and a respirator. Her serum levels of CPK were 42 times greater than the upper limits of normal. Total body irradiation (15 rad twice a week for five weeks; 150 rad total) resulted in progressive improvement, evident in the second week (vital capacity, 1.5 L). After three months the patient was discharged, and by seven months (the most recent time of observation) her vital capacity (4 L) and swallowing were normal. She was able to walk without a walker, hold her arms above her head, and transfer and totally care for herself. The prednisone, her only dysimmune medication for the time of irradiation, had been reduced gradually to 30 mg q.o.d., less than half the pretreatment dose. A circulating lymphocytopenia (about 500 mm^{-3}) accompanied the total body irradiation and has persisted (162). The patient's excellent result suggests that this new treatment for DDM/DPM merits further exploration.

In some adult patients, DDM/DPM is the first expression of an occult neoplasm. This should be sought in patients in whom onset occurs at age 30 or more; however, neoplasm is found in only a small percentage of patients. DDM/DPM associated with neoplasm responds to antidysimmune treatment, as does nonneoplastic DDM/DPM, sometimes with an excellent response that is maintained for a year or more before the underlying neoplasm is detected (although retrospective review of x-ray films may show that the neoplasm had been there throughout that time) (W.K. Engel, unpublished observations) (2). All neoplasms should be treated as such. (Except for MG associated with thymoma, the remote effects of a neoplasm on the neuromuscular system are limited to neuropathy, FMS, DDM/DPM complex [especially DDM], and atrophy of type II muscle fiber [269].) One possible mechanism of remote effect could be a molecule, such as a peptide, produced by the neoplasm to affect distant cells (a sparafucile molecule [269]).

Summary of Our Therapeutic Approach to DDM/DPM

(*1*) Prednisone plus azathioprine.

(*2*) If prednisone plus azathioprine is beneficial, withdraw the prednisone first. Maintain small dosage of azathioprine or prednisone for a long time.

(*3*) If step 1 fails, try prednisone plus cyclophosphamide or go directly to step 4.

(*4*) If step 1 or 3 fails, try long-term plasmapheresis/lymphocytopheresis (unproved). In extreme circumstances, try total body irradiation, about which we are cautiously optimistic) (162).

Some adults with DDM/DPM have very high titers of toxoplasma (W.K. Engel, M.C. Dalakas, unpublished observations) (271) without elevated antinuclear antibody or rheumatoid factor, which can give false-positive results (272). We have seen 11 such patients recently, only two of whom had signs of systemic toxoplasmosis. No parasites were evident in the muscle biopsy specimens, and antitoxoplasma treatment (a course of pyramethamine plus sulfadiazine) had no effect on muscle strength or antibody titers.

Rare cases of acute myositis in humans (273,274) have been attributed to toxoplasmosis on the basis of serologic studies but without convincing evidence of the presence of organisms; one of these patients had normal muscle (273). In another patient, recurrent toxoplasmosis was considered to be the cause of myositis, and encapsulated organisms were found in muscle (275). In contrast to the rare examples of direct parasitic myositis, we have proposed an indirect, dysimmune mechanism, as follows:

About 50% of U.S. inhabitants have serologic evidence of chronic asymptomatic toxoplasmosis (272); in addition, a relatively high percentage of humans also have been exposed to other coccidial protozoa (e.g., *Hammondia, Sarcocystis, Isospera*). For example, *Sarcocystis* is widespread in meat intended for consumption, and there is a high incidence of asymptomatic infection in meat handlers and Europeans (R. Fayer, personal communication). Infection of an intermediate host by toxoplasma or other coccidia can be acquired by ingestion of either oocysts from cat or dog feces or cysts from undercooked meat (272,276–282). In an intermediate host, coccidia schizonts move in two stages from the intestine via the blood to invade vascular endothelial cells; subsequently, their merozoites become encysted in muscle and other tissues (279–282). Since humans can be intermediate hosts for toxoplasma and other coccidia, some vascular, muscle, CNS and/or heart cells in a high percentage of the population have been invaded by the parasite, resulting in the formation of antibodies to the organisms, as evidenced by serologic studies. Therefore, we propose that, in some patients with DDM/DPM (possibly those who are genetically predisposed), the coccidial infection provoked pathogenic humoral and/or cellular immune mechanisms that were directed against vascular, muscle, and sometimes other tissues and were originally directed against either antigens of the organism or antigens the organisms altered in the invaded cells; the antigens thus were interpreted as being foreign, and the resultant immune mechanism cross-reacted against the patient's normal tissues to cause the disease. This hypothetical mechanism also might apply to other collagen-vascular diseases, such as disseminated lupus erythematosus, in which there can be false-positive titers of toxoplasma, and multiple sclerosis.

Because toxoplasmosis can sometimes cause an atypical lymphocytosis that is similar to Epstein-Barr mononucleosis (69), another possible dysimmune pathogenic mechanism in DDM/DPM could be a synergistic effect of the coccidia parasitosis with a virus (cf. 272). We feel that the possible role of coccidia-provoked dysimmune reactions in DDM/DPM and other dysimmune diseases should be explored further.

Sarcoid Myopathy

The initial clinical picture of sarcoid myopathy is similar to that of polymyositis and includes proximal muscle weakness with or without features of sarcoidosis in other systems. The muscle biopsy specimen shows features of active myopathy, perivascular mononuclear cells, and the additional presence of multinucleated giant-cell granulomas (283) although a sample of a granuloma might not be obtained in a given specimen. However, it is important not to mistake cross-sectioned regenerative muscle fibers with their multiple nuclei for multinucleated giant cells (we propose that the latter be staind strongly with nonspecific esterase because macrophages, from which they originate, do). Treatment has generally been with corticosteroids, which can be of considerable benefit (284). It has not been established whether another agent, such as azathioprine or cyclophosphamide, added to the prednisone would enhance the effectiveness of the therapy.

Vacuolar (Cabbage-Body) Myopathy

Vacuolar myopathy is a type of disease (perhaps a group of diseases) whose initial symptoms include slowly progressive muscle weakness that occurs at about age 30–70. Not only is the weakness proximal, but it also is associated with significant distal weakness, especially of the muscles of the forearm and lower leg (285–288). The disease is not hereditary. Except for neck weakness, cranial nerves are not affected, or only minimally so. Biopsy of muscle fibers reveals various irregular vacuoles, the hallmark of the disease, which ultrastructurally contain swirls and other collections of membranous material that often resemble a cross-sectioned cabbage (285,286,289). They also contain clusters of long, parallel, double-helical filaments 20 μm in "diameter" and with 100 μm periods (240,241,288,289–291). There are also some small angular fibers that suggest an aspect of denervation (63,285). There can be a mild or moderate perivascular inflammatory component with mononuclear cells in the muscle. The cause of vacuolar myopathy is not known, but it may involve a low-grade inflammatory component. Muscle fibers cultured from three patients (289) revealed viruslike structures (possibly reovirus of coxsackievirus, and not resembling experimentally produced crystallized ribosomes [292–294]). This observation raises the question of whether the cause is an indolent virus. We have tried treatment with corticosteroids and/or azathioprine, but only an occasional patient benefited significantly. On the basis of observations of tissue culture, an antiviral treatment might be appropriate; however, studies of this approach have not yet been reported.

Myositis Caused by Exogenous Organisms.
Myositis in association with known pathologic agents can be either focal or general. The infecting agents include viruses, various bacteria (e.g., tuberculi, clostridia, *Staphylococcus aureus*), fungi, and animal parasites (e.g., the roundworm *Trichinia*, the flatworm *Cysticerca*, the protozoa *Toxoplasma, Trypanosoma* and, possibly, *Sarcosporidia*). A pyogenic myositis is usually caused by *S. aureus* (295,296). *Trichina* and *Toxoplasma* myositides (106,186–189) are rarely known to infect humans, and *Trypanosoma cruzi* (especially the myopathic form) commonly infests muscle (W.K. Engel, J. A. Dvorak, unpublished observations) (297,300,301). *Sarcosporidia (Sarcocystis)* myositis is not yet known to occur in humans, although it is well known as a major or minor infestation of animal muscle (279–282). Trichinosis arises from ingestion of the meat of omnivores or carnivores (e.g., pigs, bears) that contains the nematode *Trichinella spiralis*. Gastrointestinal symptoms are followed about seven to 14 days later by fever, periorbital edema, and myalgia. There is eosinophilia, positive results on serologic tests, and sometimes positive results on muscle biopsy. Treatment usually is not satisfactory; thiabendazole must be used in the first week, but the diagnosis usually is not made until the second week. Otherwise, treatment (salicylates, daily prednisone) is given according to symptoms for the inflammatory response, self-limited to 1–2 weeks (302).

Viral myositis occurs in animals with coxsackieviruses A and B, echovirus 9 (303), Theiler's agent, EMC picornaviruses, some arboviruses, Jungblut's SK virus, avian leukosis-sarcoma virus (including cultured chick muscle [304]), and mouse C-particle-producing RNA tumor virus [retrovirus]) (i.e., host muscle is infested but not obviously damaged [305–307]) and experimentally in cultured human muscle with measles (V. Askanas, H.F. McFarland, W.K. Engel, unpublished observations). In humans, epidemic myalgia (pleurodynia, Devil's grip) probably is viral in origin because it has been associated with epidemics of coxsackievirus B, which has been isolated from muscle (308). Whether viruses plays a role in typical chronic DDM/DPM is unknown, and the triangular-lattice particles seen in DDM/DPM (241,242,309) might not be viral.

Polymyalgia Rheumatica.
Polymyalgia rheumatica is a synovitis syndrome of late middle age or older and preferentially affects women (ratio of women to men, 3:1). The condition is characterized by migratory pains in the shoulders, hip girdle, and back, sometimes with local tenderness; however, the patient often thinks that the pain and tenderness are in the muscle (295,310,311). Muscle strength, serum muscle enzymes and EMG are normal. The muscle biopsy specimen shows atrophy of type II fiber (W.K. Engel, unpublished observations) (312). The sedimentation rate is elevated (usually greater than 50 mm/hr), and results of isotope scans of the joints can be positive and diagnostic (313). Prednisone, 5–60 mg/day in single or divided doses, can provide complete relief in one to three days; the physician can convert to an alternate-day program, but this regimen usually is unsuccessful. After initial control of symptoms, the dosage probably should be reduced to as low as possible. As part of the disease, some patients develop giant-cell cranial arteritis or radiologic signs of joint damage; whether these can be prevented with prednisone treatment is uncertain (310).

Fibrositis/Fibromyositis.
We doubt that fibrositis/fibromyositis is a separate disease. Patients shown to us as typical examples had what we interpreted as arthritis, cervical spondylosis with involvement of the nerve root, "ponderous purse" disease, "compensationitis," or a combination of these. The problem infrequently seems mainly psychologically based.

Ponderous Purse Disease.
The neck, shoulder, and back pain, muscle tenderness and spasms, and secondary cervical radiculopathy in this newly recognized, highly sex-limited, autogenous disease is easily treated by eliminating the cause, which to the unwitting or unwilling patient may be more of an annoyance than a serious condition (314).

REFERENCES

1. Engel WK: Introduction to disorders of the motor neuron, nerves and related abnormalities. In: *Scientific Approaches to Clinical Neurology.* Edited by ES Goldensohn and SH Appel. Philadelphia, Lea and Febiger, 1977, pp. 1250–1321.
2. Engel WK: Introduction to the myopathies. In: *Scientific Approaches to Clinical Neurology.* Edited by ES Goldensohn and SH Appel. Philadelphia, Lea and Febiger, 1977, pp. 1555–1571.

3. Grob D: *Myasthenia Gravis.* New York, New York Academy of Sciences, 1976.
4. Rowland LP: *The Human Muscular Dystrophies.* New York, Excerpta Medica, 1977.
5. Griggs RC, Moxley RT (editors). *Advances in Neurology, vol. 17.* New York, Raven Press, 1977.
6. Aguayo AJ, Karpati G: *Current Topics in Nerve and Muscle Research.* Amsterdam, Excerpta Medica, 1979.
7. Hartog Jager WA, Bruyn GW, Heijestee APJ (editors): *Neurology. Proceedings of the 11th World Congress of Neurology.* Amsterdam, Excerpta Medica, 1978.
8. Vinken PJ, Bruyn GW, Ringel SP: *Handbook of Clinical Neurology*, vol. 41. New York, North Holland, 1979.
9. Rosenberg R: *The Treatment of Neurological Diseases.* New York, SP Medical and Scientific Books, 1979.
10. Drachman DB: Myasthenia gravis (second of two parts). N Engl J Med 298:186–192, 1978.
11. Mulder DW: *The Diagnosis and Treatment of Amyotrophic Lateral Sclerosis.* Boston, Houghton Mifflin Professional Publishers, 1979.
12. Rowland LP: Controversies about the treatment of myasthenia gravis. J Neurol Neurosurg Psychiatry 43:644–659, 1980.
13. Siegel IM: Orthopedic correction of musculoskeletal deformity in muscular dystrophy. In: *Advances in Neurology, vol. 17.* Edited by RD Griggs and RT Moxley. New York, Raven Press, 1977, pp. 343–364.
14. Siegel IM: The management of muscular dystrophy: a clinical review. Muscle and Nerve 1:453–460, 1978.
15. Vignos PJ: Rehabilitation in the myopathies. In: *Handbook of Clinical Neurology*, vol. 41, part II. Edited by PJ Vinken, GW Bruyn, and SP Ringel. New York, North Holland, 1979, pp. 197–226.
16. Hensinger RN, MacEwen GD: Spinal deformity associated with heritable neurological conditions. J Bone Joint Dis 58a:13–24, 1976.
17. Callahan A: *Reconstructive Surgery of the Eyelids and Ocular Adnexa.* Birmingham, AL, Aesculapius Publishing Co, 1966, pp. 98–99.
18. Mills CP: Dysphagia in pharyngeal paralysis treated by cricopharyngeal sphincterotomy. Lancet 1:455, 1973.
19. Engel WK, Festoff BW, Patten BM, et al: Myasthenia gravis. Ann Intern Med 81:225–246, 1974.
20. Bastron JA, Bickford RG, Brown JR, et al: *Clinical Examinations In Neurology.* Philadelphia, WB Saunders, 1963, pp. 353–354.
21. Stalberg E: Clinical electrophysiology in myasthenia gravis. J Neurol Neurosurg Psychiatry 43:622–633, 1980.
22. Lindstrom JM, Seybold ME, Lennon VA: Antibody to acetylcholine receptor in myasthenia gravis: prevalance, clinical correlates and diagnostic value. Neurology 26:1054–1059, 1976.
23. Lindstrom J, Dau P: Biology of myasthenia gravis. Ann Rev Pharmacol Toxicol 20:337–362, 1980.
24. Patten BM, Oliver KL, Engel WK: Effect of lactate infusions on patients with myasthenia gravis. Neurology 24:986–990, 1974.
25. Bender AN, Ringel SP, Engel WK: The acetylcholine receptor in normal and pathologic states: immunoperoxidase visualization of alpha-bungarotoxin binding at a light and electronmicroscopic level. Neurology 26:477–483, 1976.
26. Bender AN, Ringel SP, Engel WK, et al: Immunoperoxidase localization of alpha-bungarotoxin binding. A new approach to myasthenia gravis. Ann NY Acad Sci 274:20–30, 1976.
27. Engel AG, Santa T: Histometric analysis of the ultrastructure of the neuromuscular junction in myasthenia gravis and in the myasthenic syndrome. Ann NY Acad Sci 183:46–63, 1971.
28. Engel AG, Tsujihata M, Lindstrom JM, et al: The motor end plate in myasthenia gravis. A quantitative ultrastructural study. Ann NY Acad Sci 274:60–79, 1976.

29. Fardeau M: Normal ultrastructural aspects of human motor end-plate and its pathological modifications. In: *The Striated Muscle.* Edited by CM Pearson. Baltimore, Williams and Wilkins, 1973, pp. 342–353.

30. Fardeau M: Donnees tirees de l'examen anatomopathologique du muscle squelottique dans la myasthenie. Sem Hop Paris 9:1141–1147, 1961.

31. Lefvert AK, Bergstrom K, Matell G, et al: Determination of acetylcholine receptor antibody in myasthenia gravis: clinical usefulness and pathogenetic implications. J Neurol Neurosurg Psychiatry 41:394–403, 1978.

32. Vincent A, Newsom-Davis J: Anti-acetylcholine receptor antibodies. J Neurol Neurosurg Psychiatry 43:590–600, 1980.

33. Vincent A, Newsom-Davis J: Bungarotoxin and anti-choline receptor antibody binding to the human acetylcholine receptor. In: *Neurotoxins: Tools in Neurobiology.* Edited by B Ceccarelli and F Clementi. New York, Raven Press, 1979, pp. 269–278.

34. Lindstrom J, Campbell M, Nave B: Specificities of antibodies to acetylcholine receptors. Muscle and Nerve 1:140–145, 1978.

35. Fuchs S, Bartfeld D, Eshar Z, et al: Immune regulation of experimental myasthenia. J Neurol Neurosurg Psychiatry 43:634–643, 1980.

36. Lennon VA: Immunology of the acetylcholine receptor. Immunol Commun 4:323–344, 1976.

37. Trotter JL, Ringel SP, Cook JD, et al: Morphological and immunological studies in experimental autoimmune myasthenia gravis and myasthenia gravis. Neurology 27:1120–1124, 1977.

38. Galli M, Landi G, Restelli DL, et al: Myasthenia gravis with a monoclonal gammopathy. J Neurol Sci 45:103–108, 1980.

39. Rowland LP, Osserman EF, Scharfman WB, et al: Myasthenia gravis with a myeloma type, gamma-G (IgG) immunoglobulin abnormality. Am J Med 46:559–605, 1969.

40. Shore A, Limatibul S, Dosh H-M, et al: Identification of two serum components regulating the expression of T-lymphocyte function in childhood myasthenia gravis. N Engl J Med 301:615–629, 1979.

41. Strauss AJL, Smith CW, Cage GW: Further studies on the specificity of presumed immune associations of myasthenia gravis and consideration of possible implications. Ann NY Acad Sci 135:557–559, 1966.

42. Van der Geld HW, Strauss AJ: Myasthenia gravis: immunological relationship between striated muscle and thymus. Lancet 1:57–60, 1966.

43. McFarlin DE, Johnson JS: Studies of antimuscle factor in myasthenia gravis. II. Reactions of fragments produced by enzymatic digestion. J Immunol 106:292–294, 1971.

44. Mendell JR, Whitaker JN, Engel WK: The skeletal muscle binding site of antistriated muscle antibody in myasthenia gravis: an electron microscopic immunohistochemical study using peroxidase conjugated antibody fragments. J Immunol 1211:847–856, 1973.

45. Ringel SP, Bender AN, Engel WK, et al: Myasthenia gravis: relationship between serum factor blocking acetylcholine receptors and anti-striated-muscle antibody. Lancet 1:1388–1390, 1975.

46. Feltkamp TEW, van der Berg-Looner PM, Nihenhunis IE: Myasthenia gravis, autoantibodies and HLA antigens. Br Med J 1:131–133, 1974.

47. Nakao K, Nishitoni H, Suzuki M, et al: Antiacetylcholine receptor IgG in neonatal myasthenia gravis. N Engl J Med 297:169–170, 1977.

48. Gross WL, Kruger J, Groschel-Stewart U, et al: Studies on HLA antigens and cellular and humoral autoimmune phenomena in patients with myasthenia gravis. Clin Exp Immunol 27:48–54, 1977.

49. Herskowitz HB: Immunophysiology: cell function and cellular interactions. In: *Immunology II.* Edited by JA Bellanti. Philadelphia, WB Saunders, 1978, pp. 151–202.

50. Christadoss P, Lennon VA, David C: Genetic control of experimental autoimmune myasthenia gravis in mice. I. Lymphocyte proliferation response to acetylcholine receptor is under H-2-linked Ir gene control. J Immunol 123:2540–2543, 1979.

51. Engel WK: Myasthenia gravis, corticosteroids, anticholinesterases. Ann NY Acad Sci 274:623–630, 1976.

52. Engel WK: Dagen des oordeels: mechanisms and molecular messengers (a personal view). Arch Neurol 36:329–339, 1979.

53. Engel WK, Trotter JL, McFarlin DE, McIntosh CL: Thymic epithelial cell contains acetylcholine receptor. Lancet 1:1310–1311, 1977.

54. Dalakas MC, Engel WK, McClure J, et al: Thymosin a_1 localization in normal and myasthenia gravis thymus. N Engl J Med 19:1091–1095, 1980.

55. Engel WK: Myopathic EMG—nonesuch animal. N Engl J Med 289:485–486, 1973.

56. Simpson JA: Myasthenia gravis as an autoimmune disease: clinical aspects. Ann NY Acad Sci 135:506–516, 1966.

57. Van der Geld H, Oosterhuis HJ: Muscle and thymus antibodies in myasthenia gravis. Vox Sang 8:196–204, 1963.

58. Drachman DB: Myasthenia gravis and thyroid gland. N Engl J Med 266:330–331, 1962.

59. Penn AS, Schotland DL, Rowland LP: Immunology of muscle disease In *Immunological Disorders of the Nervous System.* Edited by LP Rowland. Baltimore, Williams and Wilkins, 1971, pp. 215–238.

60. Castleman B: The pathology of the thymus gland in myasthenia gravis. Ann NY Acad Sci 135:496–503, 1966.

61. Stump WJ, Adornato BT, Engel WK, et al: Thymectomy in myasthenia gravis (MG). Neurology 28:372, 1978.

62. Slater G, Papatestas AE, Genkins G, et al: Thymectomy in patients more than forty years of age with myasthenia gravis. Surg Gynecol Obstet 146:54–46, 1978.

63. Askanas V, Engel WK: Unpublished observations.

64. Faulkner SL, Ehyai A, Fisher RD, et al: Contemporary management of myasthenia gravis: the clinical role of early thymectomy. Ann Thorac Surg 23:348–352, 1977.

65. Twomey JJ, Lewis VM, Patten BM, et al: Myasthenia gravis, thymectomy and serum thymic hormone activity. Am J Med 66:639–643, 1979.

66. Twomey JJ, Lewis VM, Ford R, et al: An inhibitor of thymic hormone activity in serum from patients with lymphoblastic leukemia. Am J Med 68:377–380, 1980.

67. Arnason BGW: Myasthenia gravis. In: *Clinical Immunology*, vol. II. Edited by CW Parker. Philadelphia, WB Saunders, 1980, pp. 1088–1105.

68. Blatt J, Reaman G, Poplack DG: Biochemical markers in lymphoid malignancy. N Engl J Med 303:918–921, 1980.

69. Who will get leukaemia (editorial). Lancet 1:1007–1008, 1980.

70. Nakao Y, Miyazaki T, Ota K, et al: Gm allotypes in myasthenia gravis. Lancet 1:677–678, 1980.

71. Abramsky O, Brenner T, Lisak RP, et al: Significance in neonatal myasthenia gravis of inhibitory effect of amniotic fluid on binding of antibodies to acetylcholine receptor. Lancet 2:1333–1335, 1979.

72. Namba T, Brown SB, Grob D: Neonatal myasthenia gravis: report of two cases and review of the literature. Pediatrics 45:488–504, 1970.

73. Appel SH, Elias SB: Anticholine receptor antibodies in myasthenia gravis. In: *Plasmapheresis and the Immunobiology of Myasthenia Gravis.* Edited by PC Dau. Boston, Houghton Mifflin Professional Publishers, 1979, pp. 229–247.

74. Keesey J, Lindstrom J, Cokely H, et al: Anti-acetylcholine receptor antibody in neonatal myasthenia gravis. N Engl J Med 296:55–59, 1977.

75. Vincent A, Newsom-Davis J: Absence of antiacetylcholine receptor antibodies in congenital myasthenia gravis. Lancet 1:441–442, 1979.

76. Masters CL, Dawkins RL, Zilko PJ: Penicillamine-associated myasthenia gravis, antiacetylcholine receptors and antistriational antibodies. Am J Med 63:689–694, 1977.

77. Jacobus D: D-Penicillamine in the monkey. In: *Penicillin in Rheumatic Diseases.* Edited by E Munthe. Houghton Mifflin Scientific Publishers, 1976, pp. 25–40.

78. Vincent A, Newsom-Davis J, Martin A: Antiacetylcholine receptor antibodies in D-Penicillamine-associated myasthenia gravis. Lancet 1:2354, 1978.

79. Bucknall RC, Dixon ASJ, Glick EN, et al: Myasthenia gravis associated with penicillamine treatment for rheumatoid arthritis. Br Med J 1:600–602, 1976.

80. Russell AS, Lindstrom JM: Penicillamine induced myasthenia gravis associated thymectomy. J Neurol 217:133–138, 1977.

81. Patrick J, Lindstrom J: Autoimmune response to acetylcholine receptor. Science 180:871–872, 1973.

82. Lindstrom JM: The role of antibodies to the acetylcholine receptor protein and its component peptides in experimental autoimmune myasthenia gravis. In: *Plasmapheresis and the Immunobiology of Myasthenia Gravis.* Edited by PC Dau. Boston, Houghton Mifflin Professional Publishers, 1979, pp. 3–19.

83. Freeman SS, Engel AG, Drachman DB: Experimental acetylcholine blockade of the neuromuscular junction. Effects on endplate and muscle fiber ultrastructure. Ann NY Acad Sci 274:46–59, 1976.

84. Richman DP, Gomez CM, Berman PW, et al: Monoclonal anti-acetylcholine receptor antibodies can cause experimental myasthenia. Nature 296:738–739, 1980.

85. Flacke W, Caveness VS Jr, Samaha F: Treatment of myasthenia gravis with germine diacetate. N Engl J Med 275:1207, 1966.

86. Flacke W, Caveness VS Jr, Samaha F, et al: Sites of action of germine diacetate in myasthenia gravis. Trans Am Neurol Assoc 92:158, 1967.

87. Walker MB: Treatment of myasthenia gravis with physostigmine. Lancet 1:1200–1201, 1934.

88. Ringel SP, Bender AN, Festoff BW, et al: Ultrastructural demonstration and analytical application of extrajunctional receptors of denervated human and rat skeletal muscle fibres. Nature 255:730–731, 1975.

89. Rosenbaum RB, Bender AN, Engel WK: Prolonged response to edrophonium in myasthenia gravis. Trans Am Neurol Assoc 100:233–235, 1975.

90. Engel AG, Lambert EN, Tetsuji S: Long-term anticholinesterase therapy: effects on NMJ and motor end-plate fine structure. Neurology 23:1273–1281, 1973.

91. Cohen SL, Pohlmann JLW, Mikszewski J: The pharmacokinetics of pyridostigmine of myasthenia gravis. Neurology 26:536–539, 1976.

92. Merritt HH: *Textbook of Neurology,* 4th ed. Philadelphia, Lea and Febiger, 1970, p. 555.

93. *Physicians Desk Reference,* 24th ed. Oradell, NJ, Litton Publications, 1970.

94. Warmolts JR, Engel WK: Benefit from alternate-day prednisone in myasthenia gravis. N Engl J Med 286:17–20, 1971.

95. Warmolts JR, Engel WK, Whitaker JN: Remarkable benefit from alternate-day prednisone treatment in myasthenia gravis. Lancet 2:1198–1199, 1970.

96. Engel WK, DeVivo DC, Warmolts JR, et al: High-single-dose alternate-day prednisone (HSDAD-PRED) in neuromuscular diseases. In: *Proceedings of the II Internal Congress on Muscle Diseases,* Perth, Australia, 1971, p. 59.

97. Engel WK, Bornstein A, DeVivo DC, et al: High-single-dose alternate-day prednisone (HSDAD-PRED) in the treatment of the dermatomyositis/polymyositis complex. Trans Am Neurol Assoc 97:272–275, 1972.

98. von Reis G, Liljestrand A, Mattell G: Treatment of severe myasthenia gravis with large doses of corticosteroids in myasthenia gravis. Ann NY Acad Sci 183:369–374, 1971.

99. Osserman KE, Genkins G: Studies in myasthenia gravis: short-term massive corticotropin therapy. JAMA 198:699–702, 1966.

100. Grob D, Namba T: Corticotropin in generalized myasthenia gravis: effect of short, intensive courses. JAMA 198:703–707, 1966.

101. Seybold ME, Drachman DB: Gradually increasing doses of prednisone in myasthenia gravis: reducing the hazards of treatment. N Engl J Med 290:81–84, 1974.

102. Engel WK, Warmolts JR: Myasthenia gravis: a new hypothesis of the pathogenesis and a new form of treatment. Ann NY Acad Sci 183:72–78, 1971.

103. Howard FM, Duane DD, Lambert EH: Alternate-day prednisone: preliminary report of a double-blind controlled study. Ann NY Acad Sci 274:577–595, 1976.

104. Mann JD, Johns TR, Campa FJ, et al: Long-term prednisone followed by thymectomy in myasthenia gravis. Ann NY Acad Sci 274:608–622, 1976.

105. Sanders DB, Howard JR Jr, Johns TR, et al: High-dose daily prednisone in the treatment of myasthenia gravis. In: *Plasmapheresis and the Immunobiology of Myasthenia Gravis.* Edited by PC Dau. Boston, Houghton Mifflin Professional Publishers, 1979, pp. 289–306.

106. Engel WK: Diseases of the neuromuscular junction and muscle. In: *Neurohistochemistry.* Edited by C Adams. Amsterdam, Elsevier, 1965, pp. 622–672.

107. Engel WK, Brook MH: Muscle biopsy as a clinical diagnostic aid. In: *Neurological Diagnostic Techniques.* Edited by WS Field. Springfield, IL, Charles C Thomas, 1966, pp. 90–146.

108. Engel WK: Muscle biopsies in neuromuscular diseases. Pediatr Clin North Am 24:963–995, 1967.

109. Pleasure DE, Walsh GO, Engel WK: Atrophy of skeletal muscle in patients with Cushing's syndrome. Arch Neurol 22:118–125, 1970.

110. Manolagas SC, Anderson DC: Adrenal steroids and the development of osteoporosis in oophorectomised women. Lancet 2:597–600, 1979.

111. Soyka LF: Treatment of the nephrotic syndrome in childhood: use of an alternate-day prednisone regimen. Am J Dis Child 113:693, 1967.

112. Sadeghi-Nejad A, Senior B: Adrenal function, growth and insulin in patients treated with corticoids on alternate days. Pediatrics 43:277–283, 1969.

113. Reinisch JM, Simon NG, Karow WG, et al: Prenatal exposure to prednisone in humans and animals retards intrauterine growth. Science 202:436–438, 1978.

114. Patten BM, Oliver KL, Engel WK: Adverse interaction between steroid hormones and anticholinesterase drugs. Neurology 24:442–449, 1971.

115. Baxter JD, Rousseau GG: *Glucocorticoid Hormone Action. Monographs on Endocrinology,* vol. 12. Heidelberg, Springer-Verlag, 1979.

116. Cook JD, Trotter JL, Engel WK, et al: The effects of high-single-dose alternate-day prednisone on the immunological status of patients with neuromuscular diseases. Ann Neurol 3:166–176, 1978.

117. Fauci A, Dale DC: Alternate-day prednisone therapy and human lymphocyte subpopulations. J Clin Invest 55:22–32, 1975.

118. Engel WK, Cuneo RA, Levy HB: Polyinosinic-polycytidylic acid treatment of neuropathy. Lancet 1:503–504, 1978.

119. Dalakas MC, Engel WK: Chronic relapsing dysimmune polyneuropathy: Pathogenesis and treatment. Ann Neurol (Suppl) 1981 (in press)

120. Wahl SM, Rosenstreich DL: Suppression of lymphocyte function by glucocorticosteroids. In: *Mitogens in Immunology.* Edited by JJ Oppenheim and DL Rosenstreich. New York, Academic Press, 1976, pp. 537–553.

121. Blackwell GJ, Carnuccio R, DiRosa M, et al: Macrocortin: a polypeptide causing the antiphospholipase effect of glucocorticoids. Nature 287:147–149, 1980.

122. Lippman ME: Glucocorticoid receptors. In: *Hormone-Receptor Interaction. Molecular Aspects.* Edited by GS Levy. New York, Marcel Dekker, 1976, pp. 221–242.

123. Fuchs S: Immunochemical analysis of acetylcholine receptor and its relevance to specific treatment of experimental autoimmune myasthenia gravis. In: *Neurotoxins. Tools in Neurobiology.* Edited by B Ceccarelli and F Clementi. New Yorik, Raven Press 1979, pp. 279–286.

124. Fauci AS: Clinical aspects of immunosuppression: use of cytotoxic agents and cortocosteroids. In: *Immunology II.* Edited by JA Bellanti. Philadelphia, WB Saunders, 1977, pp. 740–757.

125. McMillan R, Longmire R, Yelenosky R: The effect of corticosteroids on human IgG synthesis. J Immunol 116:1592–1595, 1976.

126. Seybold ME, Lindstrom JM: Serial antiacetylcholine receptor antibody titers in patients with myasthenia gravis: effects of steroid therapy. In: *Plasmapheresis and the Immunobiology of Myasthenia Gravis.* Edited by PC Dau. Boston, Houghton Mifflin Professional Publishers, 1979, pp. 307–314.

127. Dau PC, Lindstrom JM, Cassel CK, et al: Plasmapheresis in myasthenia gravis and polymyositis. In: *Plasmapheresis and the Immunobiology of Myasthenia Gravis.* Edited by PC Dau. Boston, Houghton Mifflin Professional Publishers, 1979, pp. 229–247.

128. Wilson R, Ward MD, Johns TR: Corticosteroids: a direct effect on the neuromuscular junction. Neurology 24:1091–1095, 1974.

129. Arts WF, Oosterhuis HF: Effect of prednisone on neuromuscular blocking in mice in vivo. Neurology 25:1088–1090, 1975.

130. Leeuwin RS, Wolters ECMJ: Effects of corticosteroids on sciatic nerve–tibialis anterior muscle of rats treated with hemicholinium-3. An experimental approach to a possible mechanism of action of corticosteroids in myasthenia gravis. Neurology 27:171–177, 1977.

131. Strand FL, Stoboy H, Friedebold, et al: Effect of ACTH peptide fragment on nuscle action potentials. Lancet 2:919, 1975.

132. Wolters ECMJ, Leeuwin RS: Effect of corticosteroids on the prenic nerve–diaphragm preparation treated with hemicholinium. A possible model of myasthenia gravis. Neurology 26:574–578, 1976.

133. Levy J, Barnett Ev, MacDonald NS, et al: The effect of azathioprine on gamma globulin synthesis in man. J Clin Invest 51:2233–2238, 1971.

134. Reuther P, Fulpius BW, Mertens HG, et al: Anti-acetylcholine receptor antibody under long-term azathioprine treatment in myasthenia gravis. In: *Plasmapheresis and the Immunobiology of Myasthenia Gravis.* Edited by PC Dau, Boston, Houghton Mifflin Professional Publishers, 1979, pp. 329–342.

135. Bergsagel DE, Bailey AJ, Langley GR, et al: The chemotherapy of plasma-cell myeloma and the incidence of acute leukemia. N Engl J Med 301:743–748, 1979.

136. Azathioprine and 6-mercaptopurine for Crohn's disease (editorial). Lancet 2:298–299, 1980.

137. Kinlen LJ, Sheil AGR, Peto J, et al: Collaborative United Kingdom Australasian study of cancer in patients treated with immunosuppressive drugs. Br. Med J 2:1461–1466, 1979.

138. Mertens HG, Balzereit F, Leipert M: The treatment of severe myasthenia gravis with immunosuppressive agents. Eur Neurol 2:323–339, 1969.

139. Matell G, Bergstrom K, Franksson C, et al: Effects of some immunosuppressive procedures on myasthenia gravis. Ann NY Acad Sci 274:659–676, 1976.

140. Hertel G, Mertens HG, Reuther P, et al: The treatment of myasthenia gravis with azathioprine. In: *Plasmapheresis and the Immunobiology of Myasthenia Gravis.* Edited by PC Dau. Boston, Houghton Mifflin Professional Publishers, 1979, pp. 315–328.

141. Newsom-Davis J, Vincent A: Combined plasma exchange and immunosuppression in myasthenia gravis. Lancet 2:688, 1979.

142. Friedman OM, Myles A, Cavin M: Cyclophosphamide and related phosphoramide mustards: current status and future prospects. Adv Cancer Chemother 1:423–204, 1979.

143. Fauci AS, Doppman JL, Wolff SM: Cyclophospnamide-induced remissions in advanced polyarteritis nodosa. Am J Med 64:890–894, 1978.

144. Fauci AS, Katz P, Haynes BF, et al: Cyclophosphamide therapy of severe systemic necrotizing vasculitis. N Engl J Med 301:235–238, 1979.

145. Puri HC, Campbell RA: Cyclophosphamide and malignancy. Lancet 1:658, 1977.

146. Metzger AL, Bohan A, Goldberg LS, et al: Polymyositis and dermatomyositis: combined methotrexate and corticosteroid therapy. Ann Intern Med 81:182–189, 1974.

147. Frei E, Blum RH, Pitman SW, et al: High dose methotrexate with leucovorin rescue. Rationale and spectrum of antitumor activity. Am J Med 58:370–376, 1980.

148. Dalakas MC, Flaum M, Engel WK, et al: Successful treatment of polyneuropathy in Waldenstrom macroglobulinemia (WM): role of dysproteinemia in pathogenesis of the neuropathy. Neurology 30:428, 1980.

149. Bird AG, McLachlan SM: Cyclosporin A and Epstein-Barr virus. Lancet 2:418, 1980.

150. Isenberg DA, Snaith ML, Al-Khader AA, et al: Cyclosporin relieves arthralgia, causes angioedema. N Engl J Med 302:754, 1980.

151. Masse R, Youindou P, Dorval J-C, et al: Reversal of lupus erythematosus–like disease with danazol. Lancet 2:651, 1980.

152. Dau PC (editor): *Plasmapheresis and the Immunobiology of Myasthenia Gravis.* Boston, Houghton Mifflin Professional Publishers, 1979.

153. Wood GJ: Plasmapheresis and plasma-cholinesterase. Lancet 1:1305–1306, 1977.

154. Behan WMH, Behan PO: Immune complexes in myasthenia gravis. J Neurol Neurosurg Psychiatry 42:595–599, 1979.

155. Newsom-Davis J, Vincent A, Wilson SG, et al: Long-term effects of repeated plasma exchange in myasthenia gravis. Lancet 1:464–468, 1979.

156. Mertens HG, Hertel G: Immunosuppressive behandling der myasthenie. Med Welt 24:955–963, 1973.

157. Dau PC, Lindstrom JM, Cassel CK, et al: Plasmapheresis and immunosuppressive drug therapy in myasthenia gravis. N Engl J Med 297:1134–1140, 1977.

158. Newsom-Davis J, Wilson SG, Pinching AJ, et al: Plasmapheresis: short and long-term benefits. In: *Plasmapheresis and the Immunobiology of Myasthenia Gravis.* Edited by PC Dau. Boston, Houghton Mifflin Professional Publishers, 1979, pp. 199–208.

159. Pirofsky B, Reid RH, Bardana EJ, et al: Myasthenia gravis treated with purified antithymocyte antiserum. Neurology 29:112–116, 1979.

160. Schulz MD, Schwab RS: Results of thymic (mediastinal) irradiation in patients with myasthenia gravis. Ann NY Acad Sci 183:303–307, 1971

161. Engel WK, Dalakas MC, Lichter AS: Intractable myasthenia gravis (MG) can respond to splenic radiation (SR). Neurology 30:389, 1980.

162. Engel WK, Lichter A, Galdi A: To be published.

163. Papatestas AF, Alpert LI, Osserman KE, et al: Studies in myasthenia gravis. Effects of thymectomy. Results on 185 patients with non-thymomatous and thymomatous myasthenia gravis. Am J Med 50:465–474, 1971.

164. Genkins G, Papatestas AE, Horowitz SH, et al: Studies in myasthenia gravis: early thymectomy. Am J Med 58:517–524, 1975.

165. Slater G, Papatestas, AE, Genkins G, et al: Thymomas in patients with myasthenia gravis. Ann Surg 188:171–174, 1978.

166. Fischer KC, Schwartzman RJ: Oral corticosteroids in the treatment of ocular myasthenia gravis. Ann NY Acad Sci 274:652–658, 1976.

167. Scadding G, Thoma H, Harvard C: Myasthenia gravis: Acetylcholine receptor antibody titers after thymectomy. Br Med J 1:1512, 1977.

168. Seybold ME, Baergen RN, Nave B: Antiacetylcholine receptor antibody concentrations after thymectomy in patients with myasthenia gravis. Br Med J 2:1051–1053, 1978.

169. Rosai J, Levine GD: Tumors of the thymus. In: *Atlas of Tumor Pathology,* second series, fascicle 13. Washington, DC, AFIP, 1976.

170. Papatestas AF, Genkins G, Horowitz SH: Thymectomy in myasthenia gravis: pathogenic, clinical and electrophysiologic correlations. Ann NY Acad Sci 274:555–573, 1976.

171. Namba T, Brunner NG, Grob D: Myasthenia gravis in patients with thymoma with particular reference to onset after thymectomy. Medicine (Baltimore) 57:411–433, 1978.

172. Jaretzki A: Symposium on therapeutic controversies: myasthenia gravis. Cervical thymectomy (con). Trans Am Neurol Assoc 102:288–291, 1978.

173. Ryniewicz B, Badurska B: Follow-up study of myasthenic children after thymectomy. J Neurol 217:133–138, 1977.

174. Fonkalsrud EW, Herrmann C Jr, Mulder DG: Thymectomy for myasthenia gravis in childhood. Paediatr Univers Tokyo 18:57–68, 1977.

175. Fukuyama Y, Suzuki M, Segawa M: Studies on myasthenia gravis in childhood. Paediatr Univers Tokyo 18:57–68, 1970.

176. Hansson O, Johansson L, Stalberg E, et al: Thymectomy in juvenile myasthenia gravis. Neuropaediatrie 3:429–436, 1972.

177. Millichap JG, Dodge PR: Diagnosis and treatment of myasthenia gravis in infancy, childhood and adolescence. A study of 51 patients. Neurology 10:1007–1014, 1960.

178. Sarnat HB, McGarry JD, Lewis JE Jr: Effective treatment of infantile myasthenia gravis by combined prednisone and thymectomy. Neurology 27:550–553, 1970.

179. Seybold ME, Howard FM, Duane DD, et al: Thymectomy in juvenile myasthenia gravis. Arch Neurol 25:385–392, 1971.

180. Swaiman KF, Varco RL: Thymectomy in fulminating myasthenia gravis of childhood. Minn Med 55:809–810, 1972.

181. Molgaard HV: Assembly of immunoglobulin heavy chain genes. Nature 286:657–659, 1980.

182. Steinitz M, Izak G, Cohen S, et al: Continuous production of monoclonal rheumatoid factor by EBV-transformed lymphocytes. Nature 287:443–445, 1980.

183. Unanue ER: Cooperation between mononuclear phagocytes and lymphocytes in immunity. N Engl J Med 303:977–985, 1980.

184. Haberman PM, Green JP, Archibald C: Determinants of successful selective tracheobrachial suctioning. N Engl J Med 289:1060–1063, 1973.

185. Smith RA, Dawson A, Foroozan P: Pharmacologic and surgical modalities (commentary by Engel WK). In: *The Diagnosis and Treatment of Amyotrophic Lateral Sclerosis.* Edited by DW Mulder. Boston, Houghton Mifflin Professional Publishers, 1980, pp. 241–257.

186. Paradelis AG, Triantaphyllidis C, Giala MM: Neuromuscular blocking activity of aminoglycoside antibiotics. Methods Find Exp Clin Pharmacol 2:45–52, 1980.

187. Argov Z, Mastaglia FL: Disorders of neuromuscular transmission caused by drugs. N Engl J Med 301:409–413, 1979.

188. Hokkanen E: The aggravating effect of some antibiotics on the neuromuscular blockade in myasthenia gravis. Acta Neurol Scand 40:346–352, 1964.

189. Elmqvist D, Josefsson J-O: The nature of the neuromuscular block produced by neomycin. Acta Physiol Scand 54:105–110, 1961.

190. Farley JM, Chau HW, Narahashi T: Mechanism of neuromuscular block by streptomycin (abstract no. 1623). In: *Proceedings of the 9th Annual Meeting of the Society for Neuroscience,* Atlanta, GA, November 2–6, 1979.

191. Rowland LP: Myasthenia gravis. In: *Scientific Approaches to Clinical Neurology.* Edited by ES Goldensohn and SH Appel. Philadelphia, Lea and Febiger, 1977, pp. 1518–1554.

192. Froelich CJ, Goodwin JS, Bankhurst AD, et al: Pregnancy, a temporary fetal graft of suppressor cells in autoimmune disease. Am J Med 69:329–331, 1980.

193. Engel AG: Thyroid function with myasthenia gravis. Arch Neurol Psychiatry 4:663–665, 1961.

194. Namba T, Brown SB, Grob D: Neonatal myasthenia gravis: report of two cases and review of the literature. Pediatrics 45:488–504, 1970.

195. Dunn JM: Neonatal myasthenia. Am J Obstet Gynecol 125:265–266, 1976.

196. Engel WK, Dalakas MC: Prednisone-responsive limb-girdle syndrome. A special disorder. In: *Proceedings of the IVth International Congress on Neuromuscular Diseases.* Montreal, Canada, September 17–21, 1978.

197. Eaton LM, Lambert EH: Electromyography and electric stimulation of nerves in diseases of motor unit: observations on the myasthenic syndrome associated with malignant tumours. JAMA 163:1117–1124, 1957.

198. Lambert EH, Rooke ED, Eaton LM, Hodgson CH: Myasthenia syndrome occasionally associated with bronchial neoplasm: neurophysiological studies. In: *Myasthenia Gravis.* Edited by HR Viets. Springfield, IL, Charles C Thomas, 1961, pp. 362–410.

199. Lambert EH, Elmqvist D: Quantal components of end-plate potentials in the myasthenic syndrome. Ann NY Acad Sci 183:183–199, 1971.

200. Vroom FQ, Engel WK: Nonneoplastic steroid responsive Lambert-Eaton myasthenic syndrome. Neurology 19:281, 1961.

201. Ishikawa K, Engelhardt JK, Fujisawa T, et al: A neuromuscular transmission block produced by a cancer tissue extract derived from a patient with the myasthenic syndrome. Neurology 27:140–143, 1977.

202. Kranz HK, Caddy DJ, Williams AM, et al: Myasthenic syndrome: effect of choline, plasmapheresis and tests for circulating factor. J Neurol Neurosurg Psychiatry 43:483–488, 1980.

203. Engel AG, Lambert EH, Gomez MR: A new myasthenia syndrome with end-plate acetylcholinesterase deficiency. Small nerve terminals and reduced acetylcholine release. Ann Neurol 1:315–330, 1977.

204. Engel AG, Lambert EH, Mulder DM, et al: Investigation of 3 cases of a newly-recognized familial congenital myasthenic syndrome. Trans Am Neurol Assoc 104:8–12, 1979.

205. Cherington M: Acute muscle weakness. In: *Handbook of Clinical Neurology*, vol. 41, part II. Edited by PJ Vinken, GW Bruyn and SP Ringel. New York, North Holland, 1980, pp. 287–293.

206. Duchen LW: An electron microscopic study of the changes induced by bolulinum toxin in the motor end-plates of slow and fast skeletal muscle fibres of the mouse. J Neurol Sci 14:47–60, 1971.

207. Duchen LW: Changes in motor innervation and cholinesterase localization induced by botulinum toxin in skeletal muscle of the mouse: differences between fast and slow muscles. J Neurol Neurosurg Psychiatry 33:40–54, 1970.

208. Puggiari M, Cherington M: Botulinum and guanidine. Ten years later. JAMA 240:2277, 1978.

209. Koenig MG, Drutz PJ, Mushlin AJ: Type B botulism in man. Am J Med 42:208–219, 1967.

210. Merson MH, Hughes JM, Dowell VR, et al: Current trends in botulism in the United States. JAMA 229:1305, 1974.

211. Black RE, Gunn RA: Hypersensitivity reactions associated with botulinal antitoxin. Am J Med 69:567–570, 1980.

212. Singh YN, Marshall IG, Harvey AL: Reversal of antibiotic-induced muscle paralysis by 3,4-diaminopyridine. J Pharm Pharmacol 30:249–250, 1978.

213. Arnon SS, Midura TF, Damus K, et al: Intestinal infection and toxin production by *Clostridium botulinum* as one cause of sudden infant death syndrome. Lancet 1:1274–1276, 1978.

214. Arnon SS, Midura TF, Clay SA, et al: Infant botulism. Epidemiological, clinical and laboratory aspects. JAMA 237:1946–1951, 1977.

215. Pickett J, Berg B, Chaplin E, et al: Syndrome of botulism in infancy: clinical and electrophysiologic study. N Engl J Med 295:770–772, 1976.

216. Lee CY: Recent advances in chemistry and pharmacology of snake toxins. In: *Neurotoxins: Tools in Neurobiology*. Edited by B Ceccarelli and F Clementi. New York, Raven Press, 1979, pp. 1–16.

217. Kang S, Maelicke A: Fluorescein isothiocyanate–labeled α-cobratoxin. Biochemical characterization and interaction with acetylcholine receptor from *Electrophorus Electricus*. J Biol Chem 255:7326–7332, 1980.

218. Fritz LC, Atwood HL, Jahromi SS: Ultrastructure of lobster neuromuscular junctions treated with black widow spider venom (abstract no. 1625). In: *Proceedings of the 9th Annual Meeting of the Society for Neuroscience*. Atlanta, GA, November 2–6, 1979.

219. Wolpow R, Shahani, Zuckerman: Human ciguetera intoxication—a single-fiber study (abstract no. 14). EMG Society of Washington, D.C., September 26, 1980.

220. Wallace JF. Disorders caused by venoms, bites, and stings. In: *Harrison's Principals of Internal Medicine*. Edited by GW Thorn, RD Adams, E Braunwald, et al: New York, McGraw-Hill, 1977, pp. 732–740.

221. Liddell J, Lehmann H, Davies D, et al: Physical separation of pseudocholinesterase variants in human serum. Lancet 1:463–464, 1962.

222. Lehman H, Liddell J: Pseudocholinesterase deficiency and some other pharmacogenic disorders. In: *The Metabolic Basis of Inherited Disease*. Edited by JB Stanbury, JB Wyngaarden, and DS Frederickson. New York, McGraw-Hill, 1966, pp. 1356–1369.

223. Brody IA, Resnick JS, Engel WK: Detection of atypical cholinesterase by electrophoresis. Arch Neurol 13:126–129, 1965.

224. Kalow W, Lindsay HA: A comparison of optical and manometric methods for the assay of human serum cholinesterase. Can J Biochem Physiol 33:568, 1955.

225. Rowland LP, Christopher C, Olarte M: therapy for dermatomyositis and polymyositis. In: *Advances in Neurology*, vol. 17. Edited by RC Griggs and RT Moxley. New York, Raven Press, 1977, pp. 63–98.

226. Engel AG, Angelini C: Carnitine deficiency of human skeletal muscle with associated lipid storage myopathy: a new syndrome. Science 179:899–902, 1973.

227. Engel AG, Siekert RG: Lipid storage myopathy responsive to prednisone. Arch Neurol 27:174–181, 1972.

228. Johnson MA, Fulthorpe JJ, Hudgson P: Lipid storage myopathy: a recognizable clinicopathological entity. Acta Neuropathol 24:97–106, 1973.

229. Perkoff GT: Alcoholic myopathy. Annu Rev Med 22:125–132, 1971.

230. Engel WK: A clinical approach to the myopathies. In: *Clinical Orthopaedics and Related Research,* vol. 39. Philadelphia, JB Lippincott, 1965, pp. 6–18.

231. Engel WK: Integrative histochemical approach to the defect of Duchenne muscular dystrophy. In: *Pathogenesis of the Human Muscular Dystrophies.* Edited by JP Rowland. New York, American Elsevier, 1977, pp. 277–309.

232. Banker BQ: Dermatomyositis of childhood,. Trans Am Neurol Assoc 87:11–15, 1962.

233. Engel WK: Brief, small, abundant motor-unit action potentials. Neurology 25:173–176, 1975.

234. Engel WK, Cunningham GG: Alkaline phosphatase–positive abnormal muscle fibers of humans. J Histochem Cytochem 18:55–57, 1970.

235. Engel WK: Focal myopathic changes produced by electromyographic and hypodermic needles ('needle myopathy'). Arch Neurol 16:509–511, 1967.

236. Engel WK, Zee DS: Acupuncture myopathy (remembrance of things passed). N Engl J Med 291:801, 1974.

237. Whitaker JN, Engel WK: Vascular deposits of immunoglobulin and complement in idiopathic inflammatory myopathy. N Engl J Med 286:333–339, 1971.

238. Foidart M, Foidart J-MM, Engel WK: Collagen localization in normal and fibrotic human skeletal muscle. Arch Neurol 1980 (in press).

239. Engel WK: Duchenne muscular dystrophy: a histologically based ischemia hypothesis and comparison with experimental ischemia myopathy. In: *The Striated Muscle.* Edited by CM Pearson and FK Mostofi. Baltimore, Williams and Wilkins, 1973, pp. 453–472.

240. Sato T, Walker DL, Peters HA, et al: Chronic polymyositis and myxovirus-like inclusions: electron miscropscopic and viral studies. Arch Neurol 24:409–418, 1971.

241. Chou SM, Gutman L: Picornavirus-like crystals in subacute polyositis. Neurology 20:205–213, 1970.

242. Mastaglia FL, Walton JN: Coxsackie-like particles in skeletal muscle from a case of polymyositis. J Neurol Sci 11:593–599, 1970.

243. Tang TT, Sedinak GV, Siegesmund KA, et al: Chronic myopathy associated with Coxsackie virus type A9. N Engl J Med 292:608–611, 1975.

244. Middleton PJ, Alexander RM, Szymanski MT: Severe myositis during recovery from influenza. Lancet 2:533–535, 1970.

245. Echrengut W: Dermatomyositis and vaccination. Lancet 1:1040–1041, 1978.

246. Kass E, Straume S, Munthe E: Dermatomyositis after BCG vaccination. Lancet 1:772, 1978.

247. Schraeder PL, Peters HA, Dahl DS: Polymyositis and penicillamine. Arch Neurol 27:456–457, 1972.

248. Fontiveros ES, Cumming WJK, Hudgson P: Procainamide-induced myositis. J Neurol Sci 45:143–147, 1980.

249. Mason W, Keller E: Acute transient myositis with influenza-like illness (letter). J Pediatr 86:813–814, 1975.

250. McKinlay IA, Mitchell I: Transient acute myositis in childhood. Arch Dis Child 51:135–137, 1976.

251. Sternberg EM, Van Woert MH, Young SN, et al: Development of a scleroderma-like illness during therapy with 1-5-hydroxytryptophan and carbidopa. N Engl J Med 303:782–787, 1980.

252. Metzger AL, Singer FR, Bluestone R, et al: Failure of disodium efrodionate in calcinosis due to dermatomyositis and scleroderma. N Engl J Med 291:1284–1286, 1975.

253. Epstein O, DeVilliers D, Jain S, et al: Reduction of immune complexes and immunoglobulins induced by D-penicillamine in primary biliary cirrhosis. N Engl J Med 300:274–278, 1979.

254. Moncada S, Korbut R: Dipyridamole and other phosphodiesterase inhibitors act as antithrombotic agents by potentiating endogenous prostacyclin. Lancet 1:1286, 1978.

255. Sharma CVRK, Burleson VA, Sasahara AA: Effect of thrombolytic therapy on pulmonary-capillary blood volume in patients with pulmonary embolism. N Engl J Med 303:842–845, 1980.

256. Kula RW, Line BR, Engel WK: ^{99m}Tc-diphosphonate scanning of soft-tissues in neuromuscular diseases. In: *Proceedings of the IVth International Congress on Neuromuscular Diseases.* Montreal, Canada, September 17–21, 1978.

257. Nassim JR, Connoly CK: Treatment of calcinosis universalis with aluminum hydroxide. Arch Dis Child 45:118–121, 1970.

258. Engel WK: Investigative approach to the muscular dystrophies. In: *Advances in Neurology*, vol. 17. Edited by RC Griggs and RT Moxley. New York, Raven Press, 1977, pp. 197–116.

259. Levy RJ, Lian JB, Gallop P: Atherocalcin, a gamma-carboxyglutamic acid containing protein from atherosclerotic plaque. Biochem Biophys Res Commun 91:41–49, 1979.

260. Johnson RL, Fink CW, Ziff M: Lymphotoxin formation by lymphocytes and muscle in polymyositis. J Clin Invest 51:2435–2449, 1972.

261. Dawkins RL, Mastaglia FL: Cell-mediated cytotoxicity to muscle in polymyositis. Effect of immunosuppression. N Engl J Med 288:443–438, 1973.

262. Saunders M, Knowles M, Currie S: Lymphocyte stimulation with muscle homogenate in polymyositis and other muscle-wasting disorders. J Neurol Neurosurg Psychiatry 35:569–571, 1969.

263. Lisak RP, Zweiman B: Mitogen and muscle extract induced in vitro proliferative responses in myasthenia gravis, dermatomyositis and polymyositis. J Neurol Neurosurg Psychiatry 38:521–524, 1975.

264. Currie S, Saunders M, Nowles M: Immunological aspects of polymyositis. The in vitro activity of lymphocytes on incubation with antigen and with muscle cultures. Q J Med 157:63–84, 1971.

265. The course of necrotising vasculitis (editorial). Lancet 2:407, 1980.

266. Gottdiener JS, Sherber HS, Hawley RJ, et al: Cardiac manifestations in polymyositis. Am J Cardiol 41:1141–1149, 1978.

267. Henderson A, Cumming WJK, Williams DO, et al: Cardiac complications of polymyositis. J Neurol Sci 47:425–428, 1980.

268. Odell WD, Wolfsen AR: Hormones from tumors: are they ubiquitous? Am J Med 68:317–318, 1980.

269. Engel WK, Askanas V: Remote effects of focal cancer on the neuromuscular system. In: *Advances in Neurology.* Edited by RA Thompson and JR Green. New York, Raven Press, 1976, pp. 119–147.

270. Samuels BS, Rietschel RL: Polymyositis and toxoplasmosis. JAMA 235:60–61, 1976.

271. Kagen LJ, Kimball AC, Christian CL: Serologic evidence of toxoplasmosis among patients with polymyositis. Am J Med 56:186–191, 1974.

272. Krick JA, Remington JS: Toxoplasmosis in the adult—an overview. N Engl J Med 298:550–553, 1978.

273. Rowland LP, Greer M: Toxoplasmic polymyositis. Neurology 11:367–370, 1961.

274. Chandar K, Mair JH, Mair NS: Case of toxoplasma polymyositis. Br Med J 1:158–159, 1968.

275. Greenlee JE, Johnson WD, Campa JF, et al: Recurrent toxoplasmosis presenting as polymyositis and cerebellar ataxia. Ann Intern Med 82:367–371, 1975.

276. Feldman HA: Toxoplasmosis: an overview. Bull NY Acad Med 50:110–127, 1974.

277. Miller NL, Frenkel JK, Dubey JP: Oral infections with toxoplasma cysts and oocysts in felines, other mammals, and in birds. J Parasitol 58:928–937, 1972.

278. Teutsch SM, Juranek DD, Sulzer A, et al: Epidemic toxoplasmosis associated with infected cats. N Engl J Med 300:695–699, 1979.

279. Fayer R, Johnson AJ, Lunde M: Abortion and other signs of disease in cows experimentally infected with *Sarcocystis fusiformis* from dogs. J Infect Dis 134:624–628, 1979.

280. Leek RG, Fayer R, Johnson AJ: Sheep experimentally infected with *Sarcocystis* from dogs. I. Disease in young lambs. J Parasitol 63:642–650, 1977.

281. Leek RG, Fayer R: Sheep experimentally infected with *Sarcocystis* from dogs. II. Abortion and disease in ewes. Cornell Vet 68:108–123, 1978.

282. Fayer R: The first asexual generation in the life cycle of *Sarcocystis bovicanis.* Proc Helminth Soc Wash 44:206–209, 1977.

283. Silverstein A, Siltzbach LE: Muscle involvement in sarcoidosis. Arch Neurol 21:235–241, 1969.

284. Gardner-Thorpe C: Muscle weakness due to sarcoid myopathy. Neurology 22:917–928, 1972.

285. Askanas V, Engel WK: Diseased human muscle in tissue culture: a new approach to the pathogenesis of human neuromuscular disorders. In: *Pathogenesis of the Human Muscular Dystrophies.* Edited by LP Rowland. New York, American Elsevier, 1977, pp. 856–871.

286. Askanas V, Engel WK: Multidimensional studies of diseased human cultured muscle seeking the pathogenesis of neuromuscular diseases. In: *Neurology.* Edited by WA dens Hartog Jager, GW Bruyn, and APJ Heijstee. Amsterdam, Excerpta Medica, 1978, pp. 93–108.

287. Carpenter S, Karpati G, Heller I, et al: Inclusion body myositis: a distinct variety of idiopathic inflammatory myopathy. Neurology 28:8–17, 1978.

288. Carpenter S, Karpati G, Wolf L. Virus-like filaments and phospholipid accumulation in skeletal muscle. Neurology 20:889–903, 1970.

289. Askanas V, Engel WK: Reovirus-like particles in cultured muscle fibers of a patient with a chronic vacuolar myopathy. Neurology 28:386, 1978.

290. Askanas V: Multidimensional use of muscle tissue culture in the study of the pathogeneses of human neuromuscular disorders. In: *Proceedings of the 11th World Congress of Neurology,* Publication no. 428. Amsterdam, Excerpta Medica, 1977, pp. 76–77.

291. Askanas V, Engel WK: Normal and diseased human muscle in tissue culture. In: *Handbook of Clinical Neurology,* vol. 40, part I. Edited by PJ vinken, GW Bruyn, and SP Ringel. Boston, North Holland, 1980, pp. 183–196.

292. Barbieri M: Ribosome crystallization in homogenates and cell extracts of chick embryos. J Supramol Struct 10:349–357, 1979.

293. Barbieri M: Ribosome crystallization in nuclei of chick embryos. J Supramol Struct 10:365–375, 1979.

294. Barbieri M: The role of temperature in the crystallization of ribosomes in chick embryos. J Supramol Struct 10:359–364, 1979.

295. Hudgson P, Walton JN: Polymyositis and other inflammatory myopathies. In: *Handbook of Clinical Neurology,* vol. 14, part II. Edited by PJ Vinken, GW Bruyn, and SP Ringel. Boston, North Holland, 1980, pp. 51–93.

296. Taylor JF: Henderson BF: Tropical myositis. In: *Medicine in a Tropical Environment.* Edited by AG Shaper, JW Kibukamusoke, and MSR Hutt. London, BMA, 1972, pp. 124–146.

297. Adams RD, Denny-Brown D, Pearson CM: *Diseases of Muscle.* New York, Harper and Row, 1972.

298. Jewetz E, Nelnick JL, Adelberg EA: *Review of Medical Microbiology.* Los Altos, Lange Medical Publications, 1976.

299. Rowland LP, Greer M: Toxoplasmic polymyositis. Neurology 11:367–370, 1961.

300. Dvorak JA, Howe CL: The attraction of *Trypanosoma cruzi* to vertebrate cells in vitro. J Protozool 23:534–537, 1976.

301. Laranja FS, Dias E, Nobrega G: Chaga's disease: a clinical, epidemiologic and pathologic study. Circulation 14:1035–1060, 1956.

302. Cook JD, Haller, RG: Treatable neuromuscular diseases. In: *The Treatment of Neurological Diseases.* Edited by R Rosenberg. New York, SP Medical and Scientific books, 1979, pp. 423–455.

303. Johnson MA: Nuclear abnormalities in muscle regenerating after Echo 9 virus infection in mice. J Neurol Sci 35:117–133, 1978.

304. Engel WK, Askanas V: Overlooked avian oncornavirus in cultured muscle—functionally significant. Science 192:1251–1252, 1976.

305. Andrews JM, Gardner MB: Lower motor neuron degeneration associated with typc C RNA virus infection in mice—neuropathologic features. J Neuropathol Exp Neurol 33:285–289, 1974.

306. Gardner-Thorpe C: Muscle weakness due to sarcoid myopathy. Neurology 22:917–928, 1972.

307. Andrews JM, Andrews RL: The comparative neurology of motor neuron diseases. In: *Amyotrophic Lateral Sclerosis: Recent Research Trends.* Edited by JM Andrews, RT Johnson, and MAB Brazier. New York, Academic Press, 1976, pp. 181–216.

308. Bain HW: Epidemic pleurodynia (Bornholm's disease) due to coxsackie B5 virus: the interrelationship of pleurodynia, benign pericarditis and aseptic meningitis. Pediatrics 27:889–893, 1961.

309. Ben-Bassat M, Machtey I: Picornavirus-like structures in acute dermatomyositis. Am J Clin Pathol 58:245–249, 1971.

310. Hunder GG, Sheps SG, Allen GL, et al: Daily and alternate-day cortocosteroid regimens in treatment of giant cell arteritis. Ann Intern Med 82:613–618, 1975.

311. Bruk M: Articular and vascular manifestations of polymyalgia rheumatica. Ann Rheum Dis 26:103, 1967.

312. Brook MG, Kaplan H: Muscle pathology in rheumatoid arthritis, polymyalgia rheumatica and polymyositis. Arch Pathol 94:101–118, 1971.

313. O'Duffy JD, Wahner HW, Hunder GG: Joint imaging in polymyalgia rheumatica. Mayo Clin Proc 51:519–524, 1976.

314. Engel WK: Ponderous-purse disease. N Engl J Med 299:557, 1978.

3
Infections of the Central Nervous System

Kenneth P. Johnson

Therapy for neurologic disease has often been considered to be a discouraging field of endeavor, with the notable exception of central nervous system (CNS) infections, an area in which remarkable advances have taken place over the past century. Beginning with the successful postexposure prophylaxis of rabies virus infections, continuing through the past five decades, during which time specific treatment of bacterial meningitis with sulfa, and then antibiotic, drugs became common, proceeding further to the introduction of several antiviral vaccines, and arriving in the present, when antiviral therapy is finally becoming practical, the treatment of neurologic infections has been a succession of triumphs. Unfortunately, most viral infections and several serious bacterial infections, such as neonatal meningitis, still await adequate forms of treatment. Perhaps therapy of neurologic infections has been relatively successful because it is possible to identify a specific pathologic agent, often with great rapidity, so that treatment can be initiated almost at once. Thus, most CNS infections are rightly considered to be diagnostic and therapeutic emergencies, a concept worth repeatedly emphasizing.

This chapter will concentrate on CNS infections that affect inhabitants primarily of the temperate zones of the world and, more specifically, the United States and western Europe. There are numerous major infectious diseases of the CNS (e.g., leprosy, many types of viral encephalitis, cysticercosis, trypanosomiasis) that affect persons living in underdeveloped areas, which, for cultural, political, and economic reasons, have not been studied intensively and for which little effective therapy is available.

Bacterial infections constitute the most common and most feared yet the most treatable of all CNS infections. Acute bacterial meningitis remains a major disease problem and is best considered when classified by infectious agent and age of the host. In addition to the common bacterial agents, it is necessary to consider treatment of unusual infections, such as *Listeria* meningitis and neurosyphilis.

While measures aimed at increased public health have decreased the incidence of tuberculous meningitis markedly, the disease remains a serious problem with regard to therapy. Similar problems in diagnosis and therapy arise concerning fungal meningitis. This review will consider few epidemiologic details of such infections; rather, it will discuss standard and new forms of therapy for fungal meningitis, with a concentration on the most common treatments.

Parasitic diseases constitute some of the major CNS infectious problems throughout the world; however they are not common in the temperate zones. Nevertheless, neurologists, specialists in infectious disease, and other investigators are confronted with unusual CNS presentations of toxoplasmosis (and, in some parts of the United States, trichinosis and cysticercosis) often enough that these infections should be considered.

Viral infections of the CNS have been the focus of tremendous research interest in the last three decades; it has become evident that such infections may produce, not only acute diseases such as aseptic meningitis or encephalitis, but also chronic, latent, and slowly progressive diseases. Therapy for viral infections may require consideration of host cell metabolism, especially of replication of ribonucleic acid (RNA) and deoxyribonucleic acid (DNA). Unfortunately, the intimate association between viral and host-metabolic functions has made finding effective therapy for these diseases almost impossible. Nevertheless, some acute DNA viral infections have been successfully treated recently; in fact, one drug is licensed for the treatment of acute herpes simplex encephalitis. In the consideration of treatment of viral infections, special attention must be paid to rabies, historically a fascinating disease and one that still is encountered with distressing frequency.

The field of CNS infections is changing because use of potent therapeutic agents for neoplastic and autoimmune diseases is stripping patients of their normal immunologic defenses against infection. Opportunistic infections, which appear primarily in the immunosuppressed host, deserve consideration, since unusual pathogens of reduced virulence are often encountered, and CNS syndromes, which frequently are unfamiliar or unique, often emerge. Also the loss of synergistic effect between the host's immunologic defenses and the therapy leads to a fatal outcome.

BACTERIAL MENINGITIS

The history of therapy for the various forms of bacterial meningitis is a success story with few equals in modern medicine. Whereas patients with these diseases previously almost always died or were left with permanent CNS sequelae, rapid diagnosis and specific therapy now have allowed complete recovery in most cases. Nevertheless, mortality from bacterial meningitis still ranges between 20 and 50% (1,2) and has remained unchanged for the past 10–15 years. Therefore, rapid identification of the organism followed by specific antibiotic therapy is essential if the patient is to survive with an intact nervous system. Bacterial meningitis is common, affecting approximately five persons per 100,000 population. Most of the victims are children: approximately 15% of cases occur in infants less than one month old, 37% appear before one year of age, and 75% appear before 15 years of age. A slight preponderance for males has been noted (1). Each type of meningitis will be considered separately—neonatal forms first and those of childhood and adult life later. Unusual agents, such as *Listeria* and *Treponema pallidum,* are discussed separately.

Adequate therapy for bacterial meningitis requires that a specific etiologic diagnosis be determined as quickly as possible so that the most effective antibiotics can be given by the most efficient route (Table 1). The traditional tests for determining the etiology are assays of spinal fluid; cell count, measurement of glucose and protein, examination of stained smears for bacteria and appropriate bacteriologic cultures.

Although these tests still constitute the foundation for diagnosis, new assays also may aid in reaching a rapid, specific diagnosis. One such test is the limulus lysate assay for endotoxin in cerebrospinal fluid (CSF) (3). This test is extremely sensitive in detecting endotoxin produced by gram-negative organisms and frequently detects endotoxin several days after results of routine culture of CSF have become negative. The test is technically complicated, and both false-negative and false-positive results may occur; thus the traditional assays of spinal fluid must still be relied on for the final diagnosis.

Another useful diagnostic test in acute meningitis is counterimmunoelectrophoresis (CIE). In this test, specific bacterial antisera are reacted in agar gels with CSF that contains suspected bacterial antigens. Lines of precipitant form in the gels when the bacterial antigen reacts with specific antisera. This test usually can be performed within an hour and can give a presumptive, bacteriologically specific diagnosis. When the results are positive, CIE represents an improvement over both the endotoxin test and Gram stain of the CSF, for it can identify specific antigenic bacteria. While false-positive results rarely occur, false-negative results are more common and often relate to the specificity of the antisera used. Although both CIE and the limulus lysate assay for endotoxin can give information very rapidly, they still must be coupled with other, more conventional CSF assays in order to make a complete bacteriologic diagnosis. These tests must also include sensitivity of the cultured organism to antibiotics.

Empiric Therapy for Meningitis

Optimal antibiotic therapy for bacterial meningitis demands a knowledge of the specific infectious organism. However, at the beginning of therapy or in cases of partially treated meningitis that yield negative results on culture, therapy must be instituted rapidly on a "best guess" basis. During the first two months of life, when the likely infecting organisms include *Escherichia coli*, group B streptococci, *N. meningitidis, Diplococcus pneumoniae*, and *Listeria*, the initial drugs of choice are ampicillin, 50 mg/kg given intravenously (IV), and gentamicin, 2.5 mg/kg IV. In children between the ages of two months and 10 years, the most important organisms that cause meningitis are *Hemophilus influenzae, D. pneumoniae*, and *N. meningitidis*. For these infections, initial therapy requires ampicillin, 100 mg/kg/day IV, and cloramphenicol, 100 mg/kg/day IV. The organisms most likely to be found in otherwise healthy adults are *D. pneumoniae* and *N. Meningitidis*, both of which are best treated with penicillin G, 12–24 million units/day IV. If a brain abscess associated with secondary meningitis is suspected, penicillin G and chloramphenicol should be used to treat possible infection with *D. pneumoniae*, streptococci, or various mixed anaerobes.

Every effort should be made to culture and identify the infectious organism.

Table 1. Treatment of Bacterial Meningitis

Age Group	*Organism*	*Antibiotic and Dosage*[a]	*Route of Administration*
Newborns	Gram-negative bacilli	Ampicillin, 100 mg	IM, IV
		Gentamicin, 5–7.5 mg	IM, IV
	Group B streptococci	Penicillin G, 150,000–200,000 U/kg/day	IV
		Ampicillin, 100–200 mg	IV
	Listeria	Ampicillin, 100–200 mg	IV
	Staphylococcus aureus	Methicillin, 100–150 mg	IV
		Nafcillin, 40 mg	IV
Children and adults	*Hemophilus influenzae*	Ampicillin, 300–400 mg	IV
		Chloramphenicol, 100 mg	IV
	N. meningitidis	Penicillin G, 12 million U/day	IV
		Chloramphenicol, 100 mg	IV
	Diplococcus pneumoniae	Penicillin G, 24 million U/day	IV
		Chloramphenicol, 100 mg	IV
	Listeria	Ampicillin, 200–400 mg	IV
	S. aureus	Nafcillin, 50–150 mg	IV

[a] All dosages except penicillin G are mg/kg body weight per day.

However when this is impossible, the antibiotics listed above should be administered for a total of at least 14 days.

Neonatal Meningitis

Purulent meningitis in the newborn (less than 30 days old) continues to be a grave disease. Unfortunately, therapy has not improved remarkably during the antibiotic era. Incidence rates as high as 4–6 per 1,000 live births have been noted, and the disease is more likely to occur in infants of low birth weight or in those born after complicated pregnancies. Obstetric complications, such as prolonged rupture of the membranes, also markedly increase the risk of neonatal meningitis. The mortality from this disease, even with the best care currently available, is approximately 30% and in many hospitals is over 60%. Mortality varies widely among hospitals, suggesting that optimal care, which can reduce death in newborns, is not universally available. The long-term CNS morbidity among survivors continues to approach 50% (4).

The diagnosis of purulent meningitis in newborns is difficult. Since the disease is almost always a complication of a septicemia, prompt culture of both blood and CSF is indicated. Also, a Gram stain of peripheral blood for bacteria is a useful and productive test. The symptoms and physical signs that usually accompany acute meningitis, such as headache, fever, and nuchal rigidity, often do not appear in the newborn. Such vague signs as change in feeding habits, abdominal distention, loose stools, or unexplained seizure activity should alert the physician to the possible presence of meningitis. Changes in CSF are also different and confusing in newborns. As many as 25 white blood cells (WBCs) per mm^3 have been noted in the CSF of healthy infants, and neutrophils may predominate. CSF glucose usually is greater in newborns, and CSF protein is commonly elevated to as high as 150 mg/100 ml. During the early phases of neonatal meningitis, bacteria may be present in the CSF even though the fluid otherwise is within normal limits for that age. New diagnostic measures, such as CIE and assay for endotoxin, are useful adjuvants to Gram stains and cultures of blood and CSF (3).

In addition to specific antibiotic therapy, general supportive measures are essential. Respiratory assistance is often necessary, and fluid and electrolyte balance must be maintained. The physician must be aware that severe anemia or bacteriologic shock may occur at any time. Seizure activity is frequent and may be difficult to control.

The ultimate choice of antibiotics depends on the type and antibiotic sensitivity of the organism. However, before determination of the specific etiology, coverage with broad-spectrum antibiotics must be initiated at once. It is important to realize that newborns are physiologically unique and that multiple-system toxicity with several antibiotics may occur; thus, it is essential to provide a bacteriologically effective dose of antibiotic that is not toxic. Hepatic, renal, and peripheral-nerve toxicities are most common (4).

Initial therapy with broad-spectrum antibiotics is best achieved with a combination of an aminoglycoside (kanamycin or gentamicin) and a penicillin (most commonly ampicillin). The initial dose of kanamycin usually is 15–30 mg/kg/day. Both the aminoglycoside and the penicillin are given IM in two or three equally divided doses. Low levels of drug are recommended for infants of less than 2,000 g birth weight before seven days of age. Ampicillin, 100–200 mg/kg/day, is given IM or IV in two or three doses. It is necessary to repeat blood and CSF cultures daily to monitor the effectiveness of the therapy.

Gram-Negative Meningitis of the Newborn

Gram-negative enteric organisms, including *E. coli* and *Klebsiella,* are the most common organisms that produce acute purulent meningitis of the newborn. Although these bacteria are part of the normal flora of the mother, there is evidence that specific antigenic subtypes usually cause neonatal meningitis. Among strains of *E. coli* that produce meningitis, most contain the capsular polysaccharide antigen K1, even though more than 100 types of *E. coli* polysaccharides are known. The significance of this finding in the pathogenesis of the disease or in the consideration of useful vaccines remains to be determined.

The outcome of neonatal meningitis is directly related to the speed with which the CSF is sterilized. Nevertheless, even with optimal antibiotic therapy, gram-negative bacteria may remain in the CSF for two to three days. Once the bacteria is identified and the diagnosis is made, specific therapy consists of continuation of ampicillin, 100–200 mg/kg/day IM in two to three divided doses, plus either kanamycin, 15–30 mg/kg/day in two to three divided doses, or gentamicin 5–7.5 mg/kg/day in two to three doses. Multiple antibiotic therapy seems to be superior to the use of an aminoglycoside alone. Also, resistant strains of bacteria are less likely to emerge with this regimen. Therapy should continue for at least 14 days after sterilization of the CSF. No studies have indicated convincingly that intrathecal therapy improves the outcome.

A grave and poorly understood complication of gram-negative meningitis of the newborn is the development of ventriculitis. This complication should be considered if the clinical or bacteriologic response in the CSF is not optimal. The diagnosis of ventriculitis is made by a ventricular tap, which will show purulent ventricular fluid. Ventricular drainage and daily instillation of an appropriate antibiotic (e.g., gentamicin in a dose of 1 or 2 mg) is then necessary. When therapy seems to be adequate on the basis of clinical response and improvement of the CSF, routine tapping of the ventricles to search for ventriculitis is not recommended.

Group B Streptococcal Meningitis of the Newborn

Over the last decade, increasing numbers of cases of neonatal meningitis have been caused by group B (hemolytic) streptococci. The reason for this increase is unknown; however, in some centers, approximately one half of cases of neonatal meningitis are now caused by this organism. Interestingly, the streptococci that usually are isolated in these cases have a specific polysaccharide antigen that appears similar to the K1 antigen of *E. coli* (4). Group B streptococci usually are more susceptible to antibiotic therapy than are the gram-negative organisms, and sterilization of the CSF is often possible within 24 hours. Nevertheless, CSF evaluation is necessary and treatment should be continued for a minimum of 14 days. The antibiotics of choice are penicillin G, 150,000–200,000 units/kg in two or three divided doses, or ampicillin, 100–200 mg/kg/day in divided doses. Fortunately, serious, permanent CNS sequelae among survivors of group B streptococcal infection are less common than with infection from gram-negative organisms. Although penicillin or ampicillin therapy is usually quite effective, several cases of relapse have been reported to have followed a full course (10 to 14 days) of therapy (5); these patients required continuous observation during the follow-up period.

Other Types of Purulent Meningitis of the Newborn

Listeria monocytogenes has been recognized as a cause of abortion, intrauterine infection, and neonatal meningitis. The pathogenesis of the infection caused by this organism is unknown; however, it appears more commonly in groups of low socioeconomic status. Meningitis in the newborn usually occurs in the first week of life. As with group B streptococcal infections, the incidence of this condition appears to be increasing and may account for more than one third of cases in some series of neonatal meningitis. The disease is more benign than that caused by gram-negative organisms. The CSF may appear very benign, especially early in the disease. The recommended therapy is ampicillin, 100–200 mg/kg/day in two to three divided doses. A serious and difficult problem in therapy is meningitis caused by penicillin-resistant *Staphylococcus.* These organisms often are identified in nurseries, suggesting that the infection is spread from nursery personnel. The recommended therapy is methicillin, 100–200 mg/kg/day in two or three divided doses. Therapy must continue for at least 14–21 days.

Occasionally, *Pseudomonas* meningitis occurs in newborns. Carbenicillin, 200–400 mg/kg/day in three or four divided doses, and usually in combination with gentamicin, is recommended for at least 21 days. When it is impossible to determine the infectious organism, the initial therapy mentioned above is continued. Treatment with gentamicin or kanamycin in conjunction with ampicillin should continue for at least 14 days.

Permanent neurologic sequelae among survivors of neonatal meningitis are common, and the incidence may approach 80% after gram-negative meningitis. Disabilities include profound mental retardation, less severe defects in learning, language, or perception, seizures, deafness, spasticity, and hydrocephalus. Since such sequelae may not be apparent for several years, survivors of meningitis should be observed for prolonged periods before being assessed as normal (6).

Childhood and Adult Meningitis

Meningitis that occurs after the first month of life usually is due to one of three organisms: *H. influenzae, Neisseria meningitidis,* (meningococcus) or *D. pneumoniae* (pneumonococcus). Of these, *H. influenzae* occurs almost exclusively in patients younger than five years of age, whereas meningococcal and pneumococcal infections can occur at any age. In adults over the age of 50, and in patients with a variety of underlying diseases (e.g., immunosuppressive states, sickle-cell anemia, malnutrition, alcoholism), pneumococcal meningitis is the most common infection.

Several general therapeutic measures are necessary once the diagnosis of bacterial meningitis is considered or established. All such patients should be hospitalized at once. Nonspecific support is extremely important; measures include IV administration of fluids and electrolytes, control of seizures and/or cerebral edema, and treatment of shock. Placement of a central venous pressure line is often required. Because patients are often obtunded or even comatose, close attention must be paid to pulmonary function, skin care, and bowel and bladder control. Specific antibiotic therapy, administered IV, is mandatory as soon as possible. Unfortunately, controversy exists about the best antibiotic regimen for the various types of meningitis, and frequently a specific diagnosis is not obtainable at once. Therefore, the combination of antibiotics most likely to be effective should be administered.

H. influenzae, the most common cause of bacterial meningitis in young children, rarely produces meningitis in adolescents or adults. The organism is a pleomorphic gram-negative rod with a specific capsular polysaccharide (polyribophosphate). It is interesting that subclinical infections appear to be frequent and bactericidal antibody frequently is found in healthy children and adults. Nevertheless, high titers of such antibodies do not seem to be protective and are noted frequently in both serum and spinal fluid at the onset of *H. influenzae* meningitis. On the other hand, antipolyribophosphate antibody does appear to protect against *H. influenzae* infection in both animals and humans (2).

Ampicillin has been the standard antibiotic therapy for *H. influenzae* meningitis for many years. The drug is administered IV in a dose of 300–400 mg/kg/day in four to six divided doses. During the last decade, it has become apparent that ampicillin-resistant strains of *H. influenzae* are increasing; therefore, this drug can no longer be relied on as the sole therapeutic agent. The second most commonly recommended drug is chloramphenicol, given IV in a dose of 100 mg/kg/day in four to six divided doses. Some investigators now routinely recommend use of both drugs. Therapy should continue for 10–14 days; after this time, a repeat CSF examination is performed to monitor the effectiveness of the therapy. Comparative studies have shown that carbenicillin in comparable doses probably is as effective as ampicillin for treatment of *H. influenzae* meningitis (7).

The appearance of ampicillin-resistant strains of *H. influenzae* along with a fear of severe depression of bone marrow function with use of chloramphenicol have prompted a search for other effective forms of therapy for *H. influenzae* meningitis. Recently, an older form of combined therapy, streptomycin plus sulfisoxazole, has been recommended as an alternative (8). Streptomycin is given IV in an initial dose of 30 mg/kg/day and then intramuscularly (IM) to allow the patient freedom from constant IV fluids. Intrathecal streptomycin also is recommended during the first 24 hours. The intrathecal dose is 2 mg/kg at admission, with identical doses at 12 and 24 hours. Sulfisoxazole is given IV in an initial dose of 150 mg/kg/day, and then orally. This combination appears to be as therapeutically effective as ampicillin and chloramphenicol when given for 14 days; it has the added advantage that, in the later stages of therapy, IM and oral routes of administration can be used. Its major disadvantage is the requirement for intrathecal streptomycin therapy during the first 24 hours.

Meningococcal meningitis may develop at any age in the normal host and may appear in epidemics. *N. meningitidis* is a gram-negative, comma-shaped diplococcus that is commonly seen intracellularly, especially in neutrophils. At one time, most cases of meningococcal meningitis were caused by group A strains; however, group B, C, and Y strains are now noted more frequently, with group A causing less than 5% of cases. Group Y strains appear to cause less severe disease and cause pneumonia more frequently than meningitis (1). Petechiae or skin purpura develop in over half of the cases. Although this finding is not specific, it frequently is a useful sign.

The treatment of choice for meningococcal meningitis is penicillin G, 500,000 units/kg/day IV in eight to 12 divided doses. In patients who are allergic to penicillin, chloramphenicol, 100 mg/kg/day IV in four to six doses, is recommended. Sulfonamides, although previously used for both treatment and prophylaxis after exposure, are now seldom used, and there is evidence that group A strains are often resistant to sulfonamide drugs. Vaccines that contain purified meningococcal polysaccharides are nontoxic, useful immunizing agents and have been used especially in the military to provide protection.

D. pneumoniae is a gram-positive diplococcus that often causes a severe form of bacterial meningitis, especially in already debilitated patients. It is also the organism that produces recurrent meningitis most frequently, especially in patients with recent head trauma or an anatomic defect of the dura. Patients who develop pneumonococcal meningitis often have a predisposing pneumonia or otitis media that clearly is the source of the meningitis.

Penicillin G, 500,000 units/kg/day given every two to three hours in equally divided doses, is recommended for treatment of the disease in young children. In adolescents and adults, 24 million units/day IV in equally divided doses is recommended. In patients who are allergic to penicillin or in whom penicillin therapy is not effective, chloramphenicol, 100 mg/kg/day IV every six hours in equal doses, or erythromycin, 50–100 mg/kg/day IV at six-hour intervals, may be effective. Recently, strains of *D. pneumoniae* have been isolated that are resistant to penicillin; thus, chloramphenicol must be used whenever penicillin therapy is not effective or when sensitivity tests indicate that the strain is resistant.

Pneumonococcal meningitis may be fatal in up to 50% of patients (9). A poor outcome usually is associated with coma at the start of therapy, a relatively low white cell count in CSF, and a high titer of antigens in CSF determined by CIE. Because a poor outcome is so common, despite several modes of therapy that are very effective against pneumococcal infection in other organ systems, a vaccine for pneumococcal meningitis has been developed and licensed. The commercial vaccine contains 14 of the most common capsular antigens associated with disease-producing strains of *D. pneumoniae* and probably provides protection for more than five years. The vaccine is especially recommended for patients with chronic or debilitating disease, immunosuppressed states, sickle-cell anemia, and those over the age of 50. A single 0.5-ml subcutaneous or IM dose is recommended.

Listeria Meningitis

L. monocytogenes is a pleomorphic, gram-positive bacterium that produces a variety of clinical conditions, including granulomatosis, subacute sepsis, rare cases of endocarditis, and cutaneous infection. Although acute meningitis is the most common CNS syndrome associated with *Listeria* infection (10), rare cases of brain abscess have been reported. The meningitis is unusual in that it occurs most frequently at extremes of age or as an opportunistic infection in patients with neoplastic disease or immunosuppression. As with other types of purulent meningitis, the clinical presentation at times is subacute rather than explosive. CSF findings also may be atypical; the cell count often ranges between 50 and 1,000 cells/mm^3, and the glucose level may be normal or only slightly depressed. The level of CSF protein usually is increased. The precise diagnosis is also hampered by the frequent variation in the morphology and gram-staining properties of *L. monocytogenes.* The cultured organisms often are regarded as nonpathogenic diphtheroidlike agents and are dismissed as contaminants.

Ampicillin is the antibiotic of choice for *Listeria* meningitis. The drug is given IV in a total daily dose of 200–400 mg/kg in six or more divided doses. Therapy should continue for 12 to 14 days. Other antibiotics, such as penicillin, chloramphenicol, erythromycin, and tetracycline, also are effective when administered IV at high dosages.

Neurosyphilis

Widespread treatment of acute syphilis with antibiotics has reduced the incidence of neurosyphilis greatly. Nevertheless, occasional cases do appear and therapy is often delayed because the diagnosis is not considered. The course of syphilis is now divided into two stages: early syphilis of less than one year's duration, and syphilis of more than one year's duration which includes cardiovascular, late-benign, and neurosyphilis (11). In addition to clinical suspicion, the diagnosis is confirmed by specific serologic tests, most commonly the serum fluorescent treponemal antibody absorption (FTA-ABS) test, which measures specific antitreponemal antibodies. Therapy consists of benzathine penicillin G in a total dose of 7.2 million units, given in three weekly IM injections of 2.4 million units each. An alternative form of therapy is 9.0 million units of aqueous procaine penicillin G administered IM in daily doses of 600,000 units for 15 days. For patients who are allergic to penicillin, tetracycline hydrochloride, 500 mg, or erythromycin, 500 mg, each four times a day orally for 30 days, is acceptable. Because early neurosyphilis is frequently subclinical, it is mandatory that CSF examination be performed at the start of therapy for syphilis of more than one year's duration. In addition to assay of CSF cells and protein, it is useful to obtain a VDRL examination for CSF antibodies. The FTA-ABS test of CSF is not reliable because it merely measures small amounts of treponemal antibodies that have crossed the blood barrier into the CSF. Many investigators recommend a repeat CSF examination approximately six months after therapy for early or confirmed neurosyphilis to monitor effects of therapy.

BACTERIAL BRAIN ABSCESS AND EPIDURAL ABSCESS

Bacterial brain abscess may result from the spread of infection from adjacent structures, such as the temporal bone or middle ear; from metastatic spread from distant foci, such as the heart or lungs; or from direct contamination during penetrating head injuries or neurosurgical procedures. Numerous neurologic syndromes result from brain abscess, depending on the location of the lesion; however, the course usually is progressive and is often complicated by headache but rarely by fever. Occasionally, an abscess may rupture into the subarachnoid space and produce acute meningitis. The most common organisms found in brain abscesses are *S. aureas*, various streptococci of low virulence, and several types of anaerobic bacteria. In the neonatal period, gram-negative bacilli frequently are cultured from abscesses. Often the infections are mixed. While ultimate bacteriologic therapy depends on identification of the organisms in the abscess, initial therapy should include penicillin G, chloramphenicol, and methicillin or nafcillin (see Table 1 for appropriate dosages). With the use of the computed tomographic (CT) scan, it is possible to follow the progression of a brain abscess, and, in some cases, it has been shown clearly that antibiotic therapy alone is sufficient to control the lesion. In most cases, however, surgical drainage of the abscess in conjunction with antibiotic therapy is recommended. Controversy still exists over the relative value of simple drainage versus total excision of the abscess.

Bacterial suppuration also may develop, either beneath the dura (subdural empyema) or external to it (epidural abscess) after seeding from a previously established focus of infection. While subdural empyemas occur most commonly over the cerebral convexities and are usually secondary to infections of the paranasal sinuses or structures of the ear, epidural abscesses develop adjacent to the dura of the spinal cord and are secondary to focal infections of the skin or viscera. Cerebral subdural empyema produces compression of the brain, resulting in rapidly evolving hemiparesis, hemianopsia, or aphasia, all of which may be progressive, often accompanied by systemic toxic signs of headache, fever, and leukocytosis of the peripheral blood. Seizures may occur. Diagnosis of subdural empyema is made by cerebral angiography, CT scan, or burr holes into the lesion. Such lesions contain organisms similar to those found in brain abscesses, and mixed infections frequently are noted.

Epidural spinal abscess usually causes severe localized back pain as well as fever and leukocytosis. Percussion of the spine usually localizes the lesion, but myelography is often necessary to localize the lesion specifically enough to perform surgery. The CSF often shows an increased number of cells and protein but rarely a decrease in sugar; organisms are rarely cultured.

In both subdural empyema and epidural abscess, broad antibiotic coverage similar to that used for brain abscess is employed initially. Surgical drainage of the lesion is mandatory in both conditions, and, after identification of the organisms cultured at surgery, specific antibiotic therapy can be continued.

FUNGAL AND TUBERCULOUS INFECTIONS OF THE CNS

Fungal Meningitis

Fungal invasion of the CNS usually occurs in the setting of disseminated infection or as a result of an abnormal entry into CSF pathways (e.g., through a ventricular catheter). All CNS fungal infections are grave diseases that demand vigorous long-term treatment. Unfortunately, therapy often is unsuccessful. A poor prognosis must be expected when a CNS fungal infection is complicated by one of the following factors: lymphoreticular malignancy, high CSF pressure, low CSF glucose level or cell count, presence of fungi (especially cryptococci) on smear, and evidence of disseminated infection (12).

Numerous types of fungal infections occasionally affect the CNS. Some, such as aspergillosis and mucormycosis, are unusual; however, cryptococcosis, coccidioiodomycosis, and candidiasis occur relatively frequently, and their treatment will be discussed in detail.

Several general principles of therapy for CNS fungal infections must be followed. If possible, immunosuppressive drugs should be terminated, and catheters or shunts, which act as foreign bodies, should be removed. Intravenous therapy is almost always necessary and necessitates prolonged hospitalization. The side effects of the primary therapeutic agent, amphotericin B, are severe, so that patient monitoring must be continuous.

Cryptococcus neoformans Meningitis

The diagnosis of cryptococcal meningitis is made by evaluation of the CSF. In addition to moderate lymphocytic pleocytosis, there usually is a decrease in level of CSF glucose and an increase in total protein. Fungi may be identified by appropriate culture, India ink preparations, or identification of antigen in CSF. The primary mode of therapy is with amphotericin B, a commercially available polyene antibiotic that disrupts cellular membranes of fungi. Amphotericin B must be administered IV in an electrolyte-free solution, usually 5% dextrose in water. The usual daily dose is 0.4–6 mg/kg, infused over four to six hours. Unless the infection is overwhelming, the patient usually receives 1 mg the first day, 5 mg the second day, and then increases of 5 mg/day until the ideal daily dose is achieved. Because of the risk of permanent renal damage, a total course dose is usually between 2 and 4 g, given over several weeks or months. In order to alleviate some discomfort and side effects, a double dose every other day is sometimes adequate (13).

Reversible nephrotoxicity occurs in virtually every patient who receives the dosage recommended above. Permanent renal damage may occur with total doses of more than 3 or 4 g. In order to monitor for nephrotoxicity it is necessary to follow levels of serum creatinine and blood urea nitrogen every other day. In addition, hemoglobin, potassium, magnesium, white cell count, platelet count, and liver function studies should be done at regular intervals (14).

Side effects are very common with amphotericin B therapy. These include headache, nausea and vomiting, and fever. Generally the reactions subside with continued therapy. At times it is necessary either to reduce the dosage or add 25 mg hydrocortisone sodium succinate to the infusion solution or to treat the patient with aspirin and diphenhydramine when maximal doses of amphotericin B are first administered.

Flucytosine is another drug that is frequently administered with amphotericin B for cryptococcal meningitis. Flucytosine is a fluorinated pyrimidine that is related structurally to 5-fluorouracil. It has a narrow spectrum of activity—primarily against *C. neoformans,* some *Candida* species, and *Aspergillus.* It appears to work synergistically with amphotericin B against these agents and, in successful cases, has allowed some reduction in the dosage amphotericin B. Some strains of *Candida* are naturally resistant, and many strains of both *Candida* and *C. neoformans* develop drug resistance when flucytosine is used alone. Flucytosine is relatively free of serious side effects and can be administered orally in a dose of 150 mg/kg/day every six hours.

Coccidioidal Meningitis

Coccidioidal meningitis is a life-threatening, chronic fungal disease that, in some cases, may be controlled even though eridication of CNS effects is impossible. The primary therapeutic agent is amphotericin B, which is administered in a fashion identical to that for cryptococcal meningitis. Because amphotericin B penetrates the CSF poorly, it has often been necessary to introduce the drug intrathecally. This is done most commonly by repeated lumbar punctures. While this probably is an effective route of administration, some question has been raised about the circulation of the drug in the basal cisterns, where the disease is most active. Also, the repeated inoculation of the lumbar subarachnoid space with amphotericin B has been reported to produce a chronic arachnoiditis in some patients, limiting markedly the diffusion of the drug throughout the subarachnoid space. For these reasons, specialized methods of drug administration have been suggested and used. These include the placement of an Ommaya reservoir for direct intraventricular infusion of drug and inoculation of the cervical subarachnoid space with the drug through a lateral cervical puncture (15). It also has been shown that increased cerebral circulation from the lumbar sac can be achieved if amphotericin B is placed in a hyperbaric solution and the patient is placed in a Trendelenburg position to aid conveyance of the antibiotic from the injection site to the basal cisterns (16).

Several new experimental antibiotics have been suggested for treatment of coccidioidal meningitis. Of these, the one receiving the most interest is miconazole (17), which has been used both in cryptococcal and coccidioidal meningitis. The drug appears to have some therapeutic effect and may be quite useful, especially when amphotericin B toxicity is marked. At present, miconazole remains an experimental drug only.

Candida meningitis is infrequent and occasionally has been misdiagnosed because the fungus was thought to be a laboratory contaminant. Most cases appear to complicate conditions accompanied by marked immunosuppression or in which the subarachnoid space is violated by a foreign body, such as an intraventricular catheter. Significant control of the CNS infection often is impossible until the offending foreign body is removed. The recommended treatment in such cases is amphotericin B in small doses of 10–20 mg/day IV for 10–30 days.

Tuberculous Meningitis

Tuberculous meningitis is now an uncommon neurologic infection. The diagnosis is delayed at times because either tuberculosis is not included in the working differential diagnosis or because the usual diagnostic methods of identification of organisms in CSF smears or culture are faulty or delayed. Once the diagnosis is made, the clinician is faced with a dilemma regarding therapy because several drugs that are used produce toxicity, and because drug-resistant organisms tend to emerge.

For some time a controversy has existed about the use of adrenal corticosteroids as adjunct therapy for tuberculous meningitis. Steroids are thought to reduce the intracranial inflammatory response and thus reduce the likelihood of progressive arachnoiditis and communicating hydrocephalus. Most investigators now advocate use of oral adrenal corticosteroids during the early stages (one to two months) of therapy to prevent adhesive arachnoiditis and its complications.

Isoniazid (INH) is the primary antituberculosis drug now used and is clearly beneficial in tuberculous meningitis because of its high level of antimicrobial activity, low toxicity, and superior penetration into the CSF. The usual dose is 5–10 mg/kg/day; however, side effects such as drug-induced hepatitis and peripheral neuropathies must be considered. Pyridoxine, 25–50 mg/day, is useful as prophylaxis against peripheral neuritis. In order to reduce the emergence of resistant strains, two other drugs are commonly given concurrently. Streptomycin in a dose of 0.75–1 g/day, is given for the first two months of therapy, with constant observation for toxicity of the eighth cranial nerve. Ethambutol also may be given at a dosage of 15–30 mg/kg/day. The primary side effect of this drug is optic neuritis, which is reversible with discontinuation of therapy. Ethambutol therapy is contraindicated in patients with preexisting optic neuritis. Although toxicity is relatively low with this triad of therapeutic agents, bactericidal activity also is less than optimal, and in some cases the infection may progress.

In an effort to increase bactericidal activity, INH and either streptomycin or ethambutol can be combined with rifampin, 600 mg once a day. In children the dosage is 10–20 mg/kg body weight up to a maximum of 600 mg. Because rifampin produces hepatic damage, patients must be monitored carefully.

The third possibility is to include pyrazinamide, 20–35 mg/kg/day to a maximum of 3 g. Pyrazinamide can be administered with INH and rifampin for a maximal bactericidal dosage; however, the risk of hepatotoxicity is markedly increased when the drugs are combined.

The initial 60 days of therapy usually are crucial, and during this time, three or even four antituberculosis drugs, in addition to adrenal cortocosteroids, are recommended. Hopefully, a bactericidal drug regimen can be maintained without unacceptable toxicity and without the appearance of drug-resistant strains. Beyond the 60th day, INH should be combined with rifampin, ethambutol, or streptomycin for an additional four to six months. Finally, INH alone should be continued for a few months, for a total period of therapy of 12–18 months. Throughout this period the patient must be monitored repeatedly for drug toxicity (including hepatotoxicity), peripheral neuropathy, and optic neuropathy, as well as for complications of the infection itself, such as progressive arachnoiditis with communicating hydrocephalus.

PARASITIC INFECTIONS OF THE NERVOUS SYSTEM

A variety of parasites are known to invade the human CNS; however, few are clinically important in the United States and northern Europe. Trichinosis meningitis or encephalitis may occur after the parasites are acquired from inadequately cooked, infected pork.

Toxoplasmosis, both congenital and acquired, is the major parasitic disease of interest in the United States. *Toxoplasma gondii* is an obligate intracellular protozoan, and only one serotype of the organism has been recognized. Subclinical disease is common and is acquired primarily from consumption of poorly cooked meats or from exposure to infested animals, primarily domestic cats (18). Congenital toxoplasmosis is a direct infestation from mother to fetus and is a serious disease characterized by chorioretinitis, hydrocephalus or microcephaly, psychomotor retardation, and cerebral calcification. Acquired CNS toxoplasmosis may occur in anyone but is increasingly being recognized as an opportunistic infection of immunosuppressed patients. Toxoplasmosis has three neurologic patterns: (*1*) diffuse encephalopathy with or without seizures, (*2*) a meningoencephalitis with characteristic CSF changes, and (*3*) solitary or multiple progressive mass lesions (19).

Once CNS toxoplasmosis is suspected, two serologic studies are useful in confirming the diagnosis. These are the Sabin-Feldman dye test and the IgM indirect fluorescent antibody test (20).

Several drugs have been recommended for the treatment of CNS toxoplasmosis. The effectiveness of various preparations of tetracycline has been both advocated and questioned. Perhaps the best regimen is a combination of sulfadiazine and pyramethamine; the latter is an anti–folic acid agent that may produce thrombocytopenia and anemia when taken for prolonged periods. Sulfadiazine is given orally, 4–6 g/day for at least one month. A daily dose of 25 mg of pyramethamine for at least one month is likewise recommended.

Neurocysticercosis is the development within the CNS or meninges of cysts of the pork tapeworm, *Taenia solium.* The disease occurs after ingestion of the ova of the tapeworm, which usually are carried on poorly washed vegetables or feces-contaminated hands and is seen most commonly in patients from Latin America. The cerebral cysts may achieve a considerable size of 5–15 ml and often are multiple. Their random location within the CNS and slow development give rise to remarkably diverse neurologic syndromes, and the diagnosis is frequently missed in the United States because the condition is so rare here.

The three most common clinical syndromes associated with neurocysticercosis are increased intracranial pressure often associated with obstructive hydrocephalus, focal epilepsy, and changes in mental function, including both dementia and psychotic reactions. The disease may cause periodic bouts of severe headache in patients with papilledema. Diagnostic tests of value include a search for eosinophilia in the blood and CSF, an increase in CSF protein and immunoglobulin content, and several serologic assays, noe of which have been well standardized. Neuroradiologic procedures are of greater value and include identification of old calcified cysts in the brain or skeletal muscle, detection of cysts by cerebral angiography, pneumoencephalography, and CT scan.

No specific therapy exists for neurocysticercosis. Systemic steroids and various shunting procedures are of use in the treatment of increased intracranial pressure and hydrocephalus, and anticonvulsant medications can control some of the seizures. It sometimes is possible to remove large solitary cysts, especially in the spinal cord or along CSF pathways.

VIRAL INFECTIONS OF THE NERVOUS SYSTEM

Unfortunately therapy for neurologic viral infections is still in its infancy, and specific forms of treatment are only now beginning to emerge. Perhaps this is not too surprising, since, unlike bacteria or fungi, which are true extracellular organisms with a life cycle of their own, viruses are by definition intracellular agents with replicative cycles that are difficult to affect without affecting basic cellular functions at the same time.

Viral infections of the CNS can be classified as acute (e.g., benign aseptic meningitis, acute encephalitis) or chronic (e.g., the so-called slow virus infections of the nervous system) (Table 2). Chronic infections can be subdivided into those caused by either unconventional or conventional viruses (i.e., agents with either RNA or DNA and associated antigenic proteins). Examples of diseases caused by conventional viruses include subacute sclerosing panencephalitis (SSPE), progressive rubella panencephalitis (PRP), and progressive multifocal leukoencephalopathy (PML). Unconventional agents that produce chronic neurologic disease do not contain clearly demonstrable nucleic acid; nor do they seem to contain antigenic proteins, since no evidence of an immunologic host reaction to these agents has been demonstrated. The following discussion will be concerned with both acute and chronic diseases caused by conventional viruses, for there is no evidence that any type of therapy is beneficial for diseases caused by unconventional agents (e.g., scrapie in sheep, Creutzfeldt–Jakob disease, kuru in man).

An attack focused on replication of viral nucleic acids has been a mainstay in the search for effective antiviral agents. As mentioned earlier, all viruses contain either RNA or DNA, but never both. An effective drug that interferes with metabolism of viral RNA has yet to be produced. This may not be surprising, since any substance that interferes with replication of viral RNA would also likely affect metabolism of cellular RNA. Because constantly renewable RNA is necessary for production of proteins, almost every living cell must have relatively intact RNA metabolic machinery in order to survive. On the other hand, metabolism of DNA is intermittent and transient activity in many cells that are not actively undergoing mitosis. Therefore, substances that temporarily interfere with DNA metabolism can be used therapeutically to interfere with viral DNA metabolism. Several such agents have been tried experimentally and one drug, adenine arabinoside (Ara-A, Vidarabine), is available commercially for the treatment of herpes simplex encephalitis.

Involvement of the host immune system in antiviral prophylaxis or therapy is also possible and, in some circumstances, effective. Immunologic therapy can be classified into a number of specific mechanisms (Table 3). For instance, specific immunologic reactivity can be induced either to prevent neurologic infection or, in the case of rabies, to treat the infection in the interval between exposure and the appearance of neurologic disease (postexposure prophylaxis). Occasionally, passive immunologic therapy with specific antibodies can be used when a progressive infection involving the nervous system is anticipated or noted.

Nonspecific immunologic enhancement, as opposed to stimulation of immunologic reactivity against a specific viral antigen or agent, also can be tried. A number of substances have been described that nonspecifically stimulate the immune system, especially the cellular immune system, and there is slight evi-

Table 2. Agents That Produce CNS Infections[a]

	Acute	*Latent Recurrent*	*Slow*
CONVENTIONAL VIRAL AGENTS			
RNA viruses			
Arthropod borne	A	−	−
Polio I, II, III	A	+−	−
Coxsackie group	A	+−	−
Echo group	A	+−	−
Mumps	A–B	−	−
Rabies	A–B	−	−
Lymphocytic Choriomengitis virus	A	−	−
Measles	B	−	+
Rubella	B	−	+
Influenza	B	−	−
DNA viruses			
Herpes simplex I, II	A	+	−
Varicella zoster	A–B	+	−
Cytomegalovirus (fetus)	A	+−	
Vaccinia	B	−	−
Papova	−	−	+
UNCONVENTIONAL AGENTS (VIRUS?)			
Kuru	−	−	+
Creutzfeldt–Jakob disease	−	−	+

[a]A, active replication in CNS tissue; B, parainfectious encephalomyelitis syndrome with possible CNS replication; +, possibility of latent infection or slow disease, −, no evidence of latent or slow disease.

Table 3. Mechanisms of Antiviral Therapy

Inhibition of Nucleic Acid Metabolism
- Anti-RNA
- Anti-DNA

Immunologic Reactivity
- Specific antiviral immunity
  - Active humoral reactivity (vaccine)
  - Passive humoral reactivity (antisera)
  - Active cellular reactivity (vaccine)
- Nonspecific immune enhancement

Interferon (host cellular resistance to infection)

dence that this type of treatment does provide benefit in some infectious processes.

Study of transfer factor (TF) also has excited the hope that immunologic therapy could be induced by this novel substance. TF is a low-molecular-weight protein that is produced by lymphocytes that previously have been sensitized to a specific antigen when the cells are reexposed to that antigen. When a naive host is inoculated with TF, the immune system achieves the ability to recognize and inactivate the antigen; thus, immunologic knowledge of the antigen is transferred from one host to the other. Since TF has been well established in humans only, interspecies trials of therapy have not been possible.

In addition to the immunologic mechanisms mentioned previously there is a fascinating group of substances known collectively as interferon, which also provide protection against viral infections. When interferon is released in an infected cell, it has the ability to alter surrounding cells to make them resistant to viral infection; thus, the spread of infection from cell to cell is terminated. While the phenomenon of cell protection with interferon has been recognized for some time, practical applications of this therapeutic method in humans have been rare. Often interferon was effective only when given before the onset of the experimental infection. However, in studies of human volunteers, interferon has been used therapeutically with some success for acute pulmonary infections. Its effectiveness has not been demonstrated in neurologic infections, however. Unfortunately, interferons are highly host specific; therefore, since only human cells can be used to produce this material, it is difficult to obtain and prohibitively expensive at present.

Therapy for Acute CNS Viral Infections

Active Prophylaxis

Since specific therapy is not available for most acute viral infections of the CNS, especially those caused by RNA viruses, prophylaxis is necessary. The use of vaccines, of course, is a highly developed science and has effectively reduced the neurologic complications of a variety of infections.

Poliomyelitis is an acute, enteric infection caused by one of three small RNA viruses of the picorna group. In a small percentage of infected persons, invasion of the anterior horn cells of the spinal cord occurs, producing permanent asymmetric atrophy and paralysis. While both an injectable killed vaccine and an oral live vaccine are available, current recommendations suggest use of the live vaccine in all instances except in those with evidence of immune deficiency (21); in the latter case, the killed vaccine should be employed to prevent a chronic progressive infection. The usual schedule of administration for the live vaccine, which contains all three serotypes, is at 2, 4, and 6 months of age, with boosters at 1.5 years and at 4–6 years of age. Only rare evidence of paralytic disease with the vaccine strains has been reported, and undoubtedly the use of oral polio vaccine has effectively terminated the risk of paralytic polio in the United States. Poor compliance by some patients on this vaccination scheme has permitted occasional cases to occur in susceptible individuals, however.

A live measles virus vaccine has been distributed widely in the United States since the mid-1960s and has effectively reduced both the acute disease and its neurologic complications (22). The vaccine is administered as a single IM dose at approximately 1 year of age. The vaccine has often been ineffective when given before this age, at which time passive maternal antibodies still exist in the child's body. Rare cases of SSPE probably have occurred after exposure to measles vaccine. However, the risk of this complication is exceedingly small, whereas the risk of postinfectious encephalomyelitis after naturally occurring measles has been approximately one per 1,000 population (22).

A live mumps vaccine given IM after the age of 1 year is used widely. Complications with this vaccine are rare, even when it is given to older men without a history of natural mumps infection.

A live rubella vaccine is used in the United States for most infants of both sexes at approximately 1 year of life. A single IM dose is usually protective. The purpose of vaccinating both boys and girls is to reduce or end the possibility of widespread epidemics when there are large numbers of susceptible persons in the population. The vaccine should be considered essential for girls before puberty in order to prevent the possibility of rubella infection during pregnancy, which could result in intrauterine infection and damage to the fetus.

Passive Prophylaxis

Intramuscular administration of gammoglobulin has been recommended for susceptible individuals after exposure to a variety of acute exanthematous diseases. This is the preferred method of therapy, especially in debilitated persons in whom risk of natural infections with such viruses as measles is considered.

Hyperimmune globulin that contains antibodies to varicella zoster virus is available for passive prophylaxis of highly susceptible individuals who are exposed to chicken pox (varicella-zoster virus) or herpes zoster. This material, known as zoster immune globulin (ZIG), has been used primarily in patients with either natural or acquired immunodeficiency, in which varicella-zoster infections are known to be much more severe and to produce systemic dissemination of viral lesions (23).

Specific Antiviral Therapy

Therapy that has been proven effective has been demonstrated for only one CNS viral disease: herpes simplex encephalitis. This disease, the most common sporadic form of encephalitis recognized in the United States, is almost always caused by herpes simplex virus type I (HSV I), the agent responsible for common recurrent fever blisters. Most of the adult population have antibodies to HSV I, indicating past and often latent infection. The virus also is known to infect sensory ganglia latently, most commonly the trigeminal ganglia in humans (24). The pathogenesis of sporadic encephalitis in this setting is unknown.

HSV I is a large DNA virus. When it reaches the CNS of humans or experimental animals, it usually produces an acute necrotizing encephalitis that is characterized by hemorrhage, inflammation, necrosis, and the production of cells with nuclear eosinophilic inclusions. Although the CSF is almost invariably abnormal, with an increase in various inflammatory cells and an elevated protein level, it rarely, if ever, contains free virus. Therefore, diagnosis requires either demonstration of virus antigens or isolation of virus from fresh brain tissue obtained by cerebral biopsy. Herpes simplex encephalitis is a grave disease that ends fatally in more than 60% of cases and produces permanent neurologic sequelae in most survivors. Because of its extremely poor prognosis, major efforts have been made to find an effective therapeutic agent, including use of agents with significant toxicity.

The first antiviral therapeutic agents used in herpes simplex encephalitis were the pyrimidine nucleoside analogues idoxuridine and cytosine arabinoside. These agents inhibit both cellular and viral DNA replication in vivo as well as in vitro. Because of their toxic effect on dividing cells, these agents commonly produced hair loss, defects in intestinal mucosa and, most important, relative inhibition of bone marrow function, which produced profound leukopenia in some patients. While sporadic case reports suggested that these agents had a beneficial effect, controlled studies indicated that they were ineffective in inhibiting replication of viruses in the setting of severe toxicity (25).

Adenine arabinoside, a purine nucleoside, then was tried as a therapeutic agent for DNA viral infections in general and, more specifically, for herpes simplex encephalitis. Adenine arabinoside is given in a continuous IV infusion of 15 mg/kg/day, usually over a 12-hour period. At this dosage, the side effects seen with the previously used DNA antagonists are reduced. A double-blind study was performed that showed that, in 28 cases confirmed by brain biopsy, the mortality was reduced from 70% in the placebo-treated group to 28% in the group treated with adenine arabinoside. Further analysis of this small study group indicated that early therapy was mandatory, since patients treated after they had developed coma either died or had severe neurologic sequelae, whereas those treated before onset of coma were more likely to recover completely or at least obtain a beneficial effect (26). Adenine arabinoside has since been licensed for commercial distribution under the name of Vira-A (Parke-Davis, Morris Plains, N.J.).

Adenine arabinoside also has been used to treat herpes zoster infections in immunosuppressed patients with dissemination of disease, including invasion of the CNS. Double-blind studies have shown that herpes zoster lesions heal more rapidly with therapy with adenine arabinoside, and it is possible that such therapy can reduce or prevent dissemination and severe neurologic sequelae (27).

Postexposure Prophylaxis for Rabies

The three hallmarks of successful postexposure prophylaxis for rabies are local cleansing of the wound, passive immunization, and stimulation of an active immune response. Since certain risks are involved in each of these steps, a clear indication of need should be determined before initiation of therapy. The decision to begin postexposure prophylaxis must be made after consideration of the details of the exposure. It is important to ascertain the species of the animal involved. Among domestic animals, bites from dogs and cats usually result in a decision for treatment, although it is at least possible that other large domestic animals could accidentally be a source of virus. Wild animals are an increasing source of rabies virus in the United States; the species infected most often are skunks, foxes, raccoons, and bats. Bites from small domestic animals, such as mice, rats, hamsters, gerbils, or rabbits, almost never require rabies prophylaxis.

The second consideration is the condition of the animal, especially its behavior, at the time of bite. The third consideration is the circumstances at the time of exposure to the animal. Was the animal provoked or was the attack spontaneous? The animal's status with regard to rabies vaccination should be ascertained, and the epizootic occurrence of rabies in the area should be analyzed. Even when all these considerations have been entertained, it still may be important to proceed with postexposure prophylaxis, since recent cases of rabies in the United States were not recognized when the patient was still alive, and they occurred in persons who, at time of acute illness, were unable to give a history of exposure and who came from areas where few cases of animal rabies had been reported in previous months or years.

Local cleansing of the wound with soap and water is exceedingly important and should be done as soon as possible after exposure. If the bite was from a domestic animal, the animal should be captured at this time and quarantined for an eight- to 10-day observation period. In the case of an attack by a wild animal, an unknown domestic animal, or a domestic animal exhibiting odd behavior, passive prophylaxis should be undertaken next. Human rabies immune globulin (HRIG) is now available and should be used whenever possible. The dose is 20 international units/kg of body weight, half of which is administered around the wound and the rest given IM. This substance produces relatively few side effects. If HRIG is not available, antirabies antiserum of equine origin must be given in a dose of 40 international units/kg. Equine serum produces serum sickness in approximately 15% of children and almost half of adults; therefore, it should be avoided if possible. In addition to serum sickness, acute anaphylaxis also may occur and should be kept in mind at the time of administration.

Active rabies immunization consists of 23 doses of duck embryo vaccine (DEV), which consists of killed fixed rabies grown in duck embryo cells. DEV is given in 21 doses on 21 consecutive days, or twice a day for seven days (14 doses) and then once a day for seven more days. Booster doses should be given on the tenth and twentieth days after the last dose of the consecutive series; after the booster doses, the patient's serum should be tested for the presence of antirabies antibody. If antibody is not present, further booster doses are required. DEV usually is administered subcutaneously in the abdominal wall, buttocks, and lateral thighs. Almost always there are paresthesias and painful indurations at the injection sites, and anaphylactic reactions to products of duck eggs may occur. Recently a rabies vaccine produced in human diploid cells has been licensed and should be used if available.

Persons who are exposed to animals frequently (e.g., veterinarians, animal handlers, forestry personnel in areas of high rabies incidence) should receive preexposure prophylaxis. Two doses of DEV given subcutaneously one month apart followed by a booster six or seven months later is recommended. Neutralizing antibody develops in approximately 85% of persons on such a regimen.

Therapy for Slow Virus Infections

Three slow virus infections of the CNS caused by conventional viruses are now recognized in humans. These are SSPE, which is caused by measles virus; PRP, which is caused by rubella virus; and PML, which is almost always caused by the JC strain of papova virus. PML is an opportunistic infection that occurs primarily in patients with drug- or neoplasia-induced immunosuppression. A specific immunologic defect has not been recognized in either SSPE or PRP. Another disease, subacute measles encephalitis (SME) (28), has also been recognized recently as a slow opportunistic infection in immunosuppressed patients.

Since SSPE, PRP, and SME are all produced by RNA viruses, specific antiviral therapy is not available for treatment at present. However, several attempts have been made to stimulate host immunity in patients with these conditions. Therapies have included treatment with TF derived from lymphocytes of measles-immune patients and with several drugs (isoprinosine, tilorone) that nonspecifically enhance immunologic reactivity. Except for isolated, unconfirmed reports, these methods of therapy have not been successful. PML is produced by a small DNA virus, and experimental therapy has included the use of chemical inhibitors of DNA metabolism. In one biopsy-proved case (29), cytosine arabinoside given IV and intrathecally apparently led to remission of the disease; however, this type of treatment was unsuccessful in a number of other cases. In two additional cases of PML, treatment with adenine arabinoside was completely ineffective (30). The use of tilorone nonspecifically to enhance immunologic reactivity also has been attempted in one case. This type of therapy seemed to have led to remission of the disease (31).

REFERENCES

1. Nankervis GA: Bacterial meningitis. Med Clin North Am 58:581–592, 1974.
2. Feigin RD, Dodge PR: Bacterial meningitis: new concepts of pathophysiology and neurologic sequelae. Pediatr Clin North Am 23:541–556, 1976.
3. McCracken GH Jr: Rapid identification of specific etiology in meningitis. J Pediatr 88:706–708, 1976.
4. McCracken GH Jr: Neonatal septicemia and meningitis. Hosp Prac 10:89–97, 1976.
5. McCracken GH Jr, Feldman WE: Editorial comment. J Pediatr 89:203–204, 1976.
6. Haslam RH, Allen JR, Dorsen MM, et al: The sequelae of group B hemolytic streptococcal meningitis in early infancy. Am J Dis Child 131:845–849, 1977.
7. Overturf GD, Steinberg EA, Underman AE: Comparative trial of carbenicillin and ampicillin therapy for purulent meningitis. Antimicrob Agents Chemother 11:420–426, 1977.
8. Meade RH III: Streptomycin and sulfisoxazole for treatment of *Haemophilus influenzae* meningitis. JAMA 239:324–327, 1978.
9. Tugwell P, Greenwood EM, Warrell DA: Pneumococcal meningitis: a clinical and laboratory study. Q J Med 45:583–601, 1976.
10. Lavetter A, Leedom JM, Mathiew AW Jr, et al: Meningitis due to *Listeria monocytogenes:* a review of 25 cases. N Engl J Med 285:598–603, 1971.
11. Syphilis—CDC recommended treatment schedules, 1976. Morbid Mortal Weekly Rep 25:101–108, 1976.
12. Diamond RD, Bennett JE: Prognostic factors in cryptococcal meningitis: a study in 111 cases. Ann Intern Med 80:176–181, 1974.
13. Bennett JE: Chemotherapy of systemic mycoses. N Engl J Med 290:30–31, 1974.
14. Hermans PR: Antifungal agents used for deep-seated mycotic infections. Mayo Clin Proc 52:687–693, 1977.
15. Zivin JA: Lateral cervical puncture: an alternative to lumbar puncture. Neurology 28:616–618, 1978.

16. Alazraki NP, Fierer J, Halpern SE, et al: Use of a hyperbaric solution for administration of intrathecal amphotericin B. N Engl J Med 290:641–646, 1974.
17. Deresinski SC, Lilly RB, Levine HB, et al: Treatment of fungal meningitis with miconazole. Arch Intern Med 137:1180–1184, 1977.
18. Frenkel JK: Toxoplasma in and around us. BioScience 23:343–351, 1973.
19. Townsend JJ, Wolinsky JS, Baringer JR, et al: Acquired toxoplasmosis: a neglected cause of treatable nervous system disease. Arch Neurol 32:335–343, 1975.
20. Feldman HA: Toxoplasmosis. N Engl J Med 279:1370–1375, 1968.
21. Nightingale EO: Recommendations for a national policy on poliomyelitis vaccination. N Engl J Med 297:249–253, 1977.
22. Measles prevention. Morbid Mortal Weekly Rep 27:427–436, 1978.
23. Meyers JD, Witte JJ: Zoster-immune globulin in high-risk children. J Infect Dis 129:616–618, 1974.
24. Baringer JR: Herpes simplex virus infection of nervous tissue in animals and man. Prog Med Virol 20:1–26, 1975.
25. Boston Interhospital Virus Study Group and the NIAID-Sponsored Cooperative Antiviral Clinical Study: Failure of high-dose 5-iodo-2′-deoxyuridine in the therapy of herpes simplex virus encephalitis: evidence of unacceptable toxicity. N Engl J Med 292:599–603, 1975.
26. Whitley RJ, Soong SJ, Dolin R, et al: Adenine arabinoside therapy of biopsy-proved herpes simplex encephalitis. N Engl J Med 297:289–294, 1977.
27. Whitley RJ, Ch'ien LT, Dolin R, et al: Adenine arabinoside therapy of herpes zoster in the immunosuppressed. N Engl J Med 294:1193–1199, 1976.
28. Wolinsky JS, Swoveland P, Johnson KP, et al: Subacute measles encephalitis complicating Hodgkin's disease in an adult. Ann Neurol 1:452–457, 1977.
29. Bauer WR, Turel AP Jr, Johnson KP: Progressive multifocal leukoencephalopathy and cytarabine. JAMA 226:174–176, 1973.
30. Rand KH, Johnson KP, Rubenstein LJ, et al: Adenine arabinoside in the treatment of progressive multifocal leukoencephalopathy. Use of virus containing cells in the urine to assess response to therapy. Ann Neurol 1:456–462, 1977.
31. Selhorst JB, Ducy KF, Thomas JM, et al: PML: remission and immunologic reversals. Neurology 28:337, 1978.

4
Treatment of Dementia in Adults

Herbert R. Karp

Dementia, a deterioration or loss of intellectual function, is a manifestation of diffuse disease of the central nervous system (CNS). It often occurs in association with a systemic disease of known etiology that has pathogenic significance in relation to the dementing process. In other instances the dementia may be the result of a process of known or postulated etiology that affects the CNS either primarily or exclusively. Other dementing illnesses that affect mainly the CNS are of unknown etiology as yet. The treatment of a demented patient must be based on a correlation of the underlying pathologic changes in the brain with the clinical manifestations. This task is complicated by the fact that adult patients with dementia often have coexisting pathologic processes that by themselves may not have a direct role in the loss of intellectual function. In addition, some pathologic changes seen in the brains of demented patients are similar to those seen in elderly patients without dementia and differ in degree only.

Table 1 is a classification of dementia based on etiologic factors. In illnesses of known etiology, specific forms of treatment or prevention are available. Dementing processes of unknown etiology demand important general measures of management. In addition, there are several cardinal principles of therapy that apply equally to all patients with dementia:

1. When the brain is affected by any generalized process, it is more vulnerable to metabolic and toxic insults, including fever. Thus, careful attention must be paid to adequate respiratory function, cardiac output, fluid and electrolyte balance, and coexisting infection or other causes of fever.
2. The demented patient virtually always has problems with perception and is prone to agitation and confusion when in a strange environment or one in which sensory input is reduced. Recruiting a member of the family to sit with a patient or improving the illumination in the patient's room is often dramatically effective in restoring function. Whenever possible, demented patients are managed best in a familiar environment rather than in an extended care facility, regardless of the quality of the facility (1).
3. The effects of sedatives, tranquilizers, and antidepressant drugs on the diseased brain are unpredictable and often parodixic. Such medications may be

Table 1. Classification of Dementia in Relation to Etiologic Factors

- Dementia associated with systemic disease of pathogenetic significance
  - Multi-infarct dementia
  - Subacute combined degeneration
  - Avitaminosis (nutritional)
  - Inflammatory vascular disease
  - Remote effects of neoplasm
  - Metabolic encephalopathies
    - Dialysis dementia
    - Chronic hypoventilation
    - Uremia
    - Hypothyroidism
    - Liver
- Dementia associated with primary CNS disease of known or postulated etiology
  - Parenchymal infection
    - Viral, including PML and Jakob–Creutzfeldt disease
    - Syphilis
    - Abscess
  - Meningitis
    - Pyogenic
    - Granulomatous
    - Carcinomatous
  - Hydrocephalus dementia
  - Trauma
- Dementia associated with primary CNS disease of unknown etiology
  - Degenerative diseases
    - Alzheimer's disease (presenile dementia)
    - Pick's disease
    - Parkinson's disease
    - Progressive supranuclear palsy
  - Heredodegenerative diseases
    - Myoclonus epilepsy
    - Huntington's chorea
    - Spinocerebellar degeneration

helpful but should be used with restraint and extreme caution. General guidelines for the use of medications to relieve anxiety, improve mood, control psychotic symptoms and harmful behavior, and improve sleep are reviewed by Wells (2).

4. The aging patient, with or without dementia, who requires drugs for management of coexisting medical conditions often presents special problems with regard to drug interaction. These and other problems of the clinical pharmacology in the aged are reviewed by Bender (3).
5. Early in the course of dementia, patients frequently have insight into the fact that their intellectual function is failing. This can be devastating and can lead to profound depression and withdrawal, resulting in further limitation on intellectual function. It is at this stage that simple counseling of the patient and, more important, the family and associates can lead to restructuring of the patient's pattern of daily living so that fewer demands are made on the patient's failing function.
6. In the course of extensive evaluation of the patient to find a treatable cause of dementia, the needs of the family frequently are disregarded. A realistic assessment and prognosis are absolutely essential so that the family can make definite plans and be as supportive as possible to the patient.

Management of patients with dementia is most effective when the dementia and any associated general diseases have been identified accurately. With the advent of noninvasive diagnostic techniques, such as computerized tomography, evaluation can be done with a thoroughness that was not possible in the recent past. However, analysis of the dementing illness still depends on an orderly clinical approach.

Since demented patients are, by the very nature of their illness, unreliable observers, the history must be obtained from a qualified party, such as a family member, neighbor, or employer. In order to differentiate between the various forms of dementia, it is essential to determine the earliest manifestations of the illness and document its progression. All aspects of memory are involved in the course of dementia, in the early phase of the illness the nature of the memory loss and its relation to other cognitive functions can define the nature of the dementia. For example, loss of recent memory with relative preservation of remote memory and the ability to use stored information to solve problems is characteristic of an axial or limbic dementia, as is seen in patients with Wernicke–Korsakow disease. In contrast, impaired recent and remote memory with more prominent difficulty in problem solving and other cognitive functions is characteristic of cortical dementia, such as Alzheimer's disease. The attending physician usually can make this differentiation at the bedside by obtaining an accurate history and by adapting standard examinations of mental status to the patient's cultural and educational background.

Once the nature of the dementia has been determined, it is necessary to establish the qualitative and temporal relation of other neurologic findings to the dementing illness. Multiple episodes of acute, focal, cumulative neurologic deficits over months or years that culminate in dementia is characteristic of multi-infarct dementia. Progressive dementia over a similar period without focal deficits or with such deficits in the later stages is seen in Alzheimer's disease. In addition, workup of all patients with dementia must include a thorough search for associated systemic diseases.

By following these simple principles, the attending physician can make intelligent use of the laboratory for confirmatory data. This approach is summarized in the diagram:

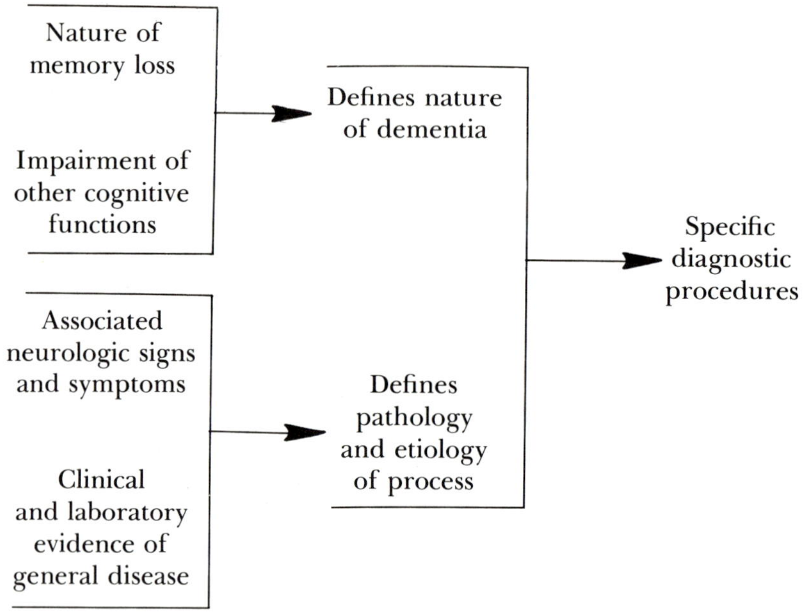

DEMENTIAS ASSOCIATED WITH SYSTEMIC DISEASE OF PATHOGENETIC SIGNIFICANCE

Multi-infarct Dementia

Multi-infarct dementia is a result of multiple infarctions in the distribution of small penetrating branches of major cerebral arteries. It is associated with the lacunar state (4). The infarctions are secondary to fibrinoid degeneration and to proliferation of small arteries secondary to hypertension.

The essential clinical features are bipyramidal disease (rigidity, increased deep-tendon reflexes, extensor plantar responses, pseudobulbar palsy, emotional lability). These signs are the culmination of a series of episodes of sudden neurologic deficit. As the number of episodes increases, the patient shows signs of progressive dementia.

There is no evidence that treatment of the hypertension has a beneficial effect on the lacunar state once the patient reaches the dementia stage. However, this form of dementia can effectively be prevented through early detection and treatment of hypertension.

Subacute Combined Degeneration

The dementia of subacute combined degeneration is usually seen in the company of symptoms and signs of posterolateral spinal cord disease and the hematologic manifestations of Addisonian anemia. However, mental and psychiatric disorders that occur alone or precede hematologic or other neurologic findings have been described (5).

In instances of pernicious anemia or other causes of vitamin B12 deficiency, appropriate therapy usually restores the blood to normal and, in most instances, controls the progression of changes in the nervous system. Although there may be an increase in reticulocytes within 48 hours after the start of therapy, the neurologic aspects do not change as quickly. Depending on their severity and duration these aspects may persist even after complete remission of the hematologic manifestations (6). In patients with CNS involvement, intramuscular (IM) injections of vitamin B12, 50 μg/day for two weeks, followed by 100 μg twice a week for eight weeks and then 100 μg monthly for life is recommended.

Dementia occasionally may be seen with folate deficiency, which also occurs in the company of megaloblastic anemia. Patients with folate deficiency should receive 20 mg folic acid per day and continue to receive 1–5 mg/day (7).

Nutritional Dementia

The principal forms of nutritional dementia are seen in patients with Wernicke–Korsakow syndrome or pellagra. Wernicke–Korsakow syndrome consists of acute onset of disturbances of eye movement, ataxia, global confusion combined with an amnestic dementia in which the defect in recent memory is disproportionate to the loss of other cognitive function. Although this condition is seen most often in alcoholics who are severely malnourished it also may be seen in any nutritionally deprived patient. Acute experiments have demonstrated clearly that the disturbances of eye movement, the acute confusion, and, to a lesser extent, the ataxia respond specifically to the administration of thiamine. The amnestic dementia is less responsive to treatment (8).

Nutritional dementia is regarded generally as a medical emergency and, once it is recognized, should be treated immediately with 50 mg thiamine intravenously (IV) and 50 mg IM. The IM dose should be repeated each day until the patient is able to resume a normal diet. The appropriate use of thiamine most often prevents progression of this aspect of the disease and may reverse many of the deficits (9). Since the patient is usually deficient in all the B vitamins, long-term management should include a balanced diet supplemented by these vitamins.

Improvement of the amnestic dementia is not immediate and is usually less complete than the recovery of eye movement and coordination. It should be emphasized, however, that partial recovery from the dementia does occur. Victor et al. (10) point out that the use of glucose or other forms of IV alimentation to treat any severely malnourished patient must always be supplemented with B vitamins; this is particularly important in alcoholics because they tend to eat foods that are low in B vitamins and high in carbohydrates, which may exhaust their existing stores of thiamine. For patients in this state, additional carbohydrates in the form of parenteral glucose may precipitate the onset of acute Wernicke's encephalopathy. Therefore, it is recommended that large doses of B vitamins be administered to all patients with disorders associated with alcohol (e.g., delirium tremens) who require parenteral glucose, even though the alcoholic-related disorder is not primarily caused by vitamin deficiency.

Pellagra, which at one time was seen in epidemic proportions in the United States, has become extremely rare as a result of the fortification of bread and cereals with vitamins. Initially, it was believed that pellagra resulted from only a deficiency of nicotinic acid. Now it is apparent that the disease also can result from a deficiency of tryptophan, the amino acid that is the precursor of nicotinic acid.

The physical signs of pellagra are highly suggestive but not necessarily diagnostic. Classically, pellagra is manifested by the "four Ds": diarrhea, dermatitis, dementia, and death. In incipient cases, skin manifestations may not be present. Neurologic signs usually appear during the phase of the disease when the skin and the gastrointestinal manifestations are very apparent. Although the neurologic findings are not specific for pellagra, the disease should be suspected in the setting of the appropriate dietary deficiency. The fasting concentration of free tryptophan in plasma of patients with pellegra has been reported to be low (11). Since pyridoxine is essential for the conversion of tryptophan to nicotinic acid, a disease state similar to pellagra may be seen in patients who receive isoniazid for the treatment of tuberculosis.

Treatment of pellagra consists of correction of water and electrolyte deficiencies and of oral administration of niacinamide, 200 mg three times a day until the acute symptoms have subsided. Niacinamide is recommended because it is free from the vasomotor effects of nicotinic acid. Occasionally it is necessary to give niacinamide IV. Since the patient with pellagra is frequently generally malnourished, other B vitamins should be given in therapeutic amounts. Demented patients usually become rational within a week unless irreversible brain damage has occurred. The polyneuritis that often is seen in this disease responds more slowly.

Systemic Lupus Erythematosus and Inflammatory Vascular Disease

Systemic lupus erythematosus very frequently involves the nervous system (12). Though CNS involvement is often seen terminally in the form of intracerebral hemorrhage or status epilepticus, it also may occur early in the disease. Convulsive disorders, dementia, and cranial neuropathies are the most common neurologic manifestations and are thought to be related to the microinfarcts that occur in the cerebral cortex and brain stem. The role of adrenocorticosteroids in the management of the neurologic manifestations remains uncertain. Some investigators consider CNS involvement to be an indication for the use of relatively high doses of corticosteroids (2 mg prednisone or prednisolone/kg body weight), with the dosage tapered and maintained at levels to control symptoms. Symptoms frequently can be controlled with 10 mg prednisone/day. Disturbances in behavior and mental function are sometimes difficult to evaluate because they may be related to the steroid therapy. If an increase in steroid dosage decreases the neurologic symptoms, then it is likely that the symptoms were due to the CNS involvement resulting from systemic erythematosus rather than to the medications.

Other vasculitides, such as polyarteritis nodosum, allergic granulomatosis, Wegener's granulomatosis, and hypersensitivity vasculitis, are less likely to involve the nervous system. Giant-cell arteritis, however, frequently involves the major branches of the aorta, including the vetebral and carotid arteries, both external and internal. Disorders of intellectual function are rare, however. Fortunately, patients with this disease respond well to relatively low doses of steroids (e.g., 30–40 mg prednisone/day). This dosage can be reduced gradually, and the patient can be maintained with 10 mg/day for an extended period.

Remote Effects of Neoplasm

Dementia has been described as one of the remote effects of carcinoma (13). Though the dementia assciated with carcinoma has been varied, it has been suggested that it is seen most frequently in patients who also had parenchymatous cerebellar degeneration. Removal of the primary neoplasm, usually located in the lungs, ovary, or breast, has resulted in some improvement in the dementia.

Metabolic Encephalopathies

The derangements of mental function seen in metabolic disorders are characterized primarily by changes in level of consciousness and behavior. Agitated confusion (delirium) is the most frequent manifestation. However, dementia, in the sense that the term is used in this chapter, may occur, particularly if the metabolic abnormality is chronic and insidiously progressive.

Progressive Dialysis Encephalopathy

Progressive dialysis encephalopathy and peripheral neuropathy are the most prominent neurologic complications of chronic dialysis. Dialysis dementia consists of intellectual impairment, stuttering, myoclonic jerks, seizures, and a characteristic electroencephalogram (EEG). Patients may complain of difficulty in concentration, reduction of attention span, and poor memory as the initial manifestations of declining intellect. As the dementing process continues it becomes global and quite severe. In its early stages, dialysis dementia usually is mild. The most characteristic abnormality is the problem with speech, which is described as hesitant, stuttering, and nonfluent. Though some workers have considered the speech abnormality to be a speech dyspraxia or dysphasia, the consensus is that it is more properly regarded as dysarthria. The EEG always shows some type of sharp or spike and slow wave activity that is paroxysmal, usually bilateral, and present either during sleep or while the patient is awake.

The current speculation regarding the pathogenesis of dialysis encephalopathy centers primarily on the role of aluminum and is based on observations of increased amounts of aluminum in the gray matter of patients with dialysis dementia. It is postulated that the excess aluminum may derive from aluminum hydroxide administered in an effort to control osteoporosis and metastatic calcification through reduction of concentrations of serum phosphate.

Another source is the excessive amounts of aluminum in tap water used for the dialysate. Additional evidence implicating aluminum is the fact that a syndrome similar to progressive dialysis encephalopathy has been reported in one patient exposed to aluminum dust.

The clinical manifestations characteristically are the worst at the end of dialysis and decrease in severity before the next dialysis is begun. There has been no apparent difference in dialysis technique, duration of dialysis, diet, serum electrolytes, creatinine, urea, or acid-base balance of patients with or without the syndrome. The hypophosphatemia induced also has been investigated and does not appear to be significant with regard to neurologic manifestations.

Treatment modalities have included increasing the frequency of dialysis, the use of corticosteroids, physostigmine, rubidium, British antilewisite, penicillamine, vitamins (including pyridoxine), and anticonvulsants (14). Favorable results in suppression of the speech difficulty and myoclonus in some patients have been reported with diazepam (15). Renal transplantation has been used as a therapeutic alternative to dialysis for patients with encephalopathy. However, there have been reports of patients who have failed to improve after successful renal transplantation. Other patients have been known to develop typical clinical and EEG findings after successful transplantation of an organ from a cadaver.

Chronic Hypoventilation

A characteristic encephalopathic picture is seen in patients with chronic hypoventilation, whether the condition be idiopathic or associated with obesity (Pickwickian syndrome). Patients experience reduced consciousness, diffuse muscle twitching, asterixis, and periodic respirations, most often the Cheyne–Stokes type. There also may be increased intracranial pressure with papilledema; this manifestation is thought to be related to increased cerebral blood flow secondary to hypoxia and hypercapnia. The encephalopathy can often be precipitated or markedly worsened by the use of sedative drugs.

Appropriate management of the encephalopathy of chronic hypoventilation consists initially of determining the reason for the impaired ventilation and beginning of appropriate corrective measures. In correcting the metabolic abnormalities it should be noted that, with the long-term retention of CO_2, the respiratory center becomes "reset" at a higher arterial P_{CO_2}. As a result, the medullary chemoreceptors may not be able to alter respiratory drive in spite of the elevated level of CO_2. Thus, the main stimulus for ventilation may be the arterial hypoxemia mediated by the peripheral chemoreceptors. Therefore, the injudicious administration of oxygen to correct the hypoxemia may lead to complete cessation of ventilation. This is followed by a further rise in P_{CO_2}, which may suppress ventilation further and also depress consciousness through its narcotic effect. This potentially catastrophic situation should be avoided through careful control of the O_2 concentrations at 24–28% and then close observation of the patient for retention of CO_2.

Uremic Encephalopathy

Nonspecific mental dullness, reduced ability to concentrate, and depressed consciousness are features of uremia. Although they frequently are associated with advanced uremia, they may be seen occasionally in patients who have only marginally elevated levels of blood urea nitrogen (BUN) on the basis of such correctable lesions as obstructive uropathy. In severe cases, hyponatremia, acidosis, and dehydration may lead to coma, which often can be reversed when the metabolic abnormalities are appropriately managed. Dementia of various degrees, depressed consciousness, myoclonic jerks, heightened neuromuscular irritability, and asterixis should alert the attending physician to the possibility that the patient's altered mental function may be due to uremia. The uremia should be treated by appropriate means, either medically or surgically. The myoclonic jerks and asterixis frequently are misinterpreted as being seizures, and patients are inappropriately treated with anticonvulsants. This can result in worsening of the neurologic manifestations.

Hypothyroidism

The alterations and mental functions associated with hypothyroidism are quite variable and usually are overshadowed by the somatic manifestations of decreased thyroid function. Nonetheless, it should be noted that permanent impairment of mental function has been reported in patients with untreated hypothyroidism. Appropriate treatment consists of the use of either of the synthetic hormones levothyroxine or liothyronine, or of liotrix (the latter is a combination of levothyroxine and liothyronine). The average daily dose for the preparations are levothyroxine, 200 μg; liothyronine, 50 μg; and liotrix, 2 units. In addition, thyroid extract of natural origin can be given in doses of 120–180 mg/day. It is recommended that restoration to the normal metabolic state should be accomplished gradually, especially in elderly patients. The optimal dosages should be based on individual clinical responses, with laboratory determinations as confirmatory tests.

Hepatic Encephalopathy

The essential elements of hepatic encephalopathy include depressed consciousness, altered intellectual function, asterixis, and EEG abnormalities. The disorder may be encountered in association with a variety of diseases that affect the liver parenchyma. It also may be seen as a complication of portal-systemic shunting. The neurologic picture is similar to that of other metabolic encephalopathies, such as chronic hypoventilation and uremia.

No single pathogenetic factor for hepatic encephalopathy has been determined. Many patients with the disease have elevated blood levels of ammonia, but substances other than ammonia probably play a role.

Patients with the chronic or recurring form of this syndrome have enlargements of protoplasmic astrocytes in the basal ganglia and the subcortical white matter. Long-standing severe hepatic encephalopathy may eventuate in non-Wilsonian hepatolenticular degeneration.

The hallmarks of treatment of hepatic encephalopathy are early recognition and prompt management. In an effort to reduce blood levels of ammonia and other postulated toxic nitrogenous substances, protein should be excluded from the diet for three to five days. As the patient improves, it may be reintroduced in increments of 10–20 g every two to four days. Laxatives should be given in order to evacuate the contents of the large bowel, which is a source of nitrogenous substances. Neomycin in oral doses of 6–12 g/day decreases the intestinal production and absorption of ammonia. It is known that respiratory alkalosis, hyponatremia, hypokalemia, anemia, infections, and hypoglycemia may potentiate the coma of hepatic encephalopathy. Therefore, these abnormalities should be corrected.

Chronic or episodic and recurrent hepatic encephalopathy may be treated effectively by protein restriction (30–40 g/day) and 2–4 g neomycin/day. Lactulose, in a concentration of 65 g/100 ml, can be given in doses of 25–30 mg three times a day. It is reported that the use of lactulose lessens the requirement for both protein restriction and neomycin, supposedly by lowering fecal pH and thus decreasing absorption of ammonia. In some instances, ileosigmoidostomy and colonic exclusion have been effective. Occasionally, in severe instances of acute hepatic coma, measures such as exchange blood transfusion, hemodialysis, plasma exchange, extracorporeal pig-liver profusion, and liver homotransplantation have been tried. L-Dopa has been reported to produce temporary improvement of neurologic function. The reader is referred to an excellent summary of hepatic encephalopathy (16).

DEMENTIA ASSOCIATED WITH PRIMARY CNS DISEASES OF KNOWN OR POSTULATED ETIOLOGY

Viral Encephalitis

Many viruses are known to affect the nervous system and produce a wide variety of clinical manifestations. Typically the disease is of gradual onset with nonspecific prodromal symptoms that most often include headache, mild fever, and other systemic manifestations, such as upper respiratory or gastrointestinal infection. Involvement of the CNS becomes apparent in altered levels of wakefulness, either restlessness or drowsiness. At this stage there is often neck stiffness, and a lumbar puncture reveals a mild increase in mononuclear cells, elevated protein, and normal glucose in the CSF. Treatment during this phase of the illness is nonspecific and consists primarily of bed rest and medications to control the patient's restlessness, malaise, and headache. Analgesics and sedatives should be used cautiously in order to avoid further depression of the level of consciousness, since this might give the false impression of progression of the primary illness.

Other viral encephalitides may produce a more fulminating form of disease that may last hours to several days. The treatment of the general aspects of this form of illness are discussed in chapter 3.

Herpes simplex encephalitis, with its predilection for involvement of the cortex and the white matter of the temporal lobes, may result in striking dementia, in either the acute or the chronic phase of the illness. Recent controlled clinical studies indicate that adenine arabinoside has reduced the mortality of encephalitis caused by herpes simplex. The effect of this medication on the morbidity and sequelae of herpes simplex is less well established. Adenine arabinoside has been shown to have antiviral activity against types I and II herpes simplex virus both in vitro and in vivo.

Adenine arabinoside has recently been released for general clinical use. Beneficial clinical effects are more likely to be seen if the medication is given early in the course of the illness. The recommended dosage is 15 mg/kg body weight per day for 10 days. The drug should be infused slowly IV over 12–24 hours. The principal adverse reactions involve the gastrointestinal tract, are relatively mild, and seldom require termination of therapy. Other, more serious reactions include mild depression of bone marrow production. Interferon, interferon inducers, and transfer factor have not been shown to have a beneficial effect. Cerebral edema is seen frequently in the acute phases of this illness and may require the use of osmotic agents. Unfortunately, successful management of patients with herpes simplex encephalitis is likely to lead to an increased number of survivors with severe dementia as their primary residual deficit.

Progressive multifocal leukoencephalopathy in patients with lymphoma, leukemia, or other illnesses characterized by abnormal immunologic responses may be associated with dementia. The presence of viral particles in the nuclei of oligodendroglia and the recovery of virus in proved cases has clearly established the viral etiology of this illness. There is one report of rather dramatic, but unfortunately temporary, improvement with the use of cytosine arabinoside (17).

Jakob-Creutzfeldt disease is a subacute, spongiform virus encephalopathy that is now clearly established to be a transmissible viral dementia. To date, however, none of the antiviral agents has been shown to have a beneficial effect on the course of this illness.

Dementia in Hydrocephalus

The classic triad of this disorder is dementia, disturbance of gait, and urinary incontinence. The illness characteristically has an indefinite onset, which, in some instances, consists of mild dementia with impairment of memory, slowness of mental and physical activity, lack of spontaneity, and easy distractibility. Unsteadiness of gait and urinary incontinence may appear later. In other instances, the gait disturbances may appear first. In most cases, the etiologic factors leading to hydrocephalus are unknown. Known causes include subarachnoid hemorrhage, cerebral trauma with subarachnoid hemorrhage, chronic meningeal infections (e.g., tuberculosis, cryptococcosis, parasitic infections). The principal pathogenetic factor is fibrosis of the leptomeninges, particularly at the incisura of the tentorium, that leads to communication of hydrocephalus and its neurologic manifestations.

Although the initial enthusiasm regarding the entity of dementia is hydrocephalus and the optimistic reports of its treatment have waned somewhat, treatment with various CSF shunting procedures has resulted in improvement for some patients. It remains important to be aware of this syndrome and the possibilities for recovery or improvement with shunting. Favorable response is more likely to be seen in patients whose hydrocephalus is secondary to a known cause. In reporting data from the literature and from personal experience, Katzman (18) found the overall incidence of positive response was much higher in patients with secondary form (64.7%) than in those with idiopathic forms (40.9%). Improvement in patients with ventricular enlargement of unknown etiology is generally slight but is best in those who have a disturbance in gait in addition to dementia. It is believed that patients with the classic syndromes including gait disturbance, dementia, with or without urinary incontinence should be considered for shunt therapy. The fact remains, however, that the frequency of a favorable response with idiopathic hydrocephalus dementia is quite low (19).

Mortality after various shunt procedures was 6–9%, and the occurrence of epidural and subdural hematoma was more than 5%. The incidence of other shunt-related complications was more than 40%. In view of the relatively high frequency of complications, some centers are exploring the alternative route of a lumbar-peritoneal shunt. The advantages of this procedure over either a ventriculoatrial or ventriculoperitoneal shunt have not yet been demonstrated. The lumbar-peritoneal shunt has the disadvantage of not being accessible for evaluation and revision if necessary.

Syphilis

Dementia may be a prominent manifestation of CNS syphilis, particularly in paretic neurosyphilis (syphilitic meningoencephalitis). In the early phase of this illness, failing memory, impaired problem-solving ability, and altered personal behavior may be the only symptoms. The underlying pathology consists of thickening of the meninges and cerebral atrophy. In addition, the inflammatory process also affects the ependyma with granular ependymitis, which often leads to hydrocephalus and an aggravation of the dementia.

Penicillin remains the treatment of choice for all varieties of neurosyphilis, including paresis. The treatment recommended by the National Communicable Disease Center Syphilis Therapy Advisory Committee for Central Nervous System Syphilis is aqueous procaine penicillin G, 600,000 units/day IM for 14 days, or aqueous penicillin G, 12–24 million units/day IV for at least 10 days. In patients with penicillin allergy, erythromycin base, stearate, or ethylsuccinate, 2 g/day for 30 days, or tetracycline hydrochloride, 2 g/day for 30 days, may be given.

It would seem logical to manage progressive hydrocephalus in a fashion similar to that for hydrocephalus dementia. However, there is insufficient experience with this form of management of neurosyphilis to make specific recommendations.

It is recommended that the CSF be reexamined six months after therapy ends. Disappearance of cells and a return of protein levels toward normal indicate a favorable response. The serologic test may remain positive, although titers will be decreased. Persistent, weakly positive serologic tests with normal cells and protein levels is not an indication for further treatment.

Brain Abscess

Early in the course of a pyogenic infection of the brain parenchyma, (the stage of so-called pyogenic cerebritis) or later, when a definite localized abscess occurs, dementia is seen occasionally as a prominent clinical manifestation. The treatment of brain abscess is discussed in Chapter 3.

Meningitis

Although pyogenic meningitis is primarily a disease of the meninges, it does involve cortical neurons to the degree that brain function is altered. Granulomatous meningeal infections, such as tuberculous or fungal infections, are more likely to produce dementia by virtue of their slowly progressive, insidious course and their tendency to affect the basilar meninges; this situation leads to communicating hydrocephalus and dementia. The same pathogenic factors may apply to carcinomatous meningitis. The reader is reminded, however, that treatment of the dementia may require a shunting procedure, and the fact that the underlying process is infectious does not contraindicate the use of these procedures.

Trauma

Trauma to the CNS may produce dementia as a result of focal lesions, particularly those with bilateral involvement of the temporal lobes or that result from communicating hydrocephalus secondary to subarachnoid hemorrhage associated with acute trauma and contusion. Long-term, recurrent, relatively minor head trauma such as might be seen in professional boxers may result in dementia (dementia pugilistica). Logically, the most effective means of treatment of each of these conditions is prevention. Treatment of hydrocephalus dementia following head trauma can often lead to dramatic restitution of intellectual function and should always be considered in a patient whose dementia is related to head trauma.

DEMENTIA ASSOCIATED WITH PRIMARY CNS DISEASES OF UNKNOWN ETIOLOGY

Alzheimer's Disease

Alzheimer's disease is the most frequent of all dementing illnesses. It is an insidiously progressive dementing process that produces prominent defects in memory and problem solving. Focal signs, if seen, appear late in the course of illness. There is widespread cortical atrophy, widening of sulci, and hydrocephalus ex vacuo. The disease remains one of unknown etiology and is not associated with systemic disease.

Recent studies of Alzheimer's disease have suggested a significant reduction in cortical choline acetyltransferase. This enzyme synthesizes the putative neurotransmitter acetylcholine. A substantial reduction in its activity could be associated with loss of synaptic acetylcholine (20). There have been attempts to counter this deficiency of central acetylcholine by inhibition of the degrading system with anticholinesterase medications, or by stimulation of the synthesizing enzymes by raising the level of substrate. The use of acetylcholine has been limited by virtue of its side effects and short duration. Lecithin, a natural source of choline, has been used, as has choline. Although the results of trials of these medications to date are inconclusive, it is encouraging that a form of treatment with some logic is being investigated.

The general principles of therapy that were presented at the beginning of this chapter are particularly helpful in managing patients with Alzheimer's disease. During the early stages of the illness, anxiety and agitation may be particularly prominent and sometimes can be managed effectively with small doses of chlordiazepoxide (Librium) or diazepam (Valium). The physician should be aware that diazepam can sometimes precipitate symptoms that suggest worsening of depression. The depressed patient with Alzheimer's disease can be helped to various degrees with nortriptyline (Aventyl), imipramine (Tofranil), amitriptyline (Elavil), or doxepin (Sinequan). Since severe depressive psychosis often mimics dementia, it has been suggested that all patients suspected of being demented should be given a trial of therapy with antidepressant medication (21).

For more severe psychotic symptoms, such as paranoia, major tranquilizers such as chlorpromazine, thioridazine, or haloperidol may be useful. Parenteral chlorpromazine frequently results in postural hypotension and should be used with extreme caution.

One of the problems encountered most frequently is insomnia and nocturnal agitation. Medications with minimal sedative effects, such as diphenhydramine hydrochloride and promethazine hydrochloride often are effective. In patients who receive chlorpromazine or other major tranquilizers, sufficient sedation may be achieved by taking a dose at bedtime.

There are several reports of ventricular shunting in patients with apparent parenchymatous degeneration of the brain. Many of these patients probably had Alzheimer's disease. Salmon (22) reported 18 patients with senile and presenile dementia who were treated with a ventriculoatrial shunt. Seven of these patients showed what was considered to be moderate or marked improvement. Shenkin and co-workers (23) noted further that cisternography, measurement of the enlarged ventricles, measurement of the callosal angle, determination of the thickness of the cortical mantle and determination of whether or not air passed over the hemisphere were not helpful in distinguishing normal-pressure hydrocephalus from Alzheimer's disease. Accordingly, these authors proposed that all patients who demonstrate senile changes that consist of either organic dementia, gait disturbance, or both should be studied for possible ventricular enlargement. If enlargement of the ventricles is demonstrated, ventricular shunting is recommended.

With the advent of computed tomographic scanning and possibly valuable information from metrizamide cisternography, it is believed that the accuracy of establishing a diagnosis of hydrocephalus dementia is increased greatly. Thus, the shunting should be reserved for situations in which the procedure is definitely likely to offer benefit.

Parkinson's Disease

A large number of patients with Parkinson's disease also have significant dementia. Treatment with L-dopa and related medications has not had a significant effect on the dementia that cannot be explained by improvement in the patient's mobility (24).

Progressive Supranuclear Palsy

The attempt to treat the motor aspects of supranuclear palsy have been of questionable benefit. The dementia that is frequently associated with this syndrome is not affected significantly by any medications tried thus far.

Heredodegenerative Diseases

Myoclonic epilepsy, Huntington's chorea, and many forms of spinal cerebellar degeneration are associated with significant dementia. The general measures outlined in the discussion of the noninherited degenerative diseases are also applicable to patients with heredodegerative diseases.

REFERENCES

1. Brody EM, Kleban M, Woldow A, et al: Survival and death in mentally impaired aged. J Chronic Dis 28:389. 1975.
2. Bender AD: Pharmacological aspects of the aging: a survey of the effect of increasing age on drug activity in adults. J Am Geriatr Soc 12:114, 1964.
3. Wells CE: Diagnostic evaluation and treatment in dementia. In: *Dementia.* Edited by CE Wells, Philadelphia. FA Davis, 1977, p. 271.
4. Hachinski VC, Lassen NA, Marshal J: Multi-infarct dementia: a cause of mental deterioration in the elderly. Lancet 2:207, 1974.
5. Strachan RW, Henderson JG: Psychiatric syndromes due to avitaminosis B12 with normal blood and marrow. Q J Med 34:303, 1965.
6. Dreyfus PN: Nutritional disorders of the nervous system. In: *Textbook of Medicine.* Edited by P Beeson and W McDermott. Philadelphia, WB Saunders, 1975, p. 710.
7. Strachan RW, Henderson JG: Dementia and folic deficiency. Q J Med 36:189, 1967.
8. Victor M: Treatment of the neurologic manifestations of alcoholism. Mod Treat 3:491, 1966.
9. Victor M, Adams RD, Collins GH: The Wernicke–Korsakoff syndrome. In: *Contemporary Neurology Series,* vol. 7. Edited by F Plum and FH McDowell. Philadelphia, FA Davis, 1971, p. 65.
10. Victor M, Adams R: *Principles of Neurology,* New York, McGraw-Hill, 1977, p. 757.
11. Mann GV, Van Itallie TB: Pellagra. In: *Harrison's Principles of Internal Medicine.* Edited by GW Thorn, RD Adams, E Braunwald, et al. New York, McGraw-Hill, 1977, p. 452.
12. Johnson RT, Richardson EP: The neurologic manifestations of systemic lupus erythematosus: a clinical-pathologic study of 24 cases and a review of the literature. Medicine (Baltimore) 77:337, 1968.
13. Brain R, Henson RA: Neurological syndrome associated with carcinoma. Lancet 2:971, 1958.
14. Lederman RJ, Henry CE: Progressive dialysis encephalopathy. Ann Neurol 4:199, 1978.
15. Nadel A, Wilson W: Dialysis encephalopathy: a possible seizure disorder. Neurology 26:1130, 1976.
16. LaMont TJ, Isselbacher KJ: Cirrhosis. *Harrison's Principles of Internal Medicine.* Edited by GW Thorn, RD Adams, E Braunwald, et al. New York, McGraw-Hill, 1977, p. 1601.

17. Conomy JP, Beard NS, Matsumoto H, et al: Cytarabine (cystosine arabinoside) treatment of progressive multifocal leukoencephalopathy: clinical course and detection of viral particles after antiviral chemotherapy. JAMA 229:1313, 1974.
18. Katzman R: Normal pressure hydrocephalus in dementia. In: *Contemporary Neurology Series,* vol. 15. Edited by F Plum and FH McDowell. Philadelphia, FA Davis, 1977, p. 69.
19. Ojemann RJ, Fischer CM, Adams RD, et al: Further experience with the syndrome 'normal' pressure hydrocephalus. J Neurosurg 31:279, 1969.
20. Perry E, Perry R, Tomlinson B: Dietary lecithin supplements in dementia of Alzheimer type (letter). Lancet 2:242, 1977.
21. Snowden J: When is dementia presenile? (letter). Br Med J 2:465, 1972.
22. Salmon JH: Senile and presenile dementia: Ventriculoatrial shunt for symptomatic treatment. Geriatrics 24:67, 1969.
23. Shenkin HA, Greenburg J, Bouzarth WF, et al: Ventricular shunting for relief of senile symptoms. JAMA 225:486, 1973.
24. Sweet JD, McDowell FH, Feigenson JP, et al: Mental symptoms in Parkinson's disease during chronic treatment with levodopa. Neurology 26:305, 1976.

5
Treatment of Peripheral Neuropathies

Robert I. Roelofs

In the consideration of the treatment of polyneuropathies, it is important to consider first the anatomy and physiology of peripheral nerves and, second, the types of signs and symptoms that diseases can produce. It is the patient's symptoms plus the findings on physical examination that generally lead to the initial diagnostic impression. Subsequent laboratory tests may then be needed to confirm the diagnosis and allow appropriate treatment to begin.

The peripheral nerves serve as a conduit for the flow of information from the central nervous system (CNS) to the periphery and from the periphery back to the CNS. Most peripheral nerves have mixed functions and carry motor, sensory, and autonomic fibers. These fibers range in size from small, poorly myelinated fibers of 1.0 to 2.0 μm to large, heavily myelinated fibers of 8–12 (up to 20) μm in cross-sectional diameter. Functionally, the poorly myelinated fibers convey pain and sensation of temperature, and the large, heavily myelinated fibers convey vibrations and sense of position, and voluntary motor activity. Autonomic fibers are generally small to intermediate in size and are relatively poorly myelinated.

Different disease processes can either attack the peripheral nerves at different places or differentially affect a part or all of the peripheral nerves. Thus, while the usual symptoms of peripheral neuropathy are symmetric, distal, sensorimotor loss, with absent or decreased reflexes, variations can occur. Patients may appear initially with a predominantly sensory neuropathy, a predominantly motor neuropathy, a disassociated sensory neuropathy with pain and temperature affected disproportionately to vibratory and position sense, or with predominantly autonomic manifestations. In addition, while the most distal portion of the peripheral nerve usually is affected first, in some entities proximal nerves are involved. In temperature-sensitive neuropathies, exposed areas of nerves in the skin are affected. In some sensory neuropathies, very proximal sensory ganglia appear to be affected primarily with a combination of sensory loss and lancinating pain. While most peripheral neuropathies are characterized by a loss of function, some are characterized predominantly by irritative effects, sometimes with pain, paresthesias and dysesthesias, and, at times, continuous motor activity (for some motor neuropathies).

The diseases to be considered here can affect the peripheral nerves singly (mononeuropathy), can affect single nerves serially (mononeuropathy multiplex), or can affect multiple nerves virtually simultaneously (polyneuropathy). Differentiation among the three groups is of importance for diagnostic and therapeutic reasons.

Pathologically, the diseases may be considered to affect peripheral nerves in two major ways: predominant involvement of the myelin sheath, or predominant involvement of the axon and its contents. Disorders that result in segmental loss of myelin around the nerve fiber are less common than those that affect the axon directly. However, because myelin has the capacity to regenerate more rapidly than the axon, diseases characterized by segmental demyelination have the potential for a more rapid recovery with fewer residua than those that affect the axon predominantly.

METABOLIC NEUROPATHIES

Diabetic Neuropathy

The clinical manifestations of diabetic neuropathy vary widely. The most common neuropathy is a distal, symmetric, sensorimotor polyneuropathy. Patients experience paresthesias and dysesthesias associated with objective sensory loss. Motor weakness is usually distal and relatively mild. In some patients, the polyneuropathy is predominantly a sensory neuropathy with little or no motor component, while in others, the sensory neuropathy may take the form of a very severe, burning, painful neuropathy that is most prominent distally. With involvement of the autonomic nervous system, postural hypotension, abnormalities in bowel or bladder function, impotence, loss of sweating, and abnormal cardiac reflexes associated with changes in position may all be seen.

The second, large group of neuropathies are the mononeuropathies and mononeuropathy multiplex. These disorders may affect the cranial nerves, usually nerves III and VI, although other cranial nerves may be involved. Other large, mixed sensorimotor nerves may be involved, which leads to the sudden onset of weakness and sensory loss in the distribution of the affected nerve. Diabetic amyotrophy, or proximal diabetic neuropathy, is marked initially by pain and discomfort in the thighs and legs in association with a progressive, predominantly proximal muscle weakness and often decreased reflexes at the knees.

The pathogenesis of the diabetic neuropathies has been discussed in several recent reviews (1–3). In many patients with mononeuropathy, or mononeuropathy multiplex, the etiology appears to be vascular secondary to nerve infarction or ischemia (4,5). A similar mechanism has been suggested for diabetic amyotrophy (6), although other authors feel that this disorder represents a metabolic change in the nerve (7).

In the symmetric, sensorimotor and autonomic neuropathies, changes in metabolism of the nerve fiber probably underly the neuropathy. Two types of metabolic change are under active investigation at present in order to determine their role in the development of neuropathies (1–3). In the first type, abnormalities in metabolism of myoinositol have been noted in experimental animals with diabetic neuropathy. In these instances, the concentration of myoinositol in the affected peripheral nerves is lower than that in normal controls (8–11). Treatment of diabetic animals with myoinositol helps to restore nerve conduction velocity to normal (9–11). The second change is one of increased shunting of sugars into the sorbitol pathway, leading to accumulation and retention of sorbitol, glucose, and fructose and a postulated increase in osmotic pressure in the Schwann cell and axon (8,9,12,13). Because this pathway is related directly to the amount of glucose that circulates in the plasma, diabetic patients with hyperglycemia have increased accumulation of sorbitol in the nerves. Further work is needed at this time to determine whether either or both of these mechanisms are critical for the development of the neuropathy.

Treatment

The most effective treatment of diabetic neuropathy available at present appears to be effective control of the diabetes. This is particularly true for individuals with newly discovered diabetes or for patients with recent onset of symptomatic polyneuropathy. In patients with longstanding diabetes with neuropathy, axonal degeneration and segmented demyelination often are prominent. These structural changes preclude rapid improvement of symptoms and may respond poorly to treatment (1,2).

Fry et al. (14) examined 490 consecutive diabetic patients in order to assess the incidence of neuropathy. Of 43 patients with polyneuropathy, 28 obtained good control of their diabetes. Good control was defined as negative results on urine glucose tests and random levels of blood sugar usually of less than 200 mg/100 ml. Of the 28 patients with good control, more than half had fair to good recovery from their polyneuropathy, while the remaining patients had poor recovery. Of the 15 patients with poor diabetic control, none had adequate recovery from their polyneuropathy. The authors stated that, although their initial clinical impression was that diabetic control had no effect on polyneuropathy, the results of the study negated this impression.

Gregersen (15) evaluated 145 diabetics on the basis of studies that used motor-nerve conduction velocities in peroneal nerves as the primary criterion for determining neuropathy. When neuropathy was examined as a function of duration of diabetes, there appeared to be a progressive decrease in motor-nerve conduction velocity, especially in young patients (aged 15–44 years). A similar reduction also was seen in patients whose disease began at an older age, although the decrease in conduction velocity was less than in the younger patients and approximated a condition that Gregerson found also to be a function of age. In a subgroup of diabetic patients in the young age group who had had diabetes for less than five years, 21 well-controlled patients had an average motor conduction velocity of 48.4 m/sec, while motor conduction velocity in the 15 poorly controlled patients was 44.3 m/sec. Of these 36 patients, 26 were selected for further study. Eleven of them were considered to have good diabetic control (i.e., mean level of blood sugar less than 140 mg/100 ml, concentration of urine sugar less than 1%). Fifteen patients with poor control were not able to meet the criteria. Of the 36 patients, the well-controlled patients had a mean motor conduction velocity of 49.5 m/sec, while the poorly controlled patients had a mean motor conduction velocity of 44.3 m/sec ($P < 0.05$). The groups were otherwise closely matched in duration of diabetes and mean age at the time of study; patients in both groups took insulin.

Ward et al. (16) used motor conduction velocity in median and lateral popliteal nerves as a criterion for determining peripheral neuropathy in a group of 39 persons with newly diagnosed diabetes. The patients were reexamined at six weeks and six months from time of diagnosis. With treatment of the diabetes, the motor conduction velocity showed improvement that was statistically significant at the six-month examination only. Graf et al. (17) also used studies of motor- and sensory-nerve conduction velocity to study the effect of various fasting levels of plasma glucose on the conduction velocities in twenty males with untreated maturity-onset diabetes from a Veteran's Administration medical center. When motor-nerve conduction velocities in median, tibial, and peroneal nerves were correlated with fasting levels of plasma glucose, the authors found progressive slowing of the velocities as glucose levels increased. These findings, however, were not noted with sensory-nerve conduction velocities.

Campbell et al. (18) studied seven diabetic patients during and after an episode of diabetic ketoacidosis. The researchers used both the conduction velocity and terminal latency of ulnar and common peroneal nerves as indices of nerve function. They studied five of the patients on day 2 of and day 6 of their hospitalizaton for acute ketoacidosis, and then at one-, two-, and three-month intervals. When the mean motor conduction velocity and terminal latency of the five patients as a group were studied, the conduction velocity of the ulnar nerve increased from 52.2 ± 6.1 m/sec on day 2 to 56.7 ± 4.9 m/sec at the end of the third month. Terminal latency of the ulnar nerve (in m/sec) decreased from 3.4 ± 0.4 to 2.9 ± 0.5 at the end of three months. Similar changes were noted in the common peroneal nerve.

These studies indicate that the degree of diabetic control can affect peripheral nerve function in diabetic persons. Although good control does not guarantee that peripheral nerve function will improve, it appears to make improvement much more likely. On the other hand, poor diabetic control is not associated with significant improvement in peripheral nerve function.

Patients with mononeuropathy, mononeuropathy multiplex, or diabetic amyotrophy probably have vascular changes in the nerve as either the primary or contributing cause of nerve dysfunction. Although peripheral nerve function tends to improve with time, in these patients, there is little evidence to suggest a direct relation between diabetic control and improvement of nerve function.

Possible Future Therapies

On the basis of experimental observations of low levels of myoinositol in the peripheral nerves of diabetic rats, and of improvement of peripheral neuropathy in rats that received supplemental myoinositol, scattered reports are beginning to appear on the use of supplemental myoinositol in patients with diabetic neuropathy. In an acute study, Salway et al. (19) gave 500 mg myoinositol orally twice a day to a small group of patients. The amplitude of the evoked motor-unit action potentials in these patients subsequently increased, although a significant change in the conduction velocity of the nerve was not noted. The patients received treatment for two weeks only; long-term results were not available.

Clements and co-workers (20) devised diets that were either low or high in myoinositol and fed them to diabetic patients who were randomized into each diet group. The patients had had symptoms of peripheral neuropathy for an average of about 18 months and had had diabetes for an average of about nine years. Dietary intake of myoinositol was about 621 mg/day on the normal diet; 440 mg/day on the low-myoinositol diet, and 1,283 mg/day on the high-myoinositol diet. Plasma concentrations of myoinositol were 38.0 μmol on the normal diet, 31.7 μmol on the low-myoinositol diet, and 45.7 μmol on the high-myoinositol diet. Patients on the low-myoinositol diet showed decreased motor-nerve conduction velocities in the median and peroneal nerves. Two of these patients discontinued the diet because of recurrent pain in the lower extremities. Conversely, sensory-nerve conduction velocities increased in patients on the high-myoinositol diets, although motor-nerve conduction velocities did not change. In addition, all but one patient on the high myoinositol diet claimed subjective improvement after at least one week of the diet. Three other patients on the high-myoinositol diet were noted to have return of their Achilles' tendon reflex. In a group of six healthy control subjects who were fed a high-myoinositol diet, median nerve sensory conduction velocities decreased slightly as compared with values on a normal diet.

Gregersen and co workers (21) studied 60 patients with diabetes of a mean duration of 11 years. The patients were randomized into two groups; one group received 3 g myoinositol/day, while the control group received a placebo. In both groups, there was about an equal incidence of clinical neuropathy. Clinical changes in the symptoms of neuropathy did not occur, and there were no quantitative changes in the threshold of vibratory perception or in motor-nerve conduction velocity of the peroneal nerves.

The possible role of supplemental myoinositol in the treatment of diabetic neuropathies remains unclear. None of the three studies described here revealed a significant effect of increased consumption of myoinositol on motor-nerve conduction velocity. It is possible, however, that the use of supplemental myoinositol can result in selective improvement in sensory nerve function. Because both excessive and insufficient amounts of myoinositol can affect peripheral nerve function adversely, future studies must be performed carefully to determine appropriate dosage, method of administration, and means of monitoring response to the drug before it becomes a practical therapeutic measure.

Attempts to alter sorbitol content in axons and Schwann cells by pharmacologic methods is just beginning. Gabbay and co-workers (22) administered an aldose-reductase inhibitor to selected patients with diabetes who also had severe peripheral neuropathy. The drug alrestatin (AY-22, 284, Ayerst) was administered intravenously (IV) in a dose of 50 mg/kg body weight daily for five days, or orally in a dose of 1 g q.i.d. for 30 days. Two patients who received the compound IV reported subjective improvement in clinical symptoms beginning two days after the start of infusions and persisting for about three weeks. Objective changes in nerve conduction velocities and neurologic function were not noted. In a 30-day oral trial in four diabetics, subjective or objective improvement in clinical symptoms did not occur; however, these patients had severe peripheral neuropathy. The authors speculate that, if the drug is to be effective in the future, it probably should be given to newly diagnosed patients with either no clinical neuropathy or minimal dysfunction.

Uremic Neuropathy

Peripheral neuropathy as a complication of chronic renal failure was not recognized until the 1960s. Since then, the disorder has been observed frequently, with about 50% of patients about to undergo hemodialysis showing signs of neuropathy (23). For unknown reasons, males are affected more frequently than females. The clinical aspects of uremic neuropathy have been reviewed recently (2,24).

Typical uremic neuropathy is a distal, symmetric sensorimotor polyneuropathy that affects the legs more than the arms. Patients may experience dysesthesias and paresthesias, with a varying number experiencing the "restless leg" syndrome. Patients also occasionally complain of burning feet. The motor weakness usually is a less prominent part of the neuropathy than the sensory dysfunction. Nevertheless, motor-nerve conduction velocity is often decreased. Deep-tendon reflexes are usually depressed or absent.

The etiology of uremic neuropathy is unclear. It probably is related to "toxins" that accumulate in the body and that are inadequately removed by hemodialysis. The "middle molecule" hypothesis suggests that molecules of a molecular weight of 300 to 2000 daltons are inadequately removed by hemodialysis and may be responsible for the neuropathy (24–26). Patients with renal failure have been noted also to have increased serum levels of myoinositol. Experimentally, rats fed a diet containing 35% myoinositol developed decreased motor-nerve conduction velocities in the sciatic nerves (27,28). More recently, Avram and coworkers (29) have raised the possibility that elevated levels of parathyroid hormone act as a neural toxin on peripheral nerves. Thomas (2), however, has refuted this hypothesis.

Treatment

Treatment of uremic neuropathy at present is based on adequate treatment of the renal failure, by either regular hemodialysis or renal transplantation. With the advent of hemodialysis, it was noted that many patients appeared to develop polyneuropathy shortly after initiation of the hemodialysis program, and physicians considered the possibility that hemodialysis was causally related to polyneuropathy. Subsequently, most studies suggested that adequate hemodialysis would either stabilize or improve the peripheral neuropathy. After the beginning of hemodialysis, symptomatic improvement for most patients occurs with a diminution in the amount of paresthesias and dysesthesias. Nielsen has also demonstrated that, along with subjective improvements in sensory function, the threshold for vibratory perception threshold, measured over the great toe, decreases with the start of hemodialysis. Before dialysis began, an abrupt increase in the threshold for vibratory perception was viewed as a warning that severe neuropathy was about to ensue (30). Although sensory symptoms improve, motor-nerve conduction velocity usually stabilizes but rarely improves significantly. Some centers have used failure of the motor-nerve conduction velocity to stabilize along with evidence of progressive slowing of conduction velocities as evidence of inadequate dialysis and of the need to increase the amount of dialysis the patient receives (31).

More consistently favorable results have been obtained in patients who have undergone successful renal transplantation. In 1962, Tyler (32) first reported clearing of symptomatic neuropathy in a pair of identical twins who underwent successful renal transplantation. In 1971, Bolton and co-workers (33) described the course of uremic neuropathy in 10 patients who underwent successful renal transplantation. Of five patients with symptomatic neuropathy, four regained complete neurologic function; the fifth patient had only partial recovery after one year. The remaining five patients had electromyographic (EMG) abnormalities but no clinical symptoms. In three of these patients, nerve conduction velocities returned to normal in four to six months (33). Nielsen was able to follow the course of a group of 27 patients who had undergone renal transplantation for about two and a half years. In those who had had successful transplantation, recovery from neuropathy followed a biphasic course. Initial improvement was marked by a reduction in the threshold for vibratory perception, followed by disappearance of sensory dysfunction occurring in the first few weeks to months after transplantation. Muscle weakness, muscle atrophy, and reflex disturbances required a much longer time to improve. The authors felt that clinical abnormalities present for six months after successful transplantation were apt to be permanent (34).

These reports and others (23) demonstrate convincingly that the peripheral neuropathy of uremia is best treated by renal transplantation. When this is not feasible, adequate hemodialysis appears to be the second best choice. In this case, the definition of adequate hemodialysis is the amount required to prevent progression of the neuropathy and provide some improvement in symptoms.

Possible Future Therapies

In a recent symposium on peripheral neuropathies held in Milan, Italy, in June 1978, attention was given to the possible role of gangliosides in the treatment of peripheral neuropathies (35). In preliminary studies, 10 patients with chronic renal failure who were treated with hemodialysis for one to nine years were given 20 mg brain cortex gangliosides/day for 30 days. All patients had clinical and EMG signs of uremic polyneuritis. Another group of 10 patients of similar age, sex, and duration of hemodialysis treatment were used as untreated controls. No information was given about the criteria for placement of the patients in the groups. Of the patients who received gangliosides, motor and sensory symptoms improved, but changes in the neuroelectric picture were not observed. No side effects of the treatment were noted (36). Although these results are intriguing, further studies are needed to determine whether the administration of brain gangliosides will ever play a role in the treatment of uremic polyneuropathy.

NEUROPATHIES IN ENDOCRINE DISEASE

Thyroid Disease

The most common peripheral nerve involvement in hypothyroidism is the carpal tunnel syndrome, which often is present bilaterally. The diagnosis is based on the usual clinical symptoms of noctural pain and discomfort, sensory loss in the median nerve distribution, and occasional weakness in the opponens pollicis muscle. The EMG often shows prolonged distal sensory or motor latencies in the median nerve distribution. With carpal tunnel syndrome associated with hypothyroidism, treatment of the underlying thyroid disease often results in resolution of the syndrome.

A diffuse, predominantly sensory distal polyneuropathy occasionally may be seen as part of hypothyroidism. If the hypothyroidism continues for a long time, the neuropathy may become more severe and result in muscle weakness and wasting. On examination, reflexes often are hypoactive or absent, with decreased sensory perception distally. In addition to EMG abnormalities that are consistent with polyneuropathy, laboratory tests may reveal an elevated level of CSF protein (37–39).

A predominantly sensory polyneuropathy also has been described in a patient with an isolated deficiency in thyrotropin hormone. On examination the patient had decreased sensation distally in the feet and hands, and decreased to absent deep-tendon reflexes distally. An EMG revealed findings of both sensory and motor neuropathy, and a muscle biopsy specimen showed groups of atrophic fibers, a finding consistent with neurogenic atrophy (40).

Treatment

Treatment of peripheral neuropathy associated with hypothyroidism, whether the hypothyroidism is due to primary dysfunction of the thyroid gland or is secondary to deficiency in thyrotopin hormone, is based on adequate replacement of the thyroid hormone. With treatment of the hypothyroidism, the symptoms of peripheral neuropathy usually respond in several weeks to several months. Use of either desiccated thyroid extract or synthetic thyroid replacement appears to be equally efficacious as far as the peripheral neuropathy is concerned.

Hyperthyroidism may be associated with proximal muscle weakness, muscle cramps, and muscle pain. However, there is little evidence to suggest that these symptoms are primarily due to peripheral nerve involvement. As with hypothyroidism, the symptoms are relieved by treatment of the hyperthyroidism, regardless of the etiology of the neuropathy.

Acromegaly

In acromegaly, as in hypothyroidism, the most common peripheral nerve involvement is carpal tunnel syndrome. In one series of 100 patients with acromegaly, 35 were found to have carpal tunnel syndrome. In these patients, treatment of the pituitary adenoma that was responsible for excessive secretion of growth hormone often resulted in relief of the symptoms of carpal tunnel syndrome (41).

More recently, Low and colleagues (42) studied 11 patients with acromegaly, eight of whom had EMG evidence of a generalized peripheral neuropathy. However, only two patients had normal results on the glucose tolerance test; the other nine showed curves that were mildly abnormal (4) or indicative of frank diabetes (5). Peripheral neuropathy was present in both patients with normal test results. The possible contribution of diabetes to the peripheral neuropathy in the other nine patients, however, is unclear. It is likely that the coexistence of the acromegaly with diabetes results in a combined metabolic insult to the peripheral nerves. The results of treatment of the pituitary adenoma and the resultant effects on the peripheral neuropathy were not reported.

According to Low and colleagues, logical treatment of peripheral neuropathy in patients with acromegaly should consist of two phases: (*1*) adequate treatment of the pituitary adenoma to suppress secretion of growth hormone, and (*2*) good control of coexisting diabetes mellitus (42).

NEUROPATHIES IN DYSPROTEINEMIA

Peripheral neuropathies have been associated with a variety of dysproteinemias, including Waldenstrom's macroglobulinemia (43), essential or secondary cryoglobulinemia (44), and other paraproteinemias (45,46). The relation between the etiology of the peripheral neuropathy and the presence of circulating serum paraproteins is not always clear. In some cases circulating paraproteins are associated with other disorders such as lymphoma or multiple myeloma, which also can be associated with peripheral neuropathy. In addition, associated amyloidosis may complicate the picture in many of these disorders. Nevertheless, enough cases exist in the literature to associate peripheral neuropathy with abnormal levels of serum paraproteins so that a causal relation probably does exist in some. This section will be devoted to the treatment of peripheral neuropathies in which the levels of paraproteins appears to be the main abnormality.

Cryoglobulinemic Neuropathy

Cryoglobulins are serum proteins that tend to precipitate from the blood during cooling. They have been associated with various connective tissue disorders, lymphomas, and plasma-cell dyscrasias. When these diseases are present, the protein abnormality is considered to be secondary cryoglobulinemia. In the absence of these conditions, the disorder is called essential cryoglobulinemia. In either case, the symptoms typically associated with cryoglobulinemia are purpuric lesions, arthralgias, occasionally renal failure, and, in some cases, peripheral neuropathy (44).

The peripheral neuropathy may be symmetric or asymmetric. It is usually a sensorimotor polyneuropathy that often is present in the same area in which the purpuric rash is seen. Progression may be relatively slow or rapid. In some patients, periods of exacerbation or worsening of symptoms coincide with exposure to cold.

The cryoglobulins are usually intact, monoclonal immunoglobulins or immunoglobulin complexes of IgG and IgM. Liver disease frequently is associated with the presence of cryoglobulins, which also are often associated with the presence of hepatitis B surface antigen and antibody. Although Levo and colleagues (47) found a strong association of hepatitis B antigen and antibody with both essential and secondary cryoglobulinemia, Popp et al. (48) found this association mainly in patients with secondary cryoglobulinemia. Levo and colleagues have speculated that cryoglobulinemia is a normal physiologic event, with the cryoglobulins removed from serum by the liver. Patients with liver disease may demonstrate incomplete removal of cryoglobulins, leading to an increased amount of circulating cryoimmunoglobulins (49).

Just as the mechanism for the development of cryoimmunoglobulinemia is unclear, so is the mechanism by which the circulating cryoglobulins result in peripheral neuropathy. Speculation has focused on vascular lesions that affect peripheral nerves either as a result of thrombotic effects or secondary to vasculitis. Pathologically, the peripheral nerves usually show Wallerian degeneration distally, with various degrees of lymphocytic infiltration.

Treatment

Treatment of essential cryoglobulinemia with regard to response of the polyneuropathy is difficult. Metzger and colleagues (50) reported one patient with cryoglobulinemic neuropathy who responded to treatment with prednisone, 60 mg q.o.d., plus cyclophosphamide, 100 mg/day. With these medications, the peripheral neuropathy gradually cleared over a period of six to 12 months. Other patients have been treated with immunosuppressants and cytotoxic agents but have showed minimal or no response. Furthermore, because the course of the neuropathy may fluctuate, it becomes difficult to know whether the improvement is a result of treatment or whether it represents a spontaneous remission.

Another logical treatment is the use of plasmapheresis. Little information is available in the literature about the response of peripheral neuropathy to plasmapheresis. However, if there is a causal relation between circulating cryoglobulins and polyneuropathy, plasmapheresis should improve neural function.

In summary, the treatment of patients with essential cryoglobulinemia associated with peripheral neuropathy should consist of corticosteroids, cytotoxic agents, and possibly plasmapheresis. Response to treatment, however, may be minimal.

Waldenström's Macroglobulinemia

In Waldenström's macroglobulinemia, an excess of circulating IgM macroglobulin is found in the blood. The disease affects mainly older persons and results in weight loss, weakness, anemia, tendency toward bleeding, and peripheral nerve involvement. A proliferation of lymphocytes is often seen, with infiltration of bone marrow, lymph nodes, and spleen. At times, macroglobulins can be found in other diseases, such as connective tissue diseases, lymphatic leukemia, carcinoma, and lymphosarcoma. The presence of circulating macroglobulins often leads to a hyperviscosity syndrome along with increased sludging of red cells.

In 1960, Logothetis et al. (43) reviewed peripheral nerve involvement in Waldenström's macroglobulinemia. A variety of abnormalities may be seen, including a distal sensorimotor polyneuropathy, mononeuritis multiplex, cranial nerve mononeuropathies, and a cauda equina syndrome. The onset is usually insidious, although there are rare reports of acute onset and resemblance to Guillain–Barré syndrome (43,51–53).

Treatment

Treatment of macroglobulinemia is difficult and often unsuccessful. Plasmapheresis has been recommended, particularly for treatment of the hyperviscosity syndrome, although the polyneuropathy may not respond at all (54). Various cytotoxic agents have been used, including chlorambucil, 16 mg/day (51); cyclophosphamide, 200 mg/day (51); and melphalan, 2 mg/day (53). These are frequently given along with prednisone, 40–80 mg/day. The response of the polyneuropathy to these measures may be minimal. Frequent blood counts are needed with use of cytotoxic agents in order to avoid significant bone marrow toxicity.

In summary, in treatment of patients with polyneuropathy secondary to Waldenström's macroglobulinemia, it is reasonable to use plasmapheresis whenever hyperviscosity exists. The use of cytotoxic agents, with or without prednisone, also can be tried. If little benefit is obtained with one drug, it probably is worthwhile to switch to another to see if the patient responds more favorably.

Polyneuropathy in Other Paraproteinemias

As noted earlier, polyneuropathy can be associated with other, apparently benign paraproteinemias (45,46). The relation between the circulating paraproteins and the development of polyneuropathy is unclear. Likewise, there appears to be little information about specific modalities of treatment. Thus, it probably is best to observe such patients carefully for subsequent development of a lymphoproliferative disorder. If the polyneuropathy is disabling, a trial of steroids, cytotoxic agents, or plasmapheresis, either sequentially or in combination, should be considered. However, little information is available to predict the success of these measures.

Polyneuropathy Secondary to Nutritional Deficiency

Victor (55) has reviewed extensively the role of vitamin deficiencies, occurring singly or multiply, in the setting of generalized nutritional deficiency and resulting in polyneuropathy. Although a number of vitamins have been associated with polyneuropathy, the clinical setting of vitamin deficiency usually is one of generally impaired nutrition; thus, the neuropathy probably is due to any of several factors. Treatment of the polyneuropathy, then, consists of therapy with multiple vitamins coupled with an adequate, balanced diet.

The clinical symptoms of most neuropathies associated with nutritional deficiency are those of distal, symmetric, sensorimotor polyneuropathy. At times, such patients may have a very unpleasant burning sensation mainly in the feet and legs and occasionally in the hands. Reflexes are hypoactive to absent distally and may be decreased proximally.

The most common polyneuropathy of nutritional deficiency is that seen in chronic alcoholism. Although alcohol may have a toxic effect on the nervous system, the polyneuropathy associated with alcoholism appears to be caused primarily by thiamine deficiency. In clinical studies, Victor and Adams (56) found that the administration of thiamine alone to alcoholics who were denied alcohol and maintained on a diet deficient in vitamin B resulted in rapid improvement of the clinical symptoms of neuropathy. It is quite likely that chronic alcoholics are deficient also in other vitamins and should be treated with large doses of multivitamin preparations and not only with thiamine.

Nutritional polyneuropathies can also result from long-term ingestion of diets deficient in one or more vitamins, in malabsorption syndromes, and in patients who previously have undergone gastrectomy. With the increased popularity of bypass procedures for treatment of obesity, it seems likely that some patients will develop deficiency states that result in polyneuropathy secondary to the surgical procedure (57).

Thiamine deficiency results in the clinical state of beri-beri. This condition is seen most commonly in chronic alcoholism but has been noted also in prisoners of war or others whose diet has been restricted severely. The symptoms of the polyneuropathy usually consist of weakness, paresthesias, and pain and often coexist with cardiac symptoms, including congestive heart failure or sudden cardiovascular collapse.

In its full-blown form, *niacin deficiency* results in pellagra. The clinical manifestations are summarized by the "three Ds": dermatitis, diarrhea, and dementia. Peripheral nerve involvement is relatively uncommon and may be secondary to other, associated vitamin deficiencies, particularly pyridoxine and thiamine deficiency. In patients with pellagra, the symptoms of peripheral neuropathy are similar to those in other vitamin deficiencies—namely, pain and tenderness in the legs, decreased sensation distally, and distal weakness.

Bean et al. (58) have linked *pantothenic acid deficiency* with sensory neuropathy in humans. Other researchers have suggested that this deficiency may be responsible for the "burning feet" syndrome in at least some cases.

Pyridoxine deficiency is seen most commonly in patients who are treated with isoniazid and have not been given pyridoxine supplements. The resulting neuropathy often begins with numbness and tingling and may progress to severe burning pain. Symptoms are most severe in the legs, and motor symptoms are relatively minor.

Vitamin B12 deficiency is associated most commonly with spinal cord dysfunction, particularly that of the posterior and lateral columns. Peripheral nerve involvement can be seen in conjunction with the spinal cord disease. Symptoms include mild, distal sensory loss, usually of position and vibratory sense more than pain and temperature sensation. Distal muscle weakness and depressed deep-tendon reflexes also may be present. Peripheral nerve dysfunction has been demonstrated on EMG and in nerve conduction studies in several series of patients (59–61). Abnormalities reported include decreased nerve action potentials, slowing of sensory-nerve conduction velocity, and evidence of denervation on EMG. Although vitamin B12 deficiency occurs as part of pernicious anemia, it is seen also in patients treated with partial or complete gastrectomy for ulcer disease. Of 223 patients treated with partial gastrectomy, 46 (21%) had a serum level of vitamin B12 of less than 200 pg/ml. Of the 46 patients, 38 were studied electrophysiologically; 13 (34%) showed evidence of peripheral nerve dysfunction (61).

Neurologic abnormalities associated with *folate deficiency* in the absence of abnormalities in vitamin B12 metabolism have been reported only recently. Patients may appear initially with peripheral neuropathy (62), evidence of myelopathy (63), or neuropsychiatric symptoms (64). The peripheral neuropathy is described as a mixed sensorimotor neuropathy that involves mainly sensory fibers and affects the legs more than the arms. In some cases the patient experiences diffuse muscle pain and restless legs. Treatment with high doses of oral folate (10–15 mg/day) resulted in slow improvement of symptoms in most patients. As improvement occurred, the dose was decreased to 5 mg/day orally (62). Patients with the restless-legs syndrome required higher doses, from 35–60 mg/day, given in part orally and in part parenterally (64).

Riboflavin deficiency is generally thought not to cause a significant peripheral neuropathy. However, Lai and Ransome (65) have described a woman with the burning-feet syndrome who responded dramatically to injections of riboflavin, 6 mg/day. The patient had evidence of malabsorption associated with low serum level of folate. Although she subsequently was given oral folic acid, her sensory symptoms improved with administration of riboflavin alone (65).

Ascorbic acid deficiency results in the clinical condition of scurvy, which often is associated with hemorrhage. Peripheral nerve involvement, if it occurs, is presumed to be secondary to hemorrhage in the nerve itself and not the result of a primary metabolic disorder of peripheral nerve function (66). Treatment consists of oral doses of vitamin C, 50–100 mg/day.

Treatment

In all the deficiency states, regardless of whether they result from single or multiple deficiencies, treatment consists of adequate replacement of the vitamins. Daily supplements of vitamin B should be given as follows: thiamine, 25 mg; niacin, 100 mg; riboflavin, 10 mg; patothenic acid, 10 mg; and pyridoxine, 5 mg (55). Folic acid, 5 mg/day, and vitamin B12, 1,000 μg IM every two to four weeks, can also be added.

In patients who may be suffering from a malabsorption syndrome, the vitamin therapy may need to be given either IV or IM. This is particularly important in patients with vitamin B12 deficiency secondary to previous gastrectomy and in patients with various malabsorption syndromes. Treatment with high doses should be continued until the patient is asymptomatic, with subsequent maintenance doses decreased to a level which keeps the patients asymptomatic.

NEUROPATHIES ASSOCIATED WITH TOXINS

A variety of substances have been shown to be toxic to the peripheral nervous system. For convenience, the resultant neuropathies can be divided into three categories: (*1*) those caused by heavy-metal intoxication; (*2*) those caused by industrial or other organic toxins; and (*3*) those secondary to drug treatment. In this section, only the effects of these various agents on the peripheral nervous system and the appropriate treatment will be considered. Although many such agents also can affect the CNS and other parts of the body, these areas will not be discussed in detail.

Neuropathies Secondary to Heavy-Metal Intoxication

Lead Intoxication

Exposure to inorganic lead often results in acute encephalopathy in children and in chronic motor neuropathy in adults. The neuropathy tends to affect the upper extremities more frequently than the lower extremities and characteristically affects the radial nerve, resulting in wrist drop. At times, weakness in the legs can result in foot drop. Sensory symptoms and findings usually are mild. In workers exposed chronically to high environmental levels of lead, a mixture of encephalopathic and neuropathic symptoms and signs may be seen (67).

Lead enters the body through inhalation or ingestion. Sources of lead include lead vapor in battery factories, ingestion of moonshine liquor that has been distilled through lead-containing pipes, leaching of lead glazes in pottery, urban dust and dirt, and exposure to lead-based paint (67–71). In adults working in areas known to be contaminated with lead, whole-blood levels of lead are used to monitor the degree of exposure. Levels of less than 40 μg lead/100 g whole blood are accepted as safe; levels of 40–80 μg/100 g are considered borderline; and levels greater than 80 μg/100 g are usually toxic. Urinary excretion of more than 150 μg/L is considered suspicious, and excretion of more than 200 μg/L in lead workers is considered dangerous. Urinary output of coproporphyrin of more than 200 μg/24 h in adults, and urinary excretion of delta-aminolevulinic acid of more than 10–20 mg/L are also evidence of lead intoxication (70).

It is not clear whether chronic exposure to low levels of lead can cause a subclinical polyneuropathy. A study by Seppalainen and co-workers (72) demonstrated mildly slowed motor-nerve conduction velocities in ulnar and median nerves in 26 patients who had been exposed to lead for various lengths of time and in whom blood levels of lead were measured regularly. In addition, nine of 11 patients who underwent EMG had abnormal results, with fibrillations found in about half. None of the patients had had documented exposure to levels of lead higher than 70 μg/100 ml whole blood (72). Subsequently, Buchthal and Behse (73) performed a similar study with 20 lead-exposed men whose blood levels of lead were higher than those of Seppalainen's subjects. None were believed to have significant evidence of peripheral neuropathy on the basis of motor-nerve conduction velocities, sensory-nerve conduction velocities, and amplitude of evoked potentials (73).

Treatment of lead intoxication depends on two factors: (*1*) removal of the patient from exposure to lead, and (*2*) chelation therapy to increase excretion of lead from the body. Although ethylendiaminetetraacetic acid and British antilewisite (BAL) have been used in patients with lead-induced neuropathy, these agents are generally reserved for the treatment of adults and children with acute lead intoxication and encephalopathy or for adults with whole-blood levels of lead of more than 100 μg/100 g (67,74). Most patients with only lead-induced neuropathies have a history of chronic lead exposure and a more slowly developing clinical picture. Treatment with penicillamine (Cuprimine) along with removal of the patient from the source of lead usually suffices. Treatment is started with 250 mg penicillamine/day for one to two weeks; the dose is increased gradually at one- to two-week intervals to a total dose of 750 mg/day. Whole-blood levels and 24-hour urinary excretion of lead should be measured regularly to monitor the effectiveness of the penicillamine. Although hard data about the recommended duration of treatment are not available, it would be reasonable to continue the drug until the 24-hour urinary excretion is within an acceptable range.

Penicillamine has been found to cause a variety of potentially serious side effects (75). Because of this, it is necessary to monitor blood counts and liver and kidney function at weekly intervals during initiation of penicillamine treatment and at monthly intervals after the treatment has been established. Generally, a one- to two-month course of penicillamine should be sufficient to decrease lead levels to normal.

Neuropathies Secondary to Arsenic Intoxication

The peripheral neuropathy of intoxication with inorganic arsenic is typically a predominantly distal sensory neuropathy that begins with mild paresthesias of the feet. In more severe cases, motor involvement may occur, with distal muscle weakness. At times, the patient may have painful paresthesias, with tenderness in the affected extremities. Intoxication with organic arsenic results more frequently in acute encephalopathy.

Along with the neurologic symptoms, patients suffering from arsenic poisoning may have nonspecific symptoms such as tiredness, fatigue, loss of appetite, diarrhea, and constipation. If the intoxication results from ingestion of a large amount of arsenic at one time, the nausea, vomiting, and diarrhea can be very severe, with associated abdominal pain and renal shutdown. In acute severe cases (76–78), dehydration, renal failure, and cardiac toxicity may combine to result in death.

Arsenic poisoning can result from the use of arsenic-containing insecticides, arsenic-containing medications (79), or compounds that contain the dye Paris green, or from industrial exposure (78). In addition, arsenic poisoning has long been a favorite method of committing homicide. When arsenic intoxication has been documented in a patient, it is prudent for health care providers to avoid ingesting samples of food brought to the patient by apparently sympathetic relatives.

Diagnosis

The diagnosis of arsenic intoxication depends on the demonstration of increased urinary excretion of arsenic in a 24-hour sample (more than 25 μg/24 hr), with additional evidence provided by examination of arsenic content in hair and fingernail samples (more than 1 μg/g for both) (80). In general, measurement of arsenic levels in blood is not useful. A mild elevation in urinary excretion of arsenic can occur in people who eat large amounts of seafood, since salt-water fish and crustaceans contain relatively high levels of arsenic. Chronic exposure to high levels of arsenic over a prolonged period may result in subclinical neuropathy in patients whose urine levels of arsenic are otherwise within an acceptable range (78).

Treatment

The cornerstone of treatment depends on the removal of the patient from the source of contamination. In patients with mild neuropathy, this measure alone is sufficient. In patients with more severe neuropathy but without significant constitutional symptoms, the correct treatment modality is less clear-cut. Patients have been treated with either BAL or penicillamine without clear evidence that these measures enhance recovery (76, 77). If penicillamine is used, it should be given in an initial dose of 250 mg/day and increased gradually to 750 mg/day over a period of four to six weeks. Although good guidelines regarding urinary excretion of arsenic are not available, it seems logical that when excretion returns to normal, penicillamine treatment can be stopped. Patients must be monitored closely for evidence of hematologic, renal, or other toxic manifestations of penicillamine (75).

In acute arsenic intoxication in which severe constitutional symptoms are found, treatment with BAL should be tried. This agent appears to be of value in the treatment of encephalopathy, although the response of the neuropathy to BAL is limited. The dosage is 2.5 mg/kg body weight, injected IM in divided doses for five to seven days. After a rest period of another five to seven days, the course is repeated. During the recovery stage, BAL treatment can be followed by oral penicillamine (76).

Mercury Intoxication

Mercury intoxication of the nervous system can occur with either elemental mercury or organic compounds of mercury. With both types of intoxication, CNS involvement is much more prevalent and severe than peripheral nervous system involvement. The neural toxicity of mercury has been reviewed recently (81–83).

Clinically, the peripheral neuropathy is most commonly a sensory neuropathy, with distal paresthesias and sensory loss. Motor involvement can occur at times. The predeliction for sensory dysfunction is seen also in experimental animals, where the dorsal-root ganglion is very sensitive to the effects of organic mercury compounds (81).

The diagnosis of acute or subacute mercury intoxication depends on the demonstration of elevated blood levels of mercury (generally more than 10 μg/100 ml blood) or increased urinary excretion of mercury (more than 20 μg/24 hr) (82). Levels of mercury in hair of more than 150 μg/g suggests exposure significant enough to cause symptoms (82).

Treatment

Most patients with mercury poisoning have only mild peripheral neuropathy, although the CNS effects may be quite severe. It is unlikely that patients will be seen with only the peripheral neuropathy as a manifestation of mercury intoxication. For those who have residual peripheral neuropathy following mercury ingestion, removal of the source of mercury is the most important therapeutic measure. If high levels of mercury are found in urine and blood, treatment with BAL in doses similar to those recommended for arsenic poisoning can be used. Penicillamine also may be an effective chelating agent, although little information is available about the effects of penicillamine on the course of the peripheral neuropathy.

Neuropathies Secondary to Industrial Toxins and Organic Compounds

A variety of compounds used in industry, plus other organic compounds, have been implicated in causing peripheral neuropathy. These include the following toxins:

1. Acrylamide
2. Carbon disulfide
3. Carbon monoxide
4. Dichlorophenoxyacetic acid (2,4-D)
5. Dimethylaminopropionitrile
6. Ethylene oxide
7. Methyl ethyl ketone (as potentiator)
8. Methyl n-butyl ketone
9. n-Hexane
10. Nitrous oxide
11. Organophosphate compounds (especially triorthocresyl phosphate [TOCP])
12. Polychlorinated biphenyls
13. Toluene
14. N-3-pyridylmethyl-N′-p-nitrophenylurea (Vacor)

Several recent articles provide details of clinical symptoms and possible pathogenetic mechanisms of neuropathy resulting from exposure to toxins (84–95). Only a few compounds, chosen because of their unusual symptoms or possible need for early, vigorous therapy during acute intoxication, will be discussed in detail.

In addition to peripheral neuropathy, many of these compounds also produce other neurologic and systemic symptoms. The severity of the reaction depends on the acuteness, duration and amount of exposure to the toxic chemical and the mode of contact. With industrial exposure, it is very common for only a small proportion of the workers to become symptomatic. The development of peripheral neuropathy in one or two workers who operate in the same work area should alert the physician to the possibility of an industrial-related illness. Large-scale screening of potentially affected employees from the same environment in a plant can then be organized with the cooperation of employees from the state health department and officials of the industry. Such screening often identifies subclinical cases.

Not all inhalation-induced neuropathies result from industrial exposure. In some cases, patients who are glue sniffers inhale volatile compounds, particularly n-hexane, toluene, and other hydrocarbons; this activity results in peripheral neuropathy as a side effect of getting high (96,97). Abuse of nitrous oxide by persons also looking for a cheap high has resulted in cases of peripheral neuropathy (98). Inhalation of mixed organic compounds including gasoline, lacquer thinner, lighter fluid, and rubber cement, also can result in peripheral nerve damage (99,100).

Treatment

For all of these toxic neuropathies, the only effective treatment is removal of the patient from the source of intoxication. Therefore, it is important for the physician who sees the patient initially to have a high index of suspicion that a toxic agent may be responsible for the neuropathy. A detailed history must be taken regarding specific compounds to which the patient was exposed. If inhalation of volatile material was done for recreational purposes, the process may require obtaining a list of ingredients from the manufacturer.

Because they produce unusual symptoms or have potential for therapy, several toxic agents and the neuropathies they cause will be described in detail.

Dimethylaminopropionitrile, a compound used in the production of polyurethane foam, has produced urinary retention. Workers who are affected most severely have abnormal findings on cystometrogram that are consistent with a neurogenic bladder. Sexual dysfunction, including impotence, is common. In addition, a mild sensory peripheral neuropathy is often found. Symptoms cleared over time when the manufacturing process was changed to avoid use of this compound (101).

Vacor Rat Killer (N-3-pyridylmethyl-N′-p-nitrophenylurea; Rohm and Haas, Philadelphia) is a relatively new rat poison. Although the manufacturer has voluntarily stopped the sale of Vacor and has recalled the existing stock from dealers, it is unclear how successful these efforts have been (102). In the meantime, many persons have attempted suicide by taking large doses of Vacor; the results have been catastrophic. The compound produces rapid destruction of pancreatic β-islet cells, resulting in initial hypoglycemia and, later, acute hyperglycemic ketoacidosis, orthostatic hypotension, peripheral neuropathy, and encephalopathy. CNS symptoms develop over hours to several days. In patients who survive acute intoxication, severe orthostatic hypotension, anorexia, and gastrointestinal hypomotility are common (103,104).

It is thought that the active ingredient in Vacor is a competitive antagonist of nicotinamide. In patients suspected or known to have ingested Vacor, rapid treatment with parenteral nicotinamide may prevent the development of severe symptoms. The recommended dosage is 100–500 mg nicotinamide IV every four to six hours, given as rapidly after ingestion as possible. In three children so treated within 30 minutes of ingestion, toxic sequelae did not occur. However, patients who were not treated for several days after ingestion had only a minimal response to the nicotinamide. Patients should not be given nicotinic acid (niacin) because it does not appear to be as effective as nicotinamide; further, the vasodilatation it produces may aggravate the symptoms of hypotension (103).

Organophosphorus-Induced Neuropathy

A variety of organophosphates are toxic to both the central and peripheral nervous systems. The acute effects are produced through inhibition of acetylcholinesterase activity, resulting in acute cholinergic poisoning. With chronic exposure, peripheral neuropathy may result, which at times is combined with CNS symptoms.

Historically, the most noted of these compounds is *triorthocresyl phosphate* (TOCP). In the 1930s, an epidemic of neurologic dysfunction occurred in the United States. Common symptoms were muscle pain, paresthesias, and distal weakness in the legs and later in the hands. Sensory abnormalities usually were minimal. In some cases, spinal cord involvement was manifested by spasticity and hyperactive reflexes. The cause of the illness was traced to the use of an alcoholic extract of ginger (Jamaica Ginger Extract [USP]) that was contaminated with TOCP. The extract was consumed by many individuals who used it as a source of alcohol during Prohibition days. Some 4,837 Americans were paralyzed, with some estimates suggesting that a total of between 20,000 and 60,000 persons were affected. The resulting impairment in gait was known as the "Jake Walk" (105). A similar outbreak apparently occurred in 1959 in Morocco, when cooking oil contaminated with aviation oil that contained 3% TOCP was sold to Moroccans. More recently, an outbreak was reported in Vietnam when Vietnamese families began to use black-market cooking oil that contained TOCP (106). TOCP is still used as a plasticizer and a high-temperature lubricant. There is no specific therapy for TOCP intoxication once the neurologic symptoms appear. Recovery is often poor and incomplete.

Other organophosphorus compounds (malathion, parathion, trichlorfon [Dipterex], are found as active ingredients in insecticides. Acute intoxication with these compounds results in a severe, acute, cholinergic crisis produced by inhibition of cholinesterase activity. Clinically, patients may appear initially with increased sweating, salivation, lacrimation, increased amounts of secretions, bradycardia, hypertension, and often severe miosis. Muscle twitching, fasciculations, cramps, and weakness also occur, with associated impaired respiration. CNS manifestations include restlessness, confusion, ataxia, generalized weakness, and possibly coma. The diagnosis depends on the history of ingestion of an organophosphate-containing compound along with demonstration of very low levels of serum and red cell cholinesterase activity.

Treatment

Treatment of acute episodes of organophosphorus-induced neuropathy is based on three modalities: (*1*) Maintenance of a patent airway, including tracheostomy or intubation, with respiratory support as needed. (*2*) Administration of atropine to block the muscarinic effects of excessive acetylcholine. Initial doses of atropine range from 1 6 mg given IV, depending on the severity of the case. Repeated doses are given at 15- to 30-minute intervals until the patient's pupils begin to dilate, the skin becomes dry and flushed, and the pulse rate increases. Further doses are repeated as necessary to maintain the atropinized state. (*3*) Pralidoxine (PAM) is given to restore cholinesterase activity. It is given in an initial dose of 1 g IV in adults or 10–12 mg/kg body weight IV slowly in infants and children. The dose can be repeated in one hour if necessary. If muscle weakness persists after the second dose, the drug can be given as an IV infusion at a rate of 0.5 g/hr (107,108).

Rarely, patients experience late onset of peripheral neuropathy after acute intoxication. Treatment of the peripheral neuropathy with PAM or atropine has been unsuccessful. The neuropathy is characterized by motor weakness distally and is often accompanied by paresthesias. If neuropathy occurs, it may persist for a prolonged period. It is unclear whether chronic, low-grade exposure to organophosphate-containing insecticides can have a cumulative effect that results in late development of a peripheral neuropathy (107,109,110).

Polyneuropathy Secondary to Drug Ingestion

As with industrial and organic toxins, a large number of drugs have been implicated in causing peripheral neuropathy. A partial list of these drugs includes:

1. Avlosulfan (Dapsone)
2. Chloramphenical
3. Cisplatinum
4. Clioquinol
5. Diphenylhydantoin
6. Disulfiram (Antabuse)
7. 5-Fluorouracil
8. Gold
9. Hexamethylmelamine
10. Hydralazine
11. Isoniazid
12. Lithium
13. Maytansine
14. Metronidazole
15. Nitrofurantoin
16. Perhexilene
17. Procainamide
18. Procarbazine
19. Sodium cyanate
20. Vincristine

The references cited in this section contain lists of other compounds reported to cause peripheral neuropathy (111,112).

In general, drug-induced peripheral neuropathies are predominantly sensory or sensorimotor. Only rarely is the neuropathy predominantly motor. Symptoms are the same as those of other peripheral neuropathies, with numbness, tingling, and paresthesias distally in the legs. Autonomic dysfunction also may occur. The mechanism by which most drug-induced neuropathies are produced is not known. With few exceptions, therapy for drug-induced neuropathy is removal of the offending agent from the patient.

Isoniazid (INH) is used commonly in the treatment of tuberculosis. It produces a peripheral neuropathy by interfering with metabolism of pyridoxine. INH is inactivated by acetylation; a portion of the population are genetically slow acetylators and more prone to neuropathy. The neuropathy can be prevented by the oral administration of pyridoxine, 50 mg/day. Once the neuropathy has developed, pyridoxine has little effect on subsequent healing.

A similar mechanism for the development of neuropathy probably applies for use of *hydralazine,* which also interferes with pyridoxine metabolism. Concurrent treatment with pyridoxine and hydralazine should prevent the neuropathy.

Disulfiram (Antabuse) is used in the treatment of chronic alcoholism. It can cause a peripheral neuropathy that is characterized by paresthesias in the feet, burning sensations, and difficulty in walking. Later the symptoms may affect the hands; weakness is a relatively minor symptom. Disulfiram is metabolized eventually to carbon disulfide, a compound also known to produce a peripheral neuropathy. Carbon disulfide in turn interferes with pyridoxine metabolism and may act as a heavy-metal chelator. The recommended treatment of patients who take disulfiram is pyridoxine, 50 mg/day, to try to prevent development of the neuropathy (113).

INFECTIOUS NEUROPATHIES

Leprosy

Leprosy is described as the most common treatable neuropathy in the world, with the disease affecting an estimated 10 to 20 million persons (114). It is endemic in many areas of the world, including Mexico, some areas of the southeastern United States, Africa, Asia, and, on the European continent, Portugal and Spain. With the large influx of refugees from Cuba, Thailand, Cambodia, and Vietnam, the likelihood of a physician in the United States seeing a patient with leprosy increases.

Leprosy is caused by *Mycobacterium leprae,* an acid-fast bacillus found in the lesions of leprosy, including skin, peripheral nerves, muscles, and other organs. The clinical disease takes one of three main forms: tuberculoid, dimorphous, and lepromatous. The difference in disease type depends on the host reaction to the bacillus rather than on differences in bacteria per se.

The tuberculoid form is most benign. It affects a localized area of skin, with neurologic changes in the same area as the skin involvement. Lepromatous leprosy is the most virulent form, with more extensive skin and neurologic involvement and greater risk of transmission to other individuals. The dimorphous form is intermediate and can change either by downgrading to the less aggressive, tuberculoid form or by upgrading to the more virulent, lepromatous form. In the dimorphous type, the host response to the infection determines the prognosis.

The hallmark of the neuropathy is dissociated sensory loss, affecting pain and temperature sensation more than other functions. The loss of pain and temperature sensation is spotty and often is most prominent in exposed areas of skin, where skin surface temperature presumably is lower (115). As the disease progresses, motor nerves may be involved, leading to weakness and muscle atrophy. Pain also may be a symptom if the nerve involvement is associated with an inflammatory nodule. With proliferation of bacilli in the nerves, especially in patients with lepromatous leprosy, nerve thickening and enlargement may occur. In contrast to amyloidosis, which also may produce dissociated sensory loss, autonomic symptoms affecting bowel and bladder function are less common in leprosy, especially early in the course of illness.

The diagnosis of leprosy depends on demonstration of the acid-fast bacillus in appropriate specimens. Skin biopsy specimens from areas of clinical involvement or from the earlobe, elbow, or knee may demonstrate the bacillus. Biopsy specimens from involved areas of peripheral nerves, muscles, and bone marrow also may demonstrate the organism (116,117).

Treatment

The treatment of leprosy requires a comprehensive approach. If the diagnosis is suspected or confirmed, local and state health departments should be notified and their aid enlisted for both evaluation of contacts and help with treatment. The Center for Disease Control in Atlanta, Georgia, should be contacted for specific recommendations of current drug dosages and use. Contractures and other physical deformities may need surgical orthopedic correction, while ocular lesions, such as keratitis, may need treatment by an ophthalmologist. Members of the household who have contact with the patient must be followed up, and prophylactic treatment should be considered for them if the patient has either the lepromatous or dimorphous form (114,118).

Dapsone is the most common drug used for treatment of leprosy. Treatment is begun at a very low dosage, 25 mg twice a week for two weeks; the dosage is increased gradually to 100 mg twice a week for tuberculoid leprosy and is continued for two years after the disease has become inactive. In dimorphous leprosy, the dosage is increased to 100 mg three to four times a week for 10 years after the disease has become inactive. In the lepromatous form, the dosage is increased gradually to 100 mg orally six times a week and continued for life. Drug resistance to dapsone has been reported and viable bacilli have been recovered from biopsy specimens after the patient has taken the drug for years (114,119).

Rifampin in doses of 600 mg/day results in rapid killing of the bacillus. However, shedding of dead bacilli from tissues may take years. Rifampin can be used in combination with dapsone, or as an alternative drug in patients with dapsone-resistant disease (120).

Acedapsone is a long-acting sulfone drug and is used in areas where leprosy is epidemic but where travel to and from a medical facility is difficult. It can be given as an injection five times per year and results in a significant decrease in cases of leprosy. It is not currently approved for use in the United States (121).

Other drugs are also being used for treatment of leprosy at present, particularly in areas of the world other than the United States. Clofazimine, 100 mg three times a week, has proved effective in clinical trials in patients with lepromatous leprosy (122).

During treatment of lepromatous leprosy, patients may experience an acute allergic reaction termed *erythema nodosum leprosum* (ENL). It usually occurs after several months of treatment and is characterized by a systemic illness with fever, malaise, hepatosplenomegaly, lymphadenopathy, and arthritis. Pathologically, the reaction is characterized by vasculitis of small and medium-sized vessels. This aspect probably represents a type of acute hypersensitivity reaction that is precipitated by release of antigens from dead bacteria (114).

When such a reaction occurs, treatment must be started immediately. Prednisone, 60 mg/day, or similar corticosteroids should be given if the reaction is severe or if it causes significant neuritis or ocular problems. General measures include bed rest, splinting, and drainage of any abscesses that occur. Thalidomide, 100–300 mg/day, is a specific treatment, and symptoms usually clear in 48 hours. If the reaction is severe and does not respond to these measures, the sulfones may need to be discontinued for a time (114).

Herpes Zoster

Herpes zoster results from reactivation of a latent varicella-zoster infection. It occurs most frequently in persons of advancing age and also with high frequency in patients with renal transplants and Hodgkin's lymphoma (5–25% of patients with Hodgkin's lymphoma develop zoster at some time during the course of their disease).

The symptoms of herpes zoster begin with localized pain, followed by an eruption of vesicular lesions in a dermatome distribution. New lesions continue to form for three or four days, while old lesions form pustules and then crusts and scabs. Generalized cutaneous dissemination occurs in about 2% of elderly persons but in about 5–15% of immunosuppressed patients. The mortality is low (0–5%) despite dissemination.

Zoster usually affects single or several adjacent dorsal-root ganglia and adjacent nerve roots. The thoracic area is affected most frequently, followed by ophthalmic division of the fifth cranial nerve. In about 30% of patients, the infection results in pain and weakness in the involved myotomes. The weakness usually improves, but the postherpetic neuralgia often remains as the main cause of morbidity (123).

Treatment

No specific, effective therapy for herpes zoster is available at present. The role of steroids in treatment is controversial. The treatment of the pain is similar to that in other painful neuropathies.

It is likely that specific antiviral treatment will be available in the future. The use of adenine arabinoside (Ara-A) in immunosuppressed patients with zoster has been shown to enhance the clearing of virus from vesicles, decrease formation of new vesicles and relieve pain acutely, with a low incidence of postherpetic neuralgia. The drug is now undergoing more clinical trials before being released for use (124).

Another compound, acyclovir (9-[2-hydroxyethoxymethyl] quanine) was given to 23 cancer patients with either herpes zoster or herpes simplex. Of seven patients with localized zoster, all received relief of pain within 24 hours of starting treatment, with no formation of new vesicles after 24 hours. This compound is being tested in England and is not yet available for general use (125).

With both adenine arabinoside and acyclovir, the earlier the treatment is started, the better the results. In addition, adenine arabinoside was more effective in younger patients (123,124).

Acute Inflammatory Polyradiculoneuropathy (Guillain–Barré Syndrome)

Guillain–Barré syndrome is an acutely or subacutely developing polyradiculoneuropathy whose hallmark is progressive motor weakness of more than one limb. Reflexes become hypoactive and then are lost. Sensory symptoms are common during the course of the disease, although severe sensory loss is less common. The disease usually progresses for a period of two to four weeks, reaches a plateau for a time, and then begins to improve. Facial weakness and other cranial nerve involvement may occur, along with autonomic dysfunction. The weakness and sensory symptoms usually are symmetric in distribution, although not necessarily in degree of involvement. After improvement begins, most patients make a functional recovery, although this may take many months.

Laboratory tests usually show an elevated level of CSF protein after the first week of symptoms, with 10 or fewer mononuclear cells per mm^3 in the spinal fluid. Electrodiagnostically, nerve conduction velocities may be slowed, distal latencies prolonged, or F-wave responses abnormal, or there may be a conduction block at some point during the illness.

The diagnosis cannot be made in the presence of other diseases known to cause polyneuropathy, such as lead intoxication, porphyria, or diphtheria. The diagnosis is in doubt if weakness is persistently asymmetric, if more than 50 white cells per mm^3 are found in the spinal fluid, or if the patient has significant CNS involvement (126).

The etiology of Guillain–Barré syndrome is unclear. It frequently follows an antecedent infection or, less commonly, surgery or other types of stress. It is marked pathologically by an inflammatory infiltrate in peripheral nerves and nerve roots in association with segmental demyelination and, in severe cases, axonal degeneration. It is generally considered to be an autoimmune disease, with tissue destruction secondary to cell-mediated responses (127).

Treatment

The mainstay of treatment is good supportive nursing care, with careful monitoring for respiratory, cardiovascular, or autonomic complications. At present, no specific drug therapy has been shown to be beneficial.

Respiratory insufficiency can develop very rapidly in severe cases of Guillain–Barré and was a common cause of mortality in the past. In patients with relatively mild weakness, close observation along with monitoring of vital capacity and tidal volume twice a day are recommended. If a decrease in vital capacity is documented, the patient should be placed in an intensive care unit and have respiratory function checked more frequently. When the vital capacity is less than three times the predicted tidal volume, the patient will be unable to cough effectively. When the vital capacity decreases to less than twice the predicted tidal volume, intubation or tracheostomy is recommended to aid ventilation. Reliance on measurements of blood gases is not recommended because younger patients with good pulmonary gas exchange may be able to maintain a normal Po_2 and Pco_2, even with a decrease in vital capacity (128). As weakness increases, the patient may suddenly decompensate and be unable to continue to ventilate adequately. Elective tracheostomy, performed in an operating room before the patient is in severe difficulty, is much more satisfactory than emergency intubation in an acutely hypoxic patient. When the patient is using a ventilator, close attention to pulmonary toilet is necessary. Optimal respiratory care requires close teamwork between respiratory therapists, pulmonary medicine specialists, and anesthesiologists.

The most common cause of mortality at present in patients with Guillain–Barré syndrome is cardiovascular collapse secondary to autonomic dysfunction. Marked swings in blood pressure with periods of hypertension or hypotension, along with cardiac arrhythmias, represent potentially life-threatening situations. Continuous electrocardiographic monitoring in an intensive care unit is necessary, along with frequent checks of blood pressure. If fluctuations in blood pressure occur, an intra-arterial line with continuous monitoring is recommended (129,130).

Episodes of significant bradycardia are usually best managed with IV atropine, with the dose titrated as needed. Patients with episodes of asystole may require installation of a demand pacemaker. Hypotension is best treated with IV fluids to expand the intravascular volume. In order to avoid reflex autonomic discharges, the patient must be handled carefully. If tracheal suctioning is needed, the procedure must be done gently with a minimum of tracheal stimulation. Because these patients are very weak, they must have their position in bed changed every one to two hours. However, these changes in position must also be done carefully in order to avoid excessive manipulation of tracheostomy tubes.

Autonomic involvement can also lead to bladder dysfunction and urine retention. If this occurs acutely, the distended bladder can produce significant reflex changes, leading to bradycardia, tachycardia, or hypertension. Urine output must be monitored, and the abdomen must be palpated to be sure that bladder distention does not occur. If retention is a problem, patients who can help support themselves can use the Crede maneuver while sitting on the commode to help empty the bladder. In a severely affected patient who is quadriplegic, temporary use of an indwelling catheter may be needed. Again, fastidious care must be taken to avoid development of significant urinary tract infection.

Because severe weakness predisposes the patient to venous stasis, thrombosis, and pulmonary emboli, the use of low-dose heparin is recommended until muscle tone returns. Care must be taken to monitor the stool for occult blood to determine whether there is gastrointestinal bleeding. At times, the stress of a severe illness associated with the autonomic dysfunction can lead to stress ulcers. Likewise, intracranial hemorrhage may occur during hypertensive episodes. Nonetheless, the incidence of pulmonary emboli in some series is significant enough that it is advisable to use prophylactic measures (129).

For the severely weak patient, the use of wrist splints, elbow and heel pads, and a foot board can help prevent the development of bed sores and flexion contractures. The patient should do passive range-of-motion exercises during the course of illness and graduate to active range-of-motion exercises as strength returns. If the patient has difficulties in swallowing, feeding via a nasogastric tube may be necessary to help maintain adequate protein and caloric intake.

Because of the probable autoimmune nature of Guillain–Barré syndrome, a variety of immunosuppressive agents have been tried in treatment of the disease. There is no consensus about the place of steroids in the treatment of Guillain–Barré syndrome. Articles that claim a beneficial effect as well as those that claim either no effect or deleterious effect exist in the literature (131–134). Similarly, a variety of immunosuppressive agents have been used with various degrees of success (135,136). The treatment modality used most recently is plasmapheresis (137–140). None of the studies of plasmapheresis in Guillain–Barré syndrome used controls, and the apparent response to plasmapheresis varied. At this time, the value of any of these modalities is unclear and must await elucidation by a well-designed, controlled clinical study.

Chronic Inflammatory and Chronic Relapsing Polyneuropathy

Chronic inflammatory polyneuropathy is a subacute to chronically progressive, predominantly motor polyneuropathy of unknown etiology. In a small percentage of cases, the disease may follow acute inflammatory polyneuropathy. The disease may begin with motor weakness or sensory symptoms and progress without significant improvement for periods of three to six months or more. Weakness eventually becomes the dominant symptom, although sensory symptoms are present. Both proximal and distal muscles may be involved, and reflexes are hypoactive or absent. Motor-nerve conduction velocities are always slowed and levels of CSF protein are elevated. Nerve biopsy specimens often show loss of large-diameter fibers, inflammatory-cell infiltrate, Wallerian degeneration, and evidence of segmental demyelination and remyelination (127,141–143).

At times remission occurs, and the patient improves spontaneously. After a period of improvement, the disease may recur, with recovery after each relapse less complete than the initial recovery. This is known as chronic relapsing neuropathy and also may occasionally follow acute inflammatory polyradiculoneuropathy. Both forms of chronic neuropathy are thought to be cell-mediated autoimmune disorders, with host factors partially responsible for the differing clinical course.

The diagnosis of chronic inflammatory or chronic relapsing polyradiculoneuropathy is based on the progressive course, absence of reflexes, elevated levels of CSF protein, and slowed motor-nerve conduction velocities. A nerve biopsy may help confirm the diagnosis (141,143–144).

Treatment

The most common treatment modality used in these disorders is prednisone (141,142,143). Both daily and alternate-day dose schedules have been used. Unless the patient is severely weak and has respiratory dysfunction or bulbar weakness, I prefer to use alternate-day prednisone from the outset. The usual dosage is 100 mg orally every other day either until the patient has reached a plateau of improvement or until three to six months of treatment have elapsed without improvement. The dosage is then tapered very slowly, and the patient's condition is observed carefully for evidence of recurrence. The usual rate of tapering prednisone is by 5 mg every two to four weeks on an alternate-day schedule.

In more severely affected patients whose respiratory status may be compromised, prednisone, 40–80 mg/day in divided doses, can be given. This dosage is continued until the patient has significant improvement and has reached a stable plateau at which time the patient is switched to an alternate-day treatment schedule. If the patient has been on daily prednisone for more than one to two weeks, the switch to alternate-day prednisone will require a period of low-dose supplemental prednisone given on one day, with the high-dose prednisone given on alternate days. Again, tapering is begun after the patient has reached a plateau and has remained there for several weeks.

A number of patients treated with steroids become quite sensitive to reduced doses of these drugs, and relapse may occur after a very small reduction in prednisone dosage. When this occurs, the dosage must be increased immediately to prevent further progression (141,143,144).

While patients take prednisone, it is advisable to give them antacids on a regular basis, along with supplemental potassium. The alternate-day regimen coupled with antacid and potassium treatment usually keeps side effects to a minimum.

During the course of treatment, some patients not only demonstrate steroid responsiveness, but also become steroid dependent. Attempts at weaning these patients from the steroids completely results in relapse, which may be more severe and of longer duration than the initial illness. As soon as a relapse occurs, prompt treatment with steroids should be instituted. In these individuals, a long-term alternate-day treatment program with prednisone can be anticipated. Many patients may require 20–30 mg prednisone every other day to maintain function (143–145).

Other immunosuppressant agents have also been used, with variable success. Frequently these drugs are coupled with prednisone, although they may be used alone. Cyclophosphamide, 1.0–3.0 mg/kg/day orally can be tried; azathioprine, 1.0–2.0 mg/kg/day orally also can be used. With both drugs, blood counts must be monitored to make sure that bone marrow suppression does not occur. The usual parameter for determining whether the dosage of immunosuppressant is adequate is the presence of leukopenia, with a white cell count in the range of 3,000–4,000 per mm^3. However, some patients with chronic inflammatory polyneuropathy respond clinically at doses lower than those needed to induce bone marrow suppression.

Plasmapheresis also has been used in chronic inflammatory and chronic relapsing polyneuropathy. In these entities, the use of plasmapheresis coupled with immunosuppression frequently results in improvement in the patient's clinical state. Plasmapheresis may need to be repeated periodically to maintain the improvement (139,146–148).

Neuropathies in Connective Tissue Disorders and Vasculitides

The clinical manifestation of peripheral nerve involvement that occurs in collagen-vascular diseases and in diseases with prominent vasculitis have been reviewed by Glaser (149) and Conn and Dyck (150). In these diseases, peripheral nerve involvement can be seen as a mononeuritis, mononeuritis multiplex, peripheral sensorimotor neuropathy, or entrapment neuropathy. The clinical aspects of the peripheral nerve involvement in these diseases will be summarized briefly.

In rheumatoid arthritis, peripheral neuropathy is usually seen only in patients with long-standing, severe rheumatoid arthritis. It often begins as a sensory neuropathy and may progress to a more severe sensorimotor neuropathy. At times mononeuritis multiplex may occur, presumably secondary to vasculitis affecting the nerve. Entrapment neuropathies may occur when there is joint swelling and inflammation; these neuropathies particularly affect the median nerve in the carpal tunnel and the ulnar nerve at the elbow.

In systemic lupus erythematosus, both generalized polyneuropathy and mononeuropathy multiplex may be seen. Either a progressive sensorimotor polyneuropathy or a neuronitis with loss of vibratory and position sense and with proximal motor weakness may occur. If mononeuritis occurs, it most frequently affects the nerves in the lower extremity, causing foot drop or lesions of the sciatic nerve. Occasionally, a picture similar to that of Guillain–Barré syndrome may be seen, with flaccid paralysis, elevated levels of CSF protein, and absence of cells in the spinal fluid.

The neuropathies seen in polyarteritis nodosa are most commonly mononeuritis multiplex. A generalized sensorimotor neuropathy may occur, occasionally with subacute to acute onset and resembling the Guillain–Barré syndrome.

Wegener's granulomatosis is often accompanied by systemic vasculitis, which may affect peripheral nerves, leading to mononeuritis multiplex. At times, cranial nerves may be affected through direct invasion of the granulomatous material from the nasopharynx back into the posterior fossa. Occasionally, a more typical, distal sensorimotor polyneuropathy may be seen.

The neuropathy in Sjögren's syndrome is usually a mild, symmetric, distal sensory neuropathy. Occasionally, an isolated trigeminal neuropathy may be seen as the only manifestation of peripheral nerve involvement. Similarly, isolated symptoms of trigeminal nerve involvement have been reported in the mixed connective tissue diseases.

A new syndrome comprised of polyneuropathy, plasma-cell dyscrasia, and endocrine disturbances has been reported recently in Japan and the United States (151,152). The disease is multisystemic in nature, with distal sensorimotor polyneuropathy, various endocrine abnormalities, edema, skin thickening and pigmentation, CNS involvement, and plasma-cell dyscrasia with monoclonal or polyclonal gammopathy. Pathologic findings showing microvascular abnormalities suggestive of vasculopathy are the rationale for including the disease in this section (152).

The pathogenesis of peripheral nerve involvement in this group of diseases is thought to be associated with vasculitis, although other contributing factors may also play a role. In systemic lupus erythematosus with severe renal disease, the effects of the uremia on peripheral nerve function may be superimposed on the vasculitis. Likewise, in rheumatoid arthritis, compression neuropathies and entrapment neuropathies may be superimposed on the peripheral nerve involvement of the arthritis. In some cases, the connective tissue diseases may be characterized by circulating paraproteins, which in turn may contribute to peripheral neuropathy.

Treatment

In general, the treatment of peripheral nerve involvement in these disorders depends on treatment of the underlying disease. Entrapment neuropathies in this setting should be handled as any other entrapment neuropathy with splints, rest, local injection of corticosteroids, and surgery if necessary. In rheumatoid arthritis, the development of significant neuropathy is usually associated with a severe disease state that necessitates the use of corticosteroids. Prednisone, 60 mg/day in divided doses, is given until symptoms decrease, at which time the prednisone dosage can be reduced gradually. Too rapid reduction in dosage may result in exacerbation of the polyneuropathy. The role of other drugs, such as penicillamine, gold, and some of the new anti-inflammatory agents, is still unclear.

In patients with polyarteritis nodosa, Wegener's granulomatosis, and systemic necrotizing vasculitis, the use of oral cyclophosphamide, 2 mg/kg body weight per day, has been reported to result in dramatic response and improvement (153–155). Other series have reported equally good results with a combination of prednisone, 1 mg/kg body weight per day, plus azathioprine, 1–2 mg/kg body weight per day (156). Prednisone alone, given on alternate days in doses of 60–100 mg, may maintain remission regardless of whether the remission was induced by prednisone or by prednisone plus a cytotoxic agent (157,158). Treatment of a patient with peripheral nerve involvement secondary to systemic vasculitis should begin with prednisone, 1–2 mg/kg body weight per day in divided doses. If a clinical response is not evident in two to four weeks, either azathioprine or cyclophosphamide, 1–2 mg/kg body weight per day, should be added, and the prednisone dosage should be switched to an alternate-day schedule. In severely ill patients, cytotoxic agents may need to be started sooner. Peripheral white cell counts should be greater than 3,000 per mm^3, with a neutrophil count greater than 1,500 per mm^3. If cyclophosphamide is used, potentially severe side effects may occur, including hemorrhagic cystitis and the late occurrence of bladder tumors (159,160).

Systemic lupus erythematosus apparently does not respond to cyclophosphamide as well as the other systemic vasculitides; therefore, treatment of lupus continues to depend on the use of prednisone. Although other immunosuppressants have been used in conjunction with prednisone, their role is still unclear (161).

The syndrome of polyneuropathy, plasma-cell dyscrasia, and endocrine abnormalities appears to respond well to low-dose prednisone or similar agents. In one patient, the use of 20 mg prednisolone/day resulted in significant improvement within two weeks of starting treatment. However, symptoms recurred about two weeks after stopping steroid treatment. It is likely that, in this illness, long-term administration of steroids is needed to ensure adequate suppression of disease (162).

Entrapment and Traumatic Neuropathies

Trauma is the most common cause of peripheral nerve dysfunction. Almost everyone has at some time experienced numbness or tingling in an extremity that usually was related to position and was relieved by moving to another position. Although patients often attribute this to "poor circulation," the tendency of an extremity to "go to sleep" is almost always related to transient compression of a peripheral nerve rather than to vascular insufficiency. These minor symptoms do not require specific therapy other than that which patients devise themselves, and the symptoms generally clear when the patient assumes a position that avoids putting strain and pressure on the nerve.

At times, a nerve may become compressed over a bony prominence or in a narrow canal with unyielding margins. The result is entrapment neuropathy. The general topic of entrapment neuropathies has been reviewed recently by Nakano (162), who has summarized the common sites and symptoms of a variety of syndromes of peripheral nerve compression. Only a few of the more common entrapment neuropathies will be discussed here, along with brief mention of some of the less common but occasionally bothersome neuropathies. The reader is referred to Nakano's article for a more complete description of this large topic.

A variety of occupations, hobbies, and systemic diseases are associated with increased likelihood of development of an entrapment neuropathy. Entrapment of the median nerve at the carpal tunnel is probably the most common entrapment syndrome. Persons in occupations that require repetitive flexion–extension movements at the wrist or that require sustained flexion (e.g., typing, playing piano or violin, operation of a jackhammer) are prone to the development of median nerve injury. Persons with systemic illnesses, such as diabetes or uremia, that may have an associated metabolic neuropathy are also more prone to compression neuropathy. Rheumatoid arthritis, hypothyroidism, primary or secondary amyloidosis, acromegaly (163), hemodialysis with placement of an arteriovenous fistula (164), mucopolysaccharidosis (165), pregnancy, and familial cases (166) have been associated with an increased incidence of carpal tunnel syndrome.

The symptoms of carpal tunnel syndrome usually are numbness and paresthesias in the first three digits of the hand; initially this symptom is intermittent but becomes continuous as the compression worsens. Weakness of the opponens pollicis muscle may occur later and cause difficulty in performance of fine movements of the thumb and forefinger. Nocturnal pain is a common symptom, with pain extending from the hand into the forearm and occasionally as far as the elbow. This may awaken the patient at night and is usually relieved by shaking the hand and wrist or changing positions. Physical examination may reveal a positive Tinel's sign (percussion of the median nerve in the carpal tunnel produces paresthesias in the appropriate areas of nerve distribution). Flexion of the wrist for two minutes (Phalen's sign) often aggravates the symptoms. Sensory examination may reveal mildly decreased pin or light-touch sensation over the first three fingers of the affected hand and occasional weakness or even atrophy in the opponens pollicis muscle.

The diagnosis of carpal tunnel syndrome can often be made on the basis of history and examination. Confirmation of the diagnosis can be made with use of electrodiagnostic studies; nerve conduction velocities show prolonged distal motor and distal sensory latencies in the appropriate areas of nerve distribution. If compression is severe enough to cause axonal disruption, examination by needle electrode will show evidence of denervation in the appropriate muscles. Because the carpal tunnel syndrome often exists bilaterally (although one side usually is more symptomatic than the other), it is advisable to perform the EMG on both sides.

The first consideration in the treatment of carpal tunnel syndrome is to rule out unrecognized accompanying medical conditions. Patients with hypothyroidism may respond quite well to simple treatment of the thyroid disease. Some patients develop the typical picture of carpal tunnel syndrome during pregnancy; however, the symptoms almost always clear after delivery. Other systemic diseases that may predispose the patient to the development of carpal tunnel syndrome may not be readily treatable. In such cases, median nerve compression requires symptomatic treatment.

In early, mild cases of carpal tunnel syndrome, the use of a wrist splint (not a cock-up splint) to hold the hand in a neutral position often provides relief of symptoms. The patient is instructed to wear it at night and for as long as is comfortable during the day. This is coupled with the use of an anti-inflammatory agent to decrease any accompanying inflammatory reaction. Although indomethacin or butazolidin can be used, I prefer to start with therapeutic doses of aspirin. In patients with more severe symptoms or in those for whom the splint fails to provide relief, surgical decompression is recommended. If the patient has evidence of denervation on EMG, decompression should be done immediately. Injection of a long-acting corticosteroid in the region of the carpal tunnel at times provides symptomatic relief for up to several months. It is my practice to go directly to surgery whenever the patient's sensory symptoms are constant and severe, distal motor or sensory latencies are prolonged more than twice the normal limit of the laboratory doing the study, or if there is evidence of denervation in the appropriate muscles.

Symptoms of ulnar neuropathy include numbness and paresthesias of the fourth and fifth fingers and the medial aspect of the hand to the wrist, along with weakness of the intrinsic muscles of the hand and loss of strength in abduction and adduction of the fingers. This commonly results from compression of the ulnar nerve at the elbow and is seen in patients who have desk jobs, who work with their elbows propped on benches, or who sit with their arms resting on an armchair for prolonged periods. Similar symptoms can at times result from compression of the ulnar nerve at the wrist, where it divides into a deep motor and superficial sensory branch. If the compression is at the wrist, the long flexor muscles of the forearm are spared. In such cases, electrodiagnostic studies are particularly important for demonstration of the site of nerve compression. If compression occurs at the elbow, patients with only minimal symptoms can avoid pressure over the elbow or use a foam-rubber doughnut over the elbow to protect the nerve. In more severe cases or in patients who have evidence of denervation in the intrinsic hand muscles, surgery is recommended either to decompress the nerve or to transpose the nerve to a position above the medial epicondyle. If compression occurs at the wrist, the use of a splint to keep the hand in a neutral position often relieves the symptoms. However, if denervation occurs or if the symptoms are chronic and continuous, exploration of the nerve and decompression are recommended.

In the lower extremities, compression of the femoral nerve, resulting in numbness over the anterior thigh and weakness in hip flexion and knee extension, has been reported in patients who receive anticoagulation therapy with development of a spontaneous hematoma (166–170). Diagnosis of the hematoma can be made by computed axial tomography. Anticoagulants must be stopped immediately and blood transfusions given, if necessary. The neuropathy usually improves spontaneously as the hematoma resorbs (170).

The common peroneal nerve or one of its branches, the superficial peroneal nerve or anterior tibial nerve, may be involved at the head of the fibula. If the common peroneal nerve is involved, weakness of dorsiflexion and eversion, and numbness along the lateral aspect of the foot and leg result. These patients walk with a foot drop and a characteristic slapping gait. If only the superficial peroneal nerve is involved, eversion is affected, with weakness of the peroneus longus and brevis muscles, and sensory loss along the lateral aspect of the foot and leg. With involvement of the anterior tibial nerve, weakness involves foot and toe dorsiflexion, although eversion remains relatively intact. Compression often occurs in patients who habitually sit with their legs crossed, with the top leg developing the neuropathy. Warning the patient to avoid sitting with legs crossed is usually sufficient to allow regeneration of the nerve. Other causes of mononeuropathy, including vasculitis, diabetes, and dysproteinemias also must be sought.

Many other peripheral nerves may be damaged by local trauma or by other types of entrapment. Frequently the damage results from specific activities and/or positions. Thus, ulnar neuropathy from compression of the ulnar nerve at the wrist is sometimes referred to as "bicyclist neuropathy" or "handlebar palsy" because it often occurs in individuals who do long-distance bicycle riding on low-handled racing bicycles (171–173). Bicyclists, particularly men who ride bicycles with narrow, hard saddles, may also develop pudendal nerve compression, which results in numbness and paresthesia in the genital area (173). The application of handcuffs may injure the superficial radial nerve, leading to numbness over the dorsal aspect of the thumb and adjacent web area (174).

Abdominal nerves may be entrapped in the rectus abdominal muscle, resulting in abdominal pain. Most commonly, the nerves that egress below the level of the umbilicus are affected. Localized tenderness over the area of nerve entrapment helps to establish the diagnosis. Infiltration of the region with lidocaine results in prompt relief of pain; relief of longer duration can be achieved by infiltration with a long-acting steroid preparation (175).

In the lower extremities, the posterior tibial nerve may be entrapped as it passes behind the medial malleolus and into the foot in the region known as the tarsal tunnel. Symptoms include pain, numbness, and tingling, along the sole of the foot and in the toes. If the medial plantar nerve is affected primarily, discomfort may involve the medial portion of the foot; if the lateral plantar nerve is affected primarily, discomfort is in the lateral aspect of the foot. Sensory loss may occur in either medial or lateral distribution, depending on the nerve branch affected. Neurodiagnostic studies will reveal increased distal motor latency in the distribution of the medial and lateral plantar nerves, with evidence of denervation in the intrinsic foot muscles, if compression has been severe enough to interrupt axonal integrity. Treatment usually requires surgical decompression of the nerve, although localized injections of cortisone in the region of entrapment may provide temporary relief (176,177).

On the anterior aspect of the foot, the anterior tarsal tunnel syndrome is produced by compression of the deep peroneal nerve under the inferior extensor retinaculum. Pain occurs over the dorsal aspect of the foot, particularly at night, with a discrete area of sensory loss over the space between the first and second toes plus weakness of the extensor digitorum brevis muscle. Treatment includes elevation of the legs at night and avoidance of wearing tight shoes. Local injections of cortisone may provide temporary relief. If conservative treatment fails, surgery is recommended for decompression of the nerve (178).

A related sensory nerve entrapment on the dorsal aspect of the foot is the musculocutaneous nerve entrapment. This is characterized by compression of the sensory musculocutaneous nerve just dorsal to the lateral malleolus. Pain is present over the dorsal aspect of the foot and is aggravated by exercise and/or at night. Local injection of cortisone in focal areas of tenderness has been reported to provide relief, although surgical decompression also may be required if drug therapy fails to relieve symptoms (179).

Although these entrapment syndromes are reported infrequently, it is quite likely that they are more common than the literature suggests. They probably are not recognized when they occur, which leads patients to undergo more extensive testing to rule out multiple sclerosis, spinal cord or CNS tumors, or other neurologic disasters.

REFERENCES

1. Thomas PK, Eliasson SG: Diabetic neuropathy. In: *Peripheral Neuropathy.* Edited by PJ Dyck, PK Thomas, and EH Lambert. Philadelphia, WB Saunders, 1975, pp. 956–981.
2. Thomas PK: Metabolic neuropathies. In: *Current Topics in Nerve and Muscle Research.* Edited by AG Aguayo and G Karpati. Amsterdam, Excerpta Medica, 1979, pp. 255–261.
3. Clements RS Jr: Diabetic neuropathy—newer concepts in etiology. Diabetes 28:604–611, 1979.
4. Raff MD, Sangalang V, Asbury AK: Ischemic mononeuropathy multiplex associated with diabetes mellitus. Arch Neurol 18:487–499, 1968.
5. Raff MD, Sangalang V, Asbury AK: Ischemic mononeuropathy and mononeuropathy multiplex in diabetes mellitus. N Engl J Med 279:17–23, 1968.
6. Asbury AK: Proximal diabetic neuropathy. Ann Neurol 2:179, 1977.
7. Chokroverty S, Reyes MG, Robino FA, et al: The syndrome of diabetic amyotrophy. Ann Neurol 2:181, 1977.
8. Gabbay KH: Role of sorbitol pathway in neuropathy. In: *Vascular and Neurological Changes in Early Diabetes.* Edited by RA Camerini-Davalos and HS Cole. New York, Academic Press, 1973, pp. 417–432.
9. Greene DA, DeJesus PV, Winegrad AI: Effects of insulin and dietary myo-inositol on impaired peripheral motor nerve conduction velocities in acute streptozotocin diabetes. J Clin Invest 55:1326–1336, 1975.
10. Winegrad AI, Greene DA: Diabetic polyneuropathy: the importance of insulin deficiency, hyperglycemia and alterations in myo-inositol metabolism in its pathogenesis. N Engl J Med 295:1416–1421, 1976.
11. Jeffreys JGR, Palmano KP, Sharma AK, et al: Influence of dietary myo-inositol on nerve conduction and inositol phospholipids in normal and diabetic rats. J Neurol Neurosurg Psychiatry 4:333–339, 1978.
12. Stewart MA, Sherman WR, Kurien MM, et al: Polyol accumulation in nerve tissue of rats with experimental diabetes and galactosemia. J Neurochem 14:1057–1066, 1967.
13. Ward JD, Baker RWP, Davis BH: Effect of blood sugar control on the accumulation of sorbitol and fructose in nervous tissue. Diabetes 21:1173–1178, 1972.

14. Fry IK, Hardwick C, Scott GW: Diabetic neuropathy: a survey and follow-up of 66 cases. Guys Hosp Rep 111:113–129, 1962.

15. Gregersen G: Diabetic neuropathy: influence of age, sex, metabolic control, and duration of diabetes on motor conduction velocity. Neurology 17:972–980, 1967.

16. Ward JD, Barnes CG, Fisher DJ, et al: Improvement in nerve conduction following treatment in newly diagnosed diabetics. Lancet 1:428–430, 1971.

17. Graf RJ, Halter JB, Halar E, et al: Nerve conduction abnormalities in untreated maturity-onset diabetes: relation to levels of fasting plasma glucose and glycosylated hemoglobin. Ann Intern Med 90:298–303, 1979.

18. Campbell IW, Fraser DM, Ewing DJ, et al: Peripheral and autonomic nerve function in diabetic ketoacidosis. Lancet 2:167–169, 1976.

19. Salway JG, Whitehead L, Finnegan JA, et al: Effect of myo-inositol on peripheral nerve function in diabetes. Lancet 2:1282–1284, 1978.

20. Clements RS Jr, Vourganti B, Kuba T, et al: Dietary myo-inositol intake and peripheral nerve function in diabetic neuropathy. Metabolism 28:477–483, 1979.

21. Gregersen G, Borsting H, Theil P, et al: Myo-inositol and function of peripheral nerves in human diabetes. Acta Neurol Scand 58:241–248, 1978.

22. Gabbay KH, Spack N, Loo S, et al: Aldose reductase inhibition: studies with alrestatin. Metabolism 28:471–476, 1979.

23. Thomas PK: Screening for peripheral neuropathy in patients treated by chronic hemodialysis. Muscle and Nerve 1:396–399, 1978.

24. Asbury AK: Uremic neuropathy. In: *Peripheral Neuropathy.* Edited by PJ Dyck, PK Thomas, and EH Lambert. Philadelphia, WB Saunders, 1975, pp. 982–992.

25. Raskin NH, Fishman RA: Neurologic disorders in renal failure. N Engl J Med 294:204–206, 1976.

26. Nolph KD: Short dialysis, middle molecules and uremia. Ann Intern Med 86:93–97, 1977.

27. Clements RS Jr, DeJesus PV Jr, Winegrad AI: Raised plasma-myo-inositol in uraemia and experimental neuropathy. Lancet 1:1137–1141, 1973.

28. DeJesus PV Jr, Clements RS Jr, Winegrad AI: Hypermyoinositolemic polyneuropathy in rats. J Neurol Sci 21:237–249, 1974.

29. Avram MM, Feinfeld DA, Huatuco AH: Search for the uremic toxin. Decreased motor-nerve conduction velocity and elevated parathyroid hormone in uremia. N Engl J Med 298:1000–1003, 1978.

30. Nielsen VK: The peripheral nerve function in chronic renal failure. VII. Longitudinal course during terminal renal failure and regular hemodialysis. Acta Med Scand 195:155–162, 1974.

31. Jebsen RH, Tenckhoff H, Honet JC: Natural history of uremic polyneuropathy and effects of dialysis. N Engl J Med 277:327–333, 1967.

32. Asbury AK, Victor M, Adams RD: Uremic polyneuropathy (discussion by HR Tyler) Trans Am Neurol Assoc 87:100–103, 1962.

33. Bolton CF, Baltzan MA, Baltzan RB: Effects of renal transplantation on uremic neuropathy. N Engl J Med 284:1170–1175, 1971.

34. Nielsen VK: The peripheral nerve function in chronic renal failure. VIII. Recovery after renal transplantation. Acta Med Scand 195:163–170, 1974.

35. Canal N: Cerebral gangliosides in the treatment of peripheral neuronal diseases (letter). Muscle and Nerve 2:238–239, 1979.

36. Fusaroli M, Catizone L, Merline L: The use of brain cortex gangliosides in patients affected by uremic neuropathy. Muscle and Nerve 1:513, 1978.

37. Fincham RW, Cape CA: Neuropathy in myxedema. Arch Neurol 19:464–466, 1968.

38. Dyck PJ, Lambert EH: Polyneuropathy associated with hypothyroidism. J Neuropathol Exp Neurol 29:631–658, 1970.

39. Shirabe T, Tawara S, Terao A, et al: Myxoedematous polyneuropathy: a light and electron microscopic study of the peripheral nerve and muscle. J Neurol Neurosurg Psychiatry 38:241–247, 1975.

40. Grabow JD, Chou SM: Thyrotropin hormone deficiency, with a peripheral neuropathy. Arch Neurol 19:284–291, 1968.

41. O'Duffy JD, Randall RV, MacCarty CS: Median neuropathy (carpal-tunnel syndrome) in acromegaly. Ann Intern Med 78:379–383, 1973.

42. Low PA, McCleod JG, Turtle JR, et al: Peripheral neuropathy in acromegaly. Brain 97:139–152, 1974.

43. Logothetis J, Silverstein P, Coe J: Neurologic aspects of Waldenström's macroglobulinemia. Report of a case. Arch Neurol 5:564–573, 1960.

44. Logothetis J, Kennedy WR, Ellington A, et al: Cryoglobulinemic neuropathy. Incidence and clinic characteristics. Arch Neurol 19:389–397, 1968.

45. Read DJ, Vanhegan RI, Mathews WB: Peripheral neuropathy and benign IgG paraproteinemia. J Neurol Neurosurg Psychiatry 41:215–219, 1978.

46. Swash M, Perrin J, Schwartz MS: Significance of immunoglobulin deposition in peripheral nerve in neuropathies associated with paraproteinemia. J Neurol Neurosurg Psychiatry 42:179–183, 1979.

47. Levo Y, Gorevic PD, Kassab HJ, et al: Association between hepatitis B virus and essential mixed cryoglobulinemia. N Engl J Med 296:1501–1504, 1977.

48. Popp JW, Dienstag JL, Wands JR et al: Essential mixed cryoglobulinemia without evidence for hepatitis B virus infection. Ann Intern Med 92:379–383, 1980.

49. Levo Y: Nature of cryoglobulinaemia. Lancet 1:285–287, 1980.

50. Metzger AL, Paulus HE, Goldberg LS: Cryoglobulinemic nephropathy and neuropathy—combined immunosuppressive and corticosteroid therapy. J Rheumatol 1:462–465, 1974.

51. Iwashita H, Argyrakis A, Lowitzch K, et al: Polyneuropathy in Waldenström's macroglobulinaemia. J Neurol Sci 21:341–354, 1974.

52. Massey W, Pleet BA, Brannon WL: Waldenström's macroglobulinemia and mononeuritis multiplex. Ann Intern Med 88:360–361, 1978.

53. Julien J, Vital C, Vallat JM, et al: Polyneuropathy in Waldenström's macroglobulinemia. Arch Neurol 35:423–425, 1978.

54. Plasmapheresis in macroglobulinaemia (comment). Lancet 2:807–808, 1977.

55. Victor M: Polyneuropathy due to nutritional deficiency and alcoholism. In: *Peripheral Neuropathy.* Edited by P Dyck, PK Thomas, and EH Lambert. Philadelphia, WB Saunders, 1975, pp. 1030–1066.

56. Victor M, Adams RD: On the etiology of the alcoholic neurologic diseases, with special references to the role of nutrition. Am J Clin Nutr 9:379–397, 1961.

57. Ciongoli AK, Posen CM: Fat malabsorption neuromyopathy. Arch Neurol 26:403–408, 1972.

58. Bean WB, Hodges RE, Daum KE: Pantothenic acid deficiency induced in human subjects. J Clin Invest 34:1073–1084, 1955.

59. Mayer RF: Peripheral nerve function in vitamin B-12 deficiency. Arch Neurol 13:355–362, 1965.

60. Lockner D, Reizenstein P, Wennberg A, et al: Peripheral nerve function in pernicious anemia before and after treatment. Acta Haematol 41:257–263, 1969.

61. Roos D: Electrophysiological findings in gastrectomized patients with low serum B 12. Acta Neurol Scand 56:247–255, 1977.

62. Botez MI, Peyronnard JM, Bachevalier J, et al: Polyneuropathy and folate deficiency. Arch Neurol 35:581–584, 1978.

63. Manzoor M, Runcle J: Folate responsive neuropathy: report of ten cases. Br Med J 1:1176–1178, 1976.

64. Botez MI, Cadotte M, Beaulieu R, et al: Neurologic disorders responsive to folic acid therapy. Can Med Assoc J 115:217–222, 1976.

65. Lai CS, Ransome GA: Burning feet syndrome. Case due to malabsorption and responding to riboflavin. Br Med J 2:151–152, 1970.

66. Hood J: Femoral neuropathy in scurvy. N Engl J Med 281:1292–1293, 1969.

67. Feldman RG, Hayes MK, Younes R, et al: Lead neuropathy in adults and children. Arch Neurol 34:481–488, 1977.

68. Lin-Fu, JS: Vulnerability of children to lead exposure and toxicity. N Engl J Med 289:1229–1233, 1973.

69. Guinee VF: Lead poisoning. Am J Med 52:283–288, 1972.

70. Browder AA, Joselow MM, Louria DB: The problem of lead poisoning. Medicine (Baltimore) 52:121–139, 1973.

71. Hammond PB: Exposure of humans to lead. Annu Rev Pharmacol Toxicol 17:197–214, 1977.

72. Seppalainen AM, Tola S, Hernberg S: Subclinical neuropathy at 'safe' levels of lead exposure. Arch Environ Health 30:180–183, 1975.

73. Buchthal F, Behse F: Electrophysiology and nerve biopsy in men exposed to lead. Br J Ind Med 36:135–147, 1979.

74. Chisolm JJ: Treatment of lead poisoning. Mod Treat 4:710–727, 1967.

75. Crawhall JC, Lecavalier D, Ryan P: Penicillamine, its metabolism and therapeutic applications: a review. Biopharm Drug Disp 1:73–95, 1979.

76. Goldstein NP, McCall JI, Dyck PJ: Metal neuropathy. In: *Peripheral Neuropathy.* Edited by PJ Dyck, PK Thomas, and EH Lambert. Philadelphia, WB Saunders, 1975, pp. 1227–1262.

77. Lequesne PM, McLeod JG: Peripheral neuropathy following a single exposure to arsenic. J Neurol Sci 32:437–451, 1977.

78. Feldman RG, Niles CA, Kelly-Hayes M, et al: Peripheral neuropathy in arsenic smelter workers. Neurology 29:939–944, 1979.

79. Robinson TJ: Arsenical polyneuropathy due to caustic arsenical paste. Br Med J 3:139, 1975.

80. Sunderman FW, Sunderman FW Jr: *Laboratory Diagnosis of Diseases Caused by Toxic Agents.* St. Louis, Warren H. Guen, 1970.

81. Chang LW: Neurotoxic effects of mercury. A review. Environ Res 14:329–373, 1977.

82. Dales LG: The neurotoxicity of alkyl mercury compounds. Am J Med 53:219–232, 1972.

83. Felton JS, Kahn E, Salick B, et al: Heavy metal poisoning: mercury and lead. Ann Intern Med 76:779–792, 1972.

84. Hopkins A: Toxic neuropathy due to industrial agents. In: *Peripheral Neuropathy.* Edited by PJ Dyck, PK Thomas, and EH Lambert. Philadelphia, WB Saunders, 1975, pp. 1207–1226.

85. Allen N: Clinical course and diagnosis of recently described toxic neuropathies. Paper presented by JN Mendell at the Annual Meeting of the American Academy of Neurology, Course No. 18: Peripheral Neuropathies, April 30, 1980.

86. Spencer PS, Sabri MI, Schaumberg HH, et al: Does a defect of energy metabolism in the nerve fiber underlie axonal degeneration in polyneuropathies? Ann Neurol 5:501–507, 1978.

87. Prockop L: Neurotoxic volatile substances. Neurology 29:862–865, 1979.

88. Schaumberg HH, Spencer PS: Toxic neuropathies. Neurology 29:429–431, 1979.

89. Schaumberg HH, Spencer PS: Toxic models of disorders of the peripheral nervous system. In: *Current Topics in Nerve and Muscle Research.* Edited by AJ Aguayo and G Karpati. Amsterdam, Excerpta Medica, 1979, pp. 265–270.

90. Spencer PS: The environmental neurotoxin. A threat and a tool. In: *Current Topics in Nerve and Muscle Research.* Edited by AJ Aguayo and G Karpati. Amsterdam, Excerpta Medica, 1979, pp. 271–273.

91. Spencer PS, Schaumberg HH: Neurotoxic chemicals as probes of cellular mechanisms of neuromuscular disease. In: *Current Topics in Nerve and Muscle Research.* Edited by AJ Aguayo and G Karpati. Amsterdam, Excerpta Medica, 1979, pp. 274–281.

92. Griffin JW, Price DL, Hoffman PN, et al: Toxic axonal neuropathies. In: *Current Topics in Nerve and Muscle Research.* Edited by AJ Aguayo and G Karpati. Amsterdam, Excerpta Medica, 1979, pp. 282–291.

93. Lampert PW, Braheny SL, Powell HC: Neuropathies caused by myelinotoxic agents. In: *Current Topics in Nerve and Muscle Research.* Edited by AJ Aguayo and G Karpati. Amsterdam, Excerpta Medica, 1979, pp. 292–298.

94. Jacobs JM: Perikaryal neurotoxins. In: *Current Topics in Nerve and Muscle Research.* Edited by AJ Aguayo and G Karpati. Amsterdam, Excerpta Medica, 1979, pp. 299–308.

95. Nicholson WJ, Moore JA (editors): *Health Effects of Hologenated Aromatic Hydrocarbons.* Ann NY Acad Sci 320:1–730, 1979.

96. Korobkin R, Asbury AK, Sumner AJ, et al: Glue-sniffing neuropathy. Arch Neurol 32:158–162, 1975.

97. Altenkirch H, Mager J, Stoltenburg G, et al: Toxic polyneuropathies after sniffing a glue thinner. J Neurol 214:137–152, 1977.

98. Sahenk Z, Mendell JR, Couri D, et al: Polyneuropathy from inhalation of N_2O cartridges through a whipped-cream dispenser. Neurology 28:485–487, 1978.

99. Prockop LD, Alt M, Tison J: 'Huffer's' neuropathy. JAMA 229:1083–1084, 1974.

100. Oh SJ, Kim JM: Giant axonal swelling in 'Huffer's' neuropathy. Arch Neurol 33:583–586, 1976.

101. Keogh, JP, Pestronk A, Wertheimer D, et al: An epidemic of urinary retention caused by dimethylaminopropionitrile. JAMA 243:746–749, 1980.

102. Chappelka R: Letter to the editor. N Engl J Med 302:1146–1147, 1980.

103. LeWitt PA: The neurotoxicity of the rat poison Vacor. N Engl J Med 302:73–77, 1980.

104. Benowitz NL, Byrd R, Schambelan M, et al: Dihydroergotamine treatment for orthostatic hypotension from Vacor rodenticide. Ann Intern Med 92:387–388, 1980.

105. Morgan JP, Tulloss TC: The Jake Walk blues. A toxicologic tragedy mirrored in American popular music. Ann Intern Med 85:804–808, 1976.

106. Dennis DT: Jake Walk in Vietnam (letter). Ann Intern Med 86:665–666, 1977.

107. Namba T, Nolte CT, Jackrel J, et al: Poisoning due to organophosphate insecticides: acute and chronic manifestations. Am J Med 50:475–492, 1971.

108. Worrell CL: The management of organophosphate intoxication. South Med J 68:335–339, 1975.

109. Takahashi K, Nakamura H, Iwata K: Ultrastructure of the peripheral nerve in polyneuropathy due to diptelex. Clin Neurol (Tokyo) 15:430–435, 1975.

110. Fukuhara N, Hoshi M, Mori S: Core/targetoid fibers and multiple cytoplasmic bodies in organophosphate neuropathy. Acta Neuropathol (Berl) 40:137–144, 1977.

111. Argov Z, Mastaglia FL: Drug-induced peripheral neuropathies. Br Med J 1:663–666, 1979.

112. Freemon FR: Causes of polyneuropathy. Acta Neurol Scand [Suppl 59]:51:7–43, 1975.

113. Major LF, Goyer PF: Effects of disulfiram and pyridoxine on serum cholesterol. Ann Intern Med 88:53–56, 1978.

114. Sabin TD, Swift TR: Leprosy. In: *Peripheral Neuropathy.* Edited by PJ Dyck, PK Thomas, and EH Lambert. Philadelphia, WB Saunders, 1975, pp. 1166–1198.

115. Sabin TD: Temperature-linked sensory loss. A unique pattern in leprosy. Arch Neurol 20:257–262, 1969.

116. Sebille A, Gray F: Electromyographic recording and muscle biopsy in lepromatous leprosy. J Neurol Sci 40:3–10, 1979.

117. Lawrence C, Schreiber AJ: Leprosy's footprints in bone marrow histiocytes. N Engl J Med 300:834–835, 1979.

118. Filice GA, Fraser DW: Management of household contacts of leprosy patients. Ann Intern Med 88:538–542, 1978.

119. Bullock WE: Immunology and the therapeutics of leprosy. Ann Intern Med 91:482–483, 1979.

120. US Leprosy Panel (US–Japan Cooperative Medical Science Program) and the Leonard Wood Memorial: Rifampin therapy of lepromatous leprosy. Am J Trop Med Hyg 24:475–484, 1975.

121. Russel DA, Shepard CC, McRae DH, et al: Acedapsone (DADDS) treatment of leprosy patients in the Karimui of Papua, New Guinea: status at six years. Am J Trop Med Hyg 24:485–495, 1975.

122. US Leprosy Panel (US–Japan Cooperative Medical Science Program) and the Leonard Wood Memorial: Spaced clofazimine therapy of lepromatous leprosy. Am J Trop Med Hyg 25:437–444, 1976.

123. Dolin R, Reichman RC, Mazur MH, et al: Herpes zoster–varicella infections in immunosuppressed patients. Ann Intern Med 89:375–388, 1978.

124. Whitley RJ, Ch'ien LT, Dolin R, et al: Adenine arabinoside therapy of herpes zoster in the immunosuppressed. N Engl J Med 294:1193–1199, 1976.

125. Selby PJ, Jameson B, Watson JG, et al: Parenteral acyclovir therapy for herpesvirus infections in man. Lancet 2:1267–1270, 1979.

126. Asbury AK, Arnason BGW, Karp HR, et al: Criteria for diagnosis of Guillain-Barré syndrome. Ann Neurol 3:565–566, 1978.

127. Arnason BGW: Inflammatory polyradiculoneuropathies. In: *Peripheral Neuropathy.* Edited by PJ Dyck, PK Thomas, and EH Lambert. Philadelphia, WB Saunders, 1975, pp. 1110–1148.

128. O'Donohue WJ Jr, Baker JP, Bell GM, et al: Respiratory failure in neuromuscular disease. Management in a respiratory intensive care unit. JAMA 235:733–735, 1976.

129. Bredin CP: Guillain-Barré syndrome: the unsolved cardiovascular problems. Ir J Med Sci 146:273–279, 1977.

130. Davies AG, Dingle AR: Observations on cardiovascular and neuroendocrine disturbance in the Guillain-Barré syndrome. J Neurol Neurosurg Psychiatry 35:176–179, 1972.

131. Swick HM, McQuillen MP: The use of steroids in the treatment of idiopathic polyneuritis. Neurology 26:205–212, 1976.

132. Marshall J: The Landry-Guillain-Barré syndrome. Brain 86:55–64, 1963.

133. Goodall JAD, Kosmidis JC, Geddes AM: Effect of corticosteroids on course of Guillain-Barré syndrome. Lancet 1:524–526, 1974.

134. Hughes RAC, Newsom-Davis JM, Perkin GD: Controlled trial of prednisolone in acute polyneuropathy. Lancet 2:750, 1978.

135. Rosen AD, Vastola EF: Clinical effects of cyclophosphamide in Guillain-Barré polyneuritis. J Neurol Sci 30:179–187, 1976.

136. Yuill GM, Swinburn WR, Liversedge LA: Treatment of polyneuropathy with azathioprine. Lancet 2:854–856, 1970.

137. Brettle RP, Gross M, Legg NJ, et al: Treatment of acute polyneuropathy by plasma exchange. Lancet 2:1100, 1978.

138. Ropper AJ, Shahani B, Huggins CE: Improvement in four patients with acute Guillain-Barré syndrome after plasma exchange. Neurology 30:361, 1980.

139. Mark B, Hurwitz BJ, Olanow CW, et al: Plasmapheresis in idiopathic inflammatory polyradiculoneuropathy. Neurology 30:361, 1980.

140. Cook JD, Tindall RAS, Walker J, et al: Plasma exchange as a treatment of acute and chronic idiopathic autoimmune polyneuropathy: limited success. Neurology 30:361, 1980.

141. Dyck PJ, Lais AC, Ohta M, et al: Chronic inflammatory polyradiculoneuropathy. Mayo Clin Proc 50:621–637, 1975.

142. Arnason BG: Polyneuritis. In: *Scientific Approaches to Clinical Neurology.* Edited by ES Goldensohn and SH Appel. Philadelphia, Lea and Febiger, 1977, pp. 1494–1509.

143. Oh SJ: Subacute demyelinating polyneuropathy responding to corticosteroid treatment. Arch Neurol 35:509–516, 1978.

144. Schwartzman RJ, Engel WK, Rapoport A: Criteria for prednisone treatment of idiopathic polyneuropathy. Neurology 27:364, 1977.

145. Austin JH: Recurrent polyneuropathies and their corticosteroid treatment. Brain 81:157–192, 1958.

146. Server AC, Lefkowith J, Braine H, et al: Treatment of chronic relapsing inflammatory polyradiculoneuropathy by plasma exchange. Ann Neurol 6:258–261, 1979.

147. Server AC, Stein SA, Braine H, et al: Experience with plasma exchange and cyclophosphamide in the treatment of chronic relapsing inflammatory polyradiculoneuropathy. Neurology 30:362, 1980.

148. Fowler H, Vulpe M, Marks G, et al: Recovery from chronic progressive polyneuropathy after treatment with plasma exchange and cyclophosphamide. Lancet 2:1193, 1979.

149. Glaser GH: Peripheral neuropathy and collagen diseases. In: *Scientific Approaches to Clinical Neurology.* Edited by ES Goldensohn and SH Appel. Philadelphia, Lea and Febiger, 1977, pp. 1510–1517.

150. Conn DL, Dyck PJ: Angiographic neuropathy in connective tissue diseases. In: *Peripheral Neuropathy.* Edited by PJ Dyck, PK Thomas, and EH Lambert. Philadelphia, WB Saunders, 1975, pp. 1149–1165.

151. Imawari M, Akatsuka N, Ishibasi M, et al: Syndrome of plasma cell dyscrasia, polyneuropathy, and endocrine disturbances. Report of a case. Ann Intern Med 81:490–493, 1974.

152. Trentham DE, Masi AI, Marker HW: Polyneuropathy and anasarca: evidence for a new connective-tissue syndrome and vasculopathic contribution. Ann Intern Med 84:271–274, 1976.

153. Fauci AS, Haynes BF, Katz P: The spectrum of vasculitis. Clinical, pathologic, immunologic, and therapeutic considerations. Ann Intern Med 89:660–676, 1978.

154. Fauci AS, Katz P, Haynes BF, et al: Cyclophosphamide therapy of severe systemic necrotizing vasculitis. N Engl J Med 301:235–238, 1979.

155. Fauci AS, Doppman JL, Wolff SM: Cyclophosphamide-induced remissions in advanced polyarteritis nodosa. Am J Med 64:890–894, 1978.

156. Pirofsky B, Bardana EJ Jr: Immunosuppressive therapy in rheumatic disease. Med Clin North Am 61:419–437, 1977.

157. Deremee RA: Letter to the editor. Ann Intern Med 90:437, 1979.

158. Deremee RA, McDonald TJ, Harrison EG Jr, et al: Wegener's granulomatosis. Anatomic correlates, a proposed classification. Mayo Clin Proc 51:777–781, 1976.

159. Plotz PH, Klippel JH, Decker JL, et al: Bladder complications in patients receiving cyclophosphamide for systemic lupus erythematosus or rheumatoid arthritis. Ann Intern Med 91:221–223, 1979.

160. Lockshin MD: Letter to the editor. N Engl J Med 301:1123, 1979.

161. Decker JL, Steinberg AD, Reinertsen JC, et al: Systemic lupus erythematosus: evolving concepts. Ann Intern Med 91:587–604, 1979.

162. Nakano KK: The entrapment neuropathies. Muscle and Nerve 1:264–279, 1978.

163. O'Duffy JD, Randall RV, MacCarty CS: Median neuropathy (carpal-tunnel syndrome) in acromegaly. A sign of endocrine overactivity. Ann Intern Med 78:379–383, 1973.

164. Warren DJ, Otieno LS: Carpal tunnel syndrome in patients on intermittent haemodialysis. Postgrad Med J 51:450–452, 1975.

165. MacDougal B, Weeks PM, Wray RC Jr: Median nerve compression and trigger finger in the mucopolysaccharidoses and related diseases. Plast Reconstr Surg 59:260–263, 1977.

166. Gray RC, Poppo MJ, Gottlieb NL: Primary familial bilateral carpal tunnel syndrome. Ann Intern Med 91:37–40, 1979.

167. Susens GP, Hendrickson CG, Mulder MJ, et al: Femoral nerve entrapment secondary to a heparin hematoma. Ann Intern Med 69:575–579, 1968.

168. Butterfield WS, Neviaser RJ, Roberts MP: Femoral neuropathy and anticoagulants. Ann Surg 176:58–61, 1972.

169. Wilbanks OL, Fuller CH: Femoral neuropathy due to retroperitoneal bleeding. Arch Intern Med 132:83–86, 1973.

170. Wells J, Templeton J: Femoral neuropathy associated with anticoagulant therapy. Clin Orthop 121:155–160, 1977.

171. Smail DF: Handlebar palsy (letter). N Engl J Med 292:322, 1975.

172. Finelli PF: Handlebar palsy (cont.) (letter). N Engl J Med 292:702, 1975.
173. Hodges SC: Handlebar palsy (cont.) (letter). N Engl J Med 292:702, 1975.
174. Dorfman LJ, Jayaram AR: Handcuff neuropathy. JAMA 239:957, 1978.
175. Doouss TW, Boas RA: The abdominal cutaneous nerve entrapment syndrome. NZ Med J 81:473–475, 1975.
176. Goodgold J, Kopell HP, Spielholz NI: The tarsal-tunnel syndrome. Objective diagnostic criteria. N Engl J Med 273:742–745, 1965.
177. Edwards WG, Lincoln CR, Bassett FH, et al: The tarsal tunnel syndrome. Diagnosis and treatment. JAMA 207:716–720, 1969.
178. Krause KH, Witt T, Ross A: The anterior tarsal tunnel syndrome. J Neurol 217:67–74, 1977.
179. Mackey D, Colbert DS, Chater EH: Musculo-cutaneous nerve entrapment. Irish J Med Sci 146:100–102, 1977.

6
Treatment of Movement Disorders

Ronald M. Kobayashi

During the past quarter century, our understanding of the role of neurotransmitters in neurologic function has increased greatly. This knowledge has served as the foundation for significant advances in neuropharmacologic treatment, and patients who suffer from movement disorders have been among the major beneficiaries of these developments.

Movement disorders may be defined operationally as abnormalities in coordinated movement or the presence of involuntary movements usually secondary to disturbed extrapyramidal function. It is acknowledged that this is a working and probably arbitrary definition that has evolved over recent years. In practical terms, these disorders include parkinsonism and various types of tremor, chorea, athetosis, ballismus, and dyskinesias.

This chapter focuses primarily on the use of drugs in the treatment of movement disorders but acknowledges the important contributions of selected surgical procedures, psychiatric care, and physical, occupational, vocational, and speech therapy. Orientation toward the use of drugs is predicated on the role, both demonstrated and postulated, of neurotransmitters in the pathogenesis of movement disorders. In many cases, our understanding of these clinical disorders is limited to recognition of the benefit of a particular drug for a particular manifestation. From these observations, certain inferences as to locus and mechanism of action seem reasonable, but direct substantive evidence may be lacking.

In almost all cases, treatment is directed against the manifestations rather than against the basic disease process; thus, it is symptomatic but not curative. Although it may not be clear whether the natural history of the disorder in a particular case is altered, functional status and quality of life certainly may be improved significantly.

The discussion of therapy for each disorder will begin with a brief summary of the important clinical features that distinguish that particular movement disturbance, since incorrect diagnosis all too often is the cause of apparent treatment failures. This chapter is intended to be practical in approach; accordingly, only drugs currently and widely available are discussed at any length. New drugs that are licensed for investigational use only are reviewed briefly.

PARKINSONISM

Treatment of parkinsonism with levodopa epitomizes more than any other neurologic disease a much-desired paradigm in clinical medicine, namely, the development of effective and rational therapy after clinical observations and laboratory investigations suggest the basic pathophysiology. After it was recognized that depletion of dopamine in the neostriatum was a fundamental aspect of parkinsonism, therapeutic trials demonstrated levodopa to be effective in treatment of the manifestations of the disease. It should be fully appreciated that this is a greatly desired but, unfortunately, seldomly achieved model of therapy flowing from basic laboratory and clinical research.

Clinical Diagnosis

The major clinical manifestations of parkinsonism are resting tremor, plastic rigidity, bradykinesia, and gait disturbance. Not only do these manifestations have special features that distinguish them from other neurologic problems, but their clinical expression often is modified by intermittence or occurrence under particular circumstances. For this reason, they require special compensation, such as scheduling of daily activities to coincide with periods of improved performance. Thus, certain patients have particular difficulty in eating or wish to receive treatment before they engage in certain social or occupational activities.

In addition to the four major manifestations, certain other clinical symptoms and signs should receive special mention with regard to diagnosis and therapy. Awareness of these symptoms may either facilitate diagnosis for the informed physician or may confuse the uninformed physician. Patients with parkinsonism may be limited significantly by sialorrhea, dysphagia, dysphonia, clumsiness of the hands or altered handwriting. Excessive drooling is frequent and has been shown to result from impaired swallowing reflexes and not from excessive production of saliva. The accompanying difficulty in swallowing results in weight loss, which in some cases may be extreme, and recurrent aspiration pneumonia. The few studies available on this clinical aspect suggest dyssynergia or incoordination of pharyngeal muscles rather than obstructive lesions. Speech may be restricted to whispering (microphonia), and slurring may be severe. Written communication may be impaired by handwriting that is stiff and slow (probably a manifestation of combined bradykinesia and rigidity) and small (micrographia). Constipation is also frequent. These less frequent, or so-called minor, manifestations may require special attention during treatment.

The major conditions in the differential diagnosis are benign essential tremor; multiple small strokes (lacunar state); cerebral atrophy resulting in rigidity, slowness, and gait disturbance; and other causes of gait disturbance, such as normal-pressure hydrocephalus.

It should be emphasized that parkinsonism is a complex of symptoms of diverse causes and not just a single disease entity. The different types may be summarized as follows:

1. Idiopathic (paralysis agitans, Parkinson's disease).
2. Postencephalitic.

3. Drug-induced.
4. Associated with systemic degeneration: progressive supranuclear palsy (Steele–Richardson–Olzewski), Shy–Drager, Striatonigral degeneration, parkinsonism–dementia–amyotrophic lateral sclerosis complex of Guam.

This classification system is important with regard to therapy because it predicts responsiveness to therapy. Three large groups emerge from this classification. The first two consist of disorders that are expected to improve with replacement of dopamine. Drug-induced cases should be treated with reduced doses of levodopa and/or use of anticholinergic antiparkinsonian drugs. The efficacy of the latter drugs is unpredictable, and if the patient responds, the improvement is likely to be unsustained or incomplete. If in doubt, a therapeutic trial should be undertaken. Failure of the patient to improve with treatment not only necessitates evaluation of the mode of administration, but also raises questions about the particular subtype of parkinsonism or the basic diagnosis.

Historical Background

Pioneering efforts to modify parkinsonism with levodopa can be reviewed in two phases. In the initial phase, Birkmayer and Hornykiewicz (1) observed definite but temporary relief of akinesia after intravenous (IV) administration of levodopa, and Barbeau (2) reported relief of rigidity after oral administration of the drug. The second phase was the clear demonstration of sustained clinical benefit by Cotzias and associates (3,4) by oral administration of what were then considered to be exceptionally high doses of the racemic mixture of D,L-dopa, using up to 16 g. This development made dopamine replacement therapy practicable. Hematologic toxicity was subsequently eliminated with the availability of the L-isomer, especially in synthetic form. Levodopa was released for general use in the 1970s, approval of Sinemet followed in 1975.

Results of Experimentation

Unquestionably, L-dopa and Sinemet are the most effective drugs available today for treatment of parkinsonism. Generally, about 50–75% of patients improve significantly.

All four major manifestations of parkinsonism are relieved with levodopa (3–10), but to different extents. Initial reports suggested that tremor was not improved, but subsequent data (7) showed that tremor was in fact improved to a greater extent than other manifestations, and a greater percentage of patients with tremor (66%) became free of that symptom (Table 1). Akinesia and postural instability improved the least, and relatively few patients actually were rid of these manifestations after two years of treatment. In a separate study, Barbeau highlighted the distinctive problems of the akinetic form of parkinsonism, suggesting a different expected course for akinetic patients (6).

Alteration of Natural History

It has often been expressed that levodopa modifies the clinical manifestations only and does not alter the natural history of parkinsonism. More recent studies,

Table 1. Effects of Two Years of Levodopa Treatment on Parkinsonism

Manifestation	*Percentage of Patients Improved*	*Percentage of Patients "Free"*
Tremor	81	66
Rigidity	56	38
Akinesia	53	15
Postural instability	38	20

SOURCE: Lee JE, Sweet RD, McDowell FH: Treatment of parkinsonism with levodopa. Ann Intern Med 75:703–708, 1971.

Table 2. Effect of Levodopa on Mortality in Patients with Parkinsonism

Study	*No. of Patients*	*No. of Deaths*	*Age at Death*	*Excess Mortality*[a]
Pre-levodopa				
Hoehn and Yahr (11)	802	340	65.9	2.9
Post-levodopa				
Sweet and McDowell (9)	100	32	73.1	1.9
Markham et al. (8)	81	10	73.5	0.8
Joseph et al. (12)	1,625			1.33
Barbeau (6)[b]	70	17	68.2	

[a] Excess mortality is defined as the ratio of the number of deaths observed to the number of deaths expected.

[b] These patients were predominantly akinetic.

however, indicate that levodopa alters the course of parkinsonism such that mortality, which was approximately 300% greater in non L-dopa treated patients as compared with the general population (11), was reduced to only 33% greater when levodopa was used. The results of these studies are summarized in Table 2.

The data of Barbeau (6) reflect predominantly akinetic patients, whose expected course appears to be worse than that of patients with other forms of parkinsonism. In summary, these data indicate that levodopa therapy does in fact prolong survival and thus alters the natural history of the disease. In their study of pre-levodopa patients, Hoehn and Yahr (11) remarked on the lack of enhanced survival as compared with mortality from parkinsonism in England a century ago (11), despite advanced medical knowledge, antibiotics, antiparkinsonian drugs, intensive care facilities, and other medical advances.

Assessment of Therapeutic Response

Before initation of treatment, therapeutic goals should be defined and clinical parameters established to assess the patient's response. The parameters should be measurable easily and quickly, and also should be manifestations that are functionally significant. Several different clinically useful notation systems are available. In my experience, a check-off format is most convenient, especially if it is accompanied by definition of the reading scale used to remind the examiner as well as to inform the reader. Figure 1 shows a modified version of such a system. Recalling the severity of a particular manifestation may be difficult when the patient is seen no more frequently than at intervals of two to six months. In some cases, a therapeutic trial with Sinemet may be undertaken when the diagnosis is unclear, but the value of the trial is lost unless a good baseline for subsequent comparison is recorded. The minimal dosage and duration of treatment I use is arbitrary—3 g levodopa for three months or three tablets of Sinemet 25/250 (i.e., 25 mg carbidopa combined with 250 mg levodopa) for one month. In both therapies, the dosage should be increased to this level gradually and maintained for the appropriate duration.

Dopamine Replacement Therapy

The rationale for levodopa therapy is based on the knowledge that, while dopamine does not pass the blood–brain barrier, its immediate precursor, levodopa, does and is converted to dopamine within the central nervous system (CNS). However, only a very small amount of administered levodopa (less than 0.1%) is actually found in the CNS. This is due to both extra-CNS decarboxylation of dopa to dopamine and methylation of dopa to methyldopa, which is stored in nonneuronal tissue, especially muscle. Enhanced conversion of dopa to dopamine in the CNS has been shown to result when levodopa is combined with an inhibitor of the decarboxylating enzyme. Sinemet combines levodopa with dopa-hydrazine (carbidopa) as the inhibitor in a fixed ratio of 10:1. Figure 2 shows the chemical structures of these agents.

After oral ingestion of levodopa, blood levels of the drug peak in one to three hours; the half-life of levodopa is 3 hours. Sinemet peaks in similar fashion but has a longer half-life (15 hours). Correlation between blood levels of levodopa and either therapeutic benefit or side effects has not been precise. What is of greatest relevancy is the neuronal levels of the drug rather than levels in peripheral blood.

It is estimated that carbidopa at a dosage of 70–100 mg/day effectively prevents decarboxylation of levodopa in the periphery. The preparation available in the United States combines levodopa with carbidopa in a fixed ratio of 10:1; Madopar, which is available outside of the United States, combines a decarboxylase inhibitor with levodopa in a ratio of 1:4.

With initiation of dopamine replacement, it is recommended that the combination of levodopa and carbidopa be used preferentially because of the following advantages (13):

1. More rapid onset of action (two weeks of Sinemit is equivalent to about six months of levodopa).
2. Reduced incidence of nausea and vomiting (15% versus 50%+).
3. Fewer tablets at longer intervals improve the likelihood of compliance.
4. Fewer cardiac arrhythmias.
5. Elimination of pyridoxine (vitamin B6)-induced deterioration.

The possible advantage of levodopa over the combination drug is a somewhat lower incidence of dyskinesias, which are involuntary movements of the choreic, dystonic, or athetotic type.

Name: ____________ Address: ____________ Telephone: ____________

RUE: Right Upper Extremity
LUE: Left Upper Extremity
RLE: Right Lower Extremity
LLE: Left Lower Extremity

PATIENT HISTORY CHART PHYSICIAN EVALUATION FORM

MEDICATION ________ Other ________

DAILY DOSE PRESCRIBED IN GRAMS

DATES									
BEFORE EXAMINATION									
AFTER EXAMINATION									

SCORES

RIGIDITY:

0 Absent
1 Slight or detectable only when activated by mirror or other movements
2 Mild to moderate
3 Marked, but full range of motion easily achieved
4 Severe, range of motion achieved with difficulty

RUE									
LUE									
NECK									
RLE									
LLE									

TREMOR:

0 Absent
1 Slight and infrequently present
2 Moderate in amplitude but present only intermittently
3 Moderate and present most of time
4 Marked in amplitude and present most of time

RUE									
LUE									
FACE, LIPS, Etc.									
RLE									
LLE									

BRADYKINESIA:

0 None
1 Minimal slowness giving movement a deliberate character; could be normal for some persons
2 Mild degree of slowness and poverty of movement which is definitely abnormal
3 Moderate slowness with occasional hesitation on initiating movement and arrests of ongoing movement.
4 Marked slowness and poverty of movement with frequent freezing and long delays in initiating movement.

GAIT DISTURBANCE:

SCORES

0 Normal walking and associated movements
1 Mild slowness or slight stiffness of one or both legs in walking
2 Walks slowly with short steps, may shuffle, but no festination or pulsion
3 Festination, pulsion and "freezing", but still freely ambulatory
4 Walks with great difficulty with festination, short steps, freezing and pulsion
5 Severe disturbance of gait, can walk only with assistance
6 Cannot walk at all, even with help

POSTURAL STABILITY: (If Romberg is normal, judge response to sudden posterior displacement produced by push on sternum).

0 Normal
1 Retropulsion, but recovers unaided
2 Absence of postural response; would fall if not caught by examiner
3 Very unstable, tends to fall spontaneously on the Romberg test
4 Unable to stand without assistance

Figure 1. Patient evaluation form for serial recording of manifestations of parkinsonism. Courtesy of Dr. P. Papavasiliou.

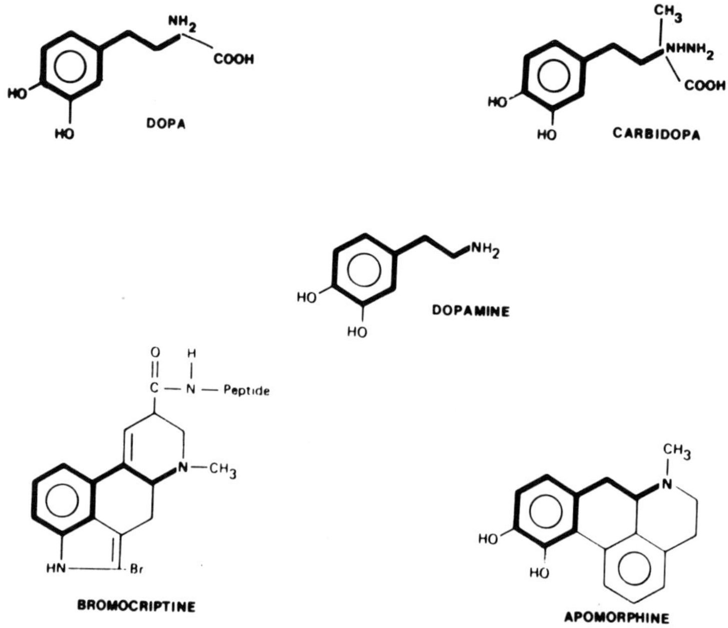

Figure 2. Chemical structures of dopamine and antiparkinsonian drugs.

It is important to appreciate two phases in the treatment of parkinsonism patient with either levodopa or Sinemet (10). When therapy is initiated in the first, or induction, phase, the objective should be to increase the dosage gradually to prevent side effects and reach the maximal dosage tolerable. For Sinemet this may require two to eight weeks, while for levodopa three to six months may be necessary. Once a therapeutic response has been obtained and stabilized, the second, or maintenance, phase is begun. During this time, it is desirable to maintain the patient on the lowest effective dosage that will reduce the occurrence of drug-induced dyskinesias; this goal actually may necessitate a reduction in dosage. Careful follow-up at intervals of three to four months or less are desirable for optimal control.

Initiation of Treatment

In patients who do not already take levodopa, treatment may be initiated with one tablet of Sinemet 10/100 (10 mg carbidopa combined with 100 mg levodopa) three times a day. Although patients often tolerate the drug better if they take it with meals, this practice is not essential. The dosage may be increased by one tablet every three to five days until the patient is taking a daily dosage of six tablets. At this point, if a further increase is desired, the larger form of Sinemet (25/250) at a dosage of one tablet three times a day is generally more convenient and is the recommended maintenance dosage. If significant residual symptoms are present, further increments of one-half to one tablet every three to five days may be added. In general, a maximum of eight tablets per day of the 25/250 size should not be exceeded, since higher doses produce toxicity without additional benefit. With this program, a therapeutic level may be reached comfortably in two to four weeks in most patients.

Levodopa is available as either capsules or tablets and in sizes of 100 mg, 250 mg, or 500 mg. The usual initial dose is 250 mg three to four times per day, taken with meals. It is much more important that levodopa be taken with food in order to minimize gastric irritation. Subsequent increases in dosage may then be instituted gradually in increments of approximately 100 to 250 mg every three to seven days. Under ordinary conditions, the maximal dosage should not exceed 8 g/day. In most patients, an increasing therapeutic response may be noticed even after several months at the same dosage, while in others, significant therapeutic response may take many months.

Pyridoxine (vitamin B6) increases the action of the decarboxylating enzyme and may either prevent or reverse the benefits of levodopa therapy. The patient should be advised to avoid taking vitamins that contain more than 10 mg vitamin B6. If the patient desires, a pyridoxine-free multivitamin (Larobec) is available.

Patients who already take levodopa may switch to Sinemet as follows. Levodopa should be discontinued after the evening dose, and Sinemet may be begun the next morning. The total amount of Sinemet chosen should be approximately one-quarter of the levodopa dosage. It should be pointed out that patients who improve satisfactorily with levodopa need not change to Sinemet.

Under certain circumstances, a combination of Sinemet and levodopa may be given concurrently. It should be remembered that one tablet of Sinemet 25/250 is equivalent to 1 g levodopa. The usual circumstance for combined therapy is in a patient in whom it is desirable to increase dopamine replacement but minimize dyskinesia.

Selection of Patients

An important perspective may be gained at this point by some general comments regarding the selection of patients for treatment. The reader may acquire a heightened appreciation of the points emphasized in this section after review of the specific features of the antiparkinsonian drugs detailed in this section.

Clearly, the most potent antiparkinsonian agent is levodopa, either alone or combined with a decarboxylation inhibitor. However, several studies indicate that, about three to five years after treatment is initiated, levodopa therapy may be associated with a variety of effects, including decline in therapeutic benefit, increase in adverse effects, fluctuation between akinesia and dyskinesia, and accelerated or irreversible dementia (5,6,14–16).

Reasonable guidelines would appear to include reservation of levodopa for patients with significant clinical symptoms that affect occupational performance, psychological well-being, and social interaction (14). Patients whose clinical manifestations are of lesser consequence should be treated with anticholinergic drugs or amantadine.

Dementia occurs in about one-quarter to one-third of patients with parkinsonism (8,16,17). Concern that levodopa increases various mental dysfunctions, (e.g., dementia, depression, mania, delirium, hallucinations, schizophrenia, hypersexuality) has been reviewed (17). However, it is likely that, in many patients, these effects are related to advanced age or are part of the degeneration associated with Parkinson's disease rather than a complication of treatment. Only when the severity of the mental effects precludes reasonable patient participation in therapy should the drug be withheld. In certain cases, specific therapy for the mental dysfunction may subsequently improve the patient's condition such that levodopa treatment can then be initiated.

Contraindications

Monoamine oxidase (MAO) inhibitors should not be given concurrently with either levodopa or Sinemet because these agents may precipitate a hypertensive crisis with serious complications. MAO inhibitors should be discontinued two weeks before the start of therapy with either levodopa or Sinemet. Phenothiazines and butyrophenones, although not contraindicated absolutely, should be used only with clear indication in patients taking dopamine replacement therapy, since these antipsychotic drugs work primarily by blocking dopamine receptors, thereby preventing improvement of the parkinsonism.

Patients with known hypersensitivity to dopamine drugs and those with narrow-angle glaucoma should not take these agents. Malignant melanoma has been reported to be activated by levodopa and presumably would also be affected by Sinemet. Both drugs should be avoided in patients with a history of melanoma or suspicious, undiagnosed skin lesions (18).

Important Drug Interactions

MAO inhibitors, which generally are administered for depression, prevent inactivation of dopamine and other catecholamines. When MAO inhibitors are combined with levodopa or Sinemet, dangerous hypertensive crises and hyperpyrexia may result. Accordingly, MAO inhibitors should be stopped two weeks before the start of dopamine replacement therapy for parkinsonism.

Simultaneous administration of phenothiazines and butyrophenones with dopamine agonists can reverse or prevent therapeutic benefit in patients with parkinsonism. There are antipsychotic drugs that work principally by blocking dopamine receptors in the CNS. Nausea or vomiting resulting from levodopa should not be treated with phenothiazines. Conversely, parkinsonism induced by these antipsychotic drugs is not responsive to dopamine replacement, since the receptors are not available for activation. Instead, either the phenothiazines should be decreased or anticholinergic drugs should be used.

Reserpine is an antihypertensive drug that works through depletion of catecholamines (including dopamine) and may cause parkinsonism. Concurrent administration with levodopa or Sinemet may inhibit therapeutic benefit in patients with parkinsonism.

Tricyclic antidepressants block the major inactivation system for dopamine. This is accomplished through reuptake of dopamine into the presynaptic neuron, thereby enhancing dopaminergic transmission. Since many patients with parkinsonism feel depressed, these agents may already have been administered before initiation of therapy with levodopa or Sinemet. Tricyclic antidepressants may be combined safely and effectively with levodopa or Sinemet with the understanding that augmentation of both benefit from and side effects of either drug may result. Thus, tricyclics may be used in some patients to improve depression as well as to enhance the antiparkinsonian effects of dopamine agonists.

Cholinergic drugs such as bethanechol should be avoided in parkinsonism patients. Often prescribed for symptomatic improvement of urine retention, these drugs antagonize the effects of levodopa and Sinemet as well as those of anticholinergics. Poor evacuation of urine may be improved by reduction of the anticholinergic dosage. On occasion, unexplained deterioration of the patient's condition may be traced to treatment with one or more of these drugs by another physician, who is unaware of their deleterious effect on the neurologic function of patients with parkinsonism.

Side Effects

Since levodopa is converted in the body to a naturally occurring neurotransmitter, the drug has multiple effects on the CNS and peripheral nervous system. It should be remembered that this drug is not a "magic bullet" whose effects on parkinsonism are limited to only those that are desired.

During the induction phase of levodopa treatment, the major side effects are gastrointestinal (nausea, vomiting, anorexia). These reactions are due in part to both central stimulation of an ill-defined medullary site and peripheral gastric irritation. Treatment of these common side effects consists of increasing the dosage of levodopa gradually and administering the medication with meals or a small snack. Increase in levodopa during the induction phase are often limited by these side effects, and one of the clear advantages of Sinemet is reduction of these reactions.

After several months of treatment, the major side effect is abnormal involuntary movement, including choreoathetosis of the limbs, facial dyskinesia, or dystonic posturing of the torso or limbs. These reactions increase significantly in proportion to the duration of treatment, and more than 75% of patients are likely to exhibit involuntary movements by two years of treatment (5,6,8–10). In principle as well as in practice, these effects can be managed by slight reduction in total daily dose as well as administration of smaller amounts at more frequent intervals. A small reduction of 100 to 250 mg of either the total daily dose of levodopa or the Sinemet equivalent is often sufficient. Reversibility is a hallmark of these involuntary movements, and their persistence after significant reduction of dosage or even cessation of therapy should raise the possibility of other conditions, such as Huntington's chorea or tardive dyskinesia of the type associated with antipsychotic drugs. Unfortunately, reduced dosage also results in reduced therapeutic benefit. In many cases, increased reliance on the anticholinergic drugs and amantadine provides a samll but noticeable measure of benefit without aggravation of the dyskinesias. Anticholinergics are especially helpful in patients taking dopamine replacement therapy for five or more years, some of whom appear to have become refractory to the therapy.

Certain patients prefer involuntary movements to parkinsonism, especially in anticipation of some activities such as shopping or an outing. It is common for such patients to take an extra amount of levodopa or Sinemet for these occasions. Other patients are extremely distressed by the dyskinesias and may actually refuse to continue treatment. In severe cases, small doses of haloperidol (Haldol) ameliorate the involuntary movements but at the expense of increasing the severity of the parkinsonism. Dimethylaminoethanol (Deanol) has been reported to benefit some patients (19,20).

Recently, valproic acid (Depakene) and baclofen (Lioresal), which augment gamma-amino butyric acid (GABA), have been released for use in other clinical conditions but may also block the dyskinesias. Furthermore, their use does not appear to reduce antiparkinsonian benefit. Baclofen, 15–80 mg/day in divided doses, may be given concurrently with levodopa or Sinemet. Valproic acid, 500-750 mg/day in divided doses, may be given in addition to dopamine replacement therapy.

Orthostatic hypotension is a frequent initial complication of antiparkinsonian therapy and may be present even in the absence of other symptoms. Only occasionally does this condition persist with continued use of levodopa or Sinemet, and it rarely is a limiting side effect. However, in instances in which symptomatic orthostatic hypotension is persistent, by simultaneous administration of fludrocortisone, (Florinef) 0.1–0.3 mg/day, may be given (21). It also is helpful to liberalize salt intake unless this is contraindicated by the presence of cardiac decompensation or fluid retention; wearing of elastic support stockings also are recommended.

Acute overdose with 100 g levodopa in one patient produced initial hypertension followed by prolonged symptomatic postural hypotension, sinus tachycardia, mental confusion, insomnia, and anorexia. The reaction resolved gradually over one week (22).

Oscillations in Performance (On-Off Effect)

Probably the most vexing problem in the treatment of parkinsonism is rapid oscillations in performance, or the "on-off" effect. This consists of episodic and sometimes rapid alternation between improved and akinetic phases (6–10, 23–28). The patient switches "off" (rigid akinetic state without dyskinesia) from a satisfactory state for a few minutes to hours. The "on" period is ushered in by severe dyskinesia and then becomes relatively symptom free. These episodes may occur many times a day; they result in greatly increased amounts of time spent in dyskinetic and parkinsonian states and less time in an improved state. These rapid oscillations have also been termed *yo-yoing* (26). A clear distinction should be made between the on-off effect and interdose or end-of-dose akinesia, and peak-dose dyskinesia, since these conditions generally are responsive to the logical adjustment in therapy. A more complicated effect has been termed *akinesia paradoxica*, or *hypotonic freezing* by Barbeau (6). This effect is characterized by abrupt onset of hypotonia and postural instability, which occurred in more than half of 80 predominantly akinetic patients after six years of therapy. Projection from present data suggests that this reaction may be at least as frequent as involuntary movements after the same amount of time.

It is estimated that the on-off phenomenon affects 10–20% of patients who take levodopa and Sinemet after an average of 28 months of therapy; however, it also may develop after only a few months (23–28). Gait disturbances and akinesia of the legs are especially prominent during the off period. Dyskinesias appear earlier and more frequently in these patients during dopamine replacement therapy (24,28). Markham (24) has highlighted two key elements in this regard. The first is loss of therapeutic efficacy, with greater variation in response from one dose to the next; the second is involuntary movements. Most authors regard on-off as due to progressive neuronal degeneration, but Barbeau (6) considered it to be a complication of levodopa treatment. The consensus points to variations in the availability of brain dopa and suggests that treatment should aim to eliminate these fluctuations.

Overall, the best therapeutic approach seems to be preferential use of Sinemet to achieve a smoother response (29), and smaller and more frequent doses, with the addition of anticholinergic drugs and short courses of amantadine. Improvement has been reported with marked reduction of total dosage for certain periods, followed by gradual increments (30) and by an increase in total daily dose (31). Continuous IV infusion of levodopa eliminated these motor fluctuations in seven parkinsonism patients with severe on-off manifestations (32); this approach supports both the general recommendations and the proposed mechanism. However, individual variations are marked, and unsatisfactory control unfortunately is prominent in many patients. These measures can be summarized as follows:

1. If the patient is taking levodopa, replace this drug with Sinemet.
2. If akinesia is predominant, increase the Sinemet dosage slightly.
3. If choreoathetosis is predominant, divide same total daily dosage of Sinemet into smaller multiple doses. If it is not effective, reduce the total daily dosage.
4. If the patient does not derive benefit from measures 1–3, take the following steps alone or in conjunction with 1–3: (*a*) add amantadine and/or anticholinergic drugs, to the reduction in total daily dosage of Sinemet; (*b*) restrict the patient's protein intake.

Nondopaminergic Drug Treatment

Anticholinergic Drugs

Before the availability of levodopa, anticholinergic drugs were the mainstay of therapy for parkinsonism. Their therapeutic effectiveness is considered to result from restoration of the cholinergic-dopaminergic balance through cholinergic blockade rather than from augmentation of dopamine. Anticholinergic drugs are useful but provide only partial improvement; they are estimated to be approximately one-quarter as effective as levodopa. Patients who are especially well suited for anticholinergic rather than dopamine agonist therapy are those with newly diagnosed parkinsonism with only mild symptoms, whose employment is not threatened and quality of life is affected minimally. The second situation in which anticholinergic therapy is appropriate is when the patient can no longer tolerate the side effects of levodopa or Sinemet, even at low dosages. Despite careful adjustment of dopamine replacement therapy, an increasing number of patients, especially those who take long-term levodopa therapy, become included in this category. Most parkinsonian patients who receive anticholinergic drugs also take either Sinemet or levodopa.

Like dopamine replacement agents, anticholinergic drugs are effective against all the manifestations of parkinsonism, but often to different extents. Sialorrhea, one of the most annoying of the minor manifestations, is particularly responsive to anticholinergic drugs. These drugs are similar to belladonna in action and side effects and were first suggested for use in this condition by Charcot in 1892. While trihexyphenidyl (Artane) is the prototype, analogues such as biperiden (Akineton), procyclidine (Kemadrin), cycrimine (Pagitane), and benztropine (Cogentin) are equally useful.

Among the major side effects of anticholinergics are blurring of vision, dryness of the mouth and throat, constipation, urinary hesitancy and retention, and mental changes such as confusion, hallucinations, and impairment of memory. More extreme cases of toxicity may result in ataxia, dysarthria, hyperthermia, and severe behavioral and cognitive disturbances that resemble those caused by atropine poisoning.

Curiously, the phenothiazine derivative ethopropazine (Parsidol) is beneficial, especially for tremor, perhaps because of its anticholinergic properties. It should be recalled that other phenothiazines are contraindicated in parkinsonism. Antihistamines such as diphenhydramine (Benadryl) also are beneficial, particularly for rigidity, and have a soothing effect on anxiety. Available drugs and their dosages are summarized in Table 3.

Amantadine

Still another effective drug is the antiviral agent amantadine (Symmetrel), which was developed for use against influenza but was noted serendipitously to ameliorate manifestations of parkinsonism (33–35). The mechanism of action is considered to be dopaminergic, but precise mechanisms have not been established. In general, one-half to two-thirds of patients improve with dosages of 200 mg/day, and maximal benefit was appreciated in the initial few days or weeks of therapy. Additional improvement may be anticipated, even if the patient is already on levodopa. No additional benefit results from daily doses of more than 200 mg, and side effects may increase at higher dosages. It is useful to add amantadine to antiparkinsonian therapy (including to levodopa or Sinemet therapy) for several weeks to months whenever enhanced therapeutic effect is desired. Unfortunately, termination of amantadine is often associated with neurologic deterioration (35). This deterioration may be managed effectively by addition of an anticholinergic drug. Serious side effects are infrequent and seem to occur particularly if the daily dosage exceeds 200 mg. Common side effects include mental symptoms (confusion, disorientation, hallucinations, depression, nervousness, insomnia), dizziness and lightheadedness, gastrointestinal symptoms (cramps, diarrhea, constipation), dryness of the mouth, edema, and livido reticularis. The actual incidence varies in the reports, and elderly patients are especially prone to the central side effects of confusion and hallucinations (half of those older than 65 years experience this effect). The peripheral side effects of edema and livido reticularis have been reported to occur in as many as one-third of patients, and women were affected twice as frequently as men (35).

Investigational and New Agents

Recent investigation has focused on the development of agents that give both sustained improvement, particularly for patients who do not respond to levodopa, and freedom from involuntary movements and oscillations in performance. In general, the chemical goal has been to activate striatal dopamine receptors directly rather than to augment dopaminergic transmission through replacement of precursors. These efforts may be regarded as a new phase of treatment with third-generation drugs.

The most extensively studied new agent is bromocriptine (bromo-alpha-

Table 3. Drugs Currently Available for Treatment of Parkinsonism

Drug	*Forms Available*	*Average Daily Dosage*
Primarily dopaminergic		
Levodopa	Tablets, capsules (100, 250, 500 mg)	3–8 g
Carbidopa/levodopa (Sinemet)	Tablets (10 mg/100 mg, 25 mg/100 mg 25 mg/250 mg)	30 mg/300 mg–150 mg/1500 mg
Amantadine (Symmetrel)	Capsules (100 mg)	200 mg
Primarily anticholinergic		
Benztropine mesylate	Syrup (50 mg/5 ml)	
(Cogentin)	Tablets (0.5, 1, 2 mg)	1–6 mg
Trihexyphenidyl (Artane)	Tablets (2, 5 mg): Timed-released capsule (5 mg) Elixir (2 mg/5 ml)	1–20 mg
Biperiden (Akineton)	Tablets (2 mg)	1–20 mg
Procyclidine (Kemadrin)	Tablets (2, 5 mg)	1–20 mg
Cycrimine (Pagitane)	Tablets (1.25, 2.5 mg)	1–20 mg
Diphenhydramine (Benadryl)	Capsules (25, 50 mg) Elixir (12.5 mg/5 ml)	25–200 mg
Ethopropazine (Parsidol)	Tablets (10, 50, 100 mg)	50–200 mg

ergocriptine) (Fig. 2), an ergot alkaloid that is licensed in the United States at present for the treatment of galactorrhea but has not been approved for use in parkinsonism. At sufficiently high dosages (50–150 mg/day), bromocriptine is effective against parkinsonism (36–42). It may be administered concurrently with levodopa or Sinemet to allow reduction of the dosages of these drugs and may benefit some patients who fail to respond to levodopa (38) but not others (39,40). Bromocriptine may also evoke a more stable response to dopamine replacement drugs (39). In addition, the drug may reduce oscillations in performance (38,39,42). Side effects include mental changes that may persist for several weeks beyond the actual period of drug administration (37, 38), dyskinesias similar to or even worse than those with levodopa (39,42), hypotension, gastrointestinal bleeding, and edema. Bromocriptine should be avoided in patients with a history of psychosis and serious cardiovascular or peptic ulcer disease. Lergotrile, a related agent, has similar efficacy but results in prominent hepatotoxicity, gastrointestinal symptoms, and hypotension. However, it is less expensive than bromocriptine (41). If bromocriptine is administered concurrently with levodopa, the levodopa dosage should be reduced by 100–500 mg for each 5–10 mg of bromocriptine (38). In some patients, doses as low as 5–10 mg may be beneficial.

Theoretically, bromocriptine has the following advantages over levodopa: (*1*) it may eliminate the competitive action of dietary amino acids; (*2*) it bypasses the need for cerebral decarboxylase activity, which has been shown to be deficient in parkinsonian striatum; and (*3*) it may activate a potentially different group of dopamine receptors than levodopa.

Another drug with dopaminergic activity is apomorphine, which resembles dopamine structurally (Fig. 2). The drug has been shown to have definite antiparkinsonian benefit, even in nonemetic doses, but it produced azotemia (43). N-propylnoraporphine, an analogue of apomorphine that produces much less nephrotoxicity, has been shown to induce significant improvement that declined gradually after several weeks. Unfortunately, the drug reproduced the same involuntary movements and on-off effect as seen with levodopa (43). Concurrent administration of Sinemet reduced or eliminated these side effects.

Oxiperomide, a new dopamine receptor antagonist, has been reported to decrease levodopa-induced dyskinesias without increasing parkinsonian manifestations (44). Broad application of this drug in a variety of movement disorders has been suggested on the basis of its observed benefits without inducing parkinsonism in Tourette's syndrome and Huntington's chorea (44). This suggests indirectly that more than one type of dopamine receptor may exist in the basal ganglia and offers the promise that selective dopamine antagonists may be developed to control involuntary movements, which are the major limitation of long-term levodopa therapy. Unfortunately, oxiperomide is not a practical drug because it causes excessive drowsiness.

Stereotaxic Surgery

Before the widespread use of levodopa, stereotaxic surgery was used extensively for treatment of parkinsonism. In a series of more than 3,000 cryothalamectomies performed for parkinsonism, Cooper (45) demonstrated that tremor and rigidity, but not akinesia and gait disturbances, may be relieved, with an operative mortality of 1.3% and temporary morbidity of 10%. At present, stereotaxic surgery is seldom undertaken and then only after extensive levodopa therapy has failed (45). The most likely candidates have predominantly or exclusively unilateral rigidity or tremor.

Summary

Over the past two decades, therapy for parkinsonism has evolved from the use of drugs with limited efficacy to rational replacement with levodopa, with improvement of both major and minor manifestations. These agents, their trade names, and their available forms and average dosages are summarized in Table 3.

In addition to drug therapy, virtually all parkinsonism patients appreciate practical advice regarding exercises, diet, and daily activities, as well as simplified explanations of the disease and how antiparkinsonian drugs should be used. The recent short book by Duvoisin (46) fulfills these needs admirably.

The following voluntary private organizations provide information to parkinsonism patients:

- American Parkinson Disease Association, Inc.
  147 East 50th Street
  New York, NY 10022

- Parkinson's Disease Foundation
  William Black Medical Research Building
  640 West 168th Street
  New York, NY 10032
- National Parkinson Foundation, Inc.
  1501 N.W. Ninth Avenue
  Miami, FL 33136
- United Parkinson Foundation
  220 South State Street
  Chicago, IL 60604

BENIGN ESSENTIAL TREMOR

Clinical Features

Benign essential tremor is a frequent cause of tremor for which effective treatment has been developed, even in the absence of any recognized neuropathology. The name accurately designates the natural course, which typically is a long period of minimal or slowly worsening tremor but without other neurologic involvement (47). Relatively little attention has been paid to this condition in recent literature, including neurology textbooks, and its actual prevalence is unknown. The condition has also been termed *senile tremor* because it frequently appears in the elderly, *familial tremor* because up to 50% of patients report a similar condition in family members, and *intention* or *action tremor* to describe its maximal expression during voluntary activity.

Clinically, the tremor is expressed maximally in such activities as raising a coffee cup, buttoning clothes, and handwriting, but it abates when the patient is at rest. Diagnostically, the major condition to be distinguished is parkinsonism. Usually the distinction is not difficult because of the other characteristic manifestations of parkinsonism, along with the pattern of maximal tremor that occurs at rest and abates during activity. However, it may be difficult to diagnose the condition in some patients, especially the elderly or those with additional conditions that produce clinical signs similar to parkinsonism. For these patients, a therapeutic trial with propranolol (Inderal) is appropriate. If they are unresponsive to propranolol, a therapeutic trial with Sinemet should be considered. The major features of the differential diagnosis are summarized in Table 4.

Intention tremor in the absence of other signs is the hallmark of this condition. Typically, the tremor is more rapid than in parkinsonism, lacks the pill-rolling quality, and is maximal during activity or with the arms held outstretched rather than at rest. The age of expression may begin in the teens and range to old age; it has no predilection for sex. Involvement of the upper limbs and especially the dominant hand is the usual distribution in tremor, but clinical examination often reveals tremor of the head, lower extremities, and nondominant hand as well. Speech also may be tremulous and needs to be differentiated from dysarthria and from the microphonia of parkinsonism.

Tremography, characterization of the tremor with clinical recording devices such as a standard EMG, has been reported (48). The study indicates that tre-

Table 4. Differential Features of Common Tremors

	Diagnosis	
Characteristic	*Essential*	*Parkinsonian*
Maximal expression	During activity (intention)	During rest
Minimal expression	During rest	During activity
Rate	Increased (6 Hz)	Decreased (3–5 Hz)
Parkinsonian manifestations	Absent	Present
Family history	Up to 50%	5–10%
Treatment	Propranolol (Inderal) Metoprolol (Lopressor) Diazepam (Valium)	Sinemet or L-dopa
Synonyms	Senile Hereditary Intention	Pill-rolling Resting

mography does not differentiate parkinsonism from benign essential tremor because the most common pattern in both conditions is an alternating pattern of firing in agonist and antagonist muscles; simultaneous firing of agonist and antagonist muscles is less common. However, the frequency of the tremor is more rapid in essential tremor (6.3 Hz) than it is in parkinsonism (4.6 Hz).

Therapy

Therapy with propranolol was initally observed serendipitously and has subsequently been demonstrated to benefit about 75% of patients (49–51). Of interest is that many patients who improve with propranolol had also noticed suppression of the tremor with alcohol. In fact, some patients have actually ascribed their alcoholism to the fact that nothing else helped the tremor. Since propranolol acts by blocking beta-adrenergic receptors, overactivity of the adrenergic nervous system in tremor is implied. Propranolol diminishes tremor amplitude but does not alter its frequency (49,51). Only rarely is the tremor totally abolished, but the amount of suppression usually is of practical benefit (49–51). Thus, with propranolol treatment patients may be able to return to their occupations and resume social and personal activities, such as writing letters or signing checks, that have become impossible because of the tremor.

The major side effects of propranolol are attributable to beta blockade. These include hypotension, bradycardia, and precipitation of bronchospasm in patients with a history of certain types of pulmonary disease. Thus, the drug is contraindicated in patients with significant asthma.

It is not clear whether the site of action of propranolol is the peripheral or the central adrenergic system. It has been argued persuasively that the action is central, since central blockade with propranolol was effective, while peripheral blockade through intra-arterial administration did not alter the amplitude of essential tremor (52). However, other workers, with use of IV intravenous propranolol, have suggested that a peripheral component is significant (53). Similarly, it has been proposed that the benefit of alcohol lies in its central rather than its peripheral mechanism (54).

For patients with bronchospastic pulmonary disease and significant essential tremor, metoprolol (Lopressor) may be considered. This drug has selective activity against $beta_1$ receptors, but not against $beta_2$ receptors, located in the lung. Recently, however, a 78-year-old man with significant chronic pulmonary disease and severe essential tremor (whose daughter was also affected) benefited significantly from metoprolol without adverse pulmonary manifestations (R. M. Kobayashi, manuscript in preparation).

Additional treatment that has been beneficial at times includes the use of sedatives such as diazepam (Valium) and reduction of anxiety-producing situations. Some patients derive benefit from the intermittent use of propranolol (e.g., before social engagements or situations in which a previously tolerable level of tremor might be intensified) rather than on continuous use.

Before and during treatment with propranolol, careful recording of blood pressure and pulse rate and a careful review of cardiac and pulmonary history are important. Propranolol should not be administered to patients with a history of cardiac decompensation, conduction defects, and severe pulmonary disease, and especially not to those with bronchospasm. In my experience, it is beneficial to follow the patient's therapeutic response on the basis of their ability to perform a semiquantitative and easily reproduced task, such as drawing five concentric circles superimposed on one drawn by the physician. The task may be timed, and the amount of tremor may be assessed during the course of treatment. Treatment with propranolol may be initiated with 10 mg t.i.d. and increased by 30 mg/day at intervals of three to five days. In general, a maximal dose of 180–240 mg is sufficient for most patients. However, it has been demonstrated that propranolol's efficacy in essential tremor depends on both the plasma level of drug and the sensitivity of the disorder in the individual patient; thus, dosages of up to 800 mg/day may be required to achieve sufficient plasma levels of propranolol (53). Although determinations of plasma levels of propranolol are not available clinically on a widespread basis, they may be helpful in guiding the therapeutic response. Until this measurement is easily obtainable, it is common practice to increase the dosage until the desired affect is achieved, while maintaining the pulse rate at more than 50 beats/min and the systolic blood pressure at more than 110 mm Hg. Perhaps more important than the basal blood pressure and pulse rate is the response to exercise. When propranolol is used to enhance therapeutic efficacy, the dosage may be increased cautiously if it is demonstrated that resting bradycardia and hypotension increase with exercise. Since often it is not possible to eliminate the tremor totally, even at high dosages, it may be more realistic to accept reduction of tremor to a level that allows resumption of previous activities.

TARDIVE DYSKINESIAS

Clinical Features

Certain abnormal involuntary movements that are termed *tardive dyskinesias* have emerged as side effects of therapy for schizophrenia with phenothiazines and butyrophenones (55,56). These dyskinesias are choreic movements that especially affect the face and oral structures and typically consist of repeated tongue protrusion, with licking of the lips, puckering and smacking of the lips, chewing movements, grunting and similar sounds, puffing of the cheeks, opening of the eyes and irregular blinking, and furrowing of the forehead. In addition, many patients also exhibit choreoathetotic movements of the limbs and trunk. These movements may be clinically indistinguishable from levodopa-induced dyskinesias; however, patients with the latter have a different drug history (which must be obtained carefully), and their dyskinesias can be reversed with reduction of levodopa. Drug-induced dyskinesias should be distinguished from Huntington's disease, Tourette's syndrome, and, infrequently, spontaneous orofacial dyskinesias.

The term *tardive dyskinesia* refers to the fact that these movements appear after prolonged and especially high-dose treatment with antipsychotic drugs and may in fact appear for the first time when the drug is tapered or discontinued. Although there is no consensus, a reasonable estimate of occurrence is in 3–6% of psychiatric patients and in 20% of elderly institutionalized patients (57). Not only are psychotic patients at risk, but also nonpsychotic patients who receive these drugs for treatment of conditions such as gastrointestinal upset or anxiety neurosis may also develop tardive dyskinesia (58). Two facets of this condition provide a sobering perspective of the significance of this problem. The first is that the number of patients likely to manifest tardive dyskinesias amount to some 10 million worldwide. The second is that reversibility is characteristic in only a minority of patients who demonstrate remission (55,56). Thus, tardive dyskinesias are the major side effects that limit the long-term use of antipsychotic drugs.

Risk Factors

Aside from the risks associated with dosage and duration of treatment, tardive dyskinesias are especially prone to develop in the elderly and in women. Drug-induced dyskinesias have been reported in 4% of men and 13% of women younger than 50 years; the incidence rose to 20% of men and 35% of women older than 50 (58). The ratio of women to men affected has been reported to be from 2:1–5:1; moreover, a higher incidence of severe cases among women than among men has been observed (56).

Virtually all antipsychotic drugs have been implicated in tardive dyskinesias, and it may be nearly impossible to determine which drug is responsible in any particular case, since multiple drugs generally are prescribed.

Although few limited neuropathologic studies have been reported, these suggest a high incidence of degeneration of the basal ganglia; however, specific features have not been documented (60).

In order to explain this disorder, a neuropharmacologic model has been postulated in which chronic, striatal, blockade of dopamine receptors induced by these drugs results in hypersensitivity of the "chemically denervated" receptors (61). This hypothesis has been demonstrated more directly in a laboratory model in which administration of haloperidol increased the number of dopamine receptors in the striatum but not in other sites, and other receptors were not altered (62,63).

Therapy

Despite the recognized association with the use of antipsychotic drugs and a reasonable pharmacologic model, it has been singularly disappointing that an effective therapy has not emerged. Thus, prevention may be the most effective means of reducing the occurrence of tardive dyskinesias. In order to accomplish this, long-term, high-dose administration of antipsychotic drugs should be avoided (especially in elderly patients) unless the need is clearly demonstrated (57,64). Drug holidays (i.e., periodic omission of antipsychotic drugs) may indicate whether continued treatment is necessary and also may reveal dyskinesia that has been masked by the drug. Early recognition may be associated with greater reversibility (65) and calls for frequent neurologic examination.

Management of tardive dyskinesias may be approached as summarized in Figure 3. Upon recognition of dyskinesia, a psychiatric decision regarding the need for continued drug treatment must be made. If continued medication is required to control psychotic behavior, a change to a drug with a low incidence of extrapyramidal side effects (e.g., thioridazine [Mellaril]) should be considered. Anticholinergic drugs given to prevent or inhibit parkinsonism appear to worsen dyskinesias and should be withdrawn (61). Routine use of anticholinergic drugs should be avoided; these agents should be given only with the emergence of symptomatic parkinsonism. At this point, further observation for three to six months is suggested, since remission of the dyskinesia may continue during this period after the medications have been stopped. Dyskinesias that persist beyond this period may then be treated with specific drugs on a therapeutic-trial basis.

Initial treatment of tardive dyskinesias previously relied on increasing the dosage of antipsychotic drug to enhance dopamine receptor blockade further. Thus, a paradox emerged in which the same group of drugs were used to treat a condition that originally was caused by those drugs. However, this approach has been shown to be of limited clinical benefit because the dyskinesias recur despite therapeutic success with higher dosages and because of an increase in drug-induced parkinsonism (66).

Multiple drugs have been reported to benefit some patients but not others; this suggests the presence of subtypes that are responsive to particular categories of drugs but refractory to others (55,56,64,67). Since therapeutic trials may be lengthy and expensive, the use of short-acting agents to "predict" response to drugs that require long treatment periods has been suggested (55,56,64,67). The drug that offers the clearest differentiation of subtypes may be physostigmine, 1.0 mg IV, plus methscopolamine, 0.75 mg IV, to block peripheral cholinergic side effects (67). Physostigmine is a cholinomimetic agent that blocks the action of acetylcholinesterase. Patients whose dyskinesias improve are more likely to respond subsequently to oral dimethylaminoethanol or to choline. In these patients, the response to diethylaminoethanol, 800 mg/day, usually is evident by one week; higher doses provide no further benefit. If physostigmine worsens the dyskinesias, the anticholinergic drug benztropine, 2 mg IV, tends to be beneficial, and dosages of diethylaminoethanol as high as 2,000 mg/day are ineffective or even detrimental. Longer periods of treatment may then be continued with oral benztropine.

It is acknowledged that such parenteral trials may not be practical or feasible

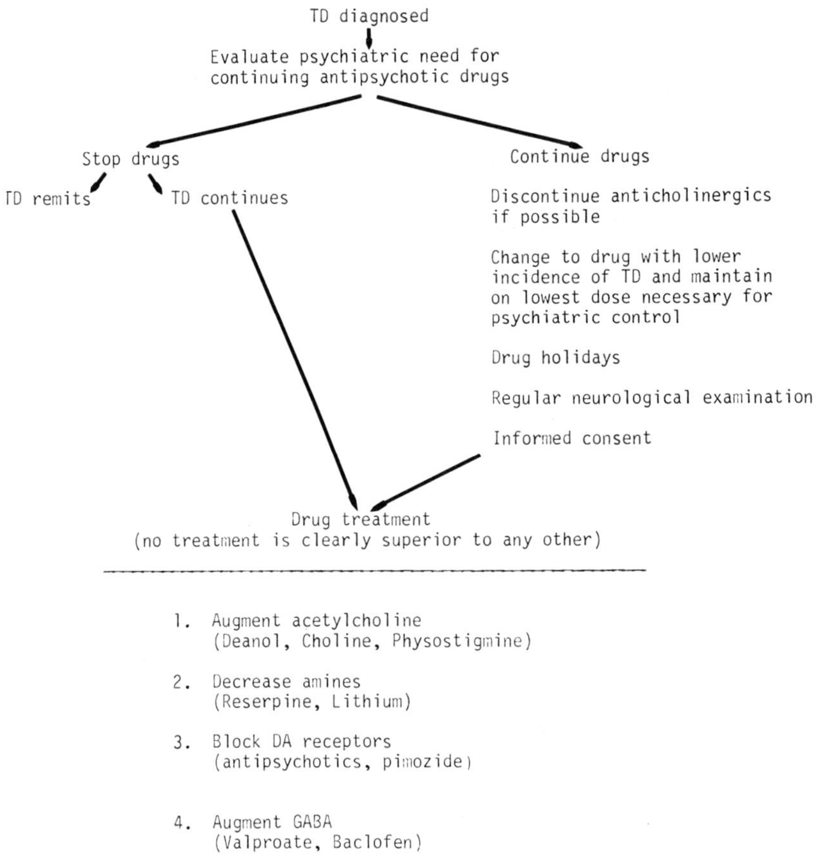

Figure 3. Management of tardive dyskinesia.

for large groups of hospitalized psychotic patients but that they do offer a rational foundation for subsequent oral therapy.

Recently, the GABA agonists sodium valproate (Depakene) and baclofen have been released for use in seizures and spasticity, respectively. They predominantly enhance levels of GABA, the major inhibitory neurotransmitter in the CNS. Encouraging results have been reported: more than 75% of patients improved with 60 mg baclofen/day (68), and 50% of patients improved with 900 mg valproate/day (69). Benefit was evident by the second week of treatment, and significant side effects were not observed. Treatment was only for a limited period, and the effects of long-term treatment have yet to be examined. Nevertheless, these agents offer the prospect of improvement without side effects, including parkinsonism or psychiatric deterioration.

HUNTINGTON'S DISEASE

Clinical Features

Huntington's disease (Huntington's chorea) is a degenerative disorder that affects the basal ganglia and cerebral cortex. The initial clinical features are progressive dementia and involuntary movements. The disease is inherited as an autosomal dominant trait but usually does not manifest until middle life; it is fatal after a progressive course of about 16 years. The involuntary movements assume a variety of forms, including chorea, athetosis, and dystonic posturing, and any part of the body may be affected. Voluntary activity and stress frequently increase the movements, although they may diminish during repose. Additional motor disturbances may include abnormal ocular movements, dysarthria, and dysphagia. Mental changes include conspicuous intellectual decline, but psychosis and profound mood changes may also be prominent. In 5–10% of patients, rigidity and bradykinesia predominate over chorea. This variant is seen most commonly when onset is during childhood or adolescence (juvenile, or Westphal, variant). Patients with this subtype also frequently exhibit seizures, and intellectual deterioration is more rapid. Involvement in other family members in an autosomal dominant pattern is the most important diagnostic feature of Huntington's disease. Thus, half the offspring would be at risk for the disease, usually at an age, unfortunately, when marriage and the birth of children have already occurred. If general questioning about similar illnesses in the family yields a negative response, specific inquiries should be made about psychiatric illnesses, early deaths (especially in psychiatric institutions), and suicide. The estimated prevalence is generally 5–10 per 100,000 population, but informal estimates suggest up to 50 per 100,000 population. Thus, in a geographic area with a population of two million inhabitants, 100–200 patients would be expected, and perhaps up to 1,000 if the higher figure is used. Clinical diagnosis may be supported by computerized tomographic scans that demonstrate atrophy of the head of the caudate nucleus. However, this method has little predictive value for patients who are at risk. These clinical features have been reviewed well (70–72).

The observation that levodopa worsens involuntary movements in Huntington's disease led to its use to detect presymptomatic patients who were at risk (73). On several grounds, including the ethical one of early detection of incurable disease, potential psychiatric impact, and uncertainty as to the reliability of prediction, this approach has not been used widely.

Neurochemical Pathology

Intensive research during the past decade has demonstrated certain neurotransmitter abnormalities in patients with Huntington's disease. Numerous investigations of drugs that would correct these defects and, hopefully, modify the inexorably fatal outcome have resulted from these findings.

The findings may be summarized as reductions of (*1*) GABA and its chief synthetic enzyme glutamic acid decarboxylase; (*2*) choline acetyltransferase, the key cholinergic synthetic enzyme, and cholinergic receptors; (*3*) serotonin receptors; (*4*) levels of angiotensin-converting enzyme; and (*5*) substance P (74). The restriction of these findings generally to the striatum and the cerebral cortex suggest that relevance and specificity are important in the pathology of the disease.

Therapy

From a functional standpoint, the observation of diminished neurotransmitter parameters has been interpreted as an alteration in the balance between these neurotransmitters and dopamine. Thus, treatment efforts have focused either on blockade of dopaminergic transmission or on augmentation of cholinergic or GABA-ergic transmission (75,76).

In current practice, the class of drugs used most extensively to suppress chorea and to some extent, psychiatric manifestations have been catecholamine-depleting and catecholamine-blocking agents. These include haloperidol (3–12 mg/day) and the phenothiazines (77–79), as well as reserpine and tetrabenazine. Tetrabenazine has fewer cardiovascular effects but is not available in the United States (80–82). Unfortunately, these drugs offer only symptomatic treatment and have little impact on the inevitable mortality as the disease progresses.

Psychiatric manifestations may predominate and are often diffiult to manage. Reactive depression is frequent, and constant supportive therapy is necessary. Tricyclic antidepressants may be helpful when depression is profound, and they are preferable to MAO inhibitors, which may worsen the dyskinesia. Severe psychotic behavior may be treated with temporary increases in the dosage of either the phenothiazines or haloperidol.

Some patients with a rigid-hypokinetic variant may improve at least temporarily with levodopa or Sinemet in dosages similar to those used in parkinsonism; however, this therapy may aggravate the chorea (83). Apomorphine has improved the chorea in some patients, suggesting preferential activation of dopamine neurons that are different from those that aggravate chorea (84). Lithium carbonate has been ineffective in treatment of the disease (85).

Cholinergic augmentation with physostigmine (86) was shown to have limited temporary benefit, while dimethylaminoethanol definitely improved five of seven patients after a short trial (87). Choline was of no benefit (88).

Stimulated by the finding that levels of GABA are diminished in Huntington's disease, trials directed toward GABA-ergic augmentation have been reported recently but have been disappointing. These include the use of dipropylacetic acid alone in juvenile patients (89) or combined with GABA in adult patients (90); muscimol (91); imidazole-4 acetic acid (92); sodium valproate (93); and L-glutamate and pyridoxine (94). Isoniazid (INH) plus pyridoxine in high doses of approximately 500–1,000 mg ameliorated involuntary movements in five of the six patients studied for four to twenty-five months (95). Further, more controlled studies are needed to assess whether the effects of diethylaminoethanol and INH are a significant advance in the search for effective treatment.

At our present level of caring for patients with Huntington's disease and their families, drugs are only one of the important treatment modalities. Equally important are a supportive attitude, explanations of the expected course that are understandable to the layperson, and genetic counseling. Evaluation of the functional stage may provide useful guidelines for the physician and the patient and family regarding capabilities for employment, financial and domestic responsibilities, activities of daily living, and whether care can be provided best at home or in an institution (96). Literature may be obtained from the Committee to Combat Huntington's Disease, Inc., Suite 2016, 250 West 57th Street, New York, NY 10019; telephone, (212) 757-0443.

GILLES DE LA TOURETTE SYNDROME

Clinical Features

Gilles de la Tourette syndrome consists of chronic involuntary movements or tics, with onset in childhood between the ages of 2 and 15. The disorder has been reviewed extensively in a comprehensive monograph (97). Both muscular and verbal tics may occur, with a fluctuating clinical course so that they may be voluntarily suppressed for brief periods or increased by stressful situations and disappear during sleep. Initial tics usually involve the eyes, head, or face; in time over half of patients exhibit eye blink, head twitch, shoulder shrug, or arm jerk. More complex muscular tics include skipping, hopping, squatting, and pelvic thrusting or tilting. Verbal tics occur in over half of the patients and include throat clearing, barks, grunts, yelps, snorts, expiratory hisses, sniffing, screaming, and coprolalia (obscenities).

Associated in about half of patients but not essential for the diagnosis are a history of hyperactivity, nonspecifically abnormal EEG, and subtle neurologic abnormalities, including an increased incidence of left-handedness. The incidence is three times as frequent in boys as in girls and is highest in Ashkenazic Jews (19–62% of patients). About 35% of patients have family members who also are affected, including both parent and child.

The fundamental disorder remains unknown, but the response to dopamine-blocking drugs such as haloperidol suggests a neurochemical defect. The disease has no relation to social class, family history of mental illness, perinatal complications, infections, trauma, or birth order. Patients with Tourette do not necessarily have an associated mental disturbance such as schizophrenia, hysteria, or obsessive-compulsive neuroses, and they have a normal distribution of intelligence.

Drug Treatment

Of the various treatments, haloperidol has produced the best overall improvement (more than 70% improvement in 75% of patients). Treatment lasting longer than six months often is required; the extended course most probably reflects the use of slow upward titration of dosage over a period of months. Improvement is sustained for years, with a median improvement of 97% for more than four years on a mean daily dose of 9.5 mg (range, 0.1–55 mg). In contrast, other methods, such as psychotherapy, hypnosis, behavior modification, or other chemotherapeutic agents, have resulted in less than a 25% improvement.

Two approaches to the therapeutic use of haloperidol have been described. For most patients the slow method is recommended because it provides sufficient opportunity for the patient to adjust to the medication and minimize its side effects; in addition, this method is accomplished easily on an outpatient basis. Initially, 0.25 mg is taken nightly and is increased by 0.25 mg every fifth day until either 70% or more improvement occurs or side effects develop, or both.

In my experience, many patients tolerate larger initial doses of haloperidol; this characteristic has the dual advantage of early symptomatic relief and of diagnostic confirmation in what amounts to a therapeutic trial. Treatment may be initiated with 0.5 mg b.i.d. daily and titrated upward at weekly intervals to achieve an optimal balance between symptomatic benefit and minimal side effects.

Rapid treatment is used only rarely, and then only in severely incapacitated patients in a hospital setting. Parenteral injections are doubled at four-hour intervals, and close supervision is essential.

Recently, cases of tardive dyskinesia arising from chronic haloperidol treatment in Tourette patients have been reported, but are unusual. This may be attributable to the young age of the patients. However, especially in adults it is conceivable that this type of involuntary movement disorder may arise from long-term high-dose use of haloperidol.

Cognitive impairment has been reported to affect all patients taking antipsychotic medication at higher than a certain dosage level; the exact dosage may vary among individual patients. This effect remains of great concern in the long-term management of Tourette patients.

Further literature may be obtained from Tourette Syndrome Association, Bell Plaza Bldg., 42–40 Bell Blvd., Bayside, NY 11361.

HEMIBALLISMUS

Clinical Features

Ballismus is the irregular proximal flinging movement of the shoulder or thigh, named from the Greek word for a throwing motion. More distal portions of the limbs also may exhibit jerking movements in typical chorea. When the arm and leg on the same side are affected by these movements, the disorder is termed *hemiballismus* and *hemichorea.* In many cases, these severely disruptive movements persist and prevent coordinated use of the limbs in activities such as driving or walking. They can lead to falls that may result in cerebral injury (e.g., subdural hematoma) or other trauma. Diagnostically and therapeutically, these movements should be distinguished from continuous partial seizures, postanoxic myoclonus, cerebellar ataxia, rubral and intention tremor, and the adventitious movements of hepatolenticular degeneration. Pathologically, hemiballismus results from involvement of the contralateral subthalamic nucleus of Luys, usually by a vascular lesion; however, thalamic and striatal lesions also have been reported. The clinical features of this disorder have been reviewed extensively (98).

Drug Treatment

Significant improvement of hemichorea and hemiballismus has been reported with the use of drugs antagonistic to dopamine, suggesting that dopaminergic overactivity is a major pathophysiologic factor. Prompt (within one week) institution of haloperidol therapy, 3–12 mg/day has been reported to reduce hemiballismus in all of eight patients studied, and only two of the eight required treatment beyond one year (99). Similarly, perphenazine (Trilafon) benefited eight patients with hemichorea, and treatment was stopped without recurrence of involuntary movements in four patients (100). The starting dosage of 12 mg/day was therapeutic in half of the patients; for the others, the dose was increased by 4 mg every three days until a response occurred. In patients with residual hemichorea and hemiballismus after treatment, a walker is recommended to prevent sudden falls caused by unexpected loss of balance.

POSTHYPOXIC INTENTION MYOCLONUS

Clinical Features

Myoclonus is a very quick, irregular muscle jerk that is more vigorous than that seen in chorea and may affect any part of the body, including limbs, trunk, or head and neck. Although diverse etiologies have been identified, one that appears with increasing frequency is caused by hypoxic effects on the CNS. This posthypoxic intention myoclonus, or Lance–Adams syndrome (101), is stimulus initiated, so that whenever voluntary activity is attempted, a disruptive train of myoclonic jerks develop that subsequently abate with cessation of activity.

Hypoxia in myoclonic patients is most commonly a sequela of cardiopulmonary arrest or drug overdose and may occur with increasing frequency as resuscitation techniques improve. Other forms of myoclonus (familial myoclonus, myoclonic epilepsy, lipidosis, leukodystrophy, Creutzfeldt–Jakob disease) must be distinguished because each has a different natural history and calls for different treatment. Generalized seizures also are present in over half of myoclonic patients.

Drug Treatment

Difficulties in treatment of myoclonus were recognized in the original comprehensive report (101), and no single drug has emerged as the agent of choice since that time. Limited benefit has been reported with diazepam, primidone (Mysoline), phenobarbital, and other anticonvulsants, and many patients have been totally unresponsive.

Clonazepam (Clonopin) resulted in significant improvement in five patients with myoclonus that was refractory to other anticonvulsants in various combinations. Therapy was initiated at 1 mg/day and was increased at two- to three-day intervals to 7–12 mg/day (102). Valproic acid is considered to mimic the effects of GABA on the CNS and has been effective in two cases (103).

A combination of 500–1,500 mg/day of 5-hydroxytryptophan (5-HTP), the immediate precursor of serotonin, and carbidopa, 100 mg/day, resulted in improvement in patients with posthypoxic myoclonus refractory to conventional agents (104,105). These therapeutic trials were based on the observation that the serotonin metabolite 5-hydroxyindoleacetic acid was reduced in the CSF of patients suffering from this syndrome. The observation coupled with the demonstrated efficacy of serotonergic augmentation in certain patients, suggests either underactivity of serotonergic neuronal systems or serotonin deficiency.

It should be understood that these agents are not widely available, that the applications described here are not FDA approved, and that side effects, especially gastrointestinal and mental ones, are frequent. Myoclonus due to other causes were not improved with this treatment (105), implying that different mechanisms may underly other myoclonias.

DYSTONIA

Clinical Features

Dystonia consists of slow, sustained, involuntary movements that result in twisting, bending, or straightening. Specific actions, such as writing or walking, may precipitate dystonia. In severe cases, fixed contractures and postural deformities result. Involvement may be either generalized or segmental (confined to one portion of the body).

Classification of the dystonias shows that some cases are primary or idiopathic, while others are symptomatic and result from encephalitis, degenerative diseases of the basal ganglia (including Wilson's disease, Huntington's disease, and Hallevorden–Spatz disease), trauma, perinatal hypoxia or intoxication. Substantial advances have been made recently in the etiology and treatment of the primary or idiopathic tortion dystonias (dystonia musculorum deformans).

The diagnosis of primary dystonia depends on the presence of dystonia plus the absence of a history of perinatal complications or conditions associated with secondary dystonia. A recent comprehensive summary of current knowledge about the dystonias may be found in the excellent volume edited by Eldridge and Fahn (106).

The onset of most cases occurs during childhood, with involvement of the legs more than the arms and trunk. More than half of patients are not able to walk five to 10 years after onset, but the illness tends to stabilize when adulthood is reached. Adult-onset cases, which are less frequent, affect the arms rather than the legs and have a more favorable outlook. Dysarthria is present in 50% of childhood-onset cases, while dysphagia is present in about 20%. Males and females are affected equally. A higher incidence among Jews has been noted, with familial involvement that indicates autosomal recessive inheritance. The age of onset for patients whose illness has progressed to generalized involvement averaged 11 years, while onset occurred at 27 years in those whose dystonia remained segmental.

Treatment

Although many drugs have been tried and none has emerged as clearly effective, four drugs deserve special mention. Carbamazepine (Tegretol) produced a good response in six of 21 patients in one series, but in another series, only one of 16 had a clear-cut benefit. Haloperidol, often in combination with other drugs, has benefited limited numbers of patients. Although baclofen improved two of 13 patients in initial reports, further studies of the drug are necessary. Perhaps the most controversial drug is L-dopa, either alone or combined with carbidopa. Early reports suggest that L-dopa offers benefit to some patients, but Cooper has cautioned against its use in children because it may worsen the dystonia (106).

Stereotaxic thalamotomy has been beneficial, especially in the extremities rather than in the trunk. Surgical treatment should be considered only after medical management has been thoroughly exhausted. In Cooper's experience with 226 patients over 20 years, about 70% had at least moderate improvement after an average of two operations per patient; the mortality for a single operation was 0.7%. In certain cases, surgical response has been very dramatic. An interval of six months between bilateral procedures is suggested to minimize voice-related complications and because benefit may be delayed for this length of time.

Sensory feedback therapy significantly has benefited the majority of seven patients; however, the initial benefit was not sustained after three months. Since this modality has provided some additional benefit, it would appear worthwhile to try this technique if it is available.

IDIOPATHIC SPASMODIC TORTICOLLIS

Clinical Features

More common than generalized dystonia musculorum deformans is idiopathic spasmodic torticollis. This disorder is characterized by restricted involvement of the neck muscles that results in intermittent turning of the head. Whether torticollis is segmental dystonia or a separate entity is debatable. As compared with patients who have dystonia musculorum deformans, patients with spasmodic torticollis are most often female, 75% have onset after 30 years of age, and the lower extremities are spared. It seems reasonable at present to distinguish the two conditions from at least the standpoint of prognosis, since initial torticollis almost never becomes generalized. In more than half of cases there may be associated mild dystonia of muscles of the shoulder, upper limbs, or neck. Most patients also exhibit tremor of the arms, head, or neck, and many have underlying degenerative disease of the cervical spine. Clinical symptoms include both head rotation and pain resulting from constant muscular contraction.

Treatment

A variety of drugs have been tried but with only limited success. In particular, these have included haloperidol and L-dopa, as well as amantadine, diazepam, baclofen, anticholinergic and antiparkinsonian drugs, and various muscle relaxants and sedatives. The associated intention tremor may improve with propranolol.

Surgical treatment of spasmodic torticollis is seldom used because bilateral operations are usually necessary and the risk of 2% mortality is difficult to justify. Sensory feedback therapy benefited more than half of 48 patients in one series, and the benefit was sutained in many.

A reasonable therapeutic approach would be a combination of symptomatic treatment of neck pain, sequential administration of various drugs for the torticollis, propranolol for tremor, and concomitant biofeedback therapy.

ACKNOWLEDGMENTS

I am indebted to my patients (especially D.C., B.E., M.G., and E.S.) for the insights they have provided and for their exemplary patience and courage, and to Cheryl Winner for typing this manuscript despite her busy schedule.

REFERENCES

1. Birkmayer W, Hornykiewicz O: Der L-3,4-Dioxyphenylalanin (=DOPA)-Effect bei der Parkinsonakinese. Wien Klin Wochenschur 73:787–788, 1961.
2. Barbeau A: Biochemistry of Parkinson's disease. In: *Proceedings of the 7th International Congress on Neurology.* Rome, Romana, 1961, p. 925.
3. Cotzias GC, Van Woert MH, Schiffer LM: Aromatic amino acids and modification of parkinsonism. N Engl J Med 276:374–379, 1967.
4. Cotzias GC, Papavasilou PS, Gellene R: Modification of parkinsonism—chronic treatment with L-dopa. N Engl J Med 280:337–345, 1969.
5. Barbeau A: L-Dopa therapy in Parkinson's disease: a critical review of nine years' experience. Can Med Assoc J 101:791–800, 1969.
6. Barbeau A: Six years of high-level levodopa therapy in severely akinetic parkinsonian patients. Arch Neurol 33:333–338, 1976.
7. Lee JE, Sweet RD, McDowell FH: Treatment of parkinsonism with levodopa. Ann Intern Med 75:703–708, 1971.
8. Markham CH, Treciokas LJ, Diamond SG: Parkinson's disease and levodopa. West J Med 121:188–206, 1974.
9. Sweet RD, McDowell FH: Five years' treatment of Parkinson's disease with levodopa. Ann Intern Med 83:456–463, 1975.
10. Yahr M: Levodopa. Ann Intern Med 83:677–682, 1975.
11. Hoehn MM, Yahr MD: Parkinsonism onset, progression, and mortality. Neurology 17:427–442, 1967.
12. Joseph C, Chassan JB, Koch ML: Levodopa in Parkinson disease: a long-term appraisal of mortality. Ann Neurol 3:116–118, 1978.
13. Marsden CD: Combined treatment with decarboxylase inhibitors. In: *The Clinical Uses of Levodopa.* Edited by G Stern. Baltimore, University Park Press, 1975, pp. 107–126.
14. Fahn S, Calne D: Considerations in the management of parkinsonism. Neurology 1:5–7, 1978.
15. Marsden CD, Parkes JD: Success and problems of long-term levodopa therapy in Parkinson's disease. Lancet 1:345–349, 1977.
16. Wolf SM, Davis RL: Permanent dementia in idiopathic parkinsonism treated with levodopa. Arch Neurol 29:276–278, 1973.
17. Sweet RD, McDowell FH, Feigenson JS, et al: Mental symptoms in Parkinson's disease during chronic treatment with levodopa. Neurology 26:305–310, 1976.
18. Lieberman AN, Shupack JL: Levodopa and melanoma. Neurology 24:340–343, 1974.
19. Miller E: Deanol in the treatment of levodopa-induced dyskinesias. Neurology 24:116–119, 1974.
20. Klawans HL, Topel JL, Bergen D: Deanol in the treatment of levodopa-induced dyskinesias. Neurology 25:290–293, 1975.
21. Hoehn MM: Levodopa induced postural hypotension. Treatment with fludrocortisone. Arch Neurol 32:50–51, 1975.
22. Hoehn MM, Rutledge CO: Acute overdose with levodopa. Neurology 25:792–794, 1975.

23. Sweet RD, McDowell FH: The on-off response to chronic L-dopa treatment of parkinsonism. Adv Neurol 5:331–338, 1974.
24. Markham CH: The on-off side-effect of L-dopa. Adv Neurol 5:387–396, 1974.
25. Yahr MD: Variations in the on-off effects. Adv Neurol 5:397–404, 1974.
26. Marsden CD, Parkes JD: 'On-off' effects in patients with Parkinson's disease on chronic levodopa therapy. Lancet 1:292–296, 1976.
27. Muenter MD, Sharpless NS, Tyce GM, et al: Patterns of dystonia ('I-D-I' and 'D-I-D') in response to L-dopa therapy for Parkinson's disease. Mayo Clin Proc 52:164–174, 1977.
28. Granerus AK: Factors influencing occurrence of 'on-off' symptoms during long-term treatment with L-dopa. Acta Med Scand 203:75–85, 1978.
29. Sweet RD, McDowell FH, Wasterlain CG: Treatment of 'on-off' effect with a dopa decarboxylase inhibitor. Arch Neurol 32:560–563, 1975.
30. Direnfeld L, Spero L, Marotta J, et al: The L-dopa on-off effect in Parkinson's disease treatment by transient drug withdrawal and dopamine receptor resensitization. Ann Neurol 4:573–575, 1978.
31. Lhermitte F, Agid Y, Signoret JL: Onset and end-of-dose levodopa-induced dyskinesias. Arch Neurol 35:261–263, 1978.
32. Shoulson I, Glaubiger GA, Chase TN: On-off response. Neurology 25:1144–1148, 1975.
33. Schwab RS, Poskanzer DC, England AC, et al: Amantadine in Parkinson's disease. JAMA 222:792–795, 1972.
34. Fahn S, Isgreen WP: Long-term evaluation of amantadine and levodopa combination in parkinsonism by double-blind crossover analysis. Neurology 25:695–700, 1975.
35. Timberlake WH, Vance MA: Four-year treatment of patients with parkinsonism using amantadine alone or with levodopa. Ann Neurol 3:119–128, 1978.
36. Gerlach J: Effect of CB 154 (2-bromo-alpha-ergocryptine) on paralysis agitans compared with madopar in a double-blind, cross-over trial. Acta Neurol Scand 53:189–200, 1976.
37. Kartzinel R, Shoulson I, Calne DB: Studies with bromocriptine. Part 2. Double-blind comparison with levodopa in idiopathic parkinsonism. Neurology 26:511–513, 1976.
38. Lieberman A, Kupersmith M, Estry E, et al: Treatment of Parkinson's disease with bromocriptine. N Engl J Med 295:1400–1404, 1976.
39. Parkes JD, Debono AG, Marsden CD: Bromocriptine in parkinsonism: long-term treatment, dose response and comparison with levodopa. J Neurol Neurosurg Psychiatry 39:1101–1108, 1976.
40. Rinne UK, Martilla R: Brain dopamine receptor stimulation and the relief of parkinsonism: relationship between bromocriptine and levodopa. Ann Neurol 4:263–267, 1978.
41. Teychenne PF, Pfeiffer RF, Bern SM, et al: Comparison between lergotrile and bromocriptine in parkinsonism. Ann Neurol 3:319–324, 1978.
42. Kartzinel R, Calne DB: Studies with bromocriptine. Part 1. 'On-off' phenomena. Neurology 26:508–510, 1976.
43. Cotzias GL, Papavasiliou PS, Tolosa ES, et al: Treatment of Parkinson's disease with aporphines. N Engl J Med 294:567–572, 1976.
44. Bedard P, Parkes JD, Marsden CD: Effect of new dopamine blocking agent (oxiperomide) on drug-induced dyskinesias in Parkinson's disease and spontaneous dyskinesias. Br Med J 1:954–956, 1978.
45. Cooper IS: Neurosurgical treatment of the dyskinesias. Clin Neurosurg 24:367–390, 1977.
46. Duvoisin R: *Parkinson's Disease. A Guide for Patient and Family.* New York, Raven Press, 1978.
47. Critchley M: Observations on essential (heredofamilial) tremor. Brain 72:113–139, 1949.
48. Kobayashi RM, Wilson JR, Seybold M: Tremography in the assessment of tremor. Bull Los Angeles Neurol Soc 43:37, 1978.
49. Winkler GF, Young RR: Efficacy of chronic propranolol therapy in action tremors of the familial, senile or essential varieties. N Engl J Med 290:984–988, 1974.

50. Tolosa ES, Loewenson RB: Essential tremor: Treatment with propranolol. Neurology 25:1041–1044, 1975.

51. Teravainen H, Fogelholm R, Larsen A: Effect of propranolol on essential tremor. Neurology 26:27–30, 1976.

52. Young RR, Growdon JH, Shahani BT: Beta-adrenergic mechanisms in action tremor. N Engl J Med 293:950–953, 1975.

53. McAllister RG, Markesbery WR, Ware RW, et al: Suppression of essential tremor by propranolol: correlation of effect with drug plasma levels and intensity of beta-adrenergic blockade. Ann Neurol 1:160–166, 1977.

54. Growdon JH, Shahani BT, Young RR: The effect of alcohol on essential tremor. Neurology 25:259–262, 1975.

55. Marsden CD, Tarsy D, Baldessarini RJ: Spontaneous and drug-induced movement disorders in psychotic patients. In: *Psychiatric Aspects of Neurological Disease.* Edited by DF Benson and D Blumer. New York, Grune and Stratton, 1975, pp. 219–266.

56. Kobayashi RM: Orofacial dyskinesia. Clinical features, mechanisms and drug therapy. West J Med 125:277–288, 1976.

57. American College of Neuropsychopharm Food and Drug Admin Task Force: Neurologic syndromes associated with antipsychotic drug use. N Engl J Med 289:20–23, 1973.

58. Klawans HL, Berger D, Bruyn GW, et al: Neuroleptic induced tardive dyskinesias in nonpsychotic patients. Arch Neurol 30:338–339, 1974.

59. Brandon S, McClelland HA, Protheroe C: A study of facial dyskinesias in a mental hospital population. Br J Psychol 118:171–184, 1971.

60. Christensen E, Moller JE, Faurbye A: Neuropathologic investigation of 28 brains from patients with dyskinesia. Acta Psychol Scand 46:14–23, 1970.

61. Klawans HL: The pharmacology of tardive dyskinesias. Am J Psychol 130:82–86, 1973.

62. Burt DB, Creese I, Snyder SH: Antischizophrenic drugs: chronic treatment elevates dopamine receptor binding in brain. Science 196:326–328, 1977.

63. Kobayashi RM, Fields JZ, Hruska RE, et al: Brain neurotransmitter receptors and chronic anti-psychotic drug treatment: a model for tardive dyskinesia. In: *Animal Models in Psychiatry and Neurology.* Edited by I Hanin and E Usdin. New York, Pergamon Press, 1977, pp. 405–409.

64. Kobayashi RM: Drug therapy of tardive dyskinesia. N Engl J Med 296:257–260, 1977.

65. Quitkin F, Rifkin A, Gochfeld L, et al: Tardive dyskinesia: are first signs reversible? Am J Psychol 134:84–87, 1977.

66. Kazamatsuri H, Chien C, Cole JO: Long-term treatment of tardive dyskinesia with haloperidol and tetrabenazine. Am J Psychol 130:479–483, 1973.

67. Casey DE, Denney D: Pharmacological characterization of tardive dyskinesia. Psychopharmacology (Berlin) 54:1–8, 1977.

68. Korsgaard S: Baclofen (Lioresal) in the treatment of neuroleptic-induced tardive dyskinesia. Acta Psychol Scand 54:17–24, 1976.

69. Linnoila M, Viukari M, Hietala O: Effect of sodium valproate on tardive dyskinesia. Br J Psychol 129:114–119, 1976.

70. Barbeau A, Chase TN, Paulson G: Huntington's chorea, 1872–1972. In: *Advances in Neurology,* vol. 1. New York, Raven Press, 1973.

71. Bruyn GW: Huntington's chorea: historical, clinical and laboratory synopsis. In: *Handbook of Clinical Neurology,* vol. 6. Edited by PJ Vinken and GW Bruyn. Amsterdam, North-Holland, 1968, pp. 298–378.

72. Shoulson I, Chase TN: Huntington's disease. Annu Rev Med 26:419–426, 1975.

73. Klawans HL, Paulson GW, Ringel SP, et al: Use of L-dopa in the detection of presymptomatic Huntington's chorea. N Engl J Med 286:1332–1334, 1972.

74. Bird ED, Iversen LL: Neurochemical findings in Huntington's chorea. In: *Essays in Neurochemistry and Neuropharmacology.* Edited by M Youdim, W Lovenberg, DF Sharman, et al. New York, John Wiley and Sons, 1977, pp. 177–193.

75. Chase TN: Rational approaches to the pharmacotherapy of chorea. In: *The Basal Ganglia.* Edited by M Yahr. New York, Raven Press, 1976, pp. 337–350.

76. Klawans HL, Weiner WJ: The pharmacology of choreatic movement disorders. Progr Neurobiol 6:49–80, 1976.

77. Divry P, Bobon J, Collard J, et al: Étude et expérimentation cliniques du R 1625 ou haloperidol, nouveau neuroleptique et neurodyseptique. Acta Neurol Belg 59:337–366, 1959.

78. Vaisberg M, Saunders JC: Treatment of dyskinesias including Huntington's chorea with thiopropazate and R-1625. Dis Nerv Syst 24:499–500, 1963.

79. Fahn S: Treatment of choreic movements with perphenazine. In: *Advances in Neurology,* vol. 1. Edited by A Barbeau, TN Chase and GW Paulson. New York, Raven Press, 1973, pp. 755–764.

80. Lazarte JA, Peterson MC, Baars CW, et al: Huntington's chorea: results of treatment with reserpine. Proc Staff Meet Mayo Clin 30:358–365, 1955.

81. McLellan DL, Chalmers RJ, Johnson RH: A double-blind trial of tetrabenazine, thiopropazate, and placebo in patients with chorea. Lancet 1:104–107, 1974.

82. Huang CV, McLeod JG, Holland RT, et al: Tetrabenazine in the treatment of Huntington's chorea. Med J Aust 1:583–584, 1976.

83. Barbeau A: L-dopa and juvenile Huntington's disease. Lancet 2:1066, 1969.

84. Tolosa ES, Sparber SB: Apomorphine in Huntington's chorea: clinical observations and theoretical considerations. Life Sci 15:1371–1380, 1974.

85. Aminoff MJ, Marshall J: Treatment of Huntington's chorea with lithium carbonate. Lancet 1:107–109, 1974.

86. Klawans HL, Rubovits R: Central cholinergic-anticholinergic antagonisms in Huntington's chorea. Neurology 22:107–116, 1972.

87. Walker JE, Hoehn M, Sears E, et al: Dimethylaminoethanol in Huntington's chorea. Lancet 1:1512–1513, 1973.

88. Growdon JH, Cohen EL, Wurtman RJ: Huntington's disease: clinical and chemical effects of choline administration. Ann Neurol 1:418–422, 1977.

89. Bachman DS, Butler IJ, McKhann GM: Long-term treatment of juvenile Huntington's chorea with dipropylacetic acid. Neurology 27:193–197, 1977.

90. Shoulson I, Kartzinel R, Chase TN: Huntington's disease: treatment with dipropylacetic acid and gamma-amino butyric acid. Neurology 26:61–63, 1976.

91. Shoulson I, Goldblatt D, Charlton M: Huntington's disease: treatment with muscimol, a GABA-mimetic drug. Ann Neurol 4:279–284, 1978.

92. Shoulson I, Chase TN, Roberts E, et al: Huntington's disease: treatment with imidazole-4-acetic acid. N Engl J Med 293:504–505, 1975.

93. Pearce I, Heathfield KWG, Pearce JMS: Valproate sodium in Huntington chorea. Arch Neurol 34:308–309, 1977.

94. Barr AN, Heinze W, Mendoza JE, et al: Long term treatment of Huntington's disease with L-glutamate and pyridoxine. Neurology 28:1280–1282, 1978.

95. Perry TL, Wright JM, Hansen S: Isoniazid therapy of Huntington disease. Neurology 29:370–375, 1979.

96. Shoulson I, Fahn S: Huntington's disease: Clinical care and evaluation. Neurology 29:1–3, 1979.

97. Shapiro AK, Shapiro ES, Brunn RD, et al: *Gilles de la Tourette Syndrome.* New York, Raven Press, 1978.

98. Meyers R: Ballismus. In: *Handbook of Clinical Neurology.* Edited by PJ Vinken and GW Bruyn. Amsterdam, North-Holland, 1968, pp. 476–490.

99. Klawans HL, Moses H, Nausieda PA, et al: Treatment and prognosis of hemiballismus. N Engl J Med 295:1348–1350, 1976.

100. Johnson WG, Fahn S: Treatment of vascular hemiballism and hemichorea. Neurology 27:634–636, 1977.

101. Lance JW, Adams RD: The syndrome of intention or action myoclonus as a sequela to hypoxic encephalopathy. Brain 86:111–136, 1963.

102. Goldberg MA, Dorman JD: Intention myoclonus: successful treatment with clonazepam. Neurology 26:24–26, 1976.

103. Fahn S: Post-anoxic action myoclonus: improvement with valproic acid. N Engl J Med 299:313–314, 1978.

104. Van Woert MH, Rosenbaum D, Howieson J, et al: Long-term therapy of myoclonus and other neurologic disorders with L-5-hydroxytryptophan and carbidopa. N Engl J Med 296:70–75, 1977.

105. Growdon JH, Young RR, Shahani B: L-5-Hydroxytryptophan in treatment of several different syndromes in which myoclonus is prominent. Neurology 26:1135–1140, 1976.

106. Eldridge R, Rahn S (editors): *Advances in Neurology*, vol. 14. New York, Raven Press, 1976.

7

Primary and Secondary Tumors of the Central and Peripheral Nervous Systems

Lawrence F. Marshall

Claudia M. Greco

Advances in neurodiagnostics, primarily the availability of computerized axial tomographic (CAT) scanning, improved neuroanesthetic techniques, and better lighting and magnification have altered dramatically the neurosurgeon's approach to tumors of the nervous system. While some tumors, such as glioblastoma multiforme, continue to resist surgical cure, other lesions heretofore thought to be unapproachable have now come into the realm of diagnosable and curable disorders.

In this chapter we will discuss the current approach to primary and metastatic neoplasms of the intracranial contents, the spinal canal, and the spinal cord. The discussion will be limited primarily to treatment, although comments will be made about new or alternative diagnostic techniques where appropriate.

INTRACRANIAL TUMORS

The diagnosis and treatment of intracranial neoplasms has been revolutionized by the introduction of CAT scanning. Not only has the CAT scanner eliminated the need for more invasive diagnostic tests in many instances, but it also has yielded a tremendous amount of information that previously was not obtainable through radionucleotide scanning, angiography, and pneumoencephalography. While each of these tests continues to have value in selected instances, CAT scanning is rapidly replacing them in most cases of suspected intracranial neoplasm. Moreover, the advent of CAT scanning has greatly reduced the importance of lumbar puncture and electroencephalography in the diagnostic evaluation of patients with suspected intracranial neoplasm.

The advantages of CAT scanning are its noninvasiveness, its high accuracy in delineating masses greater than 1 cm in size, and its ability to do scanning "cuts" to give accurate localization of intracranial neoplasms in relation to anatomic structures. The cuts can then be related to the skull, thus making surgical localization much easier. While in some instances, such as inoperable brain-stem tumors, the scanner may only allow identification of smaller tumors and observation of their inexorable course, it is likely that, as better treatment strategies for malignancies of the CNS are developed in the future, early diagnosis will become increasingly important, particularly since it is well recognized in diseases of other organs and of the central nervous system (CNS) that the smaller the neoplasm to be treated with radiation and/or chemotherapy, the greater the likelihood of long-term control or cure. In the following discussion, the treatment of brain tumors will be divided by histologic type and location, and emphasis will be placed on new approaches to the treatment of intracranial tumors.

The neoplastic processes described here are not all-encompassing. Rather, we have attempted to concentrate on primary and secondary neoplasms of the brain and spinal cord that occur most frequently. Consequently, some relatively rare tumors, such as colloid cyst of the third ventricle and choroid plexus papilloma, are treated briefly. Others, such as medulloepithelioma, are not discussed at all. Because clinical signs and symptoms of these relatively rare neoplasms do not differ remarkably from neoplasms located in the same regions of the brain, the omission of these more uncommon lesions seems appropriate.

Neuroectodermal Tumors

Astrocytomas are the most frequent primary intracranial neoplasm. Glioblastoma, its most malignant from, is found in biopsy specimens in approximately 65% of adult patients. Treatment of this tumor is no longer entirely surgical or radiotherapeutic.

The Brain Tumor Study Group has convincingly demonstrated that (*1*) bulk reduction of the tumor is of definite value in yielding prolonged and improved survival; (*2*) radiation therapy is definitely effective in improving the length and quality of survival; and (*3*) a combination of radiotherapy with a nitrosourea drug gives further improvement in survival (1). Table 1 illustrates the most recent data available from the Brain Tumor Study Group (1). It can be seen that, at one year, there is little difference in survival between patients first treated surgically and then with radiation therapy and those who were treated surgically and then with radiation therapy and chemotherapy. However, at 18 months there was a dramatic increase in the survival of patients who received chemotherapy, indicating that, at least for some patients, chemotherapy alters the natural history of the disease. If possible, therapy for patients with glioblastoma should include bulk reduction of the tumor, and radiation therapy should be delivered in a total dose of 6,000 rad to the head, 4,000 rad to the whole brain, and 2,000 rad cone down. In addition, a nitrosourea drug (BCNU, 160 mg/m^2) should be given on a six-week schedule. Although protocols using combination therapies such as procarbazine (100 mg/m^2) and vincristine (2 mg/m^2) in addition to a nitrosourea seem attractive, they do present some difficulties, particularly in patients older than 50 years of age, in whom bone marrow suppression is extremely common

Table 1. Outcome in 167 Patients Randomized to Different Postoperative Regimens (Brain Tumor Study Group)

Treatment Modality	*Median Survival (weeks)*	*Survival at 18 Months (%)*
Surgery Alone	17	0
Surgery and Radiation Therapy	38	5
Surgery and BCNU	25	5
Surgery, Radiation Therapy, and BCNU	41	23 < .01

because since patients often cannot tolerate long cycles of chemotherapy. In the future, better chemotherapeutic strategies should be possible in patients with malignant gliomas and probably will include agents other than those discussed here.

The availability of glucocorticoids has given the treating neurologist and neurosurgeon an opportunity to improve symptoms and therefore improve the quality of survival while the disease is progressing. Many patients who have severe neurologic deficit, including aphasia and hemiparesis, can return to a state of near normalcy with steroids in various dosages (up to 100 mg dexamethasone/day in four divided doses) (2). While such palliation is costly, the yield may justify the expenditure. Moreover, failure to respond to high doses of glucocorticoids also can yield information as to the prognosis. Patients who are resistant to high doses of corticosteroids usually have an extremely short course (3). While evidence from in vivo experiments that glucocorticoids have an antitumor effect is scanty, their remarkable ability to reverse progression of symptoms makes them extremely useful in the day-to-day treatment and management of patients with malignant glial tumors.

There is no definite glucocorticoid of choice for treatment of those tumors, although dexamethasone has been the most widely used drug. At present, most neurosurgeons start with dosages of approximately 16 mg/day in four divided doses. As indicated previously, the dosage can be increased up to 100 mg/day in divided doses, although this rarely is necessary. The dose of glucocorticoid should be spaced at approximately six-hour intervals unless the patient is taking diphenylhydantoin (Dilantin), in which case a four-hour schedule is preferable, since this drug appears to increase the rate of degradation of dexamethasone. The long-term objective in the treatment with corticosteroids is to find the lowest dosage that will ameliorate the symptoms. Tapering, however, must be slow, or the patient's symptoms may recur and then may not respond to reelevation of the dexamethasone dosage. In my experience, long-term complications of dexamethasone have been relatively minor, with the exception of steroid myopathy, which occasionally can be quite severe.

Benign Neuroectodermal Tumors

The treatment of astrocytomas and oligodendrogliomas that appear to be histologically benign remains an area of controversy. Grade I tumors of the cerebral cortex that can be treated by surgical extirpation should be completely removed if possible. There also is evidence to suggest that radiation therapy can significantly alter the disease course in these patients. Sheline and colleagues (4) have demonstrated a significant increase in survival in patients who receive radiation therapy as compared with those who were not irradiated. This statement appears to hold true for all grade I and II astrocytomas and supports the previous observation of Bouchard (5), who also demonstrated improved survival in low-grade tumors. The clinical presentation of these neoplasms is not markedly different from that of other intracranial masses, except that their time course is somewhat longer than that of glioblastomas, and presentation with seizures is more frequent. If such a tumor is surgically removable, we believe that surgical extirpation is definitely indicated and that extirpation should be followed with a course of radiation therapy of 6,000 rad in an attempt to achieve cure of the tumor. The role of chemotherapy in such patient is unclear. Given the agents available at present, however, it is unlikely that chemotherapy would have a significant effect, since these tumors grow rather slowly and have only a small number of cells in the proliferative pool. Therefore, they will not be very sensitive to the action of agents that affect only proliferating cells.

Cerebellar Astrocytomas

Cerebellar astrocytomas are tumors usually found in children and young adults, although they occasionally may be seen in older patients. In younger patients, the tumors tend to occur in the midline, while in adolescents they occur more commonly in the lateral lobe of the cerebellum. These children usually appear initially with symptoms identical to those of medulloblastoma, namely, obstructive hydrocephalus, gait disturbance, and papilledema on clinical examination. In most instances, optimal treatment in these children is complete surgical removal of a well-circumscribed, histologically benign-looking mass. The presence of Rosenthal fibers and the absence of mitotic figures, dense cellularity, and pleomorphism usually are indications of a benign course (juvenile type) (6). When Rosenthal fibers are not present and there is evidence of increased vascularity, increased mitotic activity, and dense cellularity (diffuse type), the tumors have a very high instance of recurrence. Therapy must be aggressive for patients with this type of tumor and should include both radical surgical removal and radiation therapy.

Ependymomas

Ependymomas comprise approximately 5% of all intracranial neuroectodermal tumors. In childhood, when they are seen most frequently, the tumor usually arises in the fourth ventricle and gives rise to symptoms by producing obstructive hydrocephalus and disturbances of the brain stem and cerebellar function. Although in adults these tumors may be seen in an infratentorial location, they are seen more frequently in the anterior or middle fossa. Again, diagnosis relies heavily on the CAT scan. The angiographic appearance of these tumors is usually nondiagnostic, and angiography usually is necessary only to delineate the tumor's vasculature better. Some surgeons operate on fourth-ventricular masses without the aid of angiography, and this appears to be a perfectly acceptable practice.

If possible, surgical removal ependymomas should be complete. This often is difficult with fourth-ventricular tumors because of their secondary attachment to the floor of the medulla. In such instances, subtotal resection with postoperative irradiation to the tumor site is appropriate (7). Ependymomas occasionally have a malignant course. In these cases, craniospinal irradiation is warranted because the tumor may spread to the cerebrospinal fluid (CSF) pathways. Although it is said that ependymomas have a marked tendency to metastasize in this way, this occurrence has been rare in our experience. Medulloblastomas, on the other hand, metastasize in this way all too frequently.

Medulloblastomas

Medulloblastomas account for approximately 5% of all intracranial tumors and for 25% of all intracranial tumors in children. Approximately one-half of medulloblastomas arise in the first decade of life, and they are seen more commonly in males. It is generally accepted that medulloblastomas arise in the cerebellum, although they often are seen in the midline and attached to the superior medullary velum. In adults, the tumor can occur in the lateral lobes of the cerebellum. In many instances, this lateral-lobe tumor has been called an embryonal sarcoma, although its histologic characteristics appear identical to those of medulloblastoma.

The diagnosis of medulloblastoma in children usually can be made by CAT scanning with contrast medium. These tumors tend to enhance dramatically. When a fourth-ventricular neoplasm is detected in a child, significant enhancement on CAT scan strongly suggests the diagnosis. Angiography occasionally is useful, but CAT scanning usually is sufficient. Plain films usually demonstrate evidence of intracranial hypertension. Almost all children with medulloblastoma have evidence of papilledema.

Controversy revolves about the treatment of these tumors in children. Raimondi and Tomita (8) maintain that complete excision combined with radiation therapy yields a longer survival than incomplete removal alone. Others maintain that the radiosensitivity of the tumor indicates that surgery should be limited to a diagnostic biopsy followed by radiation therapy. However, most surgeons at least strive to open the obstructed CSF pathways, since shunting in these children, despite the use of an indwelling filter in the shunting system, has sometimes been associated with peritoneal metastasis in the presence of a ventriculoperitoneal shunt, and with visceral and systemic metastasis when an intra-atrial shunt is used. This complication of medulloblastoma cannot be ignored, and shunting should be avoided whenever possible. Ventricular drainage can be performed before and immediately after surgery if the obstruction has not been completely removed, so that radiation therapy can be effective in resolving obstruction to CSF flow further. In instances where shunting must be done, the placement of a filtration system in the shunting apparatus is useful, although it does not give absolute ensurance against metastasis via the shunt system.

Radiation therapy for medulloblastoma remains the hallmark and cornerstone of treatment. Present radiation schemes usually consist of a dose of

4,500–5,000 rad to the brain, including the primary site, and approximately 3,500 rad to the spinal cord. Such doses yield a lower risk of tumor recurrence while they maintain a favorable benefit-to-complication ratio. In adults, the tumor behaves similarly as in children, but the results of treatment appear to be somewhat better. In one large series, mortality statistics indicate a five-year survival of approximately 30% in children and 40% in adults (9). However, a recent report of a new method of radiation therapy has suggested that higher survival and cure rates can be achieved with radiation therapy (10).

Medulloblastomas are exquisitely sensitive to chemotherapy, but remission is usually short-lived and the patient then succumbs to the disease. Agents that have been shown to be effective include the nitrosoureas, vincristine, and procarbazine. To date, controlled trials of combination therapy following surgery and radiation therapy have failed to demonstrate an improved survival.

Brain-Stem Gliomas

Brain-stem gliomas are relatively uncommon tumors that are found most often in children and young adults. They can be distinguished from ependymomas and medulloblastomas by clinical symptoms and signs, including multiple cranial-nerve palsies, a somewhat bland, pained facial expression, mixed long-tract signs, and a rather unusual gait disturbance that is not attributable to involvement of the cerebellum. CAT scanning can often distinguish this lesion from an intraventricular or extra-axial tumor, but angiography and pneumoencephalography frequently are required. When there is anterior displacement of the basilar artery against the clivus and when the angiographic choroidal point of the fourth ventricle is displaced posteriorly, the lesion must be in the pons. Posterior displacement of the fourth ventricle on pneumoencephalography to a distance of more than 4 cm from the dorsum sella in combination with anterior displacement of the basilar artery establishes the diagnosis of an intra-axial, intrapontine lesion. Exploration in children with these tumors usually is not warranted, since nothing can be accomplished surgically; in addition, clinical status may deteriorate after surgery. Radiation therapy occasionally is effective in limiting growth of the tumor, although the long-term outlook is poor.

Meningiomas

Meningiomas are generally benign intracranial tumors that comprise about 14% of all intracranial masses. They are seen most commonly in middle-aged women. In children they make up approximately 4% of intracranial tumors and more often have characteristics of malignancy. Trauma and previous irradiation to the scalp have been considered important factors in the initiation of the growth of these lesions (10).

In approximately 50% of patients, meningiomas are found in the parasagittal region. Invasion of the sagittal sinus is relatively common. The next most frequent site is the convexity, either frontally or parietally, and a less frequent site is along the sylvian fissure. Meningiomas at the base of the brain can be located within the parasellar region or along the olfactory groove or sphenoid wing.

Occasionally, meningiomas of the sheath of the optic nerve are seen. Meningiomas in the posterior fossa are much less common but are clinically significant. These tumors may appear along the tentorium or the cranial nerves, particularly the fifth, and produce symptoms that are indistinguishable from those of classic tic douloureux. Invasion of the petrous bone is relatively uncommon, but tumors may originate from the petrous bone, the sigmoid sinus, or the foramen magnum.

Meningiomas occasionally arise intraventricularly and, in patients with neurofibromatosis, may be found in the petrous bone and in other unusual locations. They are typically benign, noninvasive, and cause symptoms by compression and distortion of adjacent structures. Seizures are a relatively frequent clinical complaint but are not present in all cases. The frequency with which meningiomas tend to recur appears to be a product of both their histology and the aggressiveness with which the tumor is removed. Excluding patients with hemangiopericytic and angioblastic meningiomas, approximately 15% of patients have recurrence despite what the surgeon deems as complete removal of the tumor. In these patients, the tumor usually recurs because it has invaded the sagittal sinus and has not been recognized, is not surgically treatable, encases the carotid arteries, or invades bone at the base. With the exception of angioblastic meningiomas, the biologic behaviors of these lesions do not correlate well with their histologic appearance. There are documented cases of all histologic types spreading to the subarachnoid pathways and metastasizing outside the intracranial space. A rare form of meningioma, the so-called sarcomatous variety, is clearly a primary malignant meningeal tumor but, fortunately, is rare. As we indicated previously, angioblastic meningiomas are characterized by more aggressive activity and a much higher incidence of recurrence. The origin of these tumors remains somewhat controversial. Rubenstein (11) believes that they arise from a hemangiopericytic type of cell and thus are distinct entities that behave differently from other meningiomas.

Diagnosis

The CAT scan has contributed significantly to the diagnosis of meningiomas, particularly those in unusual locations. Plain skull radiographs usually show positive evidence in approximately 50% of patients studied prospectively and in 70% of patients studied retrospectively. Abnormal findings include calcification, enlargement of the foramen spinosum, erosion of the sella, and erosion and new bone formation along the sphenoid wing. The evaluation of a patient with meningioma is never complete without angiographic evaluation. Angiography is required both to delineate the vascular supply of the tumor and, when the tumor is located in a particular site, such as parasagittally, to demonstrate whether the tumor's blood supply is from both external carotids and whether the sinus is patent. Moreover, when the neoplasms arise at the base of the skull, they can encase major cerebral vasculature. It is imperative that the surgeon recognize this before operative intervention.

Treatment

Complete surgical removal is the treatment of choice for meningiomas. With tumors that are histologically aggressive, such as angioblastic tumors, subtotal resection can be followed with radiation therapy. In some situations, such as en plaque tumors, particularly those that involve the sphenoid bone and thus threaten blindness, radiation therapy may be useful in delaying the tumor growth, although it is not curative (12).

Pituitary Adenoma

Exciting advances in endocrinology, immunocytochemistry, and electron microscopy (13,15) have allowed earlier and more accurate diagnosis and treatment of intrasellar and suprasellar pituitary neoplasms. These advances also have contributed to increased understanding of neuraxial hormonal function. Although the technique of transsphenoidal removal of tumors has been used for almost 70 years, greater recognition of functional pituitary microadenomas has come to the fore recently. Previous studies of the incidence of secreting tumors underestimated considerably the incidence of tumors that were hormonally active. This was a product of poor correlation between the histologic and tinctorial qualities of the adenomas and their endocrine function. New advances in endocrinologic evaluation, combined with tissue analysis using immunocytochemical techniques and electron microscopy, have expanded the diagnostic capabilities. The availability of such techniques has provided a reclassification of adenomas that, although not complete, is more accurate and is based on both functional and morphologic characteristics of the tumor.

It now appears that most of what previously were called chromophobe adenomas are in fact hormonally active tumors that secrete growth hormone or prolactin. Because diagnostic evaluation and treatment of microadenomas is a relatively new area, we will discuss the subject in some detail.

The initial evaluation of patients with a suspected pituitary adenoma should include a thorough endocrinologic evaluation. Although it usually is satisfactory to assay for the hormone in question, some assessment of normal pituitary function and pituitary reserve appears to be indicated in most instances. Table 2 gives a brief summary of the diagnostic tests available (15). Neuro-ophthalmologic evaluation (at least of visual field) is always essential before surgery in patients with pituitary tumor. Wilson and Dempsey (16) reported visual field disturbances in 25% of patients, most of whom had no history of visual symptoms. Five percent of patients demonstrated abnormalities of extraocular muscle function despite lack of such symptoms on initial examination. CAT scanning is the initial neurodiagnostic procedure of choice. The role of angiography in the diagnosis of endocrine-secreting tumors that are not large remains controversial. Many surgeons experienced in transsphenoidal removal no longer carry out routine angiography in such patients, while others continue to use angiography and fractional pneumonencephalography to delineate the exact location of the cavernous carotid arteries and of suprasellar extension. For patients with large lesions on CAT scan and extension of the tumor into the middle fossa, the transsphenoidal approach for removal of such tumors usually is unacceptable unless it is performed simply to decompress the optic nerves (which is often the sole indication) and to establish a tissue diagnosis so that radiation therapy can be instituted.

Most prolactin-secreting tumors are relatively small and can be completely

Table 2. Endocrinologic Evaluation of Patients with Suspected Functional Pituitary Tumor

	Hormone				
Test for Basal Levels	*Growth Hormone*	*Prolactin*	*ACTH*	*TSH*	*LH, FSH*
Stimulation tests	Arginine	Insulin-Induced Hypoglycemia	Lysine–Vasopressin	TRH	Clomiphene
	L-Dopa	TRH	Insulin-Induced Hypoglycemia	TSH	LRH
	Insulin-induced hypoglycemia				hCG
	LRH				
	TRH				
Withdrawal of Peripheral Stimulation			Metyrapone Agents	Antithyroid	Antiandrogens
Suppression	GTT	L-Dopa	Dexamethasone	T_3 Suppression	
	Bromocriptine	Bromocriptine			

TSH, thyroid-stimulating hormone; LH, luteinizing hormone; FSH, follicle-stimulating hormone; LRH, lutein-releasing hormone; TRH, thyrotropin-releasing hormone; hCG, human chorionic gonadotropin; GTT, glucose tolerance test; T_3, triiodothyronine.

removed by the transsphenoidal approach. In patients with large pituitary tumors, particularly those that extend behind the sella and into the middle fossa, transsphenoidal surgery may still be indicated if the goals are to decompress the optic nerve and establish a tissue diagnosis. It is almost impossible to completely remove a large pituitary tumor. It also is unwise, since a combination of radiation therapy with partial excision yields long-term cure or remission of the disease in approximately 92–95% of patients (17).

The judgment as to whether a tumor should be approached by the transsphenoidal route or by the previously standard, subfrontal craniotomy is a decision that should be made by the surgeon on the basis of clinical signs and symptoms and radiologic evaluation. Particularly bulky tumors that may have cystic components are probably best managed by the standard subfrontal approach. This appears almost always to be true when the tumor extends beyond the reaches of the midline approach through the sphenoid and the sella turcica.

It is critical to remember that the most common pituitary tumors are now recognized to be functional neoplasms that secrete prolactin, growth hormone, or, occasionally, adrenocorticotropin (ACTH). Because secretory granules can be identified with hormone-specific antibodies and verified by characteristic ultrastructural appearances, the standard histologic techniques are not reliable for establishing the presence or absence of such neoplasms. It is not infrequent for surgeons to be frustrated by a pathology report that reports no evidence of neoplasm when the patient's hormonal abnormality disappears immediately after surgery, with subsequent regression of clinical symptoms (15). With increasing recognition by neuropathologists and neurosurgeons of the difficulty in establishing what appears under the microscope to be a distinct neoplasm, more attention has been given to the use of hormone-specific antibody techniques and electron microscopy as aids in establishing the tissue diagnosis. Such techniques are not yet foolproof, and verification of the clinical suspicion depends both on transsphenoidal exploration and removal of the usually identifiable adenoma and on the subsequent course of the patient.

The presence of amenorrhea and galactorrhea should always suggest the possibility of a prolactin-secreting pituitary tumor. Serum levels of prolactin can be measured accurately in many hospital laboratories. Although in most instances a lateral skull radiograph will demonstrate an enlarged or eroded sella, sellar tomography occasionally fails to demonstrate an abnormality even in the presence of a prolactin level well above normal (greater than 200 μg; upper limit of normal, 35 μg). In most such patients, exploratory transsphenoidal surgery usually demonstrates a microadenoma. The recognition that these lesions may be extremely small and are not shown to be associated with bony abnormality even with sophisticated tomographic techniques has lead to increased emphasis on the endocrinologic evaluation of patients with the classic symptoms of a prolactin-secreting lesion. In patients without visual symptoms or in whom surgery is otherwise contraindicated, bromocriptine can suppress prolactin secretion and has been reported to reduce tumor size as seen on CAT scan and to ameliorate symptoms.

Controversy exists regarding whether women with prolactin-secreting tumors who are no longer interested in bearing children should undergo transsphenoidal removal of the tumor. If galactorrhea is sufficiently disturbing to the patient, the transsphenoidal approach usually is justified, since it carries an extremely low morbidity and mortality when performed by an experienced surgeon. The natural history of small prolactin-secreting tumors is not known, but preliminary evidence suggests that their progression may often be extremely slow or that the lesions may not increase sufficiently in size to be recognized on either visual field testing or tomography of the sella. In such instances, it should be recalled that prolactin-secreting tumors can be a safe means of birth control, since they almost always produce infertility in patients with amenorrhea. Therefore, careful observation in such patients is indicated.

The role of oral contraceptives in the subsequent development of these neoplasms is undetermined, although the increased frequency of the tumors in patients who previously took oral contraceptives appears to suggest some causal relation.

The treatment of acromegaly has been altered dramatically by the availability of the transsphenoidal approach for these tumors. Endocrinologic evaluation should include measurement of basal levels of growth hormone and assay of growth hormone after some type of infusion testing and stress testing (infusion testing with either arginine or L-dopa and stress testing with insulin). The diagnosis usually can be established on clinical grounds, but the hormone baseline determination is critical to determination of the efficacy of surgical therapy. Acromegaly should be considered a disease that shortens life significantly and must be treated aggressively. If surgical removal does not result in complete restoration of growth hormone activity to normal, radiation therapy should be given to a dose of 4,500 rad, because these tumors tend to recur and because the disease frequently has characteristics of malignancy.

Recently, Tyrell et al. (18) have demonstrated that Cushing's syndrome is almost always secondary to the presence of a microadenoma composed of basophilic cells that secrete ACTH. Recognition of the role of the pituitary gland in the etiology of Cushing's syndrome has come full circle in two decades. Adrenal hyperplasia now appears almost always to be secondary to pituitary microadenoma, and the presence of elevated serum levels of ACTH can be used to establish the diagnosis. Transsphenoidal surgery is often successful in completely ameliorating both the hormonal and subsequent systemic abnormalities of the disease and results in remission of clinical symptoms and signs.

Adenomas occasionally have mixed content, most commonly prolactin and growth hormone. Ezrin et al. (19) consider approximately 25% of chromophobe adenomas to be inactive or secreting some unidentified substance. Such tumors do not react with standard hormonal antibodies and have nondiagnostic characteristics of secretory cells on electron microscopy. In the clinical setting of hormonal dysfunction, these inactive tumors, especially large ones, may produce both hormonal changes secondary to mass effect and destruction of the normal gland. They also may be recognized as space-occupying tumors that are noted incidentally in patients without clinical signs or symptoms of hormonal dysfunction but who present with headache or visual disturbance.

In children and adolescents, evaluation of pituitary function usually is triggered by concern over delayed pubescence. However, Richmond and Wilson (20) found that more than 70% of their patients appeared initially with signs of pituitary hypersecretion and growth failure. Panhypopituitarism was very uncommon in their series, and headache and visual failure were not seen frequently. It also should be emphasized that pituitary tumors appear to be somewhat more aggressive in young patients. Forty percent of patients under the age of 20 have evidence of suprasellar and parasellar extension, and they also appear to have a high incidence of recurrence. Pituitary carcinoma is rare but usually has a relatively rapid and aggressive downhill course. In patients with such tumors, the initial symptoms are almost always attributable mass effect; pituitary hypersecretion is not characteristic.

Acoustic Neuromas

There has been intense interest on the part of both neuro-otologists and neurosurgeons in the early diagnosis and treatment of acoustic neuromas. This interest has been sparked in part by the availability of new surgical techniques for removal of relatively large tumors while sparing the facial nerve and avoiding injury to the brain stem. Improved surgical techniques in the cerebellopontine angle probably have contributed more to the treatment of intracranial neoplasms than in any other region except for the sella, where the transsphenoidal technique has revolutionized the treatment of pituitary tumors.

Acoustic neuromas comprise approximately 8% of all intracranial tumors and are more common in women. A relation with von Recklinghausen's disease is well recognized and is often associated with bilateral neoplasms in the cerebellopontine angle. The initial symptoms almost always include a history of deafness and may or may not include a history of headache coupled with gait disturbance. The clinical signs frequently found on evaluation include hearing loss, depressed corneal reflex, and, if the tumor is of considerable size, gait disturbance with cerebellar dysfunction on the ipsilateral side. Severe involvement of the facial nerve before surgical intervention is uncommon in the experience of most neurosurgeons, but mild evidence of facial nerve dysfunction is often evident on clinical examination. This is true despite the fact that the tumors can grow to a huge size, with tremendous distortion of the seventh and other cranial nerves and with medical displacement of the brain stem.

The diagnosis of acoustic neuromas, when they are of small size, depends on the history of hearing loss coupled with demonstration of trumpeting of the appropriate internal acoustic meatus on polytomography of the petrous bones. Angle myelography with positive contrast agents such as Pantopaque usually delineates even relatively small lesions. CAT scanning is useful in the initial delineation of the mass, but in the presence of relatively small lesions the tumor may be obscured by adjacent bone and thus may be difficult to recognize. Angiography remains of value in presurgical evaluation of large tumors and in identification of the occasional meningioma of the cerebellopontine angle that may originate from either the dura or the tentorium.

Sophisticated techniques of audiometric testing are available for detection of disease processes that involve the eighth cranial nerve and can be used in addition to neuroradiologic procedures for detection of eighth-nerve involvement. Bekesy audiometry characteristically gives a pattern type III or IV abnormality and thus can distinguish involvement of the eighth cranial nerve from cochlear and other hearing disturbances that are not produced by eighth-nerve dysfunction. Speech discrimination is usually grossly compromised in patients with acoustic neuroma, and they often demonstrate the phenomenon known as tone decay on testing. In contrast, cochlear lesions show recruitment rather than tone decay. In addition, auditory-evoked responses of the brain stem also can be used to delineate the location of disturbances in eighth-nerve function and may contribute to the diagnosis of these tumors. Thus, this battery of tests can be used reliably to distinguish acoustic tumors from cochlear disorders, and may be helpful in establishing the diagnosis particularly in patients with small acoustic tumors. Under most circumstances, the definitive diagnosis depends on the radiologic techniques described previously.

Acoustic neuromas present a unique surgical challenge. Failure to remove the tumor completely, particularly in young patients, usually leads to recurrence and eventual demise from brain-stem distortion. Severe obstructive hydrocephalus with subsequent decompensation also can cause severe disability or death. Complete removal, particularly of large tumors, often results in facial palsy, a cosmetically unacceptable deformity. In centers where these tumors are operated on frequently, the availability of enhanced lighting and intraoperative magnification with the operating microscope has allowed for better results in removal of large tumors, with approximately 60–75% of patients being spared the facial nerve. Protection of the facial nerve remains extremely difficult for many neurosurgeons because of the anterior and superior displacement of the nerve in the presence of a large tumor. Under such circumstances, it appears that a more flexible surgical approach, such as that advocated by House and colleagues (21,22) can be particularly useful, since it allows early identification of the facial nerve and eighth nerve in the petrous bone; the nerves then can be followed into the cerebellopontine angle, and, either with this approach alone or combined with a posterior fossa approach, the neoplasm can be removed as it abuts against the brain stem. A combined approach potentially offers the advantage of a higher incidence of preservation of the facial nerve, although experience appears to be too limited at present to be certain that this is true. DiTullio and colleagues (23) have recently made a comparison of the neurosurgical and otolaryngologic approaches to acoustic neuromas. In their experience, the posterior fossa or, more accurately, the transmeatal suboccipital craniectomy appeared to offer some advantage over the translabyrinthian, middle fossa, or transsigmoidal approaches that have been advocated by otolaryngologists. Logic dictates, however, that the ability to identify the nerve early and to combine this identification with a suboccipital craniectomy would be a more rational approach than the standard suboccipital approach advocated by DiTullio.

The availability of a variety of operative approaches to these neoplasms does not appear to reflect the inadequacy of one or the other; rather, it reflects the different pathophysiologic picture that these tumors present. Because neuromas are benign tumors, the desire of the surgeon to protect the patient from severe cosmetic deformity and at the same time achieve total removal are paramount. It is hard to argue that demarcation and dissection of the facial nerve through a combined approach is not advantageous in some circumstances. In tumors that are small and in patients who have lost their hearing, identification of the facial nerve as it leaves the brain stem is usually not difficult. Under such circumstances, either the posterior fossa approach or a translabyrinthian approach can result in complete removal of the tumor with sparing of the facial nerve.

An alternative treatment for acoustic neuromas is radiofrequency ablation of the tumor, a technique developed at the Karolinski Institute in Stockholm, Sweden. This technique has been used in more than 100 patients, and although there have been more recent reports of late damage to brain-stem structures with this procedure, its value on a long-term basis remains to be proven, and trials should continue.

RADIATION-INDUCED MALIGNANCIES

The postirradiation tumor most commonly reported in humans is parasellar sarcoma following irradiation for pituitary tumor (24). Most of these tumors are fibrosarcomas, with a small number being osteogenic in nature. The tumors tend to occur after long latent periods and with intervals after radiation therapy of from 2.5 to 25 years. They are seen with radiation doses well within the accepted therapeutic ranges and thus will continue to be seen as long as radiation therapy is required for the treatment of pituitary tumors. The symptoms usually are referable to a mass effect in the sellar region and are not a product of secondary metastasis. Surgical treatment appears to be the only mode of therapy, and resection usually is limited and extremely difficult because the radiation has produced scarring and has affected adjacent vascular structures.

The incidence of astrocytomas following radiation appears to be rare. The possibility that this tumor may occasionally be induced by radiation therapy, however, is suggested by several case reports. Meningiomas have been reported after irradiation of the scalp for fungal diseases and should be treated as if they had arisen de novo (23).

Radiation Necrosis

The advent of megavoltage radiation techniques for the treatment of intracranial neoplasms and for tumors of the head and neck has had some adverse consequences for both short- and long-term survivors. Radiation necrosis of the brain, although rarely seen with doses of less than 5,000 rad, becomes increasingly common as doses in the range of 6,000–7,000 rad are used for the treatment of intracranial and head and neck neoplasms. Symptoms may develop within a few months or may not occur for years after therapy, although an interval of between six months and four to five years is most common. The basic mechanism that underlies delayed necrosis in the CNS remains unclear, although damage to the vascular network of the brain appears to be the hypothesis most consistent with these changes.

The diagnosis may be difficult to establish, particularly in patients with a previous diagnosis of cancer of the head and neck, since an area of edema, with or without enhancement, seen on CAT scanning may be thought to represent metastasis and actually represents radiation-induced change. Steroid dependency in such patients has been observed and is not helpful in determining whether the lesion is radiation induced or represents a metastatic deposit. The diagnosis depends on a high index of suspicion in patients who have received high doses of radiation to the brain. The total dose and time course of administration and the number of fractions administered are all factors in determining the likelihood of the development of radiation necrosis; however, there appears to be somewhat marked individual variability in response to doses of radiation. When progression of symptoms occurs in a patient with suspected radiation necrosis and a mass effect from the lesion, surgical excision of the necrotic tissue may be useful in alleviating the clinical symptoms.

RARE NEOPLASMS

Choroid plexus papillomas account for less than 1% of all intracranial tumors. They predominate in males and tend to be located in the left lateral ventricle, fourth ventricle, and cerebellopontine angle. They occasionally may be associated with increased CSF production, although most cause hydrocephalus by obstruction rather than by CSF production. Occasionally the tumors are malignant and behave extremely aggressively, with metastasis throughout the subarachnoid space. Leptomeningeal spread is also seen in the benign version of this lesion, although it is less common. Diagnostic procedures include CAT scanning, angiography, and, occasionally, pneumoencephalography to delineate the neoplasm better. Treatment is surgical extirpation, which often is successful.

Colloid cysts occur in the third ventricle and are almost always located anteriorly. They are considered by some physicians to be a congenital malformation rather than a true neoplasm. They tend to occur in young adults, who have an initial symptom of headache secondary to intracranial hypertension. The classic symptoms of intermittent hydrocephalus resulting from sudden obstruction of the foramen of Monro by the mobile cyst, with changes in head position, is an extremely rare occurrence in most large series (26). The tumor can be recognized on CAT scanning, where it has a particular density, and the diagnosis can often be confirmed easily by ventriculography. Surgical removal via a transfrontal transventricular approach usually allows for complete removal.

TUMORS OF THE PINEAL REGION

Tumors of the pineal region include pineal germinomas, which comprise more than one-half of these tumors; teratomas; pineal parenchymal tumors; and astrocytomas. The initial clinical picture in patients with pineal lesions is usually nonspecific. Symptoms of obstructive hydrocephalus are common, and early puberty is seen only rarely. In one-third of patients, Parinaud's syndrome (paresis of upward gaze) is seen, which indicates compression of the tectum. The diagnosis depends on recognition on neuroradiologic testing. Plain films usually are of little value, although calcification greater than usually seen in the pineal region may be noted.

Until recently, the surgical removal of tumors of the pineal region carried a considerable mortality. Surgical techniques introduced recently by Stein and others, however, have demonstrated that surgical removal of teratomas in the pineal region can be complete and that biopsy of the tumor can be done with very low risk (27). Most large centers of pediatric neurosurgery that see patients with pineal tumors now operate on these patients, at least to establish a tissue diagnosis. The atypical teratoma, or pinealoma, usually cannot be excised completely and requires radiation treatment. More aggressive tumors found in this region include pineoblastomas and pineocytomas. Patients with these tumors require radiation therapy, and there are few long-term survivors. An occasional patient with teratocarcinoma may be seen; treatment includes both surgery and radiation therapy. In a few cases, recurrences of teratocarcinoma have been treated successfully with combination chemotherapy on the basis of experience with the treatment of testicular teratomatous tumors (28).

CRANIOPHARYNGIOMAS

Craniopharyngiomas comprise approximately 3% of all intracranial neoplasms, with more than half of these tumors appearing in children. The highest incidence appears to occur in the second decade of life, and the incidence decreases with increasing age (29). There appears to be a second peak in the fourth and fifth decades of life. Craniopharyngiomas occasionally appear as a mass in the newborn. Clinical symptoms usually include visual disturbance (70%), headache (50%), and symptoms of hypogonadism (28%), polyuria (20%), and disturbances of appetite (12%) (30). An occasional patient will have other, unusual endocrinologic disturbances. In large tumors, disturbances of consciousness may be the sole initial symptom. Approximately half of children affected are of short stature and often have gonadotropin deficiency.

The diagnostic evaluation of patients with suspected craniopharyngioma has altered dramatically with CAT scanning. Although plain skull radiographs show abnormalities in 90% of children and in 60% of adults, the appearance on CAT scan can often be diagnostic. One hundred percent of tumors in children, and approximately 60% in adults demonstrate calcification. Angiography is often indicated to delineate the relation of the tumor to the supraclinoid carotid arteries, and pneumoencephalography often is of value in delineating the extent of third-ventricular extension and hypothalamic involvement.

Treatment of craniopharyngiomas remains controversial, although neurosurgeons generally agree that aggressive surgical treatment yields maximal long-term survival (31). This approach is not possible in some patients with craniopharyngioma because the neoplasm is adhered to the hypothalamus or carotid arteries. In such patients, good long-term results have been reported with a combination of subtotal resection and radiation therapy (32). While it is apparent that total resection is desirable, radical resection (particularly in the hands of an inexperienced surgeon) risks hypothalamic and endocrinologic damage. On the other hand, however, the long-term risks of radiation therapy also must be considered. These include not only endocrinologic abnormalities and damage to the optic nerve, but also vascular catastrophe with subsequent long-term deterioration of neurologic status (31).

Part of the controversy around the treatment of craniopharyngiomas is the variability in natural history. Now that hormonal replacement therapy is available, studies on the biology of this neoplasm indicate that patients who survive without recurrence after treatment might do so regardless of the treatment method (i.e., whether surgery alone or surgery plus radiation therapy are given).

Lisczak et al. (33) conducted a detailed study of the histology of craniopharyngiomas, with both light microscopy and electron microscropy. While in most patients the appearance of cells on light microscopy was homogeneous, two distinct populations of tumor cells could be identified by ultrastructural characteristics and by growth patterns in tissue culture. These cells produced two types of tumors: typical and atypical. In all patients, tumors that exhibited atypical features had more aggressive clinical behavior. Further analysis along these lines in the near future may allow more definitive statements regarding the treatment of craniopharyngiomas.

The influence of age on survival also appears to be a critical factor. Patients younger than 25 years who have craniopharyngioma survive considerably longer than those older than 25 years, especially at six or more years after radiation therapy. This observation may reflect not only the particular histologic type and intrinsic activity of the tumor, but also the fact that treatment is better tolerated by younger patients.

It must be emphasized that both posttreatment endocrinologic evaluation and pre- and postoperative glucocorticoid replacement are critical, especially in children undergoing surgery for craniopharyngioma. Hypopituitarism is almost always present in children with craniopharyngioma and must not go unrecognized.

EPIDERMOID INCLUSION CYSTS

Epidermoid inclusion cysts may arise from the same embryologic remnants as craniopharyngiomas. However, the mature histologic appearance of the cysts is somewhat different and their natural history usually somewhat more benign. Though inclusion cysts may recur if not excised completely, they are almost never aggressive as compared with craniopharyngiomas. Treatment of these tumors is complete surgical extirpation, if possible. Cyst drainage followed by radiation therapy (which decreases the secretion of cholesterollike material) is useful when complete removal cannot be achieved.

METASTATIC DISEASE

Intracerebral Metastasis

Treatment of metastatic disease to the CNS remains primarily palliative. Because systemic chemotherapy, although often successful in other organ systems, fails to produce remission of intracranial metastases, it is necessary to discuss the treatment of intracranial metastases separately.

Increased interest in the treatment of intracranial metastasis seems appropriate, since approximately 45,000 patients dying of cancer in 1977 had premorbid symptoms and signs of this process. Of these patients, approximately 60% had evidence of multiple metastasis and 40% had evidence of solitary lesions (34). Autopsy studies demonstrate a slightly higher incidence of multiple lesions. This probably reflects either the presence of small metastases beyond the resolution of current scanning devices or the development of additional lesions in the times between scanning, treatment, and death.

Meningeal carcinomatosis appears to be occurring with increasing frequency, although intraparenchymal metastases continue to represent by far the most common type of intracranial secondary deposits. The increasing frequency of meningeal carcinomatosis is particularly apparent in patients with breast carcinoma and in those who have received prophylactic or craniospinal irradiation for treatment of small-cell carcinoma of the lung and reflects the longer survival times in patients with both breast and small-cell carcinoma of the lung.

The signs and symptoms of metastatic carcinoma to the brain differ little from those of other intracranial mass lesions, although the time from onset of symptoms to diagnosis is often relatively brief. Physicians should have a high index of suspicion in patients with a previously diagnosed primary tumor, particularly if there is evidence of local spread at the time of diagnosis of breast cancer, lung cancer, or melanoma. The characteristic neurologic signs and symptoms reflect the location of the metastatic deposit. In our experience, headache is present in about 60% of patients, and symptoms such as focal weakness or behavioral or mental changes occur in approximately half of patients (35). In an additional 20% of patients, clinical examination reveals signs not present initially. Focal or generalized seizures are seen in approximately 15% of patients, and should immediately suggest metastasis in patients with a history of carcinoma. Furthermore, the presence of cranial nerve palsy in a patient with a history of cancer should always suggest the possibility of spread to the leptomeninges, especially if the neurologic deficits are multifocal and are difficult to explain on the basis of one lesion.

Diagnosis

Radionucleotide scanning and angiography were previously the mainstays of evaluation of patients with metastatic carcinoma. However, CAT scanning which is more accurate and more cost-effective, has become the procedure of choice. While other diagnostic techniques, such as pneumoencephalography and electroencephalography, may occasionally be useful, they are now of limited value. Lumbar puncture in the diagnostic workup is rarely of value, except in patients with meningeal carcinomatosis, in whom it is absolutely essential. Multiple areas of edema on a noncontrast CAT scan that enhance after injection of contrast almost always represent metastatic disease in patients with a history of cancer. In patients without such a history, metastatic disease is still the most likely diagnosis, although the possibility of parasitic or other inflammatory processes of the brain, or of progressive multifocal leukoencephalopathy, are other considerations.

When the metastasis-free interval is long in patients with a history of cancer, and if CAT scanning demonstrates a solitary lesion, a more thorough diagnostic evaluation should be performed. A single, relatively vascular metastatic deposit may look identical to a primary glioblastoma or, occasionally, to a benign meningioma. In such circumstances, angiography often is helpful in delineating further the exact location and type of intracranial lesion. It is our view, however, that surgical excision of the lesion is usually indicated in such circumstances, if possible. Such patients should be treated surgically if there are no contraindications.

Treatment

A solitary mass with no other evidence of visceral involvement is usually an indication for surgical removal, if the tumor can be excised. Under certain circumstances, long-term survival and even cure may be obtained, although in general the rate of long-term salvage has been low (less than 10%). When visceral metastases are present, a decision must be made, on the best available evidence of whether craniotomy would prolong the patient's survival life significantly and also give a respectable quality of life. Retrospective studies of patients whose initial symptoms of cerebral lesion were primarily headache and minimal neurologic disturbances and who were treated surgically or with radiation therapy, had a median survival for either treatment modality of approximately six months (36). However, a recent study of Ransohoff (37) demonstrated considerable improvement in survival in patients with solitary metastases who received combined surgery and radiation therapy. Thus, at present we favor such an approach to patients who are free of visceral metastases, particularly if the free interval is long. In our experience, treatment with dexamethasone before surgery significantly reduced morbidity and mortality associated with surgical intervention.

When the lesion does not appear to be excisable and the tissue diagnosis is dubious, needle biopsy can be performed easily under local anesthesia, with or without the aid of CAT scanning for localization. When patients are prepared properly with corticosteroids before and for a few days after biopsy, the procedure carries almost no mortality and very low morbidity. If the diagnosis of carcinoma is well established and systemic metastases are present, biopsy does not appear to be indicated. However, if the attending physician has any doubt as to the histology of the mass, tissue diagnosis is mandatory.

In patients with a short, symptom-free interval between diagnosis of the primary malignancy and the appearance of neurologic symptoms, we prefer to maintain the patients on glucocorticoids for as long as possible in order to determine whether evidence of more widespread systemic disease will appear. Surgical extirpation of a single brain mass can be carried out at a later date if it is determined that removal will give longer survival and aid in palliation.

In the treatment of solitary metastases, there is little evidence at present to support the use of adjunctive chemotherapy. The sole exception is metastatic trophoblastic disease.

Multiple Metastasis

With the rare exception of the patient who requires biopsy to establish a diagnosis, the treatment of multiple metastasis to the brain remains nonsurgical. Satisfactory palliation can be best achieved with radiation therapy and the judicious use of glucocorticoids. The Radiation Therapy Oncology Group has demonstrated that 3,000 rad given over two weeks is equivalent to 4,000 rad given over three weeks in its yield of survival (38). The former schedule is superior to a short course of high-dose therapy, as other investigators have advocated already. The median survival in patients treated with radiation therapy for multiple brain metastases is not a product of the number of metastases, but rather is related directly to the presence or absence of neurologic deficits at the time radiation therapy is begun. The median survival time of patients with minimal symptoms or no symptoms other than headache is about six months, while that of patients with significant neurologic symptoms is quite short. The addition of varying doses of glucocorticoids to radiation therapy may improve both symptoms and survival. Data suggesting that corticosteroids do not prolong survival are based on studies that used very small doses and may not be accurate.

The palliation of multiple metastases with adjunctive chemotherapy remains an attractive idea, although the value of chemotherapy in prolonging survival of patients with multiple brain metastases has yet to be demonstrated unequivocally for most cancers. Pouillart et al. (39), using a combination of adriamycin, VM-26, and CCNU in repeated cycles produced objective improvement and regression of multiple metastasis in 75% of patients with metastatic breast carcinoma, with a median survival of more than nine months. Five patients showed complete resolution of abnormalities that had been present on brain scan, and two patients are long-term survivors (39).

In a small series of patients with small cell-carcinoma of the lung who did not respond to radiation therapy and treatment with glucocorticoids, we have demonstrated objective remission with a regimen of procarbazine, 150 mg/m^2, given in two-week cycles. The fact that this agent crosses the blood–brain barrier may at least partially explain its efficacy in this disorder. Recently, Bunn et al. (40) have advocated prophylactic craniospinal irradiation and intrathecal chemotherapy in patients with small-cell bronchogenic carcinoma because this disease tends toward CNS metastasis. In our view, placement of an Ommaya reservoir or other subgaleal device that allows introduction of medication into the ventricular system without repeated lumbar puncture is preferable to intrathecal induction of agents. The placement of a permanent cannula ensures delivery of drugs to the subarachnoid space and alleviates the difficulties related to repeated puncture in an area of previous irradiation.

Metastatic melanoma to the brain has occasionally been responsive to chemotherapy. Approximately 20% of patients treated with a combination of DTIC, 250 mg/m^2 for five days, and CCNU, 100 mg/m^2 given on the first day and repeated in six-week cycles, demonstrated objective remission. The median survival varied from seven to nine months. Response can usually be predicted after the first or second course, and therapy can be terminated if the patient continues to deteriorate.

Chemotherapy for treatment of multiple metastasis has just begun. Its present relative ineffectiveness in most CNS deposits may reflect either impenetrability of the blood–brain barrier or other factors, such as "immunologic privilege" of the brain. Survival rates for patients with carcinoma and leukemia are increasing, and it is likely that CNS metastasis will become an even greater problem in determining the outcome of these diseases. Effective modalities for prophylaxis and treatment of CNS metastasis are absolutely essential if improved long-term survival is to be possible for most patients.

Leptomeningeal Carcinomatosis

Metastatic spread to the leptomeninges has attracted increasing attention in neurologic oncology. Olsen et al. (41) have emphasized that this complication of cancer is not as rare as was thought previously and is probably increasing. In the past, leptomeningeal metastasis was evident only on postmortem examination because clinicians were not attuned to the symptoms and signs. Often the only initial symptom is headache and the sole indicative finding on radiologic investigation is an enlarged ventricular system. When this occurs in patients with a history of cancer, lumbar puncture may be particularly useful in delineating the presence of other abnormalities (described later) that characterize leptomeningeal spread. It is most common for focal neurologic signs that are not explicable on the basis of one lesion to be the initial symptoms in patients with leptomeningeal spread. These symptoms may be secondary either to direct destruction of tissue or to compression ischemia or occlusion of the cerebral vasculature. Incongruous involvement of cranial nerves and spinal nerve roots that is manifested in seizures should always suggest the possibility of leptomeningeal carcinomatosis, particularly in older patients and, of course, in patients with a previous diagnosis of cancer.

The diagnosis can almost always be established on repeated examinations of the CSF. Lumbar puncture should be repeated at least four times if there has been no yield of malignant cells and diagnostic suspicion is high. Examination of the CSF usually demonstrates mild leukocytosis, slightly to severely elevated levels of protein, and some depression of CSF glucose levels, although not as low as is seen with infectious processes. When CSF cultures persistently yield negative results in the face of low CSF levels of glucose, the possibility of leptomeningeal carcinomatosis is extremely high.

Treatment

It is important to recall that leptomeningeal metastasis is a diffuse disease of the entire craniospinal axis. Previous recommendations for the use of radiation therapy to areas only from which clinical signs and symptoms emanated have yielded remarkably dismal results. Complete craniospinal irradiation to a dose of 4,000 rad has improved the outlook somewhat, but it is logical that radiation be followed by administration of intraventricular medications such as methotrexate alone in doses of 10–15 mg/m^2 or in combination with cytosine arabinoside. These medications should be delivered via ventricular cannula connected to a subcutaneous reservoir. In patients with lymphoma and breast cancer, the response to intrathecal therapy has generally been quite good. In patients with small-cell carcinoma of the lung, treatment of the meningeal spread has been relatively unrewarding. It is probable that prophylactic therapy should be begun in randomized clinical trials. Such prophylaxis should include both radiation therapy and intraventricular chemotherapy.

TUMORS OF THE SPINAL CANAL AND SPINAL CORD

Tumors of the spinal cord are much less common than those of the brain. Most large neurosurgical clinics see 10 intracranial neoplasms for each primary spinal cord tumor. Metastatic tumors of the spinal canal are seen with greater frequency and are discussed separately.

Spinal cord tumors are classified according to their location. Approximately two-thirds are located in the extramedullary space; neurilemmomas occur slightly more frequently than meningiomas, and other, rarer neoplasms make up the remainder. Intramedullary tumors in adults generally are either ependymal in origin (60%) or develop from astrocytes. In the experience of most neuropathologists, it is common to see mixed cellularity in intramedullary tumors (the tumor is named by the predominant cell type).

Symptoms and Signs

Pain and local tenderness are frequent findings in patients with spinal cord tumors. Radicular pain frequently is the first symptom and is occasionally accompanied by diffuse pain, not only within the segments supplied by the root, but also by segments in adjacent dermatomes. Initial symptoms secondary to long-tract involvement are also frequent. Patients with neoplasms located below the conus do not show evidence of involvement of the corticospinal tract; rather, they appear with symptoms of sensory and motor loss of the peripheral type. It is most common to encounter a combination of findings that indicate involvement of the roots that are located at the site of the neoplasm and to see long-tract signs in cervicothoracic tumors of the spinal cord. Intradural extramedullary tumors, such as meningioma and neurilemmoma, may occasionally demonstrate the classic findings described by Browne-Sequard. The finding of ipsilateral motor weakness with contralateral sensory loss should always suggest the possibility of spinal cord tumor, and the appropriate diagnostic studies should be performed.

One diagnostic pitfall in the recognition of spinal cord tumors is confusion of ataxic gait secondary to proprioceptic loss, resulting from involvement of the posterior columns, with cerebellar ataxia. Careful attention to the sensory examination is critical in the evaluation of patients who have what appear to be symptoms of spinal cord tumor. Although some cases of spinal cord tumor may have been diagnosed earlier as multiple sclerosis, in patients without multisystem involvement, the possibility of a spinal cord tumor must always be considered. Cervical spondylosis, particularly in older patients, is usually recognized on the basis of its typical radiographic findings and the patient's clinical history; however, an occasional spinal cord tumor, particularly of the extramedullary type, may produce symptoms identical to those of cervical spondylosis. Here, again, the diagnosis depends on appropriate radiologic investigation.

Laboratory Evaluation

The specific localization and recognition of a spinal cord tumor rests on accurate myelographic assessment. In patients with acute deterioration, we prefer to perform myelography via lateral cervical puncture at C1-2 or by cisternal puncture. In patients with a longer history of tumor, myelography from below appears to be satisfactory. Myelography may be performed either with Pantopaque, with air, or, more recently, with metrizamide. Air myelography requires the availability of polytomographic equipment but has the advantage of specifically delineating lesions in the thoracic region, a task that has been more difficult with opaque contrast agents. While myelography usually can demonstrate whether the tumor is intradural or extradural, results occasionally can be confusing. This is because when the spinal cord is flattened by an extradural mass causing dorsal or ventral compression, or when there is a large intradural mass that prevents free flow of contrast material, it may be difficult to delineate or distinguish extradural tumors from intradural tumors, particularly if only one view is seen. Usually, however, this does not present specific problems. The body scanner can be useful for identification of tumors associated with syrinx formation, but at the moment myelography appears to be more accurate and more cost-effective.

Once the diagnosis of a spinal cord tumor is made, the treatment almost always is surgical. Most meningiomas can be removed completely, particularly now that magnification and lighting are available to almost all neurosurgeons. Neurilemmomas may present more difficulty because they can be plexiform and involve a critical root in the cervical region. Under such circumstances, the surgeon must judge whether the mass effect from the lesion is sufficient to justify sacrifice of a root. Furthermore, lateral extension of neurilemmomas outside the foramina into either the thorax or the abdomen is not uncommon and usually necessitates another operation for complete removal of the lesion.

Treatment of intramedullary tumors of the spinal cord is somewhat different. Patients who have ependymomas, particularly of the myxopapillary type, often can have complete cure of their disease by surgical extirpation. However, astrocytomas of the cord or tumors of mixed cellularity—namely, ependymoma plus astrocytoma—can be impossible to remove even with microsurgical techniques, and surgery may yield only a tissue diagnosis. However, if a syrinx is suspected on the basis of myelography or CAT scanning of the spine, surgical decompression of only the cyst may be worthwhile in relieving the patient's symptoms.

Radiation Therapy

Many neurosurgeons use radiation therapy to treat intramedullary tumors of neuroectodermal origin (astrocytomas, ependymomas), particularly when the histologic grade of the spinal cord neoplasm suggests rapid growth. The presence of mitotic figures, necrosis, and other indicators of malignancy have been used as justification for radiation therapy and appear to be logical criteria. However, data are extremely limited to support the applicability and value of radiation therapy in the treatment of grade I astrocytomas of the cord that cannot be removed surgically. Because it is difficult for any neurosurgeon or group of neurosurgeons working in one institution to encounter enough benign astrocytomas in a short time, the use of radiation therapy for low-grade tumors remains strictly empirical. It is our experience that patients improve, both subjectively and objectively, after receiving radiation therapy. Whether the actual long-term process is altered is not yet clear.

Spinal Metastasis

Approximately 5% of patients with the diagnosis of carcinoma develop spinal metastases. In patients with prostatic carcinoma and other cancers that have a predilection for epidural and vertebral metastasis, the incidence of this complication appears to be increasing. This is thought to be the result of increased length of survival in these patients. It is also becoming increasingly clear that, in patients with lymphoma, alterations in the pattern of metastasis are related to the portals used for radiation therapy. Centers that see a large number of patients with Hodgkin's disease are reporting an increased incidence of cervical and lumbar epidural Hodgkin's disease, whereas, before institution of the inverted-Y port, thoracic epidural metastases were much more common.

Diagnosis

The most frequent initial symptom of metastatic disease of the spine is back pain. Approximately 30% of patients have radicular symptoms in addition to localized pain. Since approximately 65% of metastases are located in the thoracic region, there is often little weakness if the root is the only neural element involved. The predominance of metastases in the thoracic region is simply a product of the length of the canal and is not indicative of a predilection for the thoracic region. In reviewing our experience and that of others, however, it is clear that rapid deterioration in neurologic function is associated most often with metastases that occur in the regions from T-4 to T-10, an area of the spinal cord that often depends on one major feeding vessel, the artery of Adamkiewicz, for its blood supply.

In patients with a previous diagnosis of carcinoma or lymphoma, a high index of suspicion is required in order to prevent neurologic deterioration if and when spinal metastases develop. Studies of several large groups of patients have shown that response to treatment is directly proportional to the degree of neurologic deficit that is present at the time treatment is instituted. Thus, early diagnosis is mandatory if paraplegia is to be avoided in patients who already have devastating diseases.

Plain films often demonstrate abnormalities in patients with neurologic deficit and even in patients who simply have low-back pain. In the absence of changes on plain films in patients older than 50 years, even in patients with no previous diagnosis of cancer but with localized radicular pain, the diagnosis of metastatic carcinoma must be considered. Confirmation of the diagnosis rests either on bone scan if only pain is present, or on myelographic evidence to demonstrate the presence of an epidural mass.

Treatment

The goals of treatment of spinal cord metastasis are prevention of neurologic deterioration and reversal of deficits already present. As we noted previously, a critical determinant in the prediction of response to therapy is the neurologic status of the patient at the time of initial examination. It also appears, on the basis of some series, that the histologic type of tumor is a critical determinant (42).

Our scheme of treatment at present for patients with a previous diagnosis of carcinoma and with signs and symptoms of spinal cord involvement is a variation of the traditional approach of myelography followed by immediate surgical decompression. We begin by administering dexamethasone, 40 mg intravenously, and then 10 mg every six hours as maintenance therapy. We then perform myelography via C-2 puncture for localization of the lesion. Lumbar myelography is also satisfactory but may carry the increased hazard of adverse effects on CSF dynamics in a patient with evidence of cord dysfunction. Once the lesion is localized, immediate radiation therapy is instituted and chemotherapy is given if and when appropriate. Radiation therapy and chemotherapy are always guided by the tissue type of the tumor. Decompressive laminectomy is performed only in patients whose symptoms have progressed despite the treatment described above. The exception to this is patients with a previous diagnosis of adenocarcinoma or squamous cell lung carcinoma, in whom we have found this conservative medical approach to be uniformly dismal. Surgical intervention is indicated absolutely in patients who have evidence of cord compression and myelographic evidence of an extradural block but who do not have a history of carcinoma. If possible, a tissue diagnosis should be obtained at the time of decompressive laminectomy. Tumor type can guide therapy rationally. Lumbar and thoracic bony stenosis may have identical clinical pictures. Blind radiation in patients with either condition may be disastrous and should be avoided. The presence of physiologic transection of the spinal cord, of extensive visceral metastasis, or of a platelet count of less than 50,000 per mm^3 are contraindications to surgical decompression.

Patient response to chemotherapy has been varied somewhat in the treatment of spinal metastasis. Prostatic carcinoma, myeloma, and small-cell carcinoma of the lung often respond to drug therapy, while more common lung neoplasms and sarcomas have been resistant. Our experience with chemotherapy in approximately 50 patients, has resulted in a long-term ambulatory rate of more than 50%, which we believe is comparable to the best results achieved by immediate surgery. It also offers the advantage of avoiding major surgical procedures in patients who often are debilitated and in whom the incidence of surgical complications is higher than in those who undergo laminectomy for other reasons.

Recurrence of Symptoms after Therapy

It is not uncommon for symptoms to recur in patients who have undergone therapy for metastatic carcinoma to the epidural space. Therapies that can be used in such instances include further radiation therapy and, in rare instances, another surgical decompression. We have performed such a procedure in three cases, and in each case the patient regained ambulation. Patients who, for various reasons, cannot tolerate further radiation or an operation may be maintained on high dosages of dexamethasone for long periods, often with gratifying results. However, this therapy usually fails after some weeks or months, and the patient eventually becomes completely paraplegic or quadriplegic.

REFERENCES

1. Walker MD, Strike TA: An evaluation of methyl CCNU, BCNU and radiotherapy in the treatment of malignant glioma. Proc Am Assoc Cancer Res 17:163, 1976.
2. Renaudin J, Fever D, Wilson CB, et al: Dose dependency of decadron in patients with partially excised brain tumors. J Neurosurg 39:302–305, 1973.

3. Marshall LF, Langfitt TW: Needle biopsy, high-dose corticosteroids, and radiotherapy in the treatment of malignant glial tumors. In: *Modern Concepts in Brain Tumor Therapy: Laboratory and Clinical Investigation.* Edited by JC Bailar. National Cancer Institute, Monograph no. 46, 1977, pp. 157–160.
4. Leibel SA, Sheline GE, Wara WM, et al: The role of radiation therapy in the treatment of astrocytomas. Cancer 35:1551–1557, 1975.
5. Bouchard J: Central nervous system tumors. In: *Textbook of Radiotherapy*, 2nd ed. Edited by G Fletcher. Philadelphia, Lea and Febiger, 1973, pp. 366–418.
6. Gjerris F, Klinken L: Long term prognosis in children with benign cerebellar astrocytoma. J Neurosurg 49:179–184, 1978.
7. Mork SJ, Loken AC: Ependymoma: a follow up study of 101 cases. Cancer 40:907–915, 1977.
8. Raimondi AJ, Tomita T: Medulloblastoma in childhood: comparative results of partial and total resection. Child's Brain 5:310–328, 1979.
9. Quest DO, Brismo R, Artunes JC, et al: Medulloblastoma: factors influencing survival and cure. In: *Proceedings of the Trans. Amer. Assoc. Neurosurg. Meeting,* Toronto, April 1977.
10. Tokars RP, Sutton HG, Grein ML: Cerebellar medulloblastoma. Results of a new method of radiation treatment. Cancer 43:129–136, 1979.
11. Rubenstein LJ: *Tumors of the Central Nervous System. Atlas of Tumor Pathology.* Second series, fascicle 6. Washington, DC, Armed Forces Institute of Pathology, 1972, pp. 235–240.
12. Leibel SA, Wara WM, Sheline GE, et al: The treatment of meningiomas in childhood. Cancer 37:2709–2712, 1976.
13. Paiz C, Hennigan GR: Electron microscopy and histochemical correlation of human anterior pituitary cells. Am J Pathol 59:43–74, 1970.
14. Landolt AM: Ultrastructure of human sella tumors. Acta Neurochir (Wien) (Suppl 22):1–167, 1975.
15. Fahlbusch R, Marguth F: Developments in surgical treament of pituitary adenoma. Neurosurg Rev 1:2, 5–13, 1978.
16. Wilson CB, Dempsey LC: Transsphenoidal microsurgical removal of 250 pituitary adenomas. J Neurosurg 48:13–22, 1978.
17. Kramer S: Indications for, and results of, treatment of pituitary tumors by external radiation. In: *Diagnosis and Treatment of Pituitary Tumors.* Edited by PO Kohler and GT Ross. Amsterdam, Excerpta Medica, International Congress Series no. 303, 1973, pp. 217–229.
18. Tyrell JB, Brooks RM, Fitzgerald PA, et al: Cushing's disease: selective trans-sphenoidal resection of pituitary microadenomas. N Engl J Med 298:753–757, 1978.
19. Ezrin C, Horvath E, Kovacs K: The pituitary gland. In: *Endocrine Pathology Course Syllabus* for the 1977 Endocrine Pathology Course. Harvard Medical School, Boston, March 29, 1977.
20. Richmond IL, Wilson CB: Pituitary adenomas in childhood and adolescence. J Neurosurg 49:163–168, 1978.
21. House WF (editor): Transtemporal bone microsurgical removal of acoustic neuroma (monograph I). Arch Otolaryngol 80:597–756, 1964.
22. House, WF (editor): Acoustic neuroma (monograph II). Arch Otolaryngol 88:576–715, 1968.
23. DiTullio MV, Malkasian D, Rand RW: A critical comparison of neurosurgical and otolaryngological approaches to acoustic neuromas. J Neurosurg 48:1–12, 1978.
24. Powell HC, Marshall LF, Ignelzi RJ: Post-irradiation pituitary sarcoma. Acta Neuropathol 39:165–167, 1977.
25. Beller AJ, Feinsol M, Sohar A: The possible relationship between small dose irradiation to the scalp and intracranial meningiomas. Acta Neurochir (Wien) 4:135–139, 1972.
26. Little JR, MacCarty CS: Colloid cysts of the third ventricle. J Neurosurg 40:230–235, 1974.
27. Stein BM: The infratentorial supracerebellar approach to pineal lesions. J Neurosurg 35:197–202, 1971.
28. Marshall LF, Rorke LB, Schut L: Teratocarcinoma of the brain: a treatable disease. Child's Brain 5:96–102, 1979.

29. Banna M: Craniopharyngioma. Br J Radiol 49:206–233, 1976.

30. McMurry FG, Handy RW, Dohn DF, et al: Long term results in the management of craniopharyngioma. Neurosurgery 30:238–241, 1977.

31. Hoffman HJ, Hendrick EG, Humphreys RP: Management of craniopharyngioma in children. J Neurosurg 47:218–227, 1977.

32. Shanna U, Torlen PU, Saxemo KK, et al: Craniopharyngiomas treated by a combination of surgery and radiotherapy. Clin Radiol 25:13–21, 1974.

33. Lisczak T, Richards EP, Philips JP, et al: Morphological, biochemical, ultrastructural tissue culture and clinical observations of typical and aggressive craniopharyngiomas. Acta Neuropathol 43:191–203, 1978.

34. Chason JL, Walker FB, Landers JW: Metastatic carcinoma in the central nervous system and dorsal root ganglion: a prospective autopsy study. Cancer 16:781–784, 1963.

35. Marshall LF: The treatment of metastatic disease to the central nervous system and spine. In: *Surgical Oncology*. Edited by YH Pilch and TK DasGupta. New York, McGraw-Hill (in press).

36. Markesbury WR, Brooks WH, Gupta GD, et al: Treatment for patients with cerebral metastases. Arch Neurol 35:754–756, 1978.

37. Ransohoff J: Surgical management of metastatic tumors. Semin Oncol 4:81, 1977.

38. Krawer S, Hendrickson F, Zelam M, et al: Therapeutic trials in the management of metastatic brain tumors by different time/dose fraction schemes of radiation therapy. In: *Modern Concepts in Brain Tumor Therapy: Laboratory and Clinical Investigations*. Edited by JC Bailar. National Cancer Institute, Monograph no. 46, 1977.

39. Pouillart P, Mathe G, Tly TH, et al: Treatment of malignant gliomas and brain metastases in adults with a combination of adriamycin, VM 26 and CCNU. Cancer 38:1909, 1976.

40. Bunn PA, Nugent JL, Matthews MJ: Central nervous system metastasis in small cell bronchogenic carcinoma. Semin Oncology 5:31–41, 1978.

41. Olsen ME, Chernik NL, Posner JB: Infiltration of the leptomeninges by systemic cases: a clinical and pathological study. Arch Neurol 30:122, 1974.

42. Marshall LF, Langfitt TW: Combined therapy for metastatic extradural tumors of the spine. Cancer 40:2067–2070, 1977.

8
Degenerative and Hereditary Disorders

George W. Paulson

Degenerative and hereditary disorders, cannot be covered exhaustively in any one chapter or in any one monograph. Even if discussion is limited to therapy, which so often is unsatisfactory, many areas may be slighted. Numerous related topics, some of which also could be considered degenerative or hereditary, are discussed elsewhere in this text. For example, toxic and metabolic disorders, neuropathies, dementias, myopathies, seizure disorders, and even some varieties of headache have genetic significance. Unfortunately, there is no cure for most of these at present or, indeed, for most hereditary and degenerative disorders. Furthermore, even when a cure does become available, the designation of the disease may change. For example, a degenerative disorder may be considered a biochemical lesion, to be treated by internists. Recognition of the disease is important in determining the prognosis, however, and for some patients correct diagnosis implies a promise of definitive cure, now or in the future. Peripheral nerve disorders, some metabolic disorders, and similar genetic conditions will be reviewed briefly here. Pathologic features will not be emphasized in this chapter; rather, major clinical entities and treatments will be the primary focus. The outlines in Goodman's volume (1) serve as a schema for this chapter, with additional reliance on McKusick's compendium (2). References are available in these sources and in standard pediatric (3), neurology (4,5), and endocrinologic texts (6).

Genetic counseling is never easy, but some aspects are both challenging and unavoidable for any concerned clinician. The practitioner who confidently expects to obtain family data regarding hypertension, emphysema, diabetes, or alcoholism and who then uses these data to advise the patient may be appalled by a frank discussion of recessive or dominant disorders. Nevertheless, the same rules of concern for patient care apply to untreatable as well as treatable diseases. First, the diagnosis should be secure. Then the physician should consult current literature as needed, seek specialized assistance when necessary, and, finally, confer with the family and patient with compassion and skill. Expert advice is, in fact, as close as the telephone, and most major centers have special competence in genetic counseling.

Ideally, diagnosis must first be clear, even if the exact pattern of inheritance remains uncertain. In recessive disorders (e.g., Wilson's disease) siblings are at risk, whereas in dominant disorders a more vertical transmission is expected. For example, in Huntington's disease the child of an affected parent has a 50% chance of carrying the gene. The practitioner must remember, however, all members of the family, whether affected or unaffected by the disease, will worry, since they all are threatened. Variation in penetrance of many genetic disorders may lessen the severity of manifestation of the disorder from patient to patient. It is always tempting for the physician to suggest eventual or potential cure, but such prospects usually fail to materialize and may offer only false hope. Treatable disorders should always be sought first, especially when the diagnosis is uncertain.

Once the patient or family is informed of the diagnosis, they may deny it, and several conferences or the opinion of another practitioner may be required. More troublesome than denial can be the response that follows denial, that is, irritation or anger directed at family members or even at the physician. As the affected person and their family eventually accept or comprehend the situation, they move toward a rational approach to coping with the problem. During this phase, the physician may offer symptomatic relief, comfort, and moral support as well as useful general counsel. Therefore, a simple statement of diagnosis or "You have such-and-such a disease, just go home and live with it" is not only cruel (unless followed by support) but simplistic. Failure to follow the diagnosis with other assistance leads to a loss of learning for both the patient and the physician.

Details of counseling vary depending on the disorder, the intelligence and persistence of the family, and the skills of the clinician. The concept of dominant disorders should be made clear, although some families, such as those with a history of Huntington's disease, note that onset of the disorder occurs at a late age, whereas other families manifest the juvenile form of the disease. If both parents have a recessive disorder attributable to one gene locus, as in phenylketonuria or Wilson's disease, then the offspring also may have the disorder. Since such conditions are severe and rare, persons who carry the gene are not at very great risk for potentially hazardous mating. Some recessive disorders, such as albinism or varieties of deafness, may result from several genetic variants; in such cases, children of parents with two phenotypically similar conditions may not manifest the disorder. Furthermore, penetrance of the gene may modify the overt manifestations of the disorder.

Finally, counseling of family members who do not have the disease must be considered, since a major central nervous system (CNS) disorder affects everyone in the environment, often in ways more subtle than direct manifestation. The clinician who must use social services, geneticists, neurologists, and biochemists need not assume that any of these experts is superior in the overall approach to helping the family or to softening the general effects of the disease.

DISORDERS OF THE PERIPHERAL NERVES

Charcot-Marie-Tooth Disease

Peroneal muscular atrophy or Charcot-Marie-Tooth disease (CMT) has several subvarieties, as defined recently by Dyck (7), and typical cases have been found that manifest either recessive X-linked or a dominant X-linked inheritance. An autosomal recessive form also has been reported, and it can be presumed that several genetic disturbances in CMT exhibit similar phenotypic patterns of neurologic disability. Sensory and autonomic deficits have been noted in CMT disease, but the classic presentation is progressive atrophy and muscle loss. Symptoms usually appear first in the legs and later in the distal muscles of the hands. At present there is no specific therapy for any of the subtypes of CMT. In some patients, particularly those with an uncertain family history, it may be necessary to rule out spinal cord dysfunction, and a myelogram occasionally is indicated. Genetic counseling can be strengthened by use of the electromyogram (EMG) with nerve conduction, since such electrical testing may elicit evidence of a subclinical form of the disorder in family members who are still superficially unaffected.

The volume edited by Dyck et al. (8) reclassifies the hereditary motor and sensory neuropathies (HMSN) and labels classic CMT under HMSN type I (most often a dominant inherited hypertrophic neuropathy). The authors emphasize that many patients have no feeling of illness, even if they manifest classic signs of pes cavus, hammertoe, and weakness. Counseling must include both accurate assessment of the family pattern of inheritance and, if HMSN type I is recognized early in the patient's life, the useful advice regarding vocational planning. Proper supportive shoes are desirable, although braces are rarely useful in the early stages of the disorder. As disability progresses, ambulation often can be maintained by ankle supports, and some young patients with HMSN type I benefit from a triple arthrodesis, with fusion of the bones of the foot to stabilize the function of the foot and the ankle. In later stages, light braces may be required. Protection of the skin is not as important in HMSN type I as in the more profound sensory neuropathies: nor is it needed as frequently as in tabetic neuropathy. Many patients with CMT can expect to have a normal life span with modest limitation of cherished activities, and the clinician should offer an optimistic and supportive approach.

Hypertrophic Neuropathy

Dejerine and Sottas (9) have described, with repeated confirmation since, a peripheral neuropathy with palpable enlargement of the nerves. This entity has been classified as a subvariety of CMT, or HMSN type III. Hypertrophic neuropathy is inherited as a recessive disorder, and although it is a valid entity, similar thickening of the nerves can be seen in other disorders. There is no evidence at present that specific treatment is helpful for hypertrophic neuropathy, but corticosteroids have been reported to produce remission in other relapsing forms of peripheral neuropathy and have been tried in this condition as well. In hypertrophic neuropathy, as well as in most other forms of peripheral neuropathy, there is heightened vulnerability to entrapment of nerves that are at risk by virtue of location or function, such as in carpal tunnel syndrome or peroneal palsy, both of which are common forms of entrapment neuropathy. There is no evidence that systemic administration of thiamine or steroids is of help in entrapment neuropathy; nor are local injections of steroids of great benefit. In some cases, surgical decompression of the nerves may be required.

Counseling, protection of the feet, and avoidance of pressure on vulnerable peripheral nerves give benefiit to individual patients.

Hereditary Compression Syndrome

A hereditary compression syndrome has been reported in individual families (10) that manifest a tendency toward peripheral nerve palsy, particularly in the peroneal region; (e.g., bulb digger's paralysis). Inheritance may be autosomal dominant, and the major feature is heightened vulnerability to compression. Patients usually do not have other symptoms of either a classic CMT syndrome or hypertrophic neuropathy. Prevention of trauma and protection with padding are the only therapies available. There are also heredofamilial neuritides that have a brachial predilection. Some of these appear as a sporadic brachial neuritis, characterized by severe pain, weakness, and atrophy. Groups of shoulder muscles, such as the deltoid and supraspinatus muscles, are particularly vulnerable, and sensory loss is often mild. The cause of sporadic brachial neuritis is unclear, and the patient may relapse after apparent recovery. Some patients have unusual facial structure, sometimes with closely set eyes and syndactyly (11). It is possible that steroids would be helpful for some of these patients, particularly for the painful aspects of the brachial plexitis. These cases are a reminder that hereditary disorders that appear to be neuropathic are not always limited to the distal nerve endings, although in almost all other neuropathies appendicular portions such as fingers and toes are affected most severely.

Sensory Radiculopathy

In addition to predominantly motor neuropathy, sensory radiculopathy (12) may also appear. Defects of other portions of the nervous system (e.g., defective hearing) occasionally can be linked with these disorders. Some predominantly sensory disorders have an autosomal dominant inheritance and may be characterized by severe trophic ulcerations on the plantar surfaces. The ulcers tend to recur and seem to result from loss of sensation, which allows excessive and prolonged pressure. Ulcers related to such unrecognized pressure heal completely if the pressure is removed; therefore, it seems unlikely that the ulcers are caused by lack of nutritional support from the nerves. As with patients who suffer from neuropathy secondary to leprosy, a pressure boot or similar protective device that distributes weight evenly can be of benefit. There is no evidence at present that specific medications are needed or useful, although thiamine or multivitamins and an overall improvement in general nutrition can be justified.

Refsum's Disease

Refsum's disease (13,14) is less common than the subvarieties of CMT but is important because there is hope for a specific therapeutic measure. The major clinical characteristics of Refsum's disease include polyneuritis, night blindness resulting from retinitis pigmentosa, ataxia, deafness, and skin and cardiac changes. Refsum's disease is an autosomal recessive trait and is characterized by an abnormally high serum concentration of fatty acids and impairment in the oxidation of phytanic acid (15), which apparently accumulates in the tissues. The condition tends to be slowly progressive and may be ameliorated by a special diet that voids phytanic acid. The exact relation between phytanic acid and the neuropathy remains uncertain, but efforts to adhere to diet are justified. Fruit, vegetables, and butter are among foods to be avoided.

Refsum's disease is an example of a neuropathy that requires special management, such as referral to one of the few major centers that specialize in treatment of familial neuropathies. The diet, experimental therapy, and adequate counseling are beyond the capabilities of many centers. Refsum's disease demonstrates the value of the discovery of a metabolic cause, since precise identification of etiology may add opportunities for therapy to diagnostic achievements.

Progressive Sensory Neuropathy

Progressive sensory neuropathy (16,17) is usually inherited as a recessive trait, although it may have more than one pattern. From the second through the fourth decades of life, patients with sensory neuropathy experience difficulty with sensation, and patients in some family groups have spastic paraparesis in addition to profound neuropathy. At present there is no definitive therapy for this disorder. Progressive sensory neuropathy should not be confused with congenital insensitivity to pain (18), a heterogenous disorder that does not represent simply indifference to pain. Rather, there may be absence of Lissauer's tract (19) or abnormalities in the sensory end organs of the skin. Patients with congenital insensitivity to pain tend to suffer repeated damage (20) and, as with the Riley–Day syndrome (congenital dysautonomia), deserve particular instruction in self-protection. Joints can be damaged in falls, and patients often fail to give adequate attention to minor ulcerations of the skin. Education of patients with insensitivity to pain or with sensory neuropathy can forestall extreme mutilation and eventual resultant amputation. Conventional diabetes clinics may offer the best resource for such instruction.

Hereditary Amyloid Neuropathy

There are several conditions in which hereditary amyloid neuropathy (21) is found, including the subvarieties discussed by Coutinko and Andrade (22) and others. Some of these conditions have been found in people of Portuguese extraction and derive from complex genetic isolates in limited geographic areas such as the Azores. Other genetic disorders of the CNS have been reported in this population (22). Amyloid deposits in and around the peripheral nerve are not affected by medication; nor is there evidence that special attention to reduction in serum levels of lipoproteins is effective in management. However, patients with congenital amyloidosis may develop carpal tunnel syndrome or other signs of nerve entrapment, and the combination of pressure and underlying neuropathy often respond dramatically to compressive surgery.

Tangiers Disease

Tangiers disease (23), which consists of a deficiency in alpha-lipoprotein, may appear in childhood, with repeated attacks of asymmetric neuropathy, elevated levels of protein in cerebro in spinal fluid, dysesthesias or paresthesias, and distal weakness. There is no known therapy for Tangiers disease. The biochemical defects in Tangiers disease were initially discovered because enlarged yellow-orange tonsils removed in childhood were found to be laden with histiocytes and cholesterol esters. Associated corneal and arterial infiltration may occur, and corneal infiltrates may require surgical therapy. Awareness of these fat-containing histiocytes, combined with reported low levels of plasma cholesterol and low levels of high-density lipoprotein, offer the tantalizing hope of a dietary regimen for patients with this disorder in the future; at present, however, there is no specific diet that is known to be helpful.

Porphyria

It should not be necessary to confuse either amyloid neuropathy or Tangiers disease with porphyria (24). The neuropathies seen in porphyria tend to be largely motor and can be quite severe. Diagnosis is often suspected on the basis of abdominal pain, although the pain may appear first in the back. The literature has emphasized the psychologic features of the disease, and the diagnosis may be confused or delayed because of the psychic aspects. Several types of porphyria are listed in extensive medical reviews, but in many cases that are associated with neurologic complications, the complications are induced by drug therapy; thus, specific diagnosis can be very useful. Diagnosis of porphyria by the Watson–Schwartz test is well known, and this and other special tests for porphobilinogen are now available routinely in hospital laboratories. "Spontaneous" attacks of porphyria may be triggered by ingestion of barbiturates, sulfonamides, or alcohol. These agents may act by stimulating synthesis of delta-aminolevulinic acid synthetase or by altering portions of the Krebs cycle. A few patients with porphyria develop a syndrome of inappropriate secretion of antidiuretic hormone (SIADH), which requires careful water restriction. In general, however, therapy for porphyria is only supportive. Use of chelating agents has been suggested but the value of these drugs has not been proved. Diazepam (Valium), 5 mg t.i.d., may be useful in acute attacks, and phenothiazines (Thorazine), 50 mg t.i.d., may be required to manage the agitation. Propranolol (Inderal), 40 mg b.i.d., can be recommended if hypertension or tachycardia is a major feature. There is no therapy for the neuropathic aspect of the disease, but patients with episodes of respiratory failure, SIADH, or psychosis will improve with appropriate standard therapy. Administration of glucose may have a beneficial effect for some patients, and Goldberg (25) has recommended use of levulose. Pyridoxine also has been suggested, but with little proof of benefit.

Metachromatic Leukodystrophy

In metachromatic leukodystrophy (MLD), neuropathy is only one minor feature of a more general insult to nervous tissue, and there is no specific therapy for either the neuropathy or the other systemic aspects. The disorder is reviewed in the section on progressive degenerations, but awareness of the involvement of peripheral nerves in MLD may enhance diagnostic evidence seen on electromyogram (EMG) or nerve biopsy.

Many other metabolic disorders can first appear as neuropathy. This true especially of toxic states, such as those caused by the thousands of environmental substances that are potentially noxious to the CNS (26,27). One of the easiest ways to monitor the effects of these substances is to look for their effects on peripheral nerves, particularly since EMG and nerve conduction studies are simple and without significant hazard to the patient. Nonspecific measures such as protection of the extremity, bracing and support, and use of multivitamins (particularly thiamine, 50 mg b.i.d., and pyridoxine, 100 mg b.i.d.) may be considered for any of these patients. In only a few diseases with inborn errors of metabolism, such as in Refsum's disease, will definitive therapeutic or environmental measures be available to the clinician. If the toxin is exogenous and the neuropathy mild, the neuropathy usually clears after the toxin is eliminated. Some toxic neuropathies are associated with specific clinical clues, and, although recollection of these details may seem insignificant or esoteric, they help to identify the presence of genetic disorders or the role of particular toxins, thereby enabling the clinician to rule out significant treatable disease.

Diabetic Neuropathy

Diabetic neuropathy is the most common metabolic neuropathy in the Western world. Several types of diabetic neuropathy can occur, including asymmetric sensory polyneuropathy, autonomic neuropathy, mononeuropathies, and multiple mononeuropathies. Each of these deserves individual attention, although they can be mixed in a complex fashion in any one individual. Symmetric and distal neuropathies may be allieviated by adequate control of the diabetes. Since the introduction of insulin therapy there has been debate about the usefulness of therapy. Certainly neuropathy develops in some individuals as an early sign of diabetes, whereas others appear to be resistant to neuropathic disorders. In many cases of diabetic mononeuropathy it may be more helpful to determine which disorder the patient does not have. For example, search for other illnesses must be undertaken when third-nerve palsy occurs in a diabetic patient, even though diabetes may be the culprit.

Although control of the diabetes cannot guarantee freedom from neuropathy, this measure probably helps to delay the more severe change in anterior horn cells or nerves. Painful neuropathies may respond to carbamazepine (Tegretol), 200 mg t.i.d.; phenytoin (Dilantin), 100 mg t.i.d., or other anticonvulsants, but treatment is often unsatisfactory. When perforating ulcers occur, particularly over the ball of the foot, the patient must cease bearing weight in that area until the ulcer is completely clear. Education regarding care of the foot is mandatory for all such patients before the neuropathy develops. Such education deals with toe care, cleanliness, and adequate socks and shoes. The autonomic neuropathy of diabetes can lead to disturbance in sweating, pupillary disturbances, or nocturnal diarrhea. Although control of the diabetes is always the goal, it does not prevent these effects in all patients; nor is it of great benefit once nocturnal diarrhea or impotence has occurred. There have been advances in the management of impotence, most of which involve urologic intervention rather than neurologic assistance (28). Several new types of prosthetic devices may offer partial mechanical erection, a possibility that is useful for some patients. Diabetic diarrhea, which characteristically occurs at night, consists of watery stools, and measures to decrease gut motility can be considered. Dietary roughage can be limited, and diphenoxylate hydrochloride (Lomotil), 5 mg t.i.d. or before bedtime, can be helpful. The nutritional state of all diabetic patients must be maintained carefully.

One of the most common disturbances in elderly patients with diabetes is thigh pain, which may reflect involvement of the vasculature of the femoral nerve or of the lumbar plexus. Although the dull thigh pain and ophthalmoplegia of diabetes may respond somewhat to steroids, this mononeuropathy improve gradually in most instances, with or without treatment. The usefulness of vitamins in these aspects of diabetes is uncertain, but supplementary thiamine will do no harm. Although pain has been treated with chlorpromazine, thyroid hormone, salicylate, and phenytoin, these agents are usually ineffectual. Mechanical measures, such as a foot-drop brace, may be helpful for some patients, and, since these patients are vulnerable to entrapment neuropathies, surgical release of locally contused nerves may be helpful in rare cases.

Diabetic Amyotrophy

Diabetic amyotrophy has been a controversial subject in neurology, although weakness and atrophy of the thighs can occur in diabetic patients. Many cases may represent femoral neuropathy; others, deterioration of the lumbar plexus or spinal cord; and a few, microscopic damage to muscles on a metabolic, vascular, or neurologic basis. No specific therapy for diabetic amyotrophy exists, but the pain may respond to carbamazepine, 200 mg t.i.d. If this agent is continued, monitoring of blood count in the first few months is desirable. Other anticonvulsants, including phenytoin, 100 mg t.i.d., or clonazepam (Clonopin), 0.5 mg t.i.d., may also be used in a therapeutic trial.

CRANIAL NERVES

This section discusses conditions characterized by difficulty with cranial nerves. There are many congenital conditions in which defects in bone structure of the face or skull produce secondary problems with vision or functions of other cranial nerves. These conditions usually are of uncertain cause. A few result from spreading of toxins during fetal development, and some may result from the combined effects of viral disorders, toxins, and genetic susceptibility.

Cranial Nerve I

Anosmia can appear as a secondary condition in patients with Refsum's disease, diabetes, and generalized metabolic disorders. Often the cause of primary anosmia is uncertain and is not linked to systemic conditions. Exogenous and infectious factors can produce anosmia, and any neurologist may see several patients a year who have lost their sense of smell after a severe viral illness. In some persons nasal polyps lead to decreased olfaction, and removal of such polyps enhances the sense of smell. For some patients, chronic engorgement resulting from inflammatory conditions is the culprit, and a brief course of steroids can improve their sense of smell temporarily. Almost as common as any other factor is trauma which damages the cribriform plate and results in loss of the sense of smell. There is no known treatment for traumatic anosmia, but, fortunately, most patients adapt readily to loss of this sense.

A small portion of the population are markedly insensitive to various specific odors. In addition, some persons have a congenital or familial form of anosmia. Zinc sulfate has been suggested as therapy for some of these subvarieties of anosmia, although the treatment has not been confirmed adequately in the neurology literature. Dosages of zinc at 200 mg b.i.d. or t.i.d. are not harmful and may offer modest benefit in either primary or idiopathic anosmia.

Uncinate seizures may appear as disagreeable olfactory phenomena and may respond to anticonvulsants. Occasionally, olfactory phenomena such as olfactory hallucinations are the chief complaint in major psychiatric disorders. Although these conditions usually are apparent on history, a workup that includes electroencephalography and computerized tomography is indicated in many patients with olfactory complaints.

Cranial Nerve II

The number of primary difficulties in cranial nerve II is almost unlimited. In addition, there are dozens of systemic and local conditions that lead to relatively simple conditions, such as cataracts. Although cataracts can be inherited in an X-linked or autosomal recessive pattern, Sorsby (29) and others (30,31) have emphasized the dominant inheritance of many patients with congenital cataracts. Cataracts can be associated with neurologic disabilities, such as the ataxias and the cataracts found in Marinesco–Sjögren's syndrome (32). Congenital and degenerative defects of the CNS are associated frequently with cataracts in varied combinations. Choreoathetosis, telangiectasia, and polydactyly require individualized therapy. At present, there is no specific medical cure either for cataracts or for most neurologic disorders associated with them. Some cases of cataracts, such as those associated with galactosemia, may be preventable, but none are curable except by surgical removal.

Ectopia Lentis

Ectopia lentis has been reported in more than one condition with neurologic consequences. These conditions include Marfan's syndrome, homocystinuria, sulfite oxidase deficiency, and some varieties of dwarfism. Specific therapy for these entities is not available, but in conditions such as homocystinuria, various experimental therapies have been suggested. A diet low in methionine and supplemented with cystine has been suggested, along with the use of pyridoxine. Because oral contraceptives may exaggerate the tendency toward transient ischemic attacks, these agents should be avoided in patients with ectopia lentis (33). Patients with homocystinuria may have suffered major cerebrovascular accidents, retardation, or mixed neurologic problems that require individualized therapy.

Nystagmus

Nystagmus (34) is commonly inherited as an isolated trait and can be transmitted as a dominant or X-linked pattern. In addition, complex pedigrees may occur; in one usual pedigree, affected men are reported to transmit the trait to daughters, while affected women transmit it to children of either sex. Generalized albinism, which can result from a half dozen genetic patterns, or ocular albinism may be the underlying cause. Albinism affects numerous parts of the body, certain parts of the eye, and the skin. Ocular albinism can be found in regions of the retinal where the choroidal vessels are seen with the most clarity; in these areas, there may be loss of visual acuity in proportion to the extent of the pigmentary change. Many patients with congenital nystagmus are able to read and are not as retarded or as handicapped as would be expected on initial examination. There is no known therapy for nystagmus; phenytoin has been tried for this group without benefit. Some patients learn to compensate for the nystagmus, and, when the condition appears early in life, they have only the cosmetic handicap.

Night Blindness

Night blindness can be attributable to an autosomal dominant gene and has been reported to occur with extensive and varied family pedigrees. Nevertheless, the condition is not necessarily dominant and may be recessive in some families. In many patients, night blindness is not progressive. The condition usually is not relieved by vitamin A or by any other single vitamin or drug. Some patients with Waardenburg syndrome (35) have decreased vision. None of the entities are clearly treatable, but identification of the disorder may be of great value to individual families.

Retinitis Pigmentosa

A much more common problem than either nystagmus or night blindness is retinitis pigmentosa, a condition of varied etiology that can be linked to Refsum's disease, Laurence–Moon–Biedl syndrome, Bassen–Kornzweig syndrome, or cerebromacular degeneration. Retinitis pigmentosa may be noted as a secondary disturbance in patients who have seizures, retardation, deaf-mutism, or similar difficulties. There is no known treatment that prevents the development or progression of retinitis pigmentosa. Inexorable change, however, does not always occur, and the disease varies greatly among individuals with retinitis. The genetic subtype deserves recognition, since prognosis varies for each.

Lindau's Disease

Lindau's disease (36) consists of retinal angiomatosis which may be associated with hemangioblastomas of the cerebellum or other areas. Surgical removal, treatment with laser beams, or similar local ophthalmologic intervention is occasionally indicated for Lindau's disease. The disorder can have a strong inheritance pattern and may result from an autosomal dominant gene, with varying expressivity.

Color Blindness

Color blindness, particularly the X-linked variety, has been the subject of entire monographs and is not usually considered to be a major handicap. Some conditions, such as Leber's optic atrophy, also are familial and are considerably more serious than color blindness but the specific genetics of this condition is uncertain. In Leber's atrophy, environmental factors as well as genetic predisposition may play a major role. For example, smoking or prolonged exposure to toxins in the environment (e.g., cyanide products) may contribute to the ultimate severity of the optic atrophy. Each subvariety of optic atrophy deserves study in order to determine whether effects of environmental sources contribute to the generally untreatable genetic predisposition. Unilateral optic atrophy is a particularly troublesome diagnostic problem, and, unless the etiology is apparent, these cases merit consultation with a neurosurgeon to rule out tumor as the cause. Computerized tomography is needed in many cases.

Senile Macular Degeneration

Senile macular degeneration is a common disorder in which there can be profound loss of vision, particularly in relation to objects that the patient is inspecting most closely. Occasionally, this condition is familial (37). Peripheral vision may remain reasonably intact in these patients, who often ambulate safely even though they are legally blind. Since these patients have difficulty reading, which is aggravated by fatigue or in the evening, patients may benefit from special education materials, such as special books or tapes for the nonsighted. Macular degeneration can be inherited as an X-linked trait or as either a recessive or dominant characteristic. Macular dystrophy often appears without associated neurologic disease and can be identified by history, visual testing, and typical retinal changes. Many patients function quite well despite macular dystrophy, and access to competent optometric or ophthalmologic advice may help the patient cope with the disability.

Pseudopapilledema

Neurologists occasionally are confused or perplexed by pseudopapilledema, the appearance of a swollen optic disk without a true increase in intracranial pressure. Pseudopapilledema can originate from extreme myopia, can be secondary to drusen (38) in or around the disk, or can be a congenital phenomenon that is inherited in an unknown fashion. Rarely, pseudopapilledema can be confused with optic neuritis. In many cases of optic neuritis there is little or no visible change in the optic nerve head, whereas with pseudopapilledema the gross appearance of abnormality is striking in the absence of significant visual loss. Once the possibility of increased pressure has been eliminated in pseudopapilledema, there is no need for therapy. The use of computed tomography at present is reassuring in the care of these patients, but lumbar puncture may still be required for some. A knowledge of genetics can be of value for some conditions that affect the optic nerve, including tumors. Retinoblastoma can have a prominent inheritance pattern in certain families, although there may be marked variation in manifestation from family to family. A family history of retinoblastoma is an indication for serial evaluation; tumors may be detected in this way at a very early stage, and death may thus be prevented.

Cranial Nerves III and IV

Hereditary Ptosis and Ocular Motor Paralysis

There is no known treatment for hereditary ptosis (39) except for surgical elevation of the lid or the use of ophthalmic crutches for the eyelid. Some other varieties of ophthalmoplegia that are inherited in a dominant pattern are even less amenable to therapy. Ocular motor paralysis can occur as a familial trait (40) and ophthalmoplegia linked with other difficulties, such as myopia and muscle disturbances in the pharynx or elsewhere, have been discussed repeatedly. These disorders generally do not respond to treatments that are useful for myasthenia gravis.

Tolosa–Hunt Syndrome

The Tolosa–Hunt syndrome (41) consists of painful ophthalmoplegia that is sometimes related to granulomatous changes in the cavernous sinus. In most instances, the disorder responds dramatically to a brief course of steroids but may recur. Although the Tolosa–Hunt syndrome is quite distinct from the mononeuritis of diabetes that affects cranial nerve III, metabolic and tumorous conditions may be confused with this disorder. Patients with Tolosa–Hunt syndrome may be younger than those with diabetic ophthalmoplegia. Since aneurysmal problems may be difficult to distinguish from the Tolosa–Hunt syndrome, angiography is indicated for some patients. In addition to computerized tomography, angiography, and other diagnostic evaluations, a 10-day trial of prednisone or decadron can serve as a diagnostic test.

Cranial Nerve V

Tic Douloureux

Familial cases of tic douloureux have been reported (42,43), and this condition, as well as the more sporadic forms of tic douloureux, can be relieved by treatment with carbamazepine, 200 mg t.i.d., or phenytoin, 100 mg t.i.d. Clonazepam, 0.5 mg t.i.d., has also been tried with some success. Generally, tic douloureux is not a familial condition and usually appears after age 50. Atypical cases require evaluation to rule out tumor or multiple slcerosis. Tic douloureux occasionally requires surgery either to traumatize the nerve or to relieve pressure from an aberrant vessel. However, as a rule, medication with anticonvulsants is sufficient. These agents may be effective also in trigeminal neuralgia through reduction of nerve impulses.

Narcotics generally are not useful and are potentially hazardous in patients with recurring pains, such as those of trigeminal neuralgia. For a few patients, especially those with atypical facial pain, antidepressants can be tried. Surgical possibilities include traumatization of the nerve, electrical damage to the roots through surgical intervention, or nerve block through alcohol. One recent technique includes exploration of the posterior fossa in hope of relieving pressure on the nerve roots from tortuous blood vessels.

Cranial Nerve VI

Defects in cranial nerve VI, such as Duane's syndrome (44). which consists of a congenital abnormality of the nerve, are not usually associated with major problem of the CNS, and no specific therapy is known.

Cranial Nerve VII

Bell's Palsy

Bell's palsy, is one of the most common neurologic diseases that affect the cranial nerves. The site of injury is not known but may be related to pressure in the bony canal, which the seventh nerve traverses. Perhaps the size of the canal makes some individuals and some families (45) more vulnerable than others to spontaneous development of Bell's palsy. Conditions such as multiple slcerosis also may be associated with difficulties in the seventh cranial nerve. Although the literature on Bell's palsy implies strongly that steroids are useful for therapy (46), many neurologists remain skeptical even though they commonly prescribe large doses of these agents (prednisone, 60–80 mg for two weeks). Medication should be tapered at the completion of therapy. Potential side effects of steroids probably are offset by the chances for benefit, as long as the patient does not have an ear infection or herpes simplex infection that led to the palsy. Herpes simplex theoretically may spread when steroids are taken, and there is always the fear of secondary infection or of development of encephalitis with use of these drugs in patients with Bell's palsy. There are no convincing data to suggest that surgical decompression is required for Bell's palsy, despite the enthusiasm of some surgeons for this approach. If surgery is to be performed the patient probably deserves electrodiagnostic confirmation of denervation.

Melkersson's Syndrome

Melkersson's syndrome is characterized by swelling of the face or of the tongue and lips, and has been noted in association with episodic facial palsy. The mode of inheritance has not yet been defined, but the entity can be distinguished easily from congenital facial palsy and from the Möbius syndrome. Melkersson's syndrome (47) is only one variety of Bell's palsy and perhaps is triggered more clearly by allergic factors than by routine idiopathic facial palsy. Treatment is similar to that of Bell's palsy in that steroids can be recommended; surgery is rarely indicated. Even more than with Bell's palsy, mastoid films and careful general or immunologic examinations are indicated in patients with Melkersson's syndrome. Rarely is a generalized systemic immunologic disorder present, but if allergic factors are apparent, prophylactic antihistamine therapy can be tried. The condition is so uncommon that extensive evaluation with the help of immunologists may be desirable.

Cranial Nerve VIII and Hearing Problems

There are numerous conditions in childhood which can be associated with reduced hearing. These can be inherited as recessive, dominant, or even as

X-linked disorders. Subtle neurologic diseases may be associated with individual hearing problems, or there may be obvious external defects, as in the large number of conditions in which developmental defects affect the face. The latter conditions, such as Treacher–Collins syndrome, occasionally may be linked with deafness. There is no specific therapy for any of these disorders, but for some patients plastic surgery or otologic therapy is indicated.

One form of retinitis pigmentosa can be associated with deafness. Of course, both the retinitis and the deafness can appear independently, but some patients with deafness have retinitis pigmentosa, are not retarded, and do not manifest the seizures that often occur with the lipidoses. A link between profound deafness and retinitis has been noted also in Usher's syndrome. Usher's syndrome is usually reported to be a recessive trait, as in Pendred's syndrome of goiter and deafness. In both illnesses, the patient must be treated as any other individual who is deaf, with supportive educational measures to help the patient acquire social skills. The goiter and the visual problems must be treated independently but usually neither condition is lethal. One other form of deafness that may be a dominant trait and that can be life threatening is a syndrome of electrocardiographic (ECG) abnormalities, syncope, deafness, and sudden death. This syndrome has been reported frequently since the original report in 1957 by Jervell and Lange-Nielson (48). This disorder is characterized by prolongation of the Q-T interval; presumably, the patient's sudden unresponsiveness is related to the ECG change. Rarely, stenosis of the pulmonary artery and deafness also can be linked, but sudden death in that condition is not so prominent a feature as it is in Jervell's syndrome. Antiarrhythmic drugs such as propranolol may be considered when irregular pulses pose a threat. Such patients should be evaluated by a cardiologist.

Although the number of the syndromes of genetic deafness is almost overwhelming, whether they be recessive, sex linked, or autosomal dominant, they all are surveyed in standard genetics texts. One dominant form of deafness, that linked with pigmentary anomalies, should be mentioned specifically. Waardenburg identified a link among heterochromia, partial albinism with a white forelock, and overgrowth of eyebrows that are set above a peculiarly flat base of the nose. Waardenburg's syndrome is associated with deafness that may be profound. Deafness without pigmentary anomalies also has been seen, and there are several other defects of cranial nerve VIII, such as Alport's syndrome, a condition in which nephritis is linked to the deafness, that may require systemic therapy (49).

What general facts emerge about management of patients with these disorders? First almost our only treatment is concentration on diagnosis. If the diagnosis is Pendred's syndrome, then a goiter must be present or expected; if the diagnosis is Waardenburg's syndrome, then dominant transmission to offspring is possible. Efforts to provide educational resources for the deaf have undergone great change in recent years, and, in general, current goals are encouragement both of any form of communication and of as great a degree of social interaction as possible. The effects of trauma from acoustic noise also should be considered for patients who are the nearly deaf, since mild additional loss can lead to intolerable absence of perception.

PROGRESSIVE ATROPHIC DISORDERS THAT AFFECT THE ANTERIOR HORN CELL

Muscle atrophy can result from many causes. Progressive muscular atrophy and amyotrophic lateral sclerosis (ALS) were once considered to be the same disorder, but we know now that there is more than one form of ALS and that muscle atrophy can be caused by different disorders and by more than one variety of ALS.

Werdnig–Hoffmann's Syndrome

Infantile progressive muscular atrophy, or Werdnig–Hoffmann's syndrome (50), has been described for several decades. Patients usually are quite ill at the time of birth, with obvious difficulty in all muscles, loss of reflexes, and scattered fasciculations. The earlier the onset, the more severe the symptoms. At times the disorder is generalized, but often it is localized to the proximal groups. Atrophy results from disease of the anterior horn cell, as confirmed on EMG and similar studies. Patients with onset of Werdnig–Hoffmann's syndrome at or before birth usually die within the first year of life; patients with milder forms may survive to adulthood but rarely live until old age.

Fazio–Londe Syndrome and Kugelberg–Welander Syndrome

A separate disorder that appears in teenagers causes progressive bulbar parlysis and a decrease or loss of cells in most of the motor nuclei of the brain stem. This illness, the so-called Fazio–Londe syndrome, is usually inherited as a recessive trait, as is Werdnig–Hoffman's syndrome. One related disorder in the group of motor atrophies is the Kugelberg–Welander syndrome (51), which may be heterogenous in inheritance. In this disorder, disability begins between the ages of 1 and 17, with gradual onset of weakness in the proximal parts of the lower extremities and in the trunk. A waddling gait develops, and the condition, which in some cases may be dominantly inherited, is frequently slowly progressive. Distinguished from this syndrome are families with late-onset muscle atrophy, those with an uncertain genetic background, and those in whom there is exclusively bulbar or spinal atrophy. Milder forms of benign muscle atrophy, including congenital absence of muscles, have been reported by many investigators. Symptomatic therapy the only treatment that is available for any of these disorders. Protection of the respiratory system and use of braces for support may be helpful for some patients.

ALS

Hereditary ALS may affect the proximal groups of shoulder muscles, as does a more prominent, distal form of atrophy similar to that seen in ALS. ALS may progress rapidly, with overt fasciculations, hyperreflexia, and profound atrophy. Pyridostigmine bromide (Mestinon), 60 mg t.i.d., may offer modest symptomatic relief for some patients but cannot prevent the eventual terminal respiratory failure. ALS is one of the most tragic of neurologic disorders, although in a few patients the condition reaches a plateau with minimal additional deterioration. When bulbar symptoms appear, early weakness, respiratory insufficiency, and dysphagia may lead to aspiration pneumonia and a particularly poor prognosis. Measurements of respiratory function may indicate the rapid deterioration. Gastrostomies and tracheostomies have been performed in ALS patients in an effort to prolong life, but patients and physicians may elect to avoid surgery if it will only prolong distress. Needless to say, the diagnosis must be certain before the patient and family are burdened with the fear of a brief, unpleasant terminus. The physician can help by being available to provide general medical counsel.

In order to fill the treatment vacuum, numerous therapies have been suggested, including massive doses of vitamin E, snake venom, pancreatic enzymes, guanidine hydrochloride, and a host of nonspecific supportive measures. Braces and attention to muscle weakness and its secondary effects can be helpful for some patients. In most instances, these conditions are progressive and linked inexorably to gradually decreasing function and death. There is no specific therapy for any of these disorders or for most of the numerous subvarieties reviewed in recent texts of neuromuscular disease (52). The physician can advise, preserve hope and some joy in life, offer comfort, and prevent foolish expenditures on useless therapy.

AUTONOMIC NERVOUS SYSTEM

Familial dysautonomia (Riley–Day syndrome) is one of the most commonly discussed genetic entities that affect the autonomic nervous system (53,54). Patients with the Riley–Day syndrome may be mildly retarded, suffer from poor regulation of body temperature, have difficulty with postural hypotension, and manifest relative insensitivity to pain. This recessive condition is uncommon but may be associated with difficulty in coping with stress, and, perhaps, with an inappropriate response to hypoglycemic episodes. Children with this disorder have died while swimming under water and poorly tolerate either anesthesia or hyperthermia. Other than protection against these aspects of the disorder, there is no specific medical treatment. Bethanechol (Urecholine), 10 mg t.i.d., has been reported to alleviate the gastrointestinal symptoms, sweating, and enuresis. The problem with postural hypotension in this and in Shy–Drager syndrome may respond to ephedrine, 25 mgm t.i.d., or to similar medications. Rare patients require leg or body stockings or similar support measures to prevent a drop in blood pressure when in the upright position.

Apneic Episodes

Apneic episodes apparently are genetic in a few families. In early childhood, brief episodes can occur, particularly in children who were born prematurely. During these episodes there is cessation of respiration that may last up to one minute. Apneic episodes may occur particularly during the first months of life, and patients usually improve spontaneously. Cerebral hypoxia can result from the apneic episode or may, in fact, be the initial cause. Metabolic factors must be studied in some of these children. Oxygen occasionally is required and monitoring devices can be helpful in prevention of sudden death. Aminophylline has been suggested for some patients, but its efficacy has not been proved. Seizures in infancy may appear as tonic or inhibitory episodes in which respiration ceases, and electroencephalography may be desirable for some children with apnea.

The relation between apnea and the sudden infant death syndrome (SIDS) is not clear. In most cases of SIDS, there is no clear postmortem change, though minor changes in the lungs are often noted. Autonomic dysfunction or cardiac liability have been suggested, and monitoring is now considered the rule for patients with a family history of sudden death syndrome, particularly when recurrent hypoxic or apneic episodes occur. At present, no medicine is known to block these phenomena.

Breath-holding spells in infancy, which can be a familial trait, usually are benign. They occur during the same age period as febrile seizures (8 months to 5 years) but do not represent a seizural phenomenon. After a minor fall or punishment, the child seems unable to breathe or unable to catch his or her breath. Pallor or mild cyanosis can result, followed by spontaneous recovery. Classic postictal phenomena, vomiting, headaches, and lethargy are not present. The problem should be explained to the parents, and therapy usually is not required.

DISORDERS OF SPINOCEREBELLAR DEGENERATION

The most clear-cut and extreme form of spinocerebellar degeneration, and that which is best known to most physicians, is Friedreich's ataxia (55). This condition is characterized by degeneration of the sensory and motor systems, including those in the lateral and posterior spinal cord. Friedreich's ataxia appears clinically as a slowly progressive ataxic disorder. Usually of dominant inheritance, the condition is insidious but eventually becomes totally incapacitating; by early adult life, ambulation is lost. Some subvarieties of the disease, such as the Roussy–Levy syndrome, may be associated with severe tremor, and myoclonus has been reported occasionally in this condition and more frequently in a different, noncrippling variety of Friedreich's ataxia. For the attacks of vertigo seen with any ataxia, some antihistamines, such as meclizine HCl, can be considered. For tremor linked with ataxia, propranolol in doses as high as 40 mg q.i.d., may be worth a trial and can certainly be helpful occasionally. Barbeau (56) has recently suggested lecithin as temporary treatment for ataxia. Lecithin can be obtained at health food stores. It is of some value to know details of the total general physical state in ataxia because, although the frequent cardiac irregularities of Friedreich's ataxia are often innocuous, cardiac arrhythmia can be life threatening and may require therapy.

Most other spinocerebellar degenerations, such as olivopontocerebellar degeneration, vary tremendously among individual families, and there is no specific therapy for any of these conditions. Farmer and Mustian (57) have reported episodic vestibular phenomena, and recent articles have suggested that similar disorders may respond to acetazolamide (Diamox), 250 mg b.i.d. (58). It has been suggested that some types of hypersensitivity can lead to intermittent cerebellar ataxia. Another intermittent or episodic ataxic disorder, and one that is associated with abnormal erythrocytes, is the Bassen–Kornzweig syndrome. The prognosis for quality of life and ambulation is quite good for patients with this disorder. Abetalipoproteinemia is known to be associated with the syndrome. Vitamin E has been suggested as therapy (59), but at present there is no known specific treatment for either the laboratory abnormalities or the neurologic findings.

Ataxia-telangiectasia is an uncommon recessive disorder for which there is no definitive therapy (60). The progressive ataxia is not the sole neurologic disability in this condition, since spasticity also may occur. Repeated infections, especially of the sinuses and upper airways, can be crippling or lethal to patients with ataxia-telangiectasia. The immunologic defects are not amenable to specific therapy, but therapy for specific infections is helpful. Although some children with the disease manifest insulin resistance (61), flagrant clinical diabetes usually is not a problem.

FAMILIAL SPASTIC PARAPLEGIA AND RELATED DISORDERS

There is more than one condition called *familial spastic paraplegia* (62–64) and reports mention the occurrence of X-linked patterns, recessive inheritance patterns, and even a dominant inheritance pattern. Patients with juvenile onset often are reported to have been slow to begin walking and running, and hyperreflexia and extreme stiffness gradually developed. Some subvarieties of familial paraplegia include arm weakness, amyotrophy, or mental retardation. Arthritis or obesity can occur, and, in the Sjögren and Larsson syndrome, ichthyosis, mental retardation, and spasticity are linked. Some familial forms of paraplegia have been observed over many generations and a few patients have dystonia, tremor, or other disorders of the basal ganglia intermixed with spasticity. Pathologic findings have varied among the different entities that are termed *spastic paraplegia,* and pathology reports have further confirmed the presence of a heterogenous disorder rather than one single entity.

Prognosis for individuals with familial paraplegia is best judged on the basis of a detailed family history. Treatment consists of management of the individual features of the disease, including attention to the skin disorder, when it is present, and to visual defects when they are linked to paraplegia. If dystonia or increased tone is present, then an antispastic agent can be helpful. Dantrolene (Dantrium), 25 mg t.i.d., baclofen (Lioresal), 10 mg t.i.d., and various muscle relaxants have been tried. Diazepam, 5 mg t.i.d., may be the most effective drug in this group. As in the spastic form of multiple sclerosis, spinal cord stimulators and dorsal column stimulators have been investigated; these remain experimental procedures, however, and surgical intervention cannot be recommended yet. For some patients, a myelogram may be required to rule out cord compression caused by some condition that might be alleviated by surgical intervention. There is no known definitive treatment of or prophylactic therapy for the spastic paraplegias.

There is one condition that links ataxia, congenital cataracts, and retardation with ataxia: the *Marinesco–Sjögren syndrome* (65,66). This disease also can appear with bony anomalies and can be differentiated clinically from Friedreich's ataxia and similar disorders. The cataracts are managed in the same way as any other cataracts. Part of the management of each case includes an adequate genetic history and counseling, if necessary.

EXTRAPYRAMIDAL SYNDROMES

Hereditary Tremor

Essential or benign familial tremor is seen commonly in any clinic that treats parkinsonism and is one of the most common movement disorders. Although it may begin in childhood (67), it is noted more often in the middle years of life, with gradual worsening over several decades (68). Approximately one-third of patients have a family history of tremor, but the severity of the tremor differs markedly among family members. The tremor characteristically affects the head and voice and is more influenced by action than is the tremor of early parkinsonism. In general, benign tremor increases with anxiety and effort. Furthermore, the akinesia, rigidity, and reptilian facies that are typical of parkinsonism usually are absent in benign essential tremor. The pathologic basis of this disorder is uncertain, but the condition is rarely totally disabling for most individuals.

The most dramatic single treatment for benign essential tremor is a socially acceptable but medically dubious one: alcohol. Individuals may improve dramatically after only one drink, particularly just before stressful occasions. If use of alcohol becomes habitual, the tremor actually may worsen, particularly in the days just after withdrawal from excessive alcohol (69). The tremor of benign essential tremor is almost identical in pattern to that of withdrawal tremor, and this overlap is both interesting and inexplicable. It is possible that, in patients with tremor, alcohol is effective by mechanisms other than sedation; however, the biochemical basis is uncertain. Any circumstance that relaxes the patient, including proper exercise and adequate sleep, can be recommended for benign tremor without fear of harm. Furthermore, activating agents such as adrenaline, dextroamphetamine (Dexedrine), or caffeine can be deleterious for individuals with benign tremor and should be avoided.

Of particular interest in the last decade has been the use of propranolol for benign essential tremor (70,71). This agent, which may block portions of the catecholamine system, can have an effect in as many as 50% of patients; for a few, the effect is dramatic. Large dosages usually are required, with levels as high as 40 mg or more q.i.d. Propranolol is best begun cautiously and discontinued slowly because it tends to slow the heart rate and because sudden discontinuation of the drug may result in cardiac irregularities. If patients cannot tolerate propranolol, diazepam, phenobarbitol or other sedatives may be of modest value. In a few cases, stereotactic surgery can be considered.

Wilson's Disease

Progressive lenticular degeneration and cirrhosis of the liver has been known as Wilson's disease since 1912 and is an instructive disease for students of neurology and of internal medicine. The juvenile, or dystonic, variety of Wilson's disease may begin in the teenage years (72,73); when the disease begins in middle or early adult life, a coarse "wing beating" tremor is more likely. Many patients are dysarthric, and most have a change in facial expression and intellectual performance. The essentially diagnostic Kayser-Fleischer ring may be seen within the limbus of the cornea with use of a slit lamp, an ophthalmoscope, or the naked eye. This autosomal recessive disorder is significant enough to necessitate detailed family counseling and checking of siblings whenever affected individuals are found. The heterozygotes occasionally manifest aminoaciduria or low serum levels of ceruloplasmin; in these cases, measurement of uptake of radioactive copper or the use of liver biopsy to measure copper stores may be definitive in selecting persons at risk. The homozygotic individual may have high levels of copper even before classic symptoms begin (74).

Wilson's disease is related to active deposition of copper in the liver, brain, and other organs, and to basic defects that include abnormalities in serum levels of ceruloplasmin. Treatment consists of a special copper-free diet, use of absorptive agents to prevent absorption of copper from the bowl, and use of penicillamine or similar chelating agents to bind copper and increase its elimination. Penicillamine can be prescribed at a dosage of 250 mg q.i.d., with a slow increase to this level over one month. More than 2 g/day may produce signs of toxicity. The overall effect of the medication can be monitored, not only clinically, but also by measurement of the excretion of copper in the urine. If the patient cannot tolerate penicillamine, even in slowly increasing doses, because rash or leukopenia has developed, steroids can be prescribed. The therapist can consider the use of triethylenetetramine dihydrochloride, which is less generally accepted. L-dopa may offer brief relief from increased tone but does not affect the course of the disease.

Hallervorden–Spatz, Fahr's disease, and familial parkinsonism resulting from calcification of the basal ganglia are not specifically treatable, but in some cases the associated rigidity may respond to small doses of L-dopa (250 mg t.i.d.).

Dystonia Musculorum Deformans

Dystonia musculorum deformans is usually described in the texts as an autosomal recessive trait, but it also can be inherited as a less severe, dominant disorder (75). Either the severe form or the milder, dominant variety may begin insidiously in childhood with tonic posturing of a foot; by early adult life the recessive and more severe forms of the disorder are associated with total disability or death from complications of respiratory insufficiency. Surgical intervention that produces lesions in the basal ganglia or cerebellar stimulators has been popularized and can be dramatically successful in carefully selected patients. These approaches remain more experimental than therapeutic at present. On the other hand, the severe recessive form of dystonia is usually approached surgically, since dominant dystonia is rarely incapacitating. Surgery on tight tendons or contracted joints is rarely beneficial.

The biochemistry of dystonia musculorum deformans reveals suggestive abnormalities in catecholamine metabolism. This seems particularly true in patients with dominantly inherited dystonia, and whom it has been suggested that there is either an abnormality in receptor sensitivity or an oversecretion in catecholamines or dopamine by-products. Furthermore, the appearance of dystonic posturing in patients who have been treated with phenothiazines has raised the possibility that dopamine metabolism is the primary feature of these disorders. Nevertheless, the fundamental biochemical basis for dystonia remains as elusive as the causal pathology. Small doses of L-dopa, 100 mg t.i.d., may be helpful, but large doses seem only to worsen the condition. Fahn (76) recently has suggested doses of trihexyphenidyl HCl (Artane) as high as 40 mg/day, for children with dystonia, but such high levels must be achieved slowly.

Various amino acids, heroic doses of vitamins, and other therapies have been utilized by enthusiastic families, and some become fixated on certain dietary regimens. However, there is no evidence that these various therapies offer benefit.

Huntington's Disease

The major features of Huntington's disease (HD) (77) are mental changes, a dominant inheritance pattern, and choreiform movements that may begin in early adult life and usually lead to incapacity and death in 20 years. A rarer, childhood dystonic or rigid form of HD is well recognized (78), and the seizures associated with this form may require anticonvulsant medications. Patients may have either motor or mental defects but usually manifest both.

Many therapies have been tried for HD, including use of numerous tranquilizers; particularly drugs that are known to block dopamine receptors and perhaps thereby ameliorate the choreiform movements. The most popular medication in Europe for Huntington's disease is tetrabenazine; in the United States, many clinicians prescribe haloperidol (Haldol) in doses of up to 1 mg t.i.d. or chlorpromazine (Thorazine), 25 mg t.i.d. The use of cholinergic substances such as choline or lecithin has been suggested, since HD may affect both cholinergic and dopaminergic factors. A deficiency of GABA has been reported in HD, and various compounds have been used to raise the level of GABA in the brain. There is little evidence, however, that these approaches are successful in achieving this goal. Certainly, baclofen and similar GABA analogues are not clinically helpful for any patients. The concept of low GABA levels in HD led to use of isoniazid (isonicotinyl hydrazine) in doses of up to 600 mg/day (79), because isoniazid can block the aminotransferase system and theoretically could lead to a change in the GABA level in the brain. Results with isoniazid are equivocal in patients with HD. Most therapy, including isoniazid, has aimed at improvement of motor abnormalities. None of the standard therapy is purported to reverse the course of the disease or eliminate the defects in mentation.

Management of HD requires not only adequate counseling, but also an effort to alleviate the symptoms. For example, many patients with HD become depressed, and a few become combative or dangerous to their families or community. Psychotropic medications and antidepressants require assessment of the needs of each patient, both individually and through regular follow-up visits. Often, repeated visits offer a chance for unaffected family members to reveal their concerns.

HD is not discussed in studies of linkage, and major chromosomal abnormalities have not been identified. There are exciting new techniques in chromosome research that may revolutionize concepts of genetic disease; however, no linkage of HD with other genetic disorders is known at present.

MAJOR STRUCTURAL DEFECTS THAT AFFECT THE CNS

Anencephaly and Spina Bifida

Complete *anencephaly* (80,81) is not compatible with life, and most pediatricians limit supportive measures in such cases. Spina bifida, whether caused by hydrodynamic disturbance or secondary to failure of neural-tube closure, is treatable largely by surgical approaches. Antenatal diagnosis is now possible by detection of abnormally high levels of alpha fetoprotein in the amniotic fluid and perhaps also by detection of high levels of this substance in maternal serum. Spina bifida occulta usually is asymptomatic unless underlying associated abnormalities produce neurologic symptoms.

The treatment of these midline defects, including meningoceles, requires a conservative surgical approach. If the defect is very large, is not associated with potentially useful function of the legs or bladder, or is associated with other major defects, compassionate neurosurgeons may elect to withhold surgery. For infants who survive the disease, urologic attention to bladder defects is mandatory, and orthopedic specialists can help to provide braces and rehabilitative measures. Parental counseling must not be overlooked as part of therapy, since long-term management requires massive expenditure of money and concern. The optimal goal is an individual approach that tailored to the maximal potential of each child.

Arnold–Chiari malformation, with wedging of the medullary regions, usually requires surgical decompression, and a shunt may be required to treat secondary hydrocephalus.

The treatment of these disorders is largely surgical, but recent information continues to suggest that exogenous factors may contribute to production of CNS defects; therefore preventive measures may become available. Although specific toxins have not yet been identified with certainty they may represent ingested materials; infections in utero could also cause the defects. At present, definite cause for spina bifida is unknown, and a multifactorial basis is probable.

Basilar impression, an occasional defect of bone development, can be confirmed by x-ray films and may be improved dramatically by decompression of the posterior fossa (82). The Dandy–Walker syndrome (83) of posterior fossa and arachnoidal cysts of the fourth ventricles can also arise in childhood, with signs of increased pressure (84). Proper treatment is removal of the cyst or cyst walls, and, at times a shunt is required. Surgical intervention can preserve normal mentation for patients with this syndrome.

Microcephaly

Microcephaly usually is associated with low brain volume and is not due solely to craniostenosis. Microcephaly usually is linked with retardation and small stature

(85,86). Hypertonia may be present in some of these unfortunate persons, and, as new and more useful antispastic agents are developed, medication can be prescribed with little harm. Some of the more severe cerebral defects, such as lissencephaly, or microencephaly, may be associated with profound abnormalities in brain substance. No preventive measure for these disorders is known; nor is there medical therapy for the associated mental retardation.

Craniostenosis

Craniostenosis represents a complex group of disorders with no single pattern of inheritance. The genetics of craniostenosis is not well defined, but in some cases an autosomal recessive inheritance seems probable. In some patients, blindness or brain damage develops as a result of premature closing of the sutures, unless intervention is possible. Decisions regarding surgery for these children are difficult, although for some surgery can be useful for cosmetic reasons or to prevent deterioration in brain function.

Chondrodystrophy and Achondroplasia

Many disorders can lead to dwarfism, some of which are associated with nonprogressive hydrocephalus or with an insidiously progressive hydrocephalus that eventually necessitates shunting. Malformed vertebrae and osteophytes may impinge on the nerves or vessels of the spinal cord and also may call for surgical attention. Achondroplasia (87) can lead to severe spondylosis or hydrocephalus (88) and may need very extensive surgery when the cord becomes compressed.

In addition to these conditions, aqueductal stenosis can lead to hydrocephalus. Aqueductal stenosis can appear clinically in childhood or may not be noted until later in life. This developmental anomaly once was considered to be largely genetic, and, in some instances, the predisposition is clearly genetic. For example, hydrocephalus can be seen in some families as a sex-linked disorder (89). Nevertheless, it is now known that numerous conditions (including mumps, which affects the fetus in both animals and humans) can lead to ependymitis and resultant hydrocephalus. Inflammation and breakdown of the aqueductal lining of the ependymal cells produces scarring and inadequate absorption or circulation of spinal fluid. Hydrocephalus can be alleviated temporarily with acetazolamide, 250 mg b.i.d., or with similar medications; unfortunately, however, most diuretics do not offer long-lasting benefit for hydrocephalus. Shunting, with drainage of fluid by any of several new techniques, can be recommended for many patients, and, in rare instances, even removal of the choroid plexus can reduce production of cerebrospinal fluid (CSF).

Numerous other defects of midline structures can be seen in the CNS. One of these is partial agenesis of the corpus callosum. This condition can be inherited as an X-linked recessive disorder and probably represents failure in early migration and maturation. Maturational defects can be inherited genetically, and disorders of cell migration or maturation may include several conditions, such as von Recklinghausen's disease, tuberous sclerosis, and others. Several anomalous conditions of the bones of the face are inherited, such as hypertelorism and hypotelorism. Individual families may have a history of such defects, including cleft palate, deformed nose, or major brain defects underlying the bony deformities. No medical or preventive treatment for this group of diseases is known.

De Lange's Syndrome

It is easy to confuse de Lange's syndrome with dysplastic conditions that produce similar defects; certainly the symptoms and signs of de Lange's syndrome are not unique. The major features include short stature, small limbs, atypical facies, and, occasionally, an unusual cry (90). The child's eyebrows tend to be prominent and mental retardation is severe. No treatment or preventive measures for this disease are known. If phocomelia is associated, then physical therapy may be helpful for adjustment to the handicap. In contrast to thalidomide babies, many children with de Lange's syndrome are too retarded to benefit from prostheses.

Down's Syndrome

Numerous chromosomal aberrations have been reported, including problems in total number, and partial defects with replication or deletion. Neurologic aspects are common in all of these conditions, which are discussed well in the current pediatric literature. Furthermore, techniques of chromosome study and chromosome banding are progressing so fast that dozens of new and very rare syndromes are discovered each year. There is no treatment for any of the chromosomal defects, except for treatment of the symptoms, and most of the symptoms are nonspecific. For example, bony defects occasionally require management, renal problems may need corrective surgery or diagnosis by special procedures, and seizures require standard medications.

The best known of the chromosomal abnormalities is Down's syndrome, a disorder with several neurologic features (91). In addition to mental retardation, which is usually moderate to severe but not universal, approximately 20% of patients have strabismus and other anomalies related to the shape of the skull. There is laxity in the joints that may lead to dislocation at the knees and subluxation of the patella. Infection is common, and it is not rare for brain abscess or meningitis to develop in patients with Down's anomaly. Infections can also be linked with defects in cardiac formation, which of also may require intervention by a thoracic surgeon. In addition, vascular disorders can arise (92). Among the interesting, unexplained, and relatively untreatable aspects of Down's syndrome is the tendency of patients to develop Alzheimer's changes, which is diagnosed neuropathologically and manifested clinically only by premature aging in many adult patients. There are some anomalies in biochemistry and metabolism in Down's anomaly, but none requires specific therapy, and there is no proof that the frequently suggested therapy with massive doses of vitamins is of particular benefit. Seizures can be seen in up to 10% of children with Down's anomaly, but the seizure disorder usually is mild and generally responds to standard anticonvulsants. Although serotonin may lessen some of the hypotonia of Down's syndrome, it is the lowered mental state, not the reduced muscle tone, that is the major handicap; thus, serotonin is not of significant value. Surgical release of muscles and bracing have little place in Down's syndrome.

Trisomy 13–15 and 18, cri du chat syndrome, and most other chromosomal abnormalities offer no opportunity for specific therapy and are not reviewed here because detailed reports are available in the current pediatric literature.

Laurence–Moon–Biedl Syndrome

Laurence–Moon–Biedl syndrome, a recessive disorder that is not associated with major chromosomal abnormalities, is characterized by retinitis pigmentosa, sexual infantilism, polydactyly, mental deficiency, and obesity. Cardiac anomalies can occur, and deafness and diabetes mellitus may require therapy. No therapy for the retinitis pigmentosa of this condition is known; the same is true for similar conditions associated with major decline in retinal function.

Congenital Word Blindness

Congenital word blindness is considered to be a central abnormality and is not usually related to retinal defects; in fact, it may include more than one variety of dyslexia, as well as other neurologic deficits. Clumsiness, a tendency toward mirror movements, and other soft neurologic findings have been reported with the dyslexias. Dyslexia is more common in males, but the particular genetic and pathologic characteristics of dyslexia are not clear. No specific medication will improve reading or learning ability, but special educational efforts usually are desirable. Methylphenidate HCl (Ritalin), 10 mg b.i.d., and dextroamphetamine 5 mg t.i.d., are commonly prescribed for behavioral concomitants of dyslexia but have not been proved as stimuli for learning. These agents may reduce restlessness in severely hyperactive children; however, their use should not be prolonged or uninterrupted because theoretically they may affect growth.

PROGRESSIVE DISORDERS OF THE CNS

There is a bewildering series of degenerative disorders that affect white matter. These include spongy degeneration, Alexander's disease, Krabbe's disease, metachromatic leukodystrophy, Pelizaeus–Merzbacher, sudanophilic leukodystrophy, and sudanophilic leukodystrophy with adrenocortical atrophy. These entities are individually distinct clinically but are often first diagnosed pathologically. Common features for most include seizures and myoclonus, blindness, spastic paralysis, dementia, bladder insufficiency, and other neurologic dysfunction that can be associated with disorders that affect myelin.

Spongy Degeneration of the Nervous System

Spongy degeneration of the nervous system occurs early in life, with resultant optic atrophy and blindness in many cases; in addition, a spastic hyperreflexic state generally appears in late stages. CSF pressure may be elevated in these children, but CSF protein may be normal. Brain weight usually is increased, and a diffuse and rather profound spongy state is noted at autopsy. An autosomal recessive inheritance pattern usually is suggested. No therapy for this condition is known; as with other forms of spasticity, muscle relaxants can be tried, but these will not affect the course of the disease.

One other cause for diffuse enlargement of the brain is Alexander's disease, usually reported as isolated cases and of uncertain genetic origin. The condition is characterized by severe loss of myelin and secondary cavitation. No therapy for this condition is known.

Krabbe's Disease

A more frequently recognized autosomal recessive condition is globoid-cell leukodystrophy, or so-called Krabbe's disease (93). The natural history of the disorder includes onset early in life, usually in the first year, with stiffening of the legs and arching of the trunk, and gradual progression to blindness and spastic paralysis over several months. Nystagmus is common, and patients may have brief and unexplainable episodes of crying. CSF levels of protein can be increased, and beta-glucuronidase activity in CSF also may be increased. The enzyme galactosyl ceramide β-galactosidase is deficient in patients with Krabbe's disease, but there is no therapy for its replacement at present. Although research continues, there is no way known to slow the progress of this disease; however, assays of amniotic fluid may serve to predict the disease in the fetus. The seizures and extreme irritability are the greatest challenges to symptomatic management, and a combination of anticonvulsants and tranquilizers may be required.

Metachromatic Leukodystrophy

Similarly, there is no specific remedy for metachromatic leukodystrophy, which was defined initially on the basis of accumulation of acetic-acid granules that produced a metachromatic reaction. Accumulation of these granules is now known to be linked to difficulties in metabolism of aryl-sulfatase. Children with metachromatic leukodystrophy have a reduction in the enzyme cerebroside sulfatase. There is no definitive treatment for metachromatic leukodystrophy, although special diets low in vitamin A have been used in some cases. The values of these diets has not been proved, and no agent has been found that increases sulfatase activity in these patients. Autosomal recessive inheritance probably is characteristic, and genetic counseling can be useful. Although rarely used, prenatal detection may be feasible even though death generally occurs early in life. There is no way known to ameliorate the condition; the seizure activity may respond to standard therapy.

Pelizaeus–Merzbacher Disease

Pelizaeus–Merzbacher disease also affects the white matter and produces a bizarre and irregular nystagmus associated with head jerking and development of progressive neurologic deficits. In young children there is failure of neurologic development, and ambulation may be lost. In later stages, spasticity, dysarthria, and extrapyramidal symptoms appear. Less commonly, optic atrophy and deafness occur, and mentation eventually is severely impaired. The main signs indicate an irregular disturbance in the white matter, with sporadic remissions and exacerbations. In most cases, the condition seems to be inherited as an X-linked recessive disorder. The typical patchy or diffuse demyelination may be pathologically distinct from other varieties of demyelinating disorders.

No known therapy for Pelizaeus–Merzbacher disease is known, although occasional patients with seizures respond to medication. Spasticity can be very severe in the late stages, and management of this aspect is difficult. There is no explanation or cure for the basic disorder, and there is no way to predict in utero which patients will have the disease. Experience with several patients suggests that, for a time, special educational and conditioning techniques can be beneficial.

Sudanophilic Leukodystrophy and Sudanophilic Leukodystrophy with Adrenocortical Atrophy

The designation of sudanophilic leukodystrophy and sudanophilic leukodystrophy with adrenocortical atrophy probably includes a heterogenous collection of disorders that affect the white matter and begin early in life. The presence of sudan-staining breakdown products in the brain represents damage to myelin; hence, the label. The mechanism of inheritance is uncertain, and the pathology reveals widespread and diffuse loss or absence of myelin. Characteristically, subcortical U fibers are preserved. Concentrations of cholesterol esters may be increased, and it has been suggested that some distortion in the metabolism of myelin leads to the disorder. There is no metabolic therapy known for the disorder.

One subtype, sudanophilic leukodystrophy with adrenocortical atrophy (95), is a distinct entity that occurs in childhood (mostly in boys), with signs of Addison's disease that may precede the neurologic deficit. Cutaneous pigmentation and generalized weakness is the rule, but growth is not necessarily retarded. In late stages, there may be spasticity with increased reflexes plus extensor plantar reflexes and progressive tetraplegia. It has been suggested that an X-linked recessive trait accounts for the disorder. The adrenal cortex is severely atrophic at autopsy, but it is uncertain how this is linked to the neurologic deficit. No treatment for this disorder is known. Supportive management of the adrenal insufficiency may be required but does not seem to halt the damage to the CNS.

Multiple Sclerosis

Multiple sclerosis, more common than any of the conditions mentioned above, has genetic significance in that immunologic factors may predispose to the disease and siblings may be affected. Treatment of multiple sclerosis has been unsatisfactory, and a remarkable list of regimens has been suggested, including many immunologic agents, special diets, and trials of multivitamins. Antilymphocytic globulin, radiation therapy, and steroids have also been used, with the last being used at present by many clinicians, either as a short course or on an alternate-day basis. Induction of hypothermia or hyperbaria, administration of snake venom, and other dubious measures also are popular in certain areas of the United States. There is no evidence at present that any treatment influences the long-term course of the disorder, but steroids may shorten the length of exacerbations and perhaps ameliorate some of the symptoms. Surgical procedures, including dorsal column stimulators, have been used for the spasticity, but most of these operations are of dubious value in long-term management. The clinician must recognize that the concept of demyelination is relevant in many disorders. Loss of myelin may be a response to more than one insult to the CNS, and the currently accepted disease known as multiple sclerosis may eventually be shown to include more than one disorder. Each case must be assessed for possible errors in diagnosis, and hysteria, tumors at the base of the skull, and spinal cord neoplasia must be ruled out. Multiple sclerosis is discussed in other chapters and further review is not required here.

Lipidoses

Many conditions affect lipid metabolism; in fact, several disorders that are attributed conventionally to defects in myelin formation or preservation may represent a distortion in basic lipid metabolism. Although classification of the lipidoses is unsettled (96), one group of disorders that has merited special attention is the amaurotic familial idiocies. The labels of these disorders have fluctuated each decade and has included major groupings by age (e.g., congenital, infantile, late infantile, juvenile, adult). Eponyms also have been popular but most clinicians have recognized overlap among the categories described by the historically inclined clinicians. The best recognized of the group is the infantile form, or Tay–Sachs disease (GM2 gangliosidosis), which results in widespread accumulation of a glycoside characterized as a ganglioside. Progressive degeneration of cerebral function wih dementia, epilepsy, blindness, and weakness are features of this disorder. Convulsions are common and may require medication. Explosive laughter or crying, as seen in pseudobulbar palsy, also is reported. Rarely, anticonvulsants or tranquilizers may reduce the emotional incontinence. The electroencephalogram of patients with Tay–Sachs disease often shows abnormalities that may reflect the instability of the cortex.

Tay–Sachs disease is an autosomal recessive condition with complete penetrance; it is most common in people of Jewish descent. The increased incidence of many diseases in Jews from Polish, Lithuanian, and Russian areas may be a result of genetic drift, differential mutation, relatively heightened fertility of heterozygotes, or unexplained differential patterns of breeding. The ethnic linkage has led to exciting developments in prenatal genetic evaluation in subjects who may be at risk. The disorder can be diagnosed in utero by amniocentesis, massive screenings for detection of the carrier state have been successful.

One pathologic change in Tay–Sachs disease is a smaller brain size in the late stages, although in earlier phases there actually may be an appearance of cerebral swelling from the accumulation of gangliosides in nerve cells. The retina also is generally affected, and blindness in this condition does not respond to therapy. No therapy is known for this devastating disease. Anticonvulsants may soften the effects of seizures but do not change the overall prognosis.

There are several varieties of the infantile form of amaurotic idiocy, none of which respond to specific therapy. The late-infantile form consists of ataxia and cerebellar signs; with mild clonus also a common finding. This condition is also inherited as an autosomal recessive trait, usually in non–Jews. It is as devastating as Tay–Sachs disease with regard to its effects on the patient, but the decline is slower than in the infantile form and leads to death within five years. An atrophic change in the neuronal and vascular tissues of the retina can be observed, and spheroid bodies are noted pathologically in the nerve cells. There is no specific treatment for this disorder and no known measures to change the pattern of ganglioside deposition.

The juvenile form of amaurotic idiocy is more likely to be manifested by scattered retinal pigmentary changes than by cherry-red spots. Seizures, myoclonic twitching, and emotional instability are common symptoms, and the initial blindness can be so severe that patients are examined first in institutions for the blind. Later, seizures and mental deterioration cancel out many of the educational advances, and patients become helpless and demented.

There are late-life or adult forms of gangliosidosis, including some conditions in which the disease is not fatal until patients are in their twenties or thirties. None of these conditions respond to curative measures, and treatment is symptomatic.

Niemann–Pick's Disease

Niemann–Pick's disease, or sphingomyelin lipidosis, can occur in infantile, juvenile, and chronic form. Classically, the disorder begins in the sixth month of life, with arrest of development and gradual deterioration to the point of inability to sit, followed by generalized rigidity. There is a reduction in lipid levels in the white matter, although levels of sphingomyelin actually are increased in the grey matter. No specific therapy for any varieties of this disorder has yet been suggested; nor is there a therapy for Gaucher's disease, which consists of accumulation of glucocerebroside. In Gaucher's disease, which begins in the first year of life, patients may fail to thrive, then acquire bulbar signs or retroflexion, and, finally, succumb to spastic paralysis with decerebration. There may be a distortion in the cerebroside content of the brain. Renal transplantation, splenectomy, and glucocerebrosidase replacement therapy have been tried with minimal success.

Hereditary Dystopic Lipidosis

Hereditary dystopic lipidosis is also known as Fabry's disease. This is an exotic X-linked disorder characterized by accumulation of lipid material, punctate skin lesions, burning pains or paresthesias, and episodic fever. Autonomic imbalance also can occur. The ceramide that accumulates in this condition may affect intermediate-sized or small blood vessels, with severe medial hypertrophy of the vessel wall. There is no therapy known for this condition, although renal transplantation has been used to treat the renal failure. Phenytoin, 100 mg t.i.d., or carbamazepine, 200 mg t.i.d., may block the burning pains.

Infantile Necrotizing Encephalomyelopathy (Leigh's Syndrome)

Leigh's syndrome (97,98) is characterized by ataxia, muscle weakness, and ophthalmoplegia and resembles the childhood form of Wernicke–Korsakow syndrome. Hereditary factors are prominent. In Leigh's syndrome, the striking lesions have led to the use of large doses of thiamine and other vitamins to try to abort the progressive decline. There are a few reports that suggest some benefit from special dietary measures, but these results are uncertain.

Infantile Neuroaxonal Dystrophy

Infantile neuroaxonal dystrophy is an autosomal recessive degenerative disease that is characterized pathologically by focal axonal enlargment and clinically by slow progession and failure to acquire the ability to walk. An overlap between Hallervorden-Spatz disease and neuroaxonal dystrophy has been suggested. Affected children tend to be relatively unresponsive, and their brain is usually small at autopsy. Vitamin deficiency has been suggested as the cause of this disturbance, but large doses of vitamins do not eliminate the symptoms.

Mucopolysaccharidosis

There are numerous varieties of mucopolysaccharidosis (99), the most traditional of which are Hunter's and Hurler's syndromes. With as many as eight varieties of mucopolysaccharidosis, there may be various amounts of heparitin sulfate or chondroitin sulfate in the urine, as well as varied storage of mucopolysaccharidosis, sphyngolipids, or glycolysides in regions of the body or brain. In these conditions there may be changes in the cornea, in the retina, in hearing, and in any tissue that involves connective materials. Symptomatic therapy is the only goal. For example, surgical relief can be attempted for a spinal cord that is restricted by adhesive-thickened meninges.

Lipogranulomatosis

Farber et al. (100) have described an entity termed lipogranulomatosis that may be unique but that bears close resemblance to Niemann–Pick's disease. Patients have difficulty with their joints, respiratory distress, and hepatomegaly. Asthmatic breathing and other respiratory difficulties lead to increasing debility but may respond to therapy. Foam cells are noted pathologically in the heart, lungs, and joints, and a glycoprotein seems to be the cause. The genetics and pathogenesis are unknown, and there is no therapy known.

PHAKOMATOSIS

Phakomatosis implies a "cell rest," or birth mark (101), and this label has been used to cover many disorders that begin with a genetic abnormality that originates in nests of primitive cells. In addition to Lindau's disease, which has been discussed already, ataxia telangiectasis, Sturge–Weber disease, von Recklinghausen's disease, tuberous sclerosis, and other, less serious diseases are often classed among these neural ectodermal disorders.

Von Recklinghausen's Neurofibromatosis

Von Recklinghausen's neurofibromatosis has been described for years (102) and is well known to most physicians. Patients may have isolated tumors on optic nerves or on the roots of the spinal cord. Some patients have seizures and are mildly retarded, and many have characteristic cafe-au-lait spots of the skin or lipomatous skin changes. Genetic data suggests that at least 25% of patients have a family history of the disease, and it has been suggested that neurofibromatosis is a dominant disorder with incomplete penetrance. The pathology varies according to which lesion is present or which area is involved. In general, prognosis for survival is good. Gliomas of the optic nerve are one characteristic defect and often do not require surgery. Current advice suggests that surgery is not beneficial in most cases, and the lesions change so slowly that operation can be deferred. Surgery may be required occasionally for massive skin lesions or for tumors of the spinal canal, which can lead to profound or severe scoliosis and a crippling disability secondary to spinal cord compression. Part of the requirement of genetic counseling is awareness that patients with von Recklinghausen's disease are more inclined to develop tumors than the population at large, particularly in areas such as the eighth cranial nerve. There is no medication known that slows the growth of these tumors, and there is no clear biochemical explanation of the growth factors. Surgery is the generally accepted approach for local removal. Such tumors of the cerebellopontine angle may develop insidiously and should be suspected in any patient with neurofibromatosis who is becoming deaf.

Tuberous Sclerosis

Tuberous sclerosis (103) is now known to consist of much more than the classic adenoma sebaceum on the face, seizures, and retardation. Indeed, individual families may not have retardation at all, and computerized tomography may reveal asymptomatic lesions in relatives who previously were thought to be unaffected. The electroencephalographic abnormality in tuberous sclerosis has been well described and reflects the severe seizure disorder in some patients. The more frequent the seizures, the more likely the possibility of significant retardation. Seizures respond to medication, and, in rare instances, cortical excision has been performed to eliminate areas of focal involvement in the brain. Except for seizures and retardation, the single most serious neurologic problem is the development of lesions in the area of the foramen of Monro (104); these tumors require a shunt to reduce increased pressure.

Xeroderma Pigmentosum

Xeroderma pigmentosum is an autosomal recessive dermatologic disorder that is characterized by idiocy, retarded skeletal development, and microcephaly. Patients may be sensitive to sunlight, and some may have an abnormal level of porphyrin. There are numerous other diseases in which the CNS and skin difficulties are linked. These include Rud's syndrome and conditions such as Sjögren–Larssen's syndrome (discussed earlier). Each of these conditions displays carries a distinct history and prognosis, but at present there is no specific therapy for any of them.

Cutis Verticis Gyrata

Cutis verticis gyrata is a condition in which a markedly wrinkled scalp may be associated with spasticity, retardation, and seizures. The seizures (105) are mixed in type but may include some varieties of the Lennox–Gasteau syndrome of encephalopathy and a slow spike-wave pattern on electroencephalography. Some of the new medications such as valproate (Depakene), 250 mg or more t.i.d., may be of value for treatment of the seizures; ethosuximide has also been used. Dione anticonvulsants often are not useful for the seizure in this condition. There is little therapy for the spasticity or the mental retardation. Lipoid proteinosis, Blum's syndrome, and related conditions some of which are associated with retardation, are described in dermatology texts.

BRAIN TUMOR

Familial linkages of brain tumor and family constellations of cerebral aneurysm (106) can occur, but usually not together. The standard surgical approaches to each of these major problems are applicable in familial cases, and genetic ties are uncertain in most cases. Diagnostic procedures may be indicated early if there is a family history of brain tumor. Some new chemical agents are of value for long-term management of brain tumors, particularly for glioblastoma multiforme.

EPILEPSY

The familiar forms of epilepsy, such as the myoclonic disorders, hereditary myoclonus, progressive myoclonus epilepsy, and the various subvarieties, will not be discussed here, since they are covered in the chapter on convulsive disorders.

RESTLESS-LEG SYNDROME

Ekbom's description of the restless-leg syndrome (107) has been expanded by many observers, all of whom agree that this entity may exist as a manifestation of crawling or creeping sensations in the limbs, leading to restless movements. The condition may be seen in pregnancy, during dialysis, or spontaneously. Insomnia may be the major difficulty. The cause of restless-leg syndrome is obscure. In patients with associated anemia, adequate iron therapy may be of benefit. Diazepam or small doses of chlorpromazine or similar medications have been noted to be of value at times; the drugs usually are taken at bedtime.

TREATMENT OF VARIOUS SYMPTOMS

Spasticity

Spasticity, as reviewed by Calne (108), implies increased resistance to passive movement of a limb and is often linked with disorders of the pyramidal tract. Clinicians have tried to distinguish spasticity from rigidity, even though neurophysiologically there is much overlap between the two and the clinical distinction is often murky. In general, patients with spasticity display increasing tone when the limb is suddenly moved, followed by sudden release—a "clasp knife" tone. In children with cerebral palsy, the sudden stretch reflex when the limb is extended reflects this phenomenon. Rigidity is more common with extrapyramidal disorders; spasticity, with corticospinal tract disorders.

There is no clear explanation of the physiology and pharmacology that underlies spasticity. It is known that, in spasticity, activity of alpha motor neurons is altered and that transmitter function is different. It would appear logical that some drug should be able to eliminate spasticity, but, in fact, there is no completely useful therapy available at present.

The cause and treatment of spasticity should be primary or definitive, if possible. For example, administration of vitamin B12 may eliminate the increased tone of pernicious anemia with combined system degeneration. If a tumor is present in the cervical canal, removal of the tumor may improve spasticity. Whenever medical treatment is begun for spasticity, it must be recognized that most agents that relax muscle tone may be interpreted by the patient as producing weakness. In fact, for some patients with cerebral palsy, it is actually the spasticity that allows for ambulation. There is no drug known that is capable of consistently relaxing spastic limb without eliciting some complaint of weakness from patients. Baclofen, an analogue of GABA, decreases experimentally induced spasticity and has been useful for clinical spasticity (e.g., as in multiple sclerosis, which responds at times to phenytoin, carbamazepine, or clonazepam). Baclofen is absorbed readily from the gastrointestinal tract and is not given intravenously. The dose may be as high as 10 mg t.i.d. or even double, but the increase to this level should be gradual in order to lessen sedation and weakness. Nausea may occur in as many as 10% of patients who are given baclofen, but major side effects are usually minimal.

Diazepam is perhaps the drug used most commonly in the United States for relief of spasticity. Diazepam can increase the concentration of acetylcholine in the brain and inhibit the reuptake of noradrenaline or dopamine. The mechanism of relief of spasticity by diazepam is not clear, although it has been postulated that the dug may inhibit brain-stem activating systems or presynaptic or postsynaptic areas. There is no question of the therapeutic response of spasticity and flexor spasms to diazepam although no drug is ideal for these purposes. It is thought that some of the effects of diazepam occur at the spinal level; however, since it functions as a central tranquilizing agent, relief of anxiety may be the crucial factor for some patients. Public concern regarding possible habituation to diazepam has been emphasized recently in the lay literature, and some patients, therefore, are apprehensive about taking diazepam. Although few patients become formally addicted, many become habituated and, when the drug level in the body decreases, may request additional medication. Diazepam reaches its peak at approximately two to four hours after oral intake, with one component that declines rapidly and probably another, longer-lived component in blood and tissue.

The most common initial side effect of diazepam probably is sedation. The usual initial dosage is 5 mg t.i.d., which is increased to 50 mg or more per day while the spasticity is monitored. Methocarbamol (Robaxin), 500 mg t.i.d., and chlorphenesin carbamate (Maolate), 400 mg t.i.d., can reduce experimentally induced spasticity but are not generally used in the United States; therapeutic results are somewhat questionable. Another drug that is now used to treat spasticity is dantrolene, which impairs excitation and contraction coupling in skeletal muscles (109). Substantial improvement in spasticity in patients with multiple sclerosis has been reported at dosages as low as 25–50 mg three or four times a day. Because dantrolene has been reported to cause hepatotoxicity, most clinicians do not turn to this drug first and do not give more than 400 mg/day. Undoubtedly, additional medications will be suggested in time, and even medications that are considered useful for other conditions, such as benign tremor, may help individual patients with spasticity. In rare cases, the phenothiazines and propranolol may be of benefit for spasticity. Full treatment of spasticity has included injection of small doses of phenol or alcohol into the spinal canal to destroy the roots. More recently, surgical intervention with placement of a dorsal column stimulator has been studied experimentally but is not universally accepted.

Urinary Incontinence

Micturition is a complex process. It is often disturbed in the conditions reviewed here and deserves more than the few paragraphs possible in this chapter. Nevertheless, a few basic principles can be mentioned. The bladder may fail to empty because of a multitude of factors, including treatable structural ones such as urethral or prostate disease. Neurologic causes for disturbances of the urinary bladder include deafferentation, which can result in overflow incontinence and an enlarged bladder. Upper motor neuron disease can result in failure of bladder inhibition, and the bladder may become relatively hyperreflexic. Cortical deterioration also may be associated with decreased bladder inhibition. Patients may become aware of the need to urinate, but realization comes too late for halting steps to take them to a suitable area. Lower motor neuron disease can lead to a full bladder, with dilatation and dribbling; after infections, this areflexic bladder may shrink. Awareness by the physician of this wide range of bladder disturbances is mandatory as the first step toward treatment.

There is no clear-cut pharmacologic approach to all of the difficulties in micturation, and no one drug that solves every problem. One of the safest general measures is repetitive intervention with a sterile catheter; this is safer than prolonged use of an indwelling catheter. Careful avoidance of overdistention of the bladder is necessary, regardless of the fundamental mechanism of incontinence. Patients with good hand function can be instructed in self-catheterization. Such intermittent catheterization is indicated especially when there is a potential for continence. Secondly, drugs that lead to difficulty with retention of urine, including drugs used in the treatment of parkinsonism or depression, should be avoided or eliminated if possible. If the bladder is not distended, medications such as anticholinergics and atropine derivatives may relax a tonically contracted bladder. Commonly used anticholinergics include atropine, 0.25–1 mg orally three or four times a day. Urecholine (bethanechol) is another medication that is commonly used to stimulate the cholinergic system. The dosage of urecholine can be as high as 50 mg b.i.d. Bethanechol and carbachol have been used to affect the bladder through cholinergic mechanisms. In addition to atropine, other anticholinergic drugs have been tried. One of these is imipramine (Tofranil), 25 mg t.i.d., which is of particular value in enuresis. Prophylactic use of antimicrobial therapy is generally not wise but can be helpful during acute episodes of urinary retention. Large amounts of fluid intake and free drainage are required for adequate clearing of the bladder after such episodes.

Vertigo and Dizziness

Vertigo is a nonspecific symptom that can be associated with many neurologic, ophthalmologic, otologic, psychogenic, or systemic diseases. The differential diagnosis can be complex and includes common phenomena such as benign paroxysmal vertigo, which probably represents a viral disease of acute onset and is accompanied by nystagmus and nausea that are triggered by sudden postural change. Generally, benign vertigo clears rapidly. Vertigo may also originate from seizures and, in such cases, responds to specific medication. Encephalitis can occasionally lead to vertigo, and certainly labyrinthine disease can appear as dizziness.

According to Calne (108), vertigo is a hallucination of movement, and its treatment depends on the basic mechanism. However, since the mechanism frequently is obscure, it is often difficult to know how to treat this common symptom. Measures have included histamine stimulators or blockers, vasodilators, CNS stimulants, and depressants. Phenothiazines can be used, and nausea phenothiazines are of value, particularly when the vertigo is associated with nausea. Meclizine HCl (Antivert), 25 mg t.i.d., and similar antihistamines probably are the medications used most commonly; however, since acute anxiety is commonly linked with vertigo, diazepam 5 mg t.i.d., may be as valuable as any other drug that is used.

Nausea may be linked with vertigo or may be independent of it. This symptom is seen with many acute neurologic disorders. Nausea can be triggered by central phenomena, particularly those involving the chemoreceptor trigger zones or the emetic centers in the brain stem. If treatment is necessary, (sometimes nothing is required), phenothiazines probably are the most common medications. Prochlorperazine (Compazine) 5 mg intramuscularly, rectally, or orally, is often suggested as are Tigan suppositories, 200 mg as needed. Some anticholinergic and antihistaminic drugs, such as cyclizine (Marezine) and meclizine, also have been useful.

Hiccups

Hiccups is another brain-stem-mediated phenomenon that is difficult to treat. The condition usually is considered laughable until the mocker experiences it personally or until it becomes severe. Hiccups are of complex and uncertain mechanism. Occasionally, singultus can originate from abdominal distress, as from a hiatus hernia, and surgical repair is necessary. In other instances, various central lesions such as cancer or insufficiency of the basilar artery system, may be the cause. Treatment of hiccups may include simple mechanical measures, such as swallowing water or sugar, sucking a lollipop, overbreathing into a paper bag, or carbon dioxide treatment; for more severe cases, large doses of phenothiazines, such as chlorpromazine, 50 mg t.i.d., are used. Surgical intervention on the vagal nerve has been suggested but is rarely needed.

Pseudobulbar Palsy

Pseudobulbar palsy is a phenomenon that is seen commonly in persons in nursing homes and in the chronically ill, and can be noted even in children with extensive brain damage. The condition may be linked to pelvicrural contraction, or the fetal position, in which the arms and legs flexed. Similarly, patients may have a pseudoaffective hyperpathia, in that they begin to laugh or cry inappropriately whenever they are stimulated. This emotional lability is one of the most typical features of pseudobulbar palsy. With the simplest of emotional stimuli the patient weeps, often becomes red in the face, and drools. Difficulty in handling secretions, a hyperactive jaw jerk, and other signs indicate that pseudobulbar palsy is a supranuclear lesion. It is associated most commonly with bilateral cerebral disease but may be seen in numerous disorders, including ALS and multiple sclerosis.

There is no specific therapy for pseudobulbar palsy. Tranquilizers occasionally can be helpful, and anticonvulsants can be tried for some patients. Little or no research has been done on this phenomenon. The most important feature of the disorder is education of the family so that each tear or grimace of the patient is not interpreted as major emotional distress.

Insomnia and Sleep Disorders

Some persons suffer from significant insomnia, although the condition is not a common problem in clinical neurology. Numerous hypnotics have been used in treatment, and barbiturates, diazepam, chloral derivatives, and antihistamines have been used as sedatives. For patients with neurologic disease, chloral hydrate (500 mg once or twice at bedtime) probably is the safest drug. Sleep disorders are also common in phenomena such as sleep apnea or narcolepsy. Definitive diagnosis of narcolepsy can be difficult, particularly when it is combined with psychogenic problems or linked with social or cultural disturbances. For most patients, methylphenidate HCl or destroamphetamine are the most useful medications, and, for a few, dopamine derivatives or Protiptyline HCl (Vivactil), 5 mg t.i.d., can be of benefit. The latter is useful particularly when sleep apnea is combined with narcolepsy. For children and for a few adults with sleep apnea, monitoring of respiratory function is needed.

REFERENCES

1. Goodman RM: *Genetic Disorders of Man.* Boston, Little, Brown, 1970, p. 1009.
2. McKusick VA: *Mendelian Inheritance in Man.* Baltimore, Johns Hopkins University Press, 1976, p. 837.
3. Gardner LI: *Endocrine and Genetic Diseases of Childhood and Adolescence.* Philadelphia, WB Saunders, 1969, p. 1404.
4. Baker AB, Baker LH: *Clinical Neurology*, vol. 3. Hagerstown, MD, Harper and Row, 1977.
5. Pratt RTC: *The Genetics of Neurological Disorders.* London, Oxford University Press, 1965, p. 310.
6. Stanbury JB, Wyngaarden JB, Fredrickson DS: *The Metabolic Basis of Inherited Disease.* New York, McGraw Hill, 1972, p. 778.
7. Dyck PJ: Definition and basis of classification of hereditary neuropathy with neuronal atrophy and degeneration. In: *Peripheral Neuropathy*, vol. 2. Edited by PJ Dyck, PK Thomas, and EH Lambert, Philadelphia, WB Saunders, 1975, pp. 755–758.
8. Dyck PJ, Thomas PK, Lambert EH (editors): *Peripheral Neuropathy,* vols. 1 and 2. Philadelphia, WB Saunders, 1975, 2:1438.
9. Dyck PJ: Inherited neuronal degeneration and atrophy affecting peripheral motor, sensory, and autonomic neurons. In: *Peripheral Neuropathy,* vol. 2. Edited by PJ Dyck, PK Thomas, and EH Lambert. Philadelphia, WB Saunders, 1975, pp. 825–867.
10. Earl CJ, Fullerton PM, Wakefield GS, et al: Hereditary neuropathy with liability to pressure palsies, QJ Med 33:481–498, 1964.
11. Gardner JH, Maloney W: Hereditary brachial and cranial neuritis genetically linked with ocular hypotelorism and syndactyly. Neurology 18:278, 1968.
12. Denny-Brown D: Hereditary sensory radicular neuropathy. J Neurol Neurosurg Psychiatry 14:237–252, 1951.
13. Refsum S: Heredopathia atactica polyneuritiformis (Refsum's disease). In: *Peripheral Neuropathy,* vol. 2. Edited by PJ Dyck, PK Thomas, and EH Lambert. Philadelphia, WB Saunders, 1975, pp. 868–890.
14. Kolodny EH, Hass WK, Lane B, et al: Refsum's syndrome. Arch Neurol 12:583–596, 1965.
15. Richterich R, Von Mechelen P, Rossi E: Refsum's disease (heredopathia atactica polyneuritiformis): an inborn error of lipid metabolism with storage of 3, 7, 11, 15, tetramethyl hexadecanoic acid. Am J Med 39:230–236, 1965.
16. Heller IH, Robb P: Hereditary sensory neuropathy. Neurology 5:15–29, 1955.
17. Johnson RH, Spalding JMK: Progressive sensory neuropathy in children. J Neurol Neurosurg Psychiatry 27:125–130, 1964.
18. Ervin FR, Steinback RA: Hereditary insensitivity to pain. Trans Am Neurol Assoc 85:70–74, 1960.
19. Swanson AG, Buchan GC, Alvord EC Jr: Absence of Lissauer's tract and small dorsal root axons in familial, congenital, universal insensitivity to pain. Trans Am Neurol Assoc 88:99–103, 1963.
20. Magee KR: Congenital indifference to pain. Arch Neurol 9:635–640, 1963.
21. Cohen AS, Benson MD: Amyloid neuropathy. In: *Peripheral Neuropathy,* vol. 2. Edited by PJ Dyck, PK Thomas, and EH Lambert. Philadelphia, WB Saunders, 1975, pp. 1067–1091.
22. Coutinko P, Andrade C: Autosomal dominant system degeneration in Portuguese families of the Azores Islands. Neurology 28:703–709, 1978.
23. Engel WK, Dorman JD, Levy RI, et al: Neuropathy in Tangiers disease. Arch Neurol 17:1–9, 1967.
24. Ridley A: Porphyric neuropathy. In: *Peripheral Neuropathy,* vol. 2. Edited by PJ Dyck, PK Thomas, and EH Lambert. Philadelphia, WB Saunders, 1975, pp. 942–955.
25. Goldberg A: Diagnosis and treatment of the porphyrias. Proc R Soc Med 61:193–198, 1968.
26. Allen N: Chemical neurotoxins in industry and environment. Clin Neurosci 2:235–248, 1975.

27. Paulson GW: Environmental effects on the central nervous system. Environ Health Perspect 20:75–96, 1977.

28. Small MP: The small Carrion penile prosthesis. Urol Clin North Am 5(3):549–562, Oct 1978.

29. Sorsby A: *Genetics in Ophthalmology.* St. Louis, Butterworth's, 1951, p. 251.

30. Francois J: *Heredity in Ophthalmology.* St. Louis, CV Mosby, 1961, p. 731.

31. Waardenburg PJ: *Genetics and Ophthalmology,* vols. 1 and 2. Springfield, IL, Charles C Thomas, 1963, 2:1914.

32. Alter M, Talbert OR, Croffead G: Cerebellar ataxia, congenital cataracts and retarded somatic and mental maturation. Report of cases of Marinesco–Sjögren syndrome. Neurology 12:836–847, 1962.

33. Grobe H: Homocystinuria and oral contraceptives. Lancet 1:158–159, 1978.

34. Allen W: Primary hereditary nystagmus. Case study with genealogy. J Hered 33:454–456, 1942.

35. Rudolph AM: *Pediatrics.* New York, Appleton-Century-Crofts, 1977, p. 967.

36. Grossman M, Melmon KL: Von Hippel–Lindau disease. In: *Handbook Of Clinical Neurology,* vol. 24. Edited by PJ Vinken and GW Bruyn. Amsterdam, North-Holland, 1972, pp. 241–259.

37. Wright RE: Familial macular degeneration. Br J Ophthalmol 19:160–165, 1935.

38. Lorentzen SE:. Drusen of the optic disc. Acta Ophthal[Suppl]90:1–181, 1966.

39. Briggs HH: Hereditary congenital ptosis with report of 64 cases conforming to the mendelian rule of dominance. Am J Ophthalmol 2:408–417, 1919.

40. Berenberg RA, Pellock JM, DiMauro S, et al: Lumping or splitting: ophthalmoplegia plus or Kearns–Sayre syndrome. Ann Neurol 1:37–54, 1977.

41. Hunt WE, Meagher JN, LeFever HE: Painful ophthalmoplegia. Neurology 11:56–62, 1961.

42. Allan W: Familial occurrence of tic douloureux. Arch Neurol Psychiatry 40:1019–1020, 1938.

43. Auld AW, Buermann A: Trigeminal neuralgia in six members of one generation. Arch Neurol 13:194, 1965.

44. Blodi FC, Van Alleen MW, Yarbrough JC: Duane's syndrome: a brain stem lesion. Arch Ophthalmol 72:171–177, 1964.

45. Alter M: Familial aggregation of Bell's palsy. Arch Neurol 8:557–564, 1963.

46. Adour KK, Wingerd J: Idiopathic facial paralysis (Bell's palsy): factors affecting severity and outcome in 446 patients. Neurology 24:1112–1116, 1974.

47. Kunstandter RH: Melkersson's syndrome. AM J Dis Child 110:559–561, 1965.

48. Jervell A, Lange–Nielsen F: Congenital deaf-mutism, functional heart disease with prolongation of Q-T interval, and sudden death. Am Heart J 54:59, 1957.

49. Milstein JM: Abnormalities of hearing. In: *The Practice of Pediatric Neurology,* vol. 1. Edited by KF Swaiman and FS Wright. St. Louis, CV Mosby, 1975, pp. 172–180.

50. Swaiman KF: Werdnig–Hoffmann. In: *The Practice of Pediatric Neurology.* Edited by KF Swaiman and FS Wright. St. Louis, CV Mosby, 1975, 2:941–947.

51. Kugelberg E: Chronic proximal (pseudomyopathic) spinal muscular atrophy. In: *Handbook of Clinical Neurology,* vol. 22. Edited by PJ Vinken and GW Bruyn. Amsterdam, North-Holland, 1975, pp. 67–80.

52. Adams RD: *Diseases of Muscle: A Study in Pathology.* Hagerstown, MD, Harper and Row, 1975, p. 588.

53. Geltzer AI, Gluck L, Talner NS, et al: Familial dysautonomia. N Engl J Med 271:436–440, 1964.

54. Riley CM, Moore RH: Familial dysautonomia differentiated from related disorders. Pediatrics 37:435–446, 1966.

55. Barbeau A: Friedreich's ataxia 1978—an overview. Can J Neurol Sci 5:161–165, 1978.

56. Barbeau A: Phosphatidylcholine (lecithin) in neurologic disorders. Neurology 28:358, 1978.

57. Farmer TW, Mustian VM: Vestibulocerebellar ataxia. Arch Neurol 8:471–480, 1963.

58. Griggs RC, Moxley RT, Lafrance RA, et al: Hereditary paroxysmal ataxia: response to acetazolamide. Neurology 28:1259–1264, 1978.
59. Muller DP, Lloyd JK, Bird AC: Long term management of abetalipoproteinemia, possible role for vitamin E. Arch Dis Child 52:209–214, 1977.
60. Peterson RDA, Cooper MD, Good RA: Lymphoid tissue abnormalities associated with ataxia-telangiectasia. Am J Med 41:342–359, 1966.
61. Bar RS, Levis WR, Rechler MM, et al: Extreme insulin resistance in ataxia-telangiectasia. Defect in affinity of insulin receptors. N Engl J Med 298:1164–1171, 1978.
62. Schwartz GA, Lui CN: Hereditary (familial) spastic paraplegia. Further clinical and pathologic observations. Arch Neurol Psychiatry 75:144–152, 1956.
63. Haldane J: The partial sex-linkage of recessive spastic paraplegia. J Genet 41:141–147, 1941.
64. Kjellin K: Familial spastic paraplegia with amyotrophy, oligophrenia, and central retinal degeneration. Arch Neurol 1:133–140, 1959.
65. Andersen B: Marinesco–Sjögren syndrome: spinocerebellar ataxia, congenital cataract, somatic and mental retardation. Dev Med Child Neurol 7:249–257, 1965.
66. Norwood WF: The Marinesco–Sjögren syndrome. J Pediatr 65:431–437, 1964.
67. Paulson GW: Benign essential tremor in childhood. Clin Pediatr (Phila) 15:67–70, 1976.
68. Davis CH, Kunkle EC: Benign essential (heredofamilial) tremor. Arch Intern Med 87:808–816, 1951.
69. Massey EW, Paulson GW: Cause and effect in alcholic tremor. Am J Psychiatry 1572, 1978.
70. Sweet RD, Blumberg J, Lee JE, et al: Propranolol therapy of essential tremor. Neurology 24:64–67, 1974.
71. McKenney AS: The shaking patient. Diagnosis and management of tremor. Postgrad Med 61:195–199, 1977.
72. Werlin SL, Grand RJ, Perman JA, et al: Diagnostic dilemmas of Wilson's disease: diagnosis and treatment. Pediatrics 62:47–51, 1978.
73. Dobyns WB, Goldstein NP, Gordon H: Clinical spectrum of Wilson's disease (hepatolenticular degeneration). Mayo Clin Proc 54:35–42, 1979.
74. Sternlieb I, Scheinberg IH: Prevention of Wilson's disease in asymptomatic patients. N Engl J Med 278:352–359, 1968.
75. Eldridge R: The torsion dystonias: literature review and genetic and clinical studies. Neurology 20:1–78, 1970.
76. Fahn S: Treatment of dystonia with high-dosage anticholinergic medication. Paper presented at the Am Acad Neurol, Chicago, April 28, 1979.
77. Barbeau A, Chase TN, Paulson GW: *Advances in Neurology*, vol. 1. *Huntington's Chorea, 1872–1972*. New York, Raven Press, 1973, p. 826.
78. Bird M. Paulson G: The rigid form of Huntington's chorea. Neurology 21:271–276, 1971.
79. Perry TL, MacLeod P, Hansen S: Treatment of Huntington's chorea with isoniazid. N Engl J Med 297:840, 1977.
80. Book JA, Rayner S: A clinical and genetical study of anencephaly. Am J Hum Genet 2:61–84, 1950.
81. Lemire RJ, Beckwith JB, Warkany J. *Anencephaly*. New York, Raven Press 1978, p. 271.
82. Bull JWD, Nixon WLB, Pratt RTC: Radiological criteria and familial occurrence of primary basilar impression. Brain 78:229–247, 1955.
83. Scarcella G: Radiologic aspects of Dandy–Walker syndrome. Neurology 10:260–266, 1960.
84. D'Agostino AN, Kernohan JW, Brown JR: The Dandy–Walker syndrome. J Neuropathol Exp. Neurol 22:450–470, 1963.
85. Book JA, Schut JW, Reed SC: A clinical and genetical study of microcephaly. Am J Ment Defic 57:637–660, 1953.
86. Cowie V: The genetics and sub-classification of microcephaly. J Ment Defic Res 4:42–47, 1960.

87. Duvoisin RC, Yahr MD: Compressive spinal cord and root syndromes in achondroplastic dwarfs. Neurology 12:202–207, 1962.

88. Dennis JP, Rosenberg HS, Alvord EC: Megalencephaly, internal hydrocephalus, and other neurological aspects of achondroplasia. Brain 84:427–444, 1961.

89. Edwards JH, Norman RM, Roberts JM: Sex linked hydrocephalus. Arch Dis Child 36:481–485, 1961.

90. Holmes LB, Moser HW, Halldorsson S, et al: DeLange syndrome. In: *Mental Retardation.* New York, Macmillan, 1972, pp. 276–277.

91. Paulson GW, Son CD, Nance WE: Neurologic aspects of typical and atypical Down's syndrome. Dis Nerv Syst 30:632–636, 1969.

92. Fleisher GR, Bush BE, Cornfeld D: Primary internal fibroplasia in a child with Down's syndrome. Am J Dis Child 132:700–703, 1978.

93. Austin J: Studies in globoid (Krabbe) leukodystrophy. 1. The significance of lipid abnormalities in white matter in eight globoid and 13 control patients. Arch Neurol 9:207–231, 1963.

94. Zeman W, Demyer W, Falls, HF: Pelizaeus–Merzbacher disease: a study in nosology. J Neuropathol Exp Neurol 23:334–354, 1964.

95. Allen RJ: Melanodermic leukodystrophy. In: *The Practice of Pediatric Neurology.* Edited by KF Swaiman and FS Wright. St. Louis, CV Mosby, 1975, pp. 724–725.

96. Swaiman KF: Lipid diseases of the central nervous system. In: *The Practice of Pediatric Neurology.* Edited by KF Swaiman and FS Wright. St Louis, CV Mosby, 1975, pp. 397–424.

97. Leigh DN: Subacute necrotizing encephalomyelopathy in an infant. J Neurol Neurosurg Psychiatry 14:216–221, 1951.

98. Procopis PG, Turner B, Selby G: Subacute necrotizing encephalopathy in an acidotic child. J Neurol Neurosurg Psychiatry 30:349–353, 1967.

99. Swaiman KF: Mucopolysaccharidosis. In: *The Practice of Pediatric Neurology.* Edited by KF Swaiman and FS Wright. St. Louis, VS Mosby, 1975, pp. 424–436.

100. Farber S, Cohen J, Uzman LL: Lipogranulomatosis: a new lipo-glycoprotein storage disease. Mt Sinai Med J (NY) 24:816, 1957.

101. Francois J: A general introduction. In: *Handbook Of Clinical Neurology,* vol. 24. Edited by PJ Vinken and GW Bruyn. Amsterdam, North-Holland, 1972, pp. 1–18.

102. Crowe FW, Schull WJ, Neel VA: *A Clinical, Pathological and Genetic Study of Multiple Neurofibromatosis.* Springfield, IL, Charles C Thomas, 1956, p. 181.

103. Paulson GW, Lyle CB: Tuberous sclerosis. Dev Med Child Neurol 8:571–586, 1966.

104. Boesel CP, Paulson GW, Kosnik EJ, et al: Brain hamartomas and tumors associated with tuberous sclerosis. Neurosurgery 4:410–417, 1979.

105. Paulson GW: Cutis verticis gyrata and the Lennox syndrome. Dev Med Child Neurol 16:196–200, 1974.

106. Phillips RL: Familial cerebral aneurysms. Case reports. J Neurosurg 20:701–703, 1963.

107. Ekbom KA: Restless legs syndrome. Neurology 10:868–873, 1960.

108. Calne DB: *Therapeutics in Neurology.* London, Blackwell Scientific Publishing, 1975, p. 328.

109. Herman R, Mayer N, Mecomber SA: Clinical pharmaco-physiology of dantrolene sodium. Am J Phys Med 51:296–311, 1972.

9
Medical Treatment of Cerebrovascular Disease

Robert G. Siekert

Cerebrovascular disease constitutes an important and common neurologic and medical problem. On the basis of a countrywide age-adjusted incidence rate of approximately 200 strokes per 100,000 population per year, one half million strokes occur each year in the United States (1–3). Stallones's committee (1) estimated that approximately 47% die within one month after ictus; thus, a total of approximately 2.5 million persons in the United States are affected by stroke at any one time.

Fortunately, the overall mortality from stroke in the United States has been declining for the last five decades (4,5). In addition, the incidence of occurrence of all types of cerebrovascular disease also has been reported to have declined in the last 25 years (6).

Treatment for patients with cerebrovascular disease continues to be a vigorously discussed issue. Although differences of opinion exist, some consensus can be discerned. The following section will discuss general therapeutic efforts in cerebrovascular disease. Experiments with or treatments applied to animals will be mentioned only as necessary.

THERAPEUTIC CONSIDERATIONS

Objectives

The primary goal of therapy for cerebrovascular disease is prevention or reduction of cerebral damage. Toward this end, efforts are directed at all elements, including blood vessels, blood, cardiac output (circulation and pressure), and the nervous system. Specific objectives include reduction or elimination of risk factors for vascular disease, elimination of focal transient cerebral ischemic attacks, restriction of the cerebral damage, reduction in the degree or amount of damage, and rehabilitation of the patient.

Risk Factors

Kannel (7) has studied and reviewed the risk factors in stroke. The major risks are atherosclerosis, arterial hypertension, diabetes mellitus, and hyperlipidemia, when present prior to age 50 years. The degree of cerebral atherosclerotic occlusive disease and the occurrence of primary intracerebral hemorrhage are both increased proportionately to the degree of arterial hypertension. In a Veterans Administration study (8), therapeutic reduction of hypertension has reduced the incidence of stroke. Careful attention to therapy and diet in patients with diabetes mellitus and hyperlipidemia is important. Obesity, because of its aggravating effect on hypertension and diabetes, also should be considered a risk factor. Presence of left ventricular hypertrophy, ischemic heart disease (angina, myocardial infarction), congestive heart failure, and cardiac dysrhythmia are also considered risk factors (9). Smoking cigarettes is a risk factor for men, according to Kannel (7). Other less common risk factors are polycythemia vera and sickle cell disease.

Reduction or elimination of all the risks is an important element in the overall therapy of cerebrovascular disease. Evidence for the reversibility of atherosclerosis is reviewed by Armstrong (10).

Transient ischemic attacks (TIA) in themselves are considered to be a risk factor, and most studies show the incidence of subsequent cerebral infarction to be 15–40% (11–14). The greatest number of infarcts occur in the first few months after the last attack (3). After the first six months after TIA, the rate of occurrence of stroke is about 5% per year (15). After one month following a TIA, death results more frequently from myocardial infarction than from cerebral infarction (11,13). This observation prompted Toole and associates (11) to comment that TIA is a greater risk factor for cardiac disease than for cerebral disease.

Oral contraceptives also have been reported to increase the incidence of ischemic cerebrovascular disease (16,17). The actual determination of such an increase has been difficult because the incidence of stroke among women of childbearing age is low, and because there are many problems inherent in performing a statistically valid study. The collaborative study of matched controls found that the risk of thrombotic stroke in women who used birth control pills was 9.5 times greater than women who did not use the drug (17,18). On the basis of a subsequent report of that group (19) and his own observations, Horenstein (18) concluded that persons at greater risk by virtue of age, hypertension, diabetes mellitus, cardiac disease, and smoking cigarettes might reasonably be discouraged from using these agents. Further, he suggested withdrawal of the medication from other users who develop either migraine characterized by cerebral or ocular symptoms, or symptoms suggestive of TIA (18). New medications or combinations may have less risk (18).

Assessment of Treatments

Assessment of the efficacy of any treatment, whether preventive or restorative, has been very difficult in cerebrovascular disease for the following (and other) reasons:

1. Variability in the expression of potential or actual disease.
2. Disease states that form a spectrum are not easily divided and often change rapidly during observation.
3. Imprecise and inconsistently applied diagnostic criteria.
4. Variable administration of and compliance with advised (or not advised) therapeutic measures.
5. Inability to assemble, control, and study representative samples of healthy persons, of patients, and of treated and untreated victims.

Some of these difficulties are relative and others actually cannot be circumvented. An appreciation of these concepts as they apply to a particular treatment program will be of help to the practicing clinician in working with problems of individual patients.

CLASSIFICATION

The statistical frequency of different types of stroke varies on the basis of sex, race, source of sample, and criteria used for the diagnosis. On the average, community-based studies indicate that 8% of strokes are subarachnoid hemorrhage, 12% are cerebral hemorrhage, 60% are cerebral thromboembolism (of which 3–8% of the total are cardiac embolus and the remainder are thrombus), and 11% are ill-defined (2). The one-month mortality of each type is as follows: cerebral thrombosis, 27%; subarachnoid hemorrhage, 65%; cerebral hemorrhage, 83% (3).

Data on the incidence of TIAs are not included in the reports cited here because that diagnosis has been made as such only since the 1950s. Estimates of the annual incidence of TIAs vary from 31 per 100,000 population overall (20) to 1,100 per 100,000 population for people older than 52 years (21).

Since patients are observed in a clinical setting during a time course of their disease, a restructured classification based on the temporal profile of the neurologic phenomena has been proposed (22). The classification categorizes patients according to the persistence of the neurologic abnormalities rather than the type or degree of abnormalities or the pathologic substrate. The classification originally was designed to apply to all pathologic causes of cerebrovascular disease and still can be used in this way. However, in practice the scheme has been used mostly for ischemic cerebral disease, and it will be used for that purpose here.

The clinical effect of cerebral ischemia depends on the duration and degree of ischemia. Ischemia may be temporary or permanent, minimal or severe. On the one hand, when the ischemia is brief and slight, transitory disturbances of function occur without evident damage to the brain. When the ischemia is of longer duration or more severe, permanent damage to a portion or all of the brain may occur. Thus, it should be understood that the classification, which is based on persistence of neurologic deficit, is arbitrary. Further, patients may be in different categories at different times, depending on the moment in time when their disease is classified. At times, patients may be in several categories simultaneously because several different vascular phenomena are present concurrently. Despite such difficulties, however, the classification has come into common use and includes the following categories:

1. Asymptomatic cerebral atherosclerosis.
2. Focal cerebral ischemia: TIA, progressive stroke, completed stroke.

TREATMENT OF ISCHEMIC CEREBROVASCULAR DISEASE

Two main treatment programs are available to patients with various forms of ischemic disease: medical therapy (e.g., anti-platelet-aggregating therapy with platelet-suppressive agents, and anticoagulants) and surgical therapy (e.g., endarterectomy, various bypass tecniques).

Platelet-Suppressive Agents

In ischemic arterial disease, thrombi develop in response to the interaction of blood elements with an abnormal vascular surface. Since platelets play such a prominent role in the development of thrombi, the prevention of thrombi rests on inhibition of certain platelet functions, such as adhesion and aggregation (23). Although many chemical compounds inhibit various platelet functions in vitro, only a few have demonstrated potential for clinical use with regard to safety, efficacy of drug action when taken orally, sustained effect, and therapeutic benefit. Three platelet-suppressive agents are available: aspirin, dipyridamole, and sulfinpyrazone.

Although platelet-suppressive therapy is not used for this purpose, long-range inhibition of development of atherosclerosis can be derived from use of these agents. Ross and associates (24) have observed a factor that is released from platelets during clotting that stimulates the proliferation of smooth-muscle cells, the principal cells that are present in atherosclerotic areas.

Normally, circulating platelets come into contact with the subendothelial collagen at the site of damaged endothelium and adhere to these fibers. This process induces the reaction by which platelets release some of their adenosine diphosphate (ADP). ADP causes circulating platelets to adhere to platelets that already are producing an aggregate. Thrombin and platelet factor 3 lead to the deposition of fibrin. In addition, factors for prostaglandin synthesis are involved in platelet aggregation. Collagen activates phospholipase in the platelet membrane, leading to splitting of arachidonic acid from the membrane phospholipid. Prostaglandins derive from arachidonic acid. According to Didisheim and Fuster (23), prostaglandin synthetase (cyclo-oxygenase) catalyzes prostaglandin synthesis from arachidonic acid of labile endoperoxides PGG_2 and PGH_2; aspirin and sulfinpyrazone inhibit this step. The antithrombotic effect of these agents probably is attributable to the fact that platelet synthesis of thromboxane A_2, derived from PGG_2 and known to be a very potent platelet-aggregating agent, is inhibited by these two compounds.

Aspirin inhibits the collagen-induced platelet aggregation (25), blocks the release of ADP by epinephrine (26), and inhibits the collagen and ADP-induced activation of platelet factor 3 (27). As already noted, aspirin inhibits prostaglandin synthesis (28) and does not impair the thrombin-induced aggregation (29). These various effects derive from the acetyl portion of aspirin, are irreversible, and last the lifetime of the platelet (about seven to 10 days). Dipyridamole (Persantine) inhibits both the first phase of ADP-induced platelet aggregation (30) and the platelet-release reaction (26). Its action may be mediated by stimulation of platelet adenosine 3′5′-cyclic phosphate cyclic AMP. Sulfinpyrazone (Anturane) is a competitive inhibitor of platelet prostaglandin synthetase (cyclo-oxygenase) activity (31), and its action may be similar to that of aspirin. In contrast to aspirin, its effect is transient.

Use of these anti-platelet-aggregating agents is based on the belief that many TIAs are caused by emboli of platelet-fibrin aggregates breaking away from ulcerated sites in extracranial arteries. If such aggregates could be prevented, perhaps ischemic events also could be prevented. Early reports of a retrospective study of aspirin therapy by Dyken et al. (32) and of a double-blind cross-over study with sulfinpyrazone by Evans (33) indicated a significant reduction in TIAs with use of these drugs.

Aspirin

A multicenter double-blind study in the United States (34,35) has suggested that aspirin reduces the number of TIAs in this country but does not influence the incidence of cerebral infarction or death. Since some patients who were studied were chosen for surgical treatment before administration of aspirin, the design of the study may have led to distortion of the various cohorts. The multicenter Canadian study (36) concluded that aspirin (325 mg four times a day) reduces the risk of stroke or death by 48% ($P < 0.005$) in men; women did not benefit from the drug. One criticism of this study is that half the patients were excluded, about 10% for inaccurate diagnosis. Also, the lumping of end points (TIA, stroke, death) may lead to fasle conclusions, since stroke itself was hardly, if at all, reduced, and it is more common for patients who have suffered TIA or stroke to die from cardiac causes (11,13) than from stroke. Although the combination of aspirin and sulfinpyrazone (200 mg four times a day) was believed not to have offered a significant advantage, a trend of improvement was noted with this approach.

Sulfinpyrazone

Steel et al. (37) reported that the survival time of platelets was shortened in patients with TIA, and that sulfinpyrazone (400 mg/day) increased this survival time in some subjects. The frequency of TIAs decreased in half the patients who were treated with sulfinpyrazone, and the platelet survival time increased. There was no change in platelet survival time in subjects who did not experience benefit.

Dipyridamole

Dipyridamole has been studied in cardiac disease of various types but comparative studies of its use in cerebral ischemia are not available. Sullivan et al. (38) noted that the addition of dipyridamole to anticoagulant therapy in patients with prosthetic valves reduced the incidence of arterial embolic events.

The risks associated with use of these three drugs appear to be few. As is well known, aspirin irritates the stomach and duodenum, and antacid therapy may be prescribed in conjunction.

Anticoagulant Therapy

Heparin

Heparin inhibits the formation of fibrin clot by inactivating thrombin and thus preventing the conversion of fibrinogen to fibrin; heparin also inhibits the activity of serine proteases upstream in the coagulation sequence. Heparin may be administered by several methods. Opinions differ in regard to the need for and the types of laboratory control of its effects as well as to the level of anticoagulant effect necessary for prevention of thromboembolic events (39).

Continuous Intravenous Method. The continuous intravenous (IV) method uses a flow-control device or infusion pump that delivers a known volume of heparin solution (amount) over a given time. The dosage of heparin is approximately 1,000 USP units/h. A convenient method is to place 20,000 units of heparin into 1,000 ml of 5% dextrose in water. The pump is adjusted to infuse 50 ml/hr (1,000 USP units). The effect of the heparin is monitored by measurement of the activated partial thromboplastin time (APPT), with the therapeutic range (60–90 seconds) being 2–2.5 times the normal value (25–30 seconds) for the laboratory performing the tests (39,40).The APPT is checked two to three hours after the infusion begins, and the rate of infusion is adjusted accordingly. The APPT may need to be checked again in several hours but ordinarily once a day is sufficient. The concentration of the infusion mixture can be changed in response to the fluid needs of the patient. A priming dose of 5,000 units of heparin IV is administered at the start.

Intermittent Intravenous Method. Intermittent IV administration consists of injection of a bolus of heparin, usually 5,000 USP units, IV every four hours. With this schedule, monitoring of the therapy can be carried out through close clinical observation rather than through laboratory tests.

A rare patient will continue to have TIAs with this intermittent IV technique or at the therapeutic level for the continuous IV technic. In the first instance, the dosage can be increased gradually by another 2,000 or 3,000 USP units per dose; in the second, the amount infused can be increased so that the level of APPT increases to 2.5 times normal. Nonetheless, if TIAs continue to recur despite anticoagulant therapy, strong consideration should be given to surgical treatment, if the condition so warrants. Although the incidence of bleeding is reported to be lower with continuous infusion than with intermittent administration (40), I have not found the intermittent technique to cause significant bleeding or other difficulties.

When an indwelling IV needle is used, the site should be changed regularly because thrombophlebitis and infection may occur at the site after several days.

Regardless of the method of heparin administration, plans for long-term treatment should be made as soon as possible; that is either administration of coumarin drugs should be started promptly when long-term anticoagulant therapy is planned, or arteriographic study should be performed in patients in whom such study is necessary (usually as a prelude to surgery) as soon as the general status of the patient has been assessed.

Subcutaneous Small-Dose or Mini-Dose Heparin. Subcutaneous small-dose or mini-dose heparin has been advocated as prophylaxis against venous thromboembolism (41) in elderly patients who must undergo surgical procedures. In some circumstances this therapy may be useful for prevention of venous thromboembolism in patients with cerebral infarction, although its use in this setting has not been assessed.

Overdosage. Treatment of heparin overdosage depends on the urgency of the situation. The following information can help the physician to decide what measures to take in this situation.

When heparin is administered by the continuous IV method, its anticoagulant effect disappears within several hours after discontinuation of administration. When heparin is given rapidly in a single IV injection, the duration of its anticoagulant effect is related to the size of the dose. For example, the effect lasts three to four hours when 5,000 USP units are injected, and six hours when 15,000 USP units are injected (F.J. Kazmier, personal communication). When heparin is administered subcutaneously in a retarding menstrum, the anticoagulant effect may persist for 14 hours. With minimal clinical effect (e.g., hematuria), simple discontinuation of heparin will suffice. In the rare event that an antidote is required, protamine sulfate USP is effective and should be administered slowly IV. Parkin and Kvale (42) found that IV injection of protamine sulfate USP, 50 mg, within 15 minutes of an IV injection of 5,000 USP units of heparin promptly neutralized the effects of the heparin. Less protamine would be required if it is given much later after the heparin injection.

Warfarin Sodium

Oral anticoagulant agents are preferable for anticoagulant treatment that is to last longer than a week. Like other coumarin drugs, warfarin acts by depressing the hepatic synthesis of K-dependent clotting factors, causing a sequential depression of Factors VII, IX, X, and II. The degree of depression is related directly to the amount of drug given, although patients differ in the degree of their response. During initiation of therapy, daily determinations of prothrombin time usually are necessary. When heparin is administered by the intermittent technique, the determination of prothrombin time should be made at least 3.5 hours after the last heparin injection. When the continuous technique is used, the determination of prothrombin time can be made at any time, since the amount of circulating heparin introduced with this method does not influence prothrombin time greatly. With warfarin therapy, I find it helpful both to administer the drug and to measure prothrombin time at about the same time of day for each.

The dosage of warfarin should be adjusted to keep the prothrombin time at approximately two times (1.5–2.5) the normal control value for the laboratory performing the test. Institution of therapy is with a standard daily maintenance dose of 5–10 mg. Alternatively, a priming dose of 30–40 mg is given on the first day, followed on day 2 by the maintenance dose unless the prothrombin time is excessive. In most patients, satisfactory prolongation of prothrombin time is achieved in four to five days. Heparin is continued for 24 hours after therapeutic levels are reached to ensure that Factors IX and X are depressed adequately. After a week or two, when therapeutic levels of prothrombin time are steady, the frequency of their determination can be reduced gradually to about once a month. Changes in living habits should not be dramatic or abrupt without assessment of the effect on prothrombin time.

Indications. Anticoagulant therapy has been used for TIAs, progressing stroke, and cardiac embolic events (usually associated with cardiac arrhythmia). These uses will be discussed under their respective headings.

Although computerized tomography (CT) of the head and examination of cerebrospinal fluid (CSF) are not always needed in patients with TIAs, such examinations may be advisable in patients with progressing stroke or cardiac embolic events in order to assist in the diagnosis and to help exclude intracranial hemorrhage as a cause for the clinical syndrome.

Overdosage. Treatment of warfarin overdosage depends on the degree of excess and the urgency of the situation. Slightly excessive hypoprothrombinemia is treated by discontinuation of the drug or by oral administration of 5 to 10 mg of vitamin K1 (phytonadione). For significant prolongation of prothrombin time or in urgent situations (.e.g., emergency surgical procedures that require more rapid treatment) either 2.5–10 mg vitamin K1 may be given intramuscularly (IM), or 5–15 mg may be given slowly IV. Ampoules containing 1 mg and 10 mg vitamin K1 are available. If an effect is not apparent by six hours, the dose should be repeated. Prothrombin time usually returns to normal in 12–24 hours, although the vitamin K–dependent clotting factors do not return to normal for one week. Whole blood or plasma should be administered in emergencies and cases of active hemorrhage. Concentrates of vitamin K–dependent factors are available but generally are not required and carry some risk of hepatitis.

General Comment

Treatment with anticoagulant medication, particularly long-term use of coumarin drugs, requires careful observation of the patient by the responsible physician and the clear assumption of responsibility by the patient or significant relative. Of particular concern is the administration of other pharmacologic agents that perturb the effect of coumarin drugs during long-term anticoagulant therapy. Tables 1 and 2, modified from Koch–Weser (43), list some common drugs that alter the effect of warfarin and other coumarin drugs. Other reviews are available (44,45). Use of new drugs should always be considered in this light.

Contraindications to anticoagulant drugs include recent operations on the central nervous system (CNS) and the eye, active bleeding, bleeding diathesis, severe hepatic insufficiency, tube drainage of a body space, malabsorption syndrome, prolonged dietary insufficiency, and external biliary drainage. Patients with potential bleeding sites, such as duodenal ulcer, should be considered for this therapy cautiously and in light of the seriousness of the situation. A troublesome problem that can be considered a contraindication is memory deficiency in the patient or a relative.

Table 1. Inhibition of the Hypoprothrombinemic Action of Coumarin Drugs

Barbiturates
Carbamazepine
Cholestyramine
Diphenylhydantoin
Ethchlorvynol
Glutethimide
Griseofulvin
Oral Contraceptives
Rifampin
Vitamin K

SOURCE: Koch–Weser J: Drug interactions in cardiovascular therapy. Am Heart J 90:93–116, 1975.

Table 2. Enhancement of the Hypoprothrombinemic Action of Coumarin Drugs

Allopurinol
Chloral Hydrate
Clofibrate
Digoxide
Ethacrynic Acid
Nalidixic Acid
Neomycin
Nortriptyline
Phenylbutazone
Quinidine
Salicylate
Sulfonamides (long-acting)
Thyroid Drugs
Tolbutamide
Triclofos

SOURCE: Koch–Weser J: Drug interactions in cardiovascular therapy. Am Heart J 90:93–116, 1975.

Subacute bacterial endocarditis (SBE; infective endocarditis) has been considered to be a specific contraindication to anticoagulant therapy (46) because of the possibility it may cause intracranial hemorrhage or convert an infarct into hemorrhage. However, SBE itself is reported to have cerebrovascular disease in 15% of cases, 20% of which were hemorrhagic (47). In patients with transient focal cerebral symptoms associated with SBE, the incidence of bleeding was less with anticoagulant therapy than without (48). Wilson et al. (49) have noted that patients with infected prosthetic valves have fewer (8%) cerebral complications with anticoagulant therapy than without (71%), and that CNS hemorrhage occurred more frequently in patients who did not receive anticoagulants.

While insignificant bleeding, such as melena or microhematuria, may occur during long-term anticoagulant therapy, experience indicates that such instances should always be assessed carefully and not casually dismissed, since coexistent lesions often are discovered. Subdural hematoma should be considered in the elderly, even with trivial injuries or falls.

Surgical Treatment

Since Eastcott et al. (50) reported more than 25 years ago on the treatment of transient hemiplegia with carotid endarterectomy, many publications on various aspects of surgery for occlusive cerebrovascular disease have appeared. Several procedures are available. Endarterectomy is the removal of an occlusive or ulcerated lesion through an opening in the wall of the artery. Bypass grafts of synthetic tubes are used to span occluded arterial segments near the ostia of the aortic arch. A procedure described recently is the use of an artery itself to bypass an occluded segment, such as grafting the superficial temporal artery to the middle cerebral artery to bypass an occluded internal carotid artery.

Endarterectomy

Endarterectomy of the carotid artery has been the procedure performed most commonly. A recent review by West et al. (51) lists reports of large series of this operation that have been published in the last 10 years. Averaged data from these published results show the combined incidence of postoperative stroke and death to be 9.1%. A clear reduction in perioperative morbidity and mortality has occurred over this time. In surgical centers at present, these rates are on the order of 1–2%. The risks of arteriography are additional. Easton and Sherman (52) report a complication rate of 14.5% and a mortality of 6.6% in community hospitals.

The reduction in the surgical risks relates to improvement in surgical techniques, anesthesia, patient monitoring, and patient selection. The performance of the surgical procedure depends on the facilities available and on the skill and training of the attendant personnel. The surgical risks are below the estimated stroke occurrence of 5% per year over five years.

Extracranial–Intracranial Bypass Procedures

Because attempts at surgical opening of an occluded internal carotid artery have generally been unsuccessful, most patients were treated by other means, that is, by observation or anticoagulant therapy. Yasargil (53) has developed a microvascular technique for anastomosis of small vessels and has applied it to patients with cerebrovascular disease. During the last decade, the procedure has become widely used (54–56). The procedure creates a new collateral channel of the extracranial and intracranial arterial systems. The most common operation is anastomosis of the superficial temporal artery to a cortical branch of the middle cerebral artery.

Indications for the operation fall into two general categories. One is ischemic symptoms produced by inaccessible occlusive lesions and includes occlusion of the internal carotid artery, stenosis of the intracranial portion of the internal carotid artery, and occlusion or stenosis of the middle cerebral artery or of the major arteries in the vertebral basilar system. The other is prophylactic establishment of collateral flow before the treatment of the primary pathologic lesions, such as a large aneurysm or an arterial malformation.

TIAs appear to be a clear indication for bypass surgery. Less clear is the use of such surgery to prevent further infarcts in patients with a mild completed stroke. The operation does not usually reduce the disability from a mild stroke. Although some success has been noted in patients with evolving or progressing stroke (56), most investigators have not found the procedure to be of benefit; in addition, it carries a significant perioperative mortality (54). According to a cumulative review (54), TIAs are eliminated in 85–95% of patients and reduced in 5–8% of patients; cerebral infarct occurred in 3–4% during the follow-up period. A cooperative study is under way to assess the efficacy of the operation.

The graft remains patent in more than 90% of cases and may increase in size. The operative mortality is approximately 3%. In addition to cerebral infarcts, significant or fatal complications are myocardial infarction and subdural and intracerebral hemorrhage. In one series (57), intracerebral hemorrhage occurred in the area of cerebral infarction in one patient but not in another, and it was suggested that surgery be postponed until the infarct had resolved, as determined by isotopic brain scan.

Although carotid disease with TIAs is usually unilateral, bypass operation can be applied in patients with bilateral disease. An uncommon syndrome seen in patients with severe occlusive disease in both carotid arteries has been termed *orthostatic cerebral ischemia* (58,59). The symptom complex consists of syncope, confusion, dizziness, and decreased vision in an upright position; low retinal artery pressures when the patient is recumbent decrease further or disappear when the patient sits or stands. Ataxia and poor memory may persist. The positional symptoms are relieved by the surgery, and, in our experience, the remainder may improve during the ensuing months (58).

ASYMPTOMATIC PATIENTS

Persons without cerebrovascular symptoms but with evidence that may indicate a predisposition to future cerebrovascular disease can be classed as asymptomatic. The term *asymptomatic* has been applied generally to persons who are found on clinical examination to have bruits and no relevant symptoms. Rarely, a patient is noted on ocular examination to have a cholesterol embolus. Various noninvasive methods of assessing the carotid artery and circulation can identify abnormalities in asymptomatic patients.

Bruits

The finding of bruits in asymptomatic patients has been of general interest only in the last decade. Considerable controversy exists because the natural history of bruits has not been determined. In general, a bruit located over the bifurcation of the carotid artery is associated with an occlusive lesion in that region. Arteriography is required to assess the underlying lesion. Arteriography discloses normal vessels and no explanation for the bruits in about 5% of cases (60), and Ackerman (61) reports that one third of patients with severe stenosis (to less than 2 mm open) do not have bruits. An occluded internal carotid artery will not have a bruit, although a stenotic associated external carotid may have one.

A universal opinion on the treatment of asymptomatic bruits is lacking, since the risk-benefit ratio of study and treatment is uncertain. However, reports indicate a clear trend toward study and treatment. Wolf and associates (62) conclude from the Framingham study that the incidence of bruits increases with age and that "carotid bruit makes a significant contribution to stroke risk" even when other factors are taken into account by multivariate analysis. Thrombotic stroke, however, often occurred in other vascular territory.

Thompson and associates (63) compared the results of endarterectomy and no treatment over a 10-year period in patients with asymptomatic carotid bruits. They found that patients who did not have surgery had seven times as many nonfatal cerebral strokes as the endarterectomized patients, although the incidence of fatal cerebral infarction was equal in the two groups. The operative mortality was zero, and the operative morbidity was 1%.

When a bruit is discovered during a general examination, the finding should be earmarked for a treatment plan and not dismissed. Such treatment may include periodic observation, noninvasive assessment, medical therapy, arteriography, and appropriate surgical procedures.

Retinal Emboli

The presence of a cholesterol embolus in a retinal arteriole indicates an proximal ulcerative lesion in the carotid system, almost always near the carotid bifurcation. Cholesterol emboli discovered incidentally are classified as asymptomatic. Although no data exist on the natural history of these emboli, the same treatment plan as for bruits should be applied. When a retinal embolus is present along with an asymptomatic bruit, surgical or long-term anticoagulant therapy should be strongly considered.

Fibrin-platelet emboli also arise in ulcerated lesions and are observed rarely. These emboli cause obscuration of vision. Treatment should be carried out with IV heparin therapy until a long-term treatment program is established.

Noninvasive Studies

Because arteriography is cumbersome and has some minor risks, other methods of assessing the cerebral circulation have been sought. Such tests are useful but do not replace arteriography. Ackerman (61) divides these noninvasive methods into direct and indirect tests.

The direct tests are techniques for study of the carotid artery by the analysis of bruits and by imaging. Analysis of bruits (phonoangiography) depends on the presence of a bruit, which is absent in approximately one-third of patients who have a severe carotid stenosis. B-scan systems and continuous or pulsed-wave Doppler devices construct an image of the carotid artery which can display significant narrowing but cannot distinguish virtual from actual occlusion or identify ulcerated lesions and minimal narrowing.

Indirect methods assess orbital and cerebral circulation by measuring ophthalmic artery pressures and the direction of blood flow in the periorbital arteries. These techniques do not identify ulcerative lesions or carotid artery stenosis of less than 60%. They usually identify stenosis of more than 90% although occasional false results may occur. Such examinations usually have been done in patients with ischemic symptoms who are destined for arteriography. The usefulness of these tests when used for screening for carotid occlusive disease in asymptomatic patients has not been determined.

TRANSIENT FOCAL CEREBRAL ISCHEMIC ATTACKS

Since a TIA increases the likelihood of subsequent cerebral infarct, with a risk of 25–40% occurring in five years, 50% of these in the first year and 20% in the first month (13), it is important to devise a treatment plan for these patients. Some authors (11) have questioned the efficacy of any treatment. Elements to consider in planning therapy for patients with TIA include the following: (*1*) the interval between the most recent attack and the examination; (*2*) the presence of abnormalities on neurovascular study (e.g., bruits over relevant arterial pathways, cholesterol emboli in the retinal arterioles, abnormalities on noninvasive strudies); and (*3*) generally good health, particularly with regard to cardiac status (e.g., no angina, no recent myocardial infarction). The risk of cerebral infarction is greatest the more recent the last attack. If the attack was within recent months, the patient should be placed in this hospital and IV heparin therapy administered until a decision is made concerning long-term treatment. If the last attack occurred more than three months earlier, pertinent investigation can be accomplished without beginning heparin therapy.

Three specific long-term treatments have been proposed: anti-platelet-aggregating agents, anticoagulants, and surgery. Patients with TIA are divided into two groups; those in whom the carotid arterial system is affected, and those in whom the vertebral-basilar arterial system is affected. The approach to each is somewhat different.

Carotid System TIA

The symptoms of carotid TIA are the swift onset of one or more of the following: motor deficits on one side (weakness, paralysis, or clumsiness of one or both limbs); unilateral sensory deficits (numbness or paresthesias of one or both limbs or the face); speech or language deficit of aphasic type; visual deficit in one eye or a part of one eye (amaurosis fugax); and homonymous hemianopsia. Physical abnormalities, when present, include bruits over the involved carotid bifurcation and cholesterol emboli in the ipsilateral optic fundus. Special noninvasive tests for carotid atherosclerosis may show abnormalities.

Anti-platelet-aggregating drugs, anticoagulant treatment, and surgery have been reported to be of value in these patients. Aspirin, alone or in combination with sulfinpyrazone, has been suggested as a long-term treatment for men with TIA (34–36). Since this therapy is without significant risk, it can be given either as the first treatment in all cases, with the option to change if ineffectual, or as the only treatment regardless of the occurrence of further TIAs. Aspirin was not found to be of benefit in women (36).

Anticoagulant therapy can be used for a short time (e.g., six months) or for an indefinite period. Anticoagulants have been used in the treatment of TIAs for some 20 years. Differences of opinion exist as to its value in the prevention of cerebral infarction. Several reviewers (64,65) doubt its value. Millikan and McDowell (66) believe that such treatment is beneficial. In my experience (67), anticoagulant therapy is associated with the cessation or reduced numbers of TIAs and with reduced incidence of cerebral infarction.

Surgical therapy also has been advised in patients with a surgically correctable lesion and should be considered hospitals with appropriate personnel and facilities. The general condition of the patient is an important element, particularly with regard to ischemic cardiac disease. A recent myocardial infarction or active and severe angina are relative contraindications to surgical therapy; minimal angina can be accommodated. Riles et al. (68) have reported the occurrence of postoperative myocardial infarction to be 0.5% in patients without previous heart disease and 4.9% in those with such disease. If the general condition of the patient is satisfactory, arteriography is performed to assess the arterial lesion and its location so that appropriate surgery can be planned. Some physicians perform arteriography in patients who have evidence of arterial abnormalities on clinical examination (including noninvasive tests). However, since such evidence is not diagnostic, there is a trend toward performing arteriography in all patients with TIA and, if a surgical lesion is found, to perform appropriate surgery. I believe that, in the presence of bruits over the carotid bifurcation, reduced retinal artery pressure, or cholesterol emboli in the retina, arteriography and surgery should be considered strongly.

Arteriography should examine all four cerebral vessels to identify the source of the arterial insufficiency. At present, this is usually accomplished by the transfemoral aortic route rather than by injection of the brachial and left common carotid arteries. Arterial abnormalities that may be associated with carotid transient ischemic attacks include various degrees of stenosis of the internal carotid artery, with or without ulcerative lesions; occlusion of the internal carotid artery; flat, ulcerated plaques of the internal carotid; stenosis or occlusion of the external carotid artery; and stenosis or occlusion of the middle cerebral artery (69). Various combinations of these arterial lesions may be found in the two internal and in the common carotid arteries. Arteriographic abnormalities are found in more than half of patients with TIA and may be present in more than 90% of patients with abnormalities on other tests. Most authorities who find a lesion on the symptomatic side of more than 75% stenosis advise its removal by endarterectomy. An occluded internal carotid artery or an affected middle cerebral artery can be bypassed by anastomosis of the superficial temporal and middle cerebral arteries. Lesser degrees of stenosis or flat ulcers are recommended for repair by some authorities, while others believe that anticoagulant therapy achieves the same result as surgery (Sundt, personal communication).

When both carotid arteries are stenotic, the symptomatic one is repaired first; the opposite, asymptomatic carotid can be repaired in a month or not at all. If one carotid is stenotic and the other occluded, bypass on the side of the occlusion can be done first, even if this side is not symptomatic. (The treatment proposals here are from my own experience; no controlled studies exist). A chronically occluded internal carotid artery cannot be opened by direct operation. In patients who have occluded common carotid, brachiocephalic, or subclavian arteries, surgical bypass of the lesion with a synthetic tube can be done.

Before surgery, measurements of baseline arterial should be recorded by noninvasive techniques, since a sudden reduction in pressure after surgery indicates an occluded internal carotid artery. This artery needs immediate reopening by removal of the clot. Postoperatively, aspirin, 650 mg b.i.d., may be considered for long-term use in men.

In patients who are judged not to be a satisfactory operative risk or who do not have an identifiable lesion on arteriography, anticoagulant therapy should be considered. Oral administration of coumarin drugs is used, and the therapy is monitored by measurement of the prothrombin time, which is kept at 1.5–2 times the normal control value. Some investigators believe that therapy for six months is all that is required, while others continue the medication indefinitely. The potential (although minimal) for untoward bleeding, including intracranial hemorrhage, exists with this medication. Recently, aspirin has been advised for long-term treatment of men with TIAs. This may be substituted for the anticoagulant therapy or may follow a six-month course of anticoagulant therapy; I prefer the latter program. Gastric and duodenal ulcers are the side effects of aspirin, and the likelihood of their occurrence may be lessened by antacids. Overall, the risk of bleeding is minimal.

Combined carotid and coronary atherosclerosis is to be expected, since atherosclerosis is a generalized, multifocal disease. When patients about to undergo coronary bypass procedures are found to have a bruit or to have had TIAs, some authors suggest carotid angiography before coronary bypass (70). Following this plan, Mehigan et al. (70) reported that 12% of coronary bypass candidates required carotid angiography, and half of them had significant extracranial lesions. The authors suggest simultaneous repair of the carotid and of the coronary lesions in patients at high risk (i.e., with unstable angina), and a staged repair, with the carotid operation first and the coronary bypass one week later, in patients with stable angina. Goldstone (71) would rely on results of noninvasive methods of evaluation of the carotid artery, (e.g., oculoplethysmography, Doppler studies) rather than on the presence of bruits.

Ennix et al. (72) believe patients with primary carotid disease who also have symptomatic coronary arterial disease should have simultaneous repair of both systems. According to some authors (70), patients with only TIA should be subjected to stress tests (treadmill) to identify who has coronary artery lesions that may be amenable to bypass.

There is no uniform approach to the problems of these patients, all of whom could have lesions in both the carotid and coronary circulations. Examination and history will define those who require study for the secondary problem. Full angiographic screening of all patients with symptoms in only one area appear to be impractical.

From the foregoing discussion, one can conclude that the therapeutic approach to patients with carotid TIA varies considerably. While it is possible to adopt either the view that all patients need arteriography and surgical treatment for a suitable lesion or the view that they do not need treatment at all, my own approach is to consider several factors. The greater the number or frequency of attacks, the more recent the last spell, the younger the physiologic age of the patient, the least significant the medical (cardiac) disease, and the presence on clinical examination of extracranial arterial disease, the more I favor a surgical approach. Because of its convenience over time and the relatively low morbidity and mortality of surgical therapy, most patients now qualify for arteriography. In nonsurgical patients, anticoagulant therapy should be used for at least six months.

Vertebral-Basilar TIA

The symptoms of vertebral-basilar TIA are the swift onset of one or more of the following: motor deficit (weakness, paralysis, clumsiness, or ataxia of any combination of the four limbs); sensory deficit (numbness or paresthesia of one or more limbs or the face, particularly on both sides of the mouth); visual loss in both eyes (complete or partial in both eyes, or homonymous hemianopsia); and disequilibrium without vertigo. The symptoms disappear in minutes or hours. The occurrence of diplopia with any of these symptoms is very supportive of the diagnosis (22). Physical abnormalities include unequal blood pressure in the two upper limbs and bruits over the supraclavicular fossa. Since patients with vertebral-basilar TIA are less likely to have operable lesions than those with carotid TIA, arteriography generally is not performed. In the presence of supraclavicular bruits, arteriography may be considered because operative intervention can be done at or near the origin of the subclavian artery. Some workers (73) assert that operation on an occlusive lesion in the carotid artery reduces attacks in patients with vertebral-basilar TIAs; others (74) conclude that this approach has no therapeutic value. In the presence of occlusion of an inaccessible portion of the vertebral artery, an extracranial-to-intracranial shunt, with anastomosis of the occipital artery to the posterior inferior cerebellar artery, may be performed. This treatment is relatively new and the risks are as yet unknown. In general, I prefer to use anticoagulant therapy for at least six months in patients with vertebral-basilar TIA. In men, aspirin can be used instead of or after the anticoagulant treatment.

Reversal of blood flow in the verebral artery (subclavian-steal syndrome) has been treated with a shunt from the corresponding common carotid artery to the subclavian artery distal to its occlusion. Since many of patients with this condition also have multiple atherosclerotic lesions, consideration should be given to surgical repair of them if any surgical procedure is performed. Alternatively, anticoagulant therapy for six months or longer may be used.

PROGRESSING STROKE

Patients with a focal cerebral ischemic lesion whose manifestations are gradually increasing in degree over a period of four to six hours (rarely longer) should be considered for immediate treatment. The condition is uncommon, and other causes, such as intracranial hemorrhage, abscess, and neoplasm, must be eliminated. Computerized tomographic (CT) and examination of CSF are helpful in making the diagnosis. In some instances arteriography is needed for diagnostic purposes. Anticoagulant therapy has been considered the treatment of choice as soon as the diagnosis is established. After the patient has had a week of stabilized course, a plan for long-term treatment is necessary. Progressing stroke is divided into two categories: carotid and vertebral.

Patients with mild neurologic deficit (carotid) can be considered for either medical or surgical therapy. Medical therapy is long-term anticoagulant treatment. In patients considered for surgery, arteriography is carried out seven to 10 days after the neurologic abnormalities cease progressing and appropriate surgery is performed as described in the section on carotid TIA. In severely damaged patients, I believe that medical treatment is preferable to surgery. Long-term (six months or more) therapy with anticoagulants followed by aspirin (in men) is advised.

Patients with progressing stroke of the vertebral-basilar system usually are treated medically and in the same way as patients with progressing stroke of the carotid system.

COMPLETED STROKE

Patients with a completed infarct present a variety of problems—as a consequence of other, associated illnesses, in the degree of neurologic deficit, and the amount of time between the stroke and examination. Approximately 15–20% of patients die during the first month after a cerebral infarct, and one half of these die in the first week (15).

In general, patients with minimal neurologic deficit do not require specific therapy for this event. Long-term prevention of further cerebral infarctions has not been studied, no doubt because of the problems in defining a sample suitable for study. Aspirin or other anti-platelet-aggregation agents can be recommended. In the past I have not advocated anticoagulant treatment of completed stroke because of the risk of intracerebral hemorrhage. At present, the ability to rule out either silent hemorrhage or a hemorrhagic infarct by CT scan provides the opportunity to review this therapy, particularly in patients whose neurologic deficit worsens in increments during the first few days after the original ictus but remains relatively minimal. Patients with a mild deficit can be considered for arteriography and prophylactic surgery after 6 months.

Surgical therapy has been used as a long-term prophylactic treatment for patients with minor neurologic deficit and is included frequently in reports of patients with TIAs or carotid disease. When evidence of occlusive carotid disease, is present on clinical examination, arteriography and surgical therapy can be considered. At least one week should elapse so that the infarct will heal before the occlusive lesion is opened fully.

General Care

During the period immediately after a severe or catastrophic infarction, general care of the patient is most important. Specific therapy to prevent extension of the infarct or to revascularize the marginal zone is not available. The following discussion will deal with specific aspects of general care for stroke patients.

Respiratory care includes moistening of the inspired air, frequent tracheal suctioning, and, in more severely affected patients, respiratory assistance. For care of the skin, the patient should be turned from one side to the other at two-hour intervals. Padding on pressure points and careful cleansing of the skin, particularly after evacuation of the bowels, are necessary. Daily IV feeding with 1,500 ml of 5% dextrose and 500 ml of 5% dextrose in normal saline should suffice at first. Appropriate replacement or adjustment of electrolytes in the blood also should be carried out. For incontinent patients, use of a condom or an indwelling catheter will keep the skin dry. Antibiotics should be administered for urinary antisepsis, pneumonia, or infections after identification of the specific organism. Passive movement of the paralyzed extremities should be started promptly. The head of the bed should be raised gradually over one to two days, and the patient should sit in bed and in a chair and be walking as soon as possible. Avoidance of long periods of recumbency will prevent orthostatic hypotension.

In patients with a severe or catastrophic stroke, arteriography is rarely necessary and then only for diagnosis, since surgery is not indicated. Therapy with anticoagulants platelet inhibitors do not offer any benefit for the cerebral lesion.

Steroid therapy has been used in acute cerebral infarction, and the evidence available suggests that it is ineffectual for routine use (75). An early study (76) found that treatment with cortisone, 300 mg/day, did not alter the mortality rate of patients with cerebral infarction. Immediately after diagnosis, Bauer and Tellez (77) administered dexamethasone, 12 mg IV and 1 mg IM, followed by 1 mg every six hours for 72 hours, and then in decreasing amounts for the next seven days. They found that this therapy offered no benefit. Recent observations have confirmed their results (78). Although dexamethasone has been of value in reducing (often very quickly) the edema seen with cerebral neoplasms, in my experience the drug has not been successful in achieving this in patients with cerebral infarcts. This is because the edema probably differs in the two conditions.

Some investigators (79,80) have reported glycerol to be of benefit in patients with acute cerebral infarcts as compared with untreated persons. Other authors (81) who used dexamethasone-treated patients as controls found no benefit from glycerol.

Gilroy and associates (82) have reported that dextran 40 reduces mortality and enhances the quality of survival in patients with acute cerebral infarction. They instituted treatment with a dose of 500 ml administered rapidly IV in one hour; therapy was then continued with 500 ml every 12 hours for 72 hours. This treatment has not been widely used.

In double-blind studies, ornithine alpha-ketoglutarate (83) and naftidrofuryl (84) have been reported to be of benefit by reducing residual deficit in patients with cerebral infarcts. Further study of these agents is desirable.

Since autoregulation is lost in the area in and near a cerebral infarction, treatment to increase blood flow in that region by constriction of flow by hypocapnia elsewhere in the brain was studied in alternate patients by Christensen el al. (85). The investigators induced prolonged artificial hyperventilation, and the patients were treated with penobarbital and curare. The hypocapnia treatment was not effectual in aiding the clinical course or reducing the mortality, however. The patients who did not receive artificial hyperventilation or barbiturate actually fared slightly better in their clinical course, but the results were not significantly better than those of the patients with barbiturate, hyperventilation, normocapnia, and curare. Although this experiment is not specific for barbiturate therapy, it indicates that, at least with our current knowledge, the apparent efficacy of barbiturate therapy in animals cannot be transferred exactly to humans for either focal ischemia (86–88) resulting from cerebral infarction or for global ischemia (89,90) resulting from cardiorespiratory emergencies.

Lacunar Infarcts

In recent years, Fisher (91) has popularized several well-delineated acute stroke syndromes called *lacunar infarcts.* These infarcts result from occlusions of small hyalinized arteries in patients with hypertension (91). Accurate diagnosis generally is easy, and extensive study is not needed. Pure motor hemiplegia (92) is weakness or paralysis of the face, arm, and/or leg on one side without sensory, visual, or language deficit. Pure sensory stroke (93) consists only of altered sensation on one side of the person. Ataxic hemiparesis (94) is only weakness and cerebellar ataxia of the affected limbs. The importance of lacunar infarcts derives from their favorable outcome without treatment. Fisher's advice that anticoagulant therapy is not required because the prognosis is good is significant, since a recent study by Weisberg (95) with CT scans on the syndrome of pure motor hemiplegia disclosed that silent hemorrhage may mimic a lacunar infarct (see discussion on completed infarct).

Cerebellar Infarcts

Cerebellar infarcts are characterized by abrupt onset of nausea and vomiting, and truncal and limb ataxia. CSF is clear, and CT scanning is normal or shows evidence of an infarct. Patients with mild deficits require no treatment. Should edema occur in the next few days as manifested by signs of brain-stem compression, including peripheral facial palsy and ipsilateral gaze paralysis, leading to obstruction and respiratory failure, surgical decompression of the posterior fossa is recommended (96,97).

Fibromuscular Dysplasia

Fibromuscular dysplasia of the cerebral vessels is treated according to the concepts described in the section on atherosclerotic ischemic disease. In addition to medical therapy with anticoagulant drugs, surgical resection or dilatation of the involved segments has been described (98). Paulson (99) believes that patients should avoid antiovulant drugs (estrogen) and ergot preparations.

Moyamoya

Moyamoya is a rare, chronic, occlusive disease of unknown cause that is characterized by severe stenosis or occlusion of the distal carotid arteries, lack of filling of the anterior and middle cerebral arteries, and a fine telangiectatic network of vessels in the basal portion of the brain. The condition is manifested by fixed or transient ischemic symptoms. The diagnosis is made by findings on arteriogram. Noting that medical treatments have not been of value, Karasawa and associates (100), have reported on 13 patients with carotid bypass procedures (primarily anastomosis of the superficial temporal artery to the middle cerebral artery). Nine of the 13 patients experienced no more TIAs (or only one) or infarcts after surgery.

Sickle-Cell Disease

Occlusive and hemorrhagic cerebral vascular lesions are known to be common in patients with sickle-cell disease. Children are particuarly vulnerable and are at greatest risk before adolescence. Patients who suffer an initial stroke apparently are more likely to have recurrent strokes. For those who have suffered a cerebral lesion, appropriate general care should be given. In the past, results of prophylactic treatment have been disappointing.

Transfusion or infusions of fresh whole blood or fresh red cells has been suggested recently by Russell and associates (101) and offers great promise. One or two units of red blood cells are administered every month to keep the level of hemoglobin greater than 10 g/100 ml and the concentration of hemoglobin-S less than 30%. With this therapy, serial angiograms in several patients showed disappearance of an occlusive lesion.

CEREBRAL EMBOLISM OF CARDIAC ORIGIN

Although the cause of most instances of focal cerebral ischemia is embolic (from carotid or other large-vessel atherosclerosis; i.e., artery to artery), cerebral embolism has been attributed historically to a cardiac source. Various types of cardiac disease give rise to embolic material, which commonly travels to the CNS. The clinical neurologic picture varies in the degree and duration of ischemic deficit. Treatment is designed to prevent such cerebral embolization.

Atrial Fibrillation

Atrial fibrillation associated with rheumatic heart disease, particularly with mitral stenosis, predisposes the patient to cerebral emboli and infarction (102). Long-term anticoagulant therapy has been recommended and reduces the incidence of cerebral emboli significantly (103). The long-term treatment for chronic atrial fibrillation, presumably of atherosclerotic cause, is not as clear. When atrial fibrillation is discovered independently of any cerebral lesion, anticoagulant therapy may be instituted. There has been controversy over when to begin anticoagulation once a cerebral event has occurred. Meyer and colleagues (104) suggest waiting three weeks, while others (105) suggest waiting 48 hours. I have waited one week, or longer if the CSF contains more than 50 red cells per mm^3. The cerebral infarction itself is not affected by anticoagulant therapy, since treatment is only for prophylaxis against further infarction.

SBE

SBE may be the source of cerebral emboli that cause infarction or bleeding, and appropriate antimicrobial therapy should be given. Anticoagulant therapy generally has been thought to be contraindicated in these patients because it may cause bleeding; this opinion may be changing, however, although a consensus has not yet been reached. In patients with infective endocarditis who develop neurologic symptoms, CSF examination and CT scan should be performed. When the deficit is minor and there is no evidence of intracranial bleeding, anticoagulant therapy may be considered after a wait, as for atrial fibrillation. Patients with severe deficits should not be treated with anticoagulant drugs. In patients with intracranial bleeding, arteriography may disclose a mycotic aneurysm that can be treated surgically.

Wilson and associates (106) currently recommend continuation of anticoagulant therapy in patients with infected prosthetic valves. Cerebral complications were 8% in patients so treated and 71% in patients who were not anticoagulated. CNS hemorrhage actually occurred more frequently in patients who were not anticoagulated than in those who were. Should an intracranial lesion occur while the patient is on anticoagulant therapy, the therapy should be discontinued until it can be determined whether bleeding has occurred (W. R. Wilson, personal communication).

Myxoma

Myxoma of the heart, which usually occurs in young women, may appear as transient episodes of cerebral dysfunction, including syncope. Diagnosis is made by echocardiography. Treatment consists of complete excision of the tumor, including the pedicle, under the cardiopulmonary bypass. Results of this surgery generally are satisfactory (107,108).

Mitral Valve Prolapse

Mitral valve prolapse is seen in approximately 6% of individuals, almost all women. In some 10% of patients with this condition various neurologic abnormalities, including TIA or cerebral infarct (109,110) appear. An embolic cause is proposed on the basis of history and angiographic findings of multiple arterial lesions. Watson (111) has reported that, in eight patients with TIA, only one episode occurred with aspirin treatment and no attacks occurred with anticoagulant treatment (111).

VASCULITIS

Vasculitis is a pathologic process characterized by inflammation and necrosis of blood vessels. Since any size or type of blood vessel in any organ can be affected, neurologic manifestations are common. Although there is some overlap between the several different diseases in the broad spectrum of vasculitis, Wegener's granulomatosis, periarteritis nodosa, and temporal arteritis usually can be recognized. The current treatment has been reviewed by Fauci et al. (112), and much of the following discussion is based on their report.

Temporal arteritis is treated with corticosteroid therapy. Fauci and colleagues (112) suggest that treatment "begin with 40 to 60 mg per day of prednisone followed by gradual tapering to a maintenance dose of 7.5 mg to 10 mg per day, with careful attention to readjustment of dosage if symptoms recur" (p. 669). They note that many authors suggest treatment be continued for one to two years. Should the erythrocyte sedimentation rate increase, the amount of drug can be increased.

Wegener's granulomatosis, which has an active but stable clinical course, should be treated with cyclophosphamide (112). The dosage schedule is 1–2 mg/kg body weight per day. The initial dosage is maintained for two weeks and, if favorable clinical response is seen, is kept at this level, with readjustment to maintain a total leukocyte count of more than 3,000 per m^3 and a total neutrophil count of at least 1,000 per mm^3. If the clinical response is not favorable, the daily dose should be increased by 25 mg and be kept at this level for an additional two weeks. "This rate of increment should be continued until evidence of clinical response is seen or until drug toxicity, such as leukopenia, occurs" (p. 671).

Another type of Wegener's granulomatosis is fulminant vasculitis, which often includes cerebral vasculitis and rapidly progressive peripheral neuropathy. The therapy recommended for fulminant vasculitis is cyclophosphamide, 4 mg/kg body weight per day, administered either orally or IV for three days. This is followed by a rapid reduction in dosage during the next three days until a dosage of 1–2 mg/kg body weight is reached (110). This dosage is maintained in the same manner as for the nonfulminant form. Cyclophosphamide therapy should be continued for one year after the disappearance of all traces of active disease, which can be monitored by the erythrocyte sedimentation rate.

Patients who cannot tolerate cyclophosphamide because of severe leukopenia or hemorrhagic cystitis, or young women who are unwilling to accept the ovarian damage associated with cyclophosphamide, can take azathioprine as an alternate cytotoxic agent, although experience indicates that it is not as effective as cyclophosphamide.

Periarteritis nodosa, although previously treated simply with corticosteroids, has responded to cyclophosphamide in the same dosages as listed for stable Wegener's granulomatosis. Cyclophosphamide, alone or in combination with corticosteroids, is recommended (110).

Takayasu's arteritis may be treated with surgical bypass, either of the great vessels or the carotid (113). Anticoagulant therapy may be used for transient attacks. Corticosteroid therapy has not been shown to improve the condition of these patients.

MEDICAL TREATMENT OF INTRACRANIAL HEMORRHAGE

Subarachnoid Hemorrhage

In the past, some support for medical (i.e., nonsurgical) treatment of subarachnoid hemorrhage (SAH) from ruptured berry aneurysms of cerebral arteries has been expressed (114). My impressison is that surgical therapy (direct intracranial procedure) is increasingly favored by most physicians who prescribe therapy for such patients, particularly patients who have minimal neurologic involvement, namely, grades 1, 2, and 3 of Botterell (115). The surgical therapist is aware that waiting to operate three or more weeks after bleeding results in a lower surgical risk yet the surgeon is anxious to prevent the potential devastation of rebleeding and of infarction which commonly occur in the 14 days of watchful waiting after the initial bleeding. Delayed ischemia occurs in the first week after bleeding or after an intracranial procedure (116). With microsurgical techniques, excellent anesthesia with controlled hypotension, and previous placement of extracranial-intracranial bypass when required have made direct attack on the offending lesion less risky than in the past. While guidelines for deciding between medical and surgical therapy and at what point the latter should be carried out, are not precise, a surgical therapy should be strongly considered except in severely damaged patients. Medical management can be used either in conjunction with (i.e., needing) or in place of surgical therapy. There is a trend to perform surgical procedures earlier than in previous years, as soon as possible after the bleeding in some instances. Hori and Suzuki (116a) report no post-operative deaths in patients operated within 48 hours after bleeding. The basic premise of medical therapy is bed rest.

The method used in the Cooperative Aneurysm Program is reported by Nibbelink (117). The following features were included:

1. Hospitalization for at least three weeks, with bed rest early with subdued lighting and stimulation.
2. Head of the bed elevated no more than 30° during the first week; after first week, if necessary, patient can be helped to bedside commode.
3. Patient can turn in bed but not sit or feed self.
4. Regulation of bowel movements with stool softeners.
5. Maintenance of adequate airway and oxygenation.
6. Prophylaxis of seizures by administration of diphenylhydantoin, 100 mg t.i.d.
7. Administration of paraldehyde, phenobarbital, or chloral hydrate if sedation is required for restlessness.
8. Fluid intake of 1,800–2,000 ml/24 hr.
9. Intake of 1,000 calories/24 hr.
10. Condom drainage in men and catheter drainage in women, for patients with incontinence.
11. Analgesia by administration of acetylsalicylic acid, codeine, or meperidene HCl.
12. No agents, such as osmotic diuretics, corticosteroids or similar medications.
13. Appropriate treatment for hypertension.
14. Appropriate nursing care, with regular assessment of vital and neurologic signs.

Bed rest is the feature common to all plans, although the length of time varies; it may be as long as six weeks in some plans (118). Surgical therapy may then be applied. The routine prophylaxis against seizures is not used universally, although anticonvulsant treatment is instituted whenever seizure activity occurs.

Coexisting hypertension should be treated appropriately. In addition, the cooperative plan (117) suggests hypotensive therapy until a moderate degree of response is achieved. Blood pressure is reduced by use of drugs familiar to the attending physician. Depending on baseline levels of systolic blood pressure, the goals in blood pressure are as follows:

1. 20% reduction when actual blood pressure is less than 140 mm Hg.
2. 25% reduction when blood pressure is between 140 and 180 mm Hg.
3. 30% reduction when blood pressure exceeds 180 mm Hg.

Slosberg (119) has suggested a more severe reduction in blood pressure, to a level 30 mm Hg greater than the critical level, which is defined as the level at which symptoms of brain ischemia appear (e.g., dizziness, poor vision, disorientation). This treatment has not been used widely.

Two specific complications of aneurysmal hemorrhage are rebleeding and spasm. The former has been treated by antifibrinolytic therapy, while treatment for the latter remains dubious.

Antifibrinolytic Therapy

Because the highest incidence of rebleeding occurs between six and 11 days after the initial bleeding, which is coincident with the period when fibrinolysis is most active, antifibrinolytic therapy has been suggested for ruptured aneurysms (120). The strength of the thrombus in an experimental aneurysm model has been demonstrated to be stronger after antifibrinolytic therapy with ε-aminocaproic acid (EACA) or tranexamic acid (121).

In the cooperative study on SAH (122), patients who were treated with the bed-rest regime had a rebleeding rate of 20.9% at 14 days after the most recent bleeding and a mortality of 20.9% by the end of the 14-day period. In patients treated with antifibrinolytic therapy, the rebleeding rate was 12.7% at 14 days and mortality was 11.4% by the end of 14 days after the most recent bleeding. Patients who receive EACA, 30 g/day IV appeared to be in better condition than those who received a lower dosage or a similar one by the oral route. Nibbelink (122) states that the best results are obtained with the following regimen: 18 g EACA in 400 ml 5% dextrose in water every 12 hours in a continuous IV infusion for 10 days; then oral therapy of 3 g every two hours. This dosage is maintained until surgery is performed. If surgery is not performed, the therapy should be continued for three weeks after the most recent bleeding; then the dose is reduced to 2 g every two hours for three days, and then to 1 g every two hours for three days. After this the medication is discontinued.

A recent report by Chowdhary and colleagues (123) on treatment of SAH with EACA gives a rebleeding rate of only 4% in patients treated with the drug and 27% in patients not treated with the drug. The early mortality was 1% in treated and 12% in untreated patients. Park (124) has reported an increased incidence of post-SAH communicating hydrocephalus, from 16% before EACA therapy to 43% after EACA therapy became available.

Nibbelink (122) reported that some investigators gave tranexamic acid, 8–16 g/24 hr IV, followed (time not stated) by an oral preparation. Tranexamic acid, which is another antifibrinolytic agent, has been reported to be useful in treatment of SAH (125–127). Maurice-Williams (127) randomly divided 50 low-risk patients with ruptured aneurysm into control and treated groups. Both groups were given with bed rest and sedation; the treated group also received tranexamic acid twice a day. Maurice-Williams concluded that rebleeding was higher (56%) in the control group than in the treated group (24%); with fatal rebleeding in the two groups was 40% and 12%, respectively. In this study, the survival rate in nonoperated patients was 42% (8 of 19) in the control group and 81% (13 of 16) in the treated group. Fibrin-degradation products (FDP) can be measured in the CSF and generally are normal (i.e., absent) a few days after the start of therapy. Delayed progressive neurologic deterioration was associated with a secondary rise in CSF FDP in patients who already were obtunded and in whom large clots did not dissolve. The incidence of communicating hydrocephalus apparently was not increased during the time of observation.

van Rossum et al. (128) concluded that tranexamic acid was of no value in prevention of rebleeding or reduction of mortality (twenty-two percent of their patients did not undergo angiography because of their poor condition or because of the effects of anticoagulant therapy. An additional 22% did not have an aneurysm on angiography. These factors may have a bearing on the interpretation of their results.) They studied 51 patients in double-blind fashion. Of the drug-treated group (26 patients), five (19%) had episodes of rebleeding (four fatal). Of the control group (25), four (16%) had episodes of rebleeding (three fatal). This difference is not significant. In another large, recent series, antifibrinolytic therapy was not used (129).

Antispasmodic Therapy

Perhaps as many as one third of patients with SAH suffer from vasospasm which causes focal or diffuse ischemia (116). Treatment for this condition has not been clearly effectual.

Because it dilates peripheral arteries, isoproterenol was used in conjunction with lidocaine, which reduces the accompanying cardiac irregularities. The preliminary results were encouraging (130). Zervas (131) administered reserpine and kanamycin, which reduce vasospasm by reducing serotonin. He reported that deaths from spasm was 40% in untreated subjects and 12% in treated subjects.

Nitroglycerin has been noted to reduce vasospasm in experimental studies (132) and R.M. Crowell (personal communication) reported similar findings in one patient.

PARENCHYMATOUS HEMORRHAGE

Spontaneous acute cerebral and cerebellar hemorrhage are treated according to the general principles for ill patients. Under certain circumstances surgical therapy is useful. In the past, diagnosis depended on the finding of bloody CSF and the clinical picture. CT scanning enables the diagnosis to be made with greater precision.

Cerebellar hemorrhage presents as an acute symptom complex of varying degrees of severity. Nausea and vomiting, headache, dizziness, and truncal ataxia occur early; ataxic gait and limbs on one side with ipsilateral peripheral facial palsy, ipsilateral gaze palsy, and nystagmus are found (133). Stupor and coma may supervene in several days, or patients may have stupor and signs of brain-stem dysfunction, particularly external ophthalmoplegia. Early evacuation of the hemorrhage has been recommended (133). Patients with moderate deficits and stable course can be treated with general care and do not require an operation.

Cerebral hemorrhage appears as an acute symptom complex, also of varying degree, consisting of focal cerebral deficits and headache. The bleeding usually is located in the basal ganglia and frequently causes severe neurologic loss, including stupor and coma. Occasionally the hemorrhage lies near the surface of the cerebrum and can be surgically drained. Generally, only supportive medical care is required.

REHABILITATION

For all patients who suffer a stroke, the need for rehabilitation must be reviewed and appropriate plans made. It is asserted that rehabilitation is effective (135,136). Since the manifestations of stroke vary, so must the rehabilitation requirements of different patients. For patients with minimal neurologic deficit, little or no rehabilitation is required, and perhaps only a review of employment requirements is needed. For patients with more severe deficits, such as hemiplegia, rehabilitation should aim to return the patient to as close to the prestroke status as possible. Of particular importance is independence in walking and in the activities of daily living.

Rehabilitation measures should start as soon as possible after the occurrence of cerebral infarction or hemorrhage. Passive movements of the affected limbs and proper positioning at rest are instituted. Each joint is put through its range of movement at least three times a day. When the medical conditions are stabilized, plans for a more formal rehabilitation program should be formulated. A stroke rehabilitation program is an ideal goal and should be considered in most hospitals. The type of unit, the location, the goals, and the comprehensiveness will vary from hospital to hospital as dictated by need and resources. Whether a hospital should or should not have a "stroke unit" is a local option. Patients who are critically ill can be cared for as easily in a general medical intensive care unit as in one directed solely toward management of patients with cerebral lesions. Similarly, during prolonged rehabilitation, stroke patients can reside in a mixed medical ward, in a rehabilitation ward with patients who have various disabilities, or in a stroke unit.

The most important factor for successful therapy is the personnel and their dedication. Many individuals participate in the care and rehabilitation of stroke patients. Responsibility must be clearly defined and, in my opinion, is best handled by a physician, since these patients have medical needs other than those related to stroke. A successful program is based on clear communication between therapists and the patient and family, with continuous participation of all parties.

When available, a physiatrist prescribes and supervises specialized treatment. Ideally, the physiatrist will be associated with a physical therapy technologist, who will perform day to day retraining and carry out recommended therapeutic program. The program should deal with such aspects of daily living as transfers (e.g., from bed to chair), dressing, use of a wheelchair and walking (alone or aided). Feigenson (135) reports that, on discharge from a rehabilitation unit, approximately 85% of patients are ambulatory and about 55% are independent in self-care.

Rehabilitation must be applied with a clear understanding of goals and what can reasonably be expected.

REFERENCES

1. Stallones RA, Dyken ML, Fang HCH, et al: Epidemiology for stroke facilities planning. Stroke 3:360–371, 1972.
2. Kurtzke JF: Epidemiology of cerebrovascular disease. In: *Cerebrovascular Survey Report for Joint Council Subcommittee on Cerebrovascular Disease, NINCDS and NHLI, PHS*. Edited by RG Siekert, Whiting Press, Rochester, MN, 1976, pp. 213–242.
3. Whisnant JP, Fitzgibbons JP, Kurland LT, et al: Natural history of stroke in Rochester, Minnesota, 1945 through 1954. Stroke 2:11–12, 1971.
4. Soltero I, Liu K, Cooper R, et al: Trends in mortality from cerebrovascular disease in the United States, 1960 to 1975. Stroke 9:549–555, 1978.
5. Haberman S, Capildeo R, Rose FC: The changing mortality of cerebrovascular disease. Q J Med 47:71–88, 1978.
6. Garraway WM, Whisnant JP, Furland AJ, et al: The declining incidence of stroke. N Engl J Med 300:449–452, 1979.
7. Kannel WB: Current status of the epidemiology of brain infarction associated with occlusive arterial disease. Stroke 2:295–318, 1971.
8. Veterans Administration Cooperative Study Group on Antihypertensive Agents: Effects of treatment on morbidity in hypertension: results in patients with diastolic blood pressures averaging 115 through 129 mm Hg. JAMA 202:1028–1034, 1967.
9. American Heart Association, Council on Cerebrovascular Disease: Risk factors in stroke due to cerebral infarction. Stroke 2:423–428, 1971.
10. Armstrong ML: Evidence of regression of atherosclerosis in primates and man. Postgrad Med J 52:456–461, 1976.
11. Toole JF, Yuson CP, Janeway R, et al: Transient ischemic attacks: a prospective study of 225 patients. Neurology 28:746–753, 1978.
12. Siekert RG, Millikan CH, Whisnant JP: Anticoagulant therapy in intermittent cerebrovascular insufficiency. Follow-up data. JAMA 176:19–22, 1961.
13. Cartlidge NEF, Whisnant JP, Elveback LR: Carotid and vertebral-basilar transient cerebral ischemic attacks: a community study, Rochester, Minnesota. Mayo Clin Proc 52:117–120, 1977.
14. Baker RN, Ramseyer JC, Schwartz WS: Prognosis in patients with transient cerebral ischemic attacks. Neurology 18:1157–1165, 1968.
15. Matsumoto N, Whisnant JP, Kurland LT, et al: Natural history of stroke in Rochester, Minnesota, 1955 through 1969: an extension of a previous study, 1945 through 1954. Stroke 4:20–29, 1973.
16. Vessey MP, Doll R: Investigation of relation between use of oral contraceptives and thromboembolic disease: a further report. Br Med J 2:651–657, 1969.
17. Collaborative Group for the Study of Stroke in Young Women: Oral contraception and increased risk of cerebral ischemia or thrombosis. N Engl J Med 288:871–878, 1973.
18. Horenstein S: Oral contraceptives, stroke, and related phenomena (parts I and II). Curr Conc Cerebrovasc Dis Stroke 10:25–33, 1975.
19. Collaborative Group for the Study of Stroke in Young Women: Oral contraceptives and stroke in young women: associated risk factors. JAMA 23:718–722, 1975.
20. Whisnant JP, Matsumoto N, Elveback LR: Transient cerebral ischemic attacks in a community, Rochester, Minnesota, 1955 through 1969. Mayo Clin Proc 48:194–198, 1973.
21. Friedman GD, Wilson WS, Mosier JM, et al: Transient ischemic attacks in a community. JAMA 210:1428–1434, 1969.
22. Committee on Cerebrovascular Diseases: A classification and outline of cerebrovascular diseases II. Stroke 6:564–616, 1975.
23. Didisheim P, Fuster V: Actions and clinical status of platelet-suppressive agents. Semin Hematol 15:55–72, 1978.

24. Ross R, Glomset J, Harker L: Response to injury and atherogenesis. Am J Pathol 86:675–684, 1977.
25. Weiss HJ, Aledort LM: Impaired platelet/connective-tissue reaction in man after aspirin ingestion. Lancet 2:495–497, 1967.
26. Zucker MB, Peterson J: Effect of acetylsalicylic acid, other nonsteroidal anti-inflammatory agents and dipyridamole on human platelets. J Lab Clin Med 76:66–75, 1970.
27. Weiss HJ, Aledort LM, Kochwa S: The effect of salicylates on the hemostatic properties of platelets in man. J Clin Invest 47:2169–2180, 1968.
28. Smith JB, Willis AL: Aspirin selectively inhibits prostaglandin production in human platelets. Nature 231:235, 1971.
29. al-Mondhiry H, Marcus AJ, Spaet TH: On the mechanism of platelet function inhibition by acetylsalicylic acid. Proc Soc Exp Biol Med 133:632–636, 1970.
30. Emmons PR, Harrison MJG, Honour AJ, et al: Effect of dipyradamole on human platelet behaviour. Lancet 2:603–606, 1965.
31. McDonald JWD, Ali M, Nagai GR, et al: Inhibition of platelet prostaglandin synthetase and platelet release reaction of sulfinpyrazone. Blood 46:1033, 1975.
32. Dyken ML, Kolar OJ, Jones FH: Differences in the occurrence of carotid transient ischemic attacks associated with antiplatelet aggregation therapy. Stroke 4:732–736, 1973.
33. Evans G: Effect of drugs that suppress platelet surface interaction on incidence of amaurosis fugax and transient cerebral ischemia. Surg Forum 23:239–241, 1972.
34. Fields WS, Lemak NA, Frankowski RF, et al: Controlled trial of aspirin in cerebral ischemia. Stroke 8:301–316, 1977.
35. Fields WS, Lemak NA, Frankowski RF, et al: Controlled trial of aspirin in cerebral ischemia. II. Surgical group. Stroke 9:309–319, 1978.
36. Canadian Cooperative Study Group: A randomized trial of aspirin and sulfinpyrazone in threatened stroke. N Engl J Med 299:53–59, 1978.
37. Steele P, Carroll J, Overfield D, et al: Effect of sulfinpyrazone on platelet survival time in patients with transient cerebral attacks. Stroke 8:396–398, 1977.
38. Sullivan JM, Harken DE, Gorlin R: Pharmacologic control of thromboembolic complications of cardiac-valve replacement. N Engl J Med 284:1391–1394, 1971.
39. Salzman EW, Dykin D, Shapiro RM, et al: Management of heparin therapy. Controlled prospective trial. N Engl J Med 292:1046–1050, 1975.
40. Glazier, RL, Crowell EB: Randomized prospective trial of continuous vs. intermittent heparin therapy. JAMA 236:1365–1367, 1976.
41. Wessler S: Prevention of venous thromboembolism by low-dose heparin: a 1976 status report. Mod Concepts Cardiovasc Dis 9:105–109, 1976.
42. Parkin TW, Kvale WF: Neutralization of the anticoagulant effects of heparin with protamine (salmine). Am Heart J 37:338–342, 1949.
43. Koch–Weser J: Drug interactions in cardiovascular therapy. Am Heart J 90:93–116, 1975.
44. O'Reilly RA, Aggeler PM: Determinants of the response to oral anticoagulant drugs in man. Pharmacol Rev 22:35–96, 1970.
45. MacLeod SM, Sellers EM: Pharmacodynamic and phamacokinetic drug interactions with coumarin anticoagulants. Drugs 11:461–470, 1976.
46. Douglas AS: *Anticoagulant Therapy.* Oxford: Blackwell Scientific Publications, 1964, p. 249.
47. Jones HR Jr Siekert RG, Geraci JE: Neurologic manifestations of bacterial endocarditis. Ann Intern Med 71:21–28, 1969.
48. Siekert RG, Jones HR Jr: Transient cerebral ischemic attacks associated with subacute bacterial endocarditis. Stroke 1:178–183, 1970.
49. Wilson WR, Geraci JE, Danielson GK, et al: Anticoagulant therapy and central nervous system complications in patients with prosthetic valve endocarditis. Circulation 57:1004–1007, 1978.
50. Eastcott HG, Pickering GW, Rob CG: Reconstruction of internal carotid artery in a patient with intermittent attacks of hemiplegia. Lancet 2:994–996, 1954.

51. West H, Burton R, Roon AJ, et al: Comparative risk of operation and expectant management for carotid artery disease. Stroke 10:117–121, 1979.

52. Easton JD, Sherman DG: Stroke and mortality rate in carotid endarterectomy: 228 consecutive operations. Stroke 8:565–568, 1977.

53. Yasargil MG: Anastomosis between the superficial temporary artery and a branch of the middle cerebral artery. In: *Microsurgery Applied to Neurosurgery.* Edited by MG Yasargil, Stuttgart, George Thieme Verlag, 1969, pp. 105–115.

54. Samson DS, Boone S: Extracranial-intracranial (EC-IC) arterial bypass: past performance and current concepts. Neurosurgery 3:79–86, 1978.

55. Spetzler RF: Extracranial-intracranial arterial anastomosis for cerebrovascular disease. Surg Neurol 11:157–161, 1979.

56. Reichman OH: Extracranial-intracranial arterial anastomosis. In: *Cerebral Vascular Diseases: Ninth Conference.* Edited by JP Whisnant and BA Sandok. New York, Grune and Stratton, 1975, pp. 175–185.

57. Hodge CJ, Gross CE: Cerebral revascularization. Acta Neurochir (Wien) 44:115–130, 1978.

58. Sundt TM Jr, Siekert RG, Piepgras DG, et al: Bypass surgery for vascular disease of the carotid system. Mayo Clin Proc 51:677–692, 1976.

59. Caplan LR, Sergay S: Positional cerebral ischaemia. J Neurol Neurosurg Psychiatry 39:385–391, 1976.

60. Ziegler DK, Zileli T, Dick A, et al: Correlation of bruit over carotid artery with angiographically demonstrated lesions. Neurology 21:860–865, 1971.

61. Ackerman RH: A perspective on non-invasive diagnosis of carotid disease. Neurology 29:615–622, 1979.

62. Wolf PA, Kannel WB, Gordon T, et al: Asymptomatic arotid bruit and risk of stroke: the Framingham study (abstract). Fourth Joint Meeting on Stroke and Cerebral Circulation. Stroke 10:96, 1979.

63. Thompson JE, Patman RD, Talkington CM: Asymptomatic carotid bruit: long-term outcome of patients having endarterectomy compared with unoperated controls. Ann Surg 188:308–316, 1978.

64. Cervantes FD, Schneiderman LJ: Anticoagulants in cerebrovascular disease: a critical review of studies. Arch Intern Med 135:875–877, 1975.

65. Brust JCM: Transient ischemic attacks: natural history and anticoagulation. Neurology 27:701–707, 1977.

66. Millikan CH, McDowell FH: Treatment of transient ischemic attacks. Stroke 9:299–308, 1978.

67. Siekert RG, Whisnant JP, Millikan CH: Surgical and anticoagulant therapy of occlusive cerebral vascular disease. Ann Intern Med 58:637–641, 1963.

68. Riles TS, Kopelman I, Imparato AM: Myocardial infarction following carotid endarterectomy: a review of 683 operations. Surgery 85:249–252, 1979.

69. Siekert RG, Reagan TJ: Clinical and pathologic correlations in ischemic cerebrovascular disease. Cardiovasc Clin 5:311–325, 1973.

70. Mehigan JT, Buch WS, Pyskin RD, et al: A planned approach to coexistent cerebrovascular disease in coronary artery bypass candidates. Arch Surg 112:1403–1409, 1977.

71. Goldstone J: Discussion. In Mehigan JT, Bush WS, Pyskin RD: A planned approach to coexistent cerebrovascular disease in coronary artery bypass candidates. Arch Surg 112:1403–1409, 1977.

72. Ennix CL Jr, Lowrie GM, Morris GL Jr, et al: Improved results of carotid endarterectomy in patients with symptomatic coronary disease: an analysis of 1546 consecutive carotid operations. Stroke 10:122–125, 1979.

73. Ford JJ Jr, Baker WH, Ehrenhaft JL: Carotid endarterectomy for nonhemispheric transient ischemic attacks. Arch Surg 110:1314–1317, 1975.

74. McNamara JO, Heyman A, Silver D, et al: The value of carotid endarterectomy in treating transient cerebral ischemia of the posterior circulation. Neurology 27:682–684, 1977.

75. Anderson DC, Cranford RE: Corticosteroids in ischemic stroke. Stroke 10:68–71, 1979.

76. Dyken M, White PT: Evaluation of cortisone in the treatment of cerebral infarction. JAMA 162:1531–1534, 1956.
77. Bauer RB, Tellez H: Dexamethasone as treatment in cerebrovascular disease. 2. A controlled study in acute cerebral infarction. Stroke 4:547–555, 1973.
78. Mulley G, Wilcox RG, Mitchell JRA: Dexamethasone in acute stroke. Br Med J 2:994–996, 1978.
79. Meyer JS, Charney JZ, Rivera VM, et al: Treatment with glycerol of cerebral oedema due to acute cerebral infarction. Lancet 2:993–997, 1971.
80. Mathew NT, Meyer JS, Rivera VM: Double-blind evaluation of glycerol therapy in acute cerebral infarction. Lancet 2:1327–1329, 1972.
81. Gilsanz V, Rebollar JL, Buencuerpo J, et al: Controlled trial of glycerol versus dexamethasone in the treatment of cerebral oedema in acute cerebral infarction. Lancet 1:1049–1051, 1975.
82. Gilroy J, Barnhart MI, Meyer JS: Treatment of acute stroke with dextran 40. JAMA 210:293–298, 1969.
83. Woolard ML, Pearson RM, Dorf D, et al: Controlled trial of ornithine alpha ketoglutarate (OAKG) in patients with stroke. Stroke 9:218–222, 1978.
84. Admani AK: New approach to treatment of recent stroke. Br Med J 2:1678–1679, 1978.
85. Christensen MS, Paulson OB, Olesen J, et al: Cerebral apoplexy (stroke) treated with or without prolonged artificial hyperventilation. 1. Cerebral circulation, clinical course, and cause of death. Stroke 4:568–619, 1973.
86. Levy DE, Brierley JB: Delayed pentobarbital administration limits ischemic brain damage in gerbils. Ann Neurol 5:59–64, 1979.
87. Mosley JI, Laurent JP, Molinari GF: Barbiturate attenuation of the clinical course and pathologic lesions in a primate stroke model. Neurology 25:870–874, 1975.
88. Michenfelder JD, Milde JH, Sundt TM Jr: Cerebral protection by barbiturate anesthesia. Use after middle cerebral artery occlusion in Java monkeys. Arch Neurol 33:345–350, 1976.
89. Yatsu FM, Diamond I, Graziano C, et al: Experimental brain ischemia: protection from irreversible damage with a rapid-acting barbiturate (methohexitol). Stroke 3:726–732, 1972.
90. Nemoto EM, Kofke WA, Kessler P, et al: Studies on the pathogenesis of ischemic brain damage and the mechanism of its amelioration by thiopental. Acta Med Scand 57[Suppl 64]:72–73, 1977.
91. Fisher CM: The arterial lesions underlying lacunes. Acta Neuropathol (Berl) 12:1–15, 1969.
92. Fisher CM, Curry HB: Pure motor hemiplegia of vascular origin. Arch Neurol 13:30, 1965.
93. Fisher CM: Pure sensory stroke involving face, arm and leg. Neurology 15:76, 1965.
94. Fisher CM: Ataxic hemiparesis: a pathologic study. Arch Neurol 35:126–128, 1978.
95. Weisberg LA: Computed tomography and pure motor hemiparesis. Neurology 29:490–495, 1979.
96. Sypert GW, Alvord EC Jr: Cerebellar infarction: clinicopathological study. Arch Neurol 32:357–363, 1975.
97. Feely MP, Dempsey PJ: Acute cerebellar infarction—a surgical emergency (abstract). Stroke 9:96, 1978.
98. Paulson GW, Boesel CP, Evans WE: Fibromuscular dysplasia. Arch Neurol 35:287–290, 1978.
99. Paulson GW: Fibromuscular dysplasia, antiovulant drugs and ergot preparations. Stroke 9:172, 1978.
100. Karasawa J, Kikuchi H, Furuse S, et al: Treatment of moyamoya disease with STA–MCA anastomosis. J Neurosurg 49:679–688, 1978.
101. Russell MO, Goldberg HI, Reis L, et al: Transfusion therapy for cerebrovascular abnormalities in sickle cell disease. J Pediatr 88:382–387, 1976.
102. Wolf PA, Dawber TR, Thomas HE Jr, Kannel WB: Epidemiologic assessment of chronic atrial fibrillation and risk of stroke: the Framingham study. Neurology 28:973–977, 1978.
103. McDevitt E: Treatment of cerebral embolism. Mod Treatment 2:52, 1965.

104. Meyer JS, Charney JZ, Rivera VM, et al: Cerebral embolization: prospective clinical analysis of 42 cases. Stroke 2:541–554, 1971.

105. Carter AB: Prognosis of cerebral embolism. Lancet 2:514–519, 1965.

106. Wilson WR, Geraci JE, Danielson GK, et al: Anticoagulant therapy and central nervous system complications in patients with prosthetic valve endocarditis. Circulation 57:1004–1007, 1978.

107. Desousa AL, Muller J, Campbell RL, et al: Atrial myxoma: a review of the neurological complications, metastases, and recurrences. J Neurol Neurosurg Psychiatry 41:1119–1124, 1978.

108. Arnar O, Schmidt WR, Garamella JJ, et al: Left atrial myxoma: surgical experience. Minn Med 61:532–533, 1978.

109. Barnett HJM, Jones MW, Boughner DR, et al: Cerebral ischemic events associated with prolapsing mitral valve. Arch Neurol 33:777–782, 1976.

110. Hirsowitz GS, Saffer D: Hemiplegia and the billowing mitral leaflet syndrome. J Neurol Neurosurg Psychiatry 41:381–383, 1978.

111. Watson RT: TIA stroke, and mitral valve prolapse. Neurology 29:886, 1979.

112. Fauci AS, Haynes BF, Katz P: The spectrum of vasculitis: clinical, pathologic, immunologic, and therapeutic considerations. Ann Intern Med 89:660–676, 1978.

113. Lande A, Bard R, Bole P, et al: Aortic arch syndrome (Takayasu's arteritis). Arteriographic and surgical considerations. J Cardiovasc Surg (Torino) 19:507–513, 1978.

114. McKissock W, Richardson A, Walsh L: 'Anterior communicating' aneurysms: trial of conservative and surgical treatment. Lancet 1:873–876, 1965.

115. Botterell EH, Lougheed WM, Scott JW, et al: Hypothermia and interruption of carotid or carotid and vertebral circulation in the surgical management of intracranial aneurysms. J Neurosurg 13:1–42, 1956.

116. Fisher CM, Robertson GH, Ojemann RG: Cerebral vasospasm after ruptured aneurysm—the clinical manifestations. Neurosurgery 1:245–248, 1977.

116a. Hori S, Suzuki J: Early intracranial operations for ruptured aneurysms. Acta Neurochirurgica 46:93–104, 1979.

117. Nibbelink DW, Torner JC, Henderson WG: Intracranial aneurysms and subarachnoid hemorrhage—report on a randomized treatment study. IV–A. Regulated bed rest. Stroke 8:202–218, 1977.

118. Post KD, Flamm ES, Goodgold A, et al: Ruptured intracranial aneurysms: case morbidity and mortality. J Neurosurg 46:290–295, 1977.

119. Slosberg P: Hypotensive therapy of acute intracranial hemorrhage: further studies. Mt Sinai J Med (NY) 26:553–561, 1959.

120. Norlen G, Thulin CA: Experiences with epsilon-aminocaproic acid in neurosurgery. Neurochirurugica (Stuttg) 10:81–86, 1967.

121. Patterson RH, Harpel P: The effect of epsilon-aminocaproic acid and tranexamic acid on thrombus size and strength in a simulated arterial aneurysm. J Neurosurg 34:363–371, 1971.

122. Nibbelink DW, Torner JC, Henderson WG: Intracranial aneurysms and subarachnoid hemorrhage. A cooperative study. Antifibrinolytic therapy in recent onset subarachnoid hemorrhage. Stroke 6:622–629, 1975.

123. Chowdhary UM, Carey PC, Hussein MM: Prevention of early recurrence of spontaneous subarachnoid hemorrhage byepsilon-aminocaproic acid. Lancet 1:741–743, 1979.

124. Park BE: Spontaneous subarachnoid hemorrhage complicated by communicating hydrocephalus: epsilon-aminocaproic acid as a possible predisposing factor. Surg Neurol 11:73–80, 1979.

125. Tovi D, Nilsson JM, Thulin C-A: Fibrinolysis and SAH inhibitory effect of tranexamic acid. Acta Neurol Scand 48:.393–402, 1972.

126. Maurice-Williams RS: Prolonged antifibrinolysis: an effective non-surgical treatment for ruptured intracranial aneurysms. Br Med J 1:945–947, 1978.

127. Fodstad H, Liliquist B, Schannong M, et al: Tranexamic acid in the preoperative management of ruptured intracranial aneurysms. Surg Neurol 10:9–15, 1978.

128. van Rossum J, Wintzen AR, Endtz LJ, et al: Effect of tranexamic acid on rebleeding after subarachnoid hemorrhage: a double-blind controlled clinical trial. Ann Neurol 2:242–245, 1977.

129. Sundt TM Jr, Whisnant JP: Subarachnoid hemorrhage from intracranial aneurysms: surgical management and natural history of disease. N Engl J Med 299:116–122, 1978.

130. Sundt TM Jr, Onofrio BM, Merideth J: Treatment of cerebral vasospasm from subarachnoid hemorrhage with isoproterenol and lidocaine hydrochloride. J Neurosurg 38:557–560, 1973.

131. Zervas N: Medical News Section. JAMA 240:2143, 1978.

132. Kistler JP, Lees RS, Candia G, et al: Intravenous nitroglycerin in experimental cerebral vasospasm. A preliminary report. Stroke 10:26–29, 1979.

133. Ott KH, Kasess C, Ojemann RG, et al: Cerebellar hemorrhage: diagnosis and treatment: a review of 56 cases. Acta Neurol 31:160–167, 1974.

134. Greenberg J, Shubick D, Shenkin H: Acute hydrocephalus in cerebellar infarct and hemorrhage. Neurology 29:409–413, 1979.

135. Feigenson JS, McCarthy ML, Meese PD, et al: Stroke rehabilitation: factors predicting outcome and length of stay—an overview. NY State J Med 77:1426–1430, 1977.

136. Feigenson JS: Stroke rehabilitation: effectiveness, benefits, and cost. Stroke 10:1–4, 1979.

10

Demyelinating Diseases

William A. Sibley

There is no therapy generally accepted for diseases that attack primarily the myelin sheath with relative sparing of axons. However, drug therapy has some effect on the course of these illnesses, at least in the acute stages, and a variety of new treatments are being evaluated. At the present stage of our knowledge, a regimen can be devised that will help many patients tolerate the effects of illness; such regimens include efforts to influence natural history, treat complications, maintain mobility, and deal with emotional and social problems. Multiple sclerosis (MS) is the diagnosis in the vast majority of patients with demyelinating disease and will be the subject of most of this review.

MULTIPLE SCLEROSIS

Natural Course

In approximately two-thirds of cases, MS assumes a course of exacerbation and remission in the early years. Complete improvement is almost universal after the first attack in MS patients; substantial improvement, usually beginning within 30–60 days after the onset of new symptoms, is also common with subsequent attacks. In time, however, improvement tends to be less complete, and eventually most patients—approximately 60% of this subgroup—enter a slowly progressive phase. About one-third of MS patients never have distinct exacerbations or remissions, and the disease progresses slowly from the start. Many of these patients have onset of illness after age 40 (1).

About 25% of patients have a form of illness that has been called *benign MS*. Among these patients are a number who continue in a typical exacerbation-remission pattern, but who recover well from each attack and never become seriously disabled. Others in this category have only two or three attacks of MS in a lifetime and recover from each. The benign designation also includes patients in whom all disease activity seems to cease before significant disability is manifest. The proportion of patients with relatively benign MS is reflected in the statistics of Bauer (2), who reported on the working capacity of 800 MS patients. After 20 years of illness, 28% were still actively employed.

Series of cases that include patients in the early years of the illness often report exacerbation rates of 0.5–1 attacks per patient per year. Later in the illness, exacerbations are either less frequent or more difficult to detect clinically. Thus, in the middle years of illness, attack rates of less than 0.5 per patient per year are common. In a large clinic population that includes patients with both early and advanced disease, the average exacerbation rate is similar to that in our clinic—about 0.25 attacts per patient per year.

Evaluation of Therapy

Clinical Evaluation

Theoretically, an ideal treatment of MS would prevent the exacerbations and halt progression in all stages of the illness. However, it probably would not alleviate symptoms that had been present continuously for longer than two years; such long-standing deficits are probably the result of irreversible changes in the nervous system and usually do not remit under any circumstances (3). It is likely that symptoms of shorter duration would be improved by a curative agent, but it should be emphasized that the ideal therapy would be recognized primarily by its ability to prevent worsening.

On the other hand, a totally ineffective therapy that is given to patients with recent exacerbation will be associated with marked improvement. Thus, in the National Cooperative ACTH Study in the United States, about 70% of patients with recent worsening improved with placebo treatment (4).

It is evident, therefore, that the recognition of a partially effective treatment is especially difficult in MS and requires the use of control subjects. The controls should be from the same geographic area, be of the same age, have essentially the same degree of disability, and should have been ill for about the same length of time as the treated patients. In practice, this is accomplished by randomized admission of patients to the control and treated groups. Treated and control subjects then are observed for various periods with use of standardized methods of clinical evaluation and scoring forms, until statistically significant conclusions can be reached.

The difficulties involved in undertaking such a controlled treatment trial are many. Unless the therapeutic agent is extremely effective (which has not yet been achieved), large numbers of patients have to be studied; this often means a cooperative effort involving many different centers, Such efforts are time consuming and expensive and require frequent communication among centers to ensure that uniform methods of clinical evaluation are being used (5). In spite of these problems, however, one must count among the recent advances a widespread recognition that controlled treatment trials are essential to definitive evaluation of therapy for MS. It has now been demonstrated that large-scale controlled trials can be successful, even in a disease as variable as MS (4).

An alternative to the controlled trial of therapy, which is more suitable for pilot studies in smaller groups of patients, is testing of the ability of an agent to prevent exacerbations. This method has the disadvantage of not recognizing treatments that may be modestly effective and probably would not be considered suitable if there were compelling theoretical reasons to expect benefit. However, if the empirical search for an effective remedy is to continue, this method is certainly preferred. If agents that are shown incapable of preventing worsening were discarded and not regarded as suitable for repeated uncontrolled trials, then a larger number of potential therapies could be screened in a reasonable time. This method of evaluation should become increasingly useful as laboratory monitoring of disease activity becomes available.

Laboratory Evaluation

Only recently have laboratory methods become available that may make it possible to quantitate the activity of MS. McPherson et al. (6) reported a radioimmunoassay of cerebrospinal fluid (CSF) for myelin basic protein (MBP) that distinguished MS from most other neurologic diseases. Cohen et al. (7) have recently reported that almost all neurologic diseases that are not demyelinating, all healthy persons, and have CSF levels of less than 6 ng/ml; patients with MS in exacerbation usually have levels greater than 15 ng/ml; and patients in the slowly progressive phase of the illness have levels in an intermediate range (6–14 ng/ml). Technical difficulties in the accurate performance of the tests have limited their general availability; however, as these problems are overcome, the ability of a potential therapeutic agent to depress CSF levels of MBP and maintain them in a normal range might become an important adjunct to clinical evaluation.

Computerized tomography (CT) of the brain in 49 patients with MS reported by Radue and Kendall (8) revealed a normal study in 43%, cerebral atrophy in 35%, and MS plaques in 23%. It is not clear how many of these patients had symptoms suggesting recent activity. The authors emphasize that contrast enhancement is important in the identification of MS lesions, which they found to be most numerous in the parietal white matter and in the periventricular areas. Both low-attenuation lesions and isodense plaques may enhance with iodide contrast medium. A number of other reports during the past year suggest that new, often contrast-enhancing lesions may appear in the cerebral white matter concurrently with clinical evidence of other new lesions in brain stem or spinal cord, confirming a well-known tendency for new lesions to occur simultaneously in several different areas (9–14).

Figure 1 reproduces the CT scan of a 52-year-old patient with far-advanced MS of 20 years' duration (Kurtzke disability status score, 8); five days before the first CT scan, she developed a new internuclear ophthalmoplegia, indicating a lesion in the pons; a contrast-enhancing right periventricular lesion is also evident on the first scan. The latter lesion no longer enhanced in a repeat scan 32 days later, but an area of low density persisted; more importantly, on the repeat scan a new enhancing lesion was seen adjacent to the superior surface of the posterior body of the left lateral ventricle. This patient did not receive corticosteroids or other treatment.

Further studies are needed to determine how often such evidently active lesions appear in MS patients and whether they can be monitored directly by CT scanning. It is not clear what the natural time course of such enhancing lesions is;

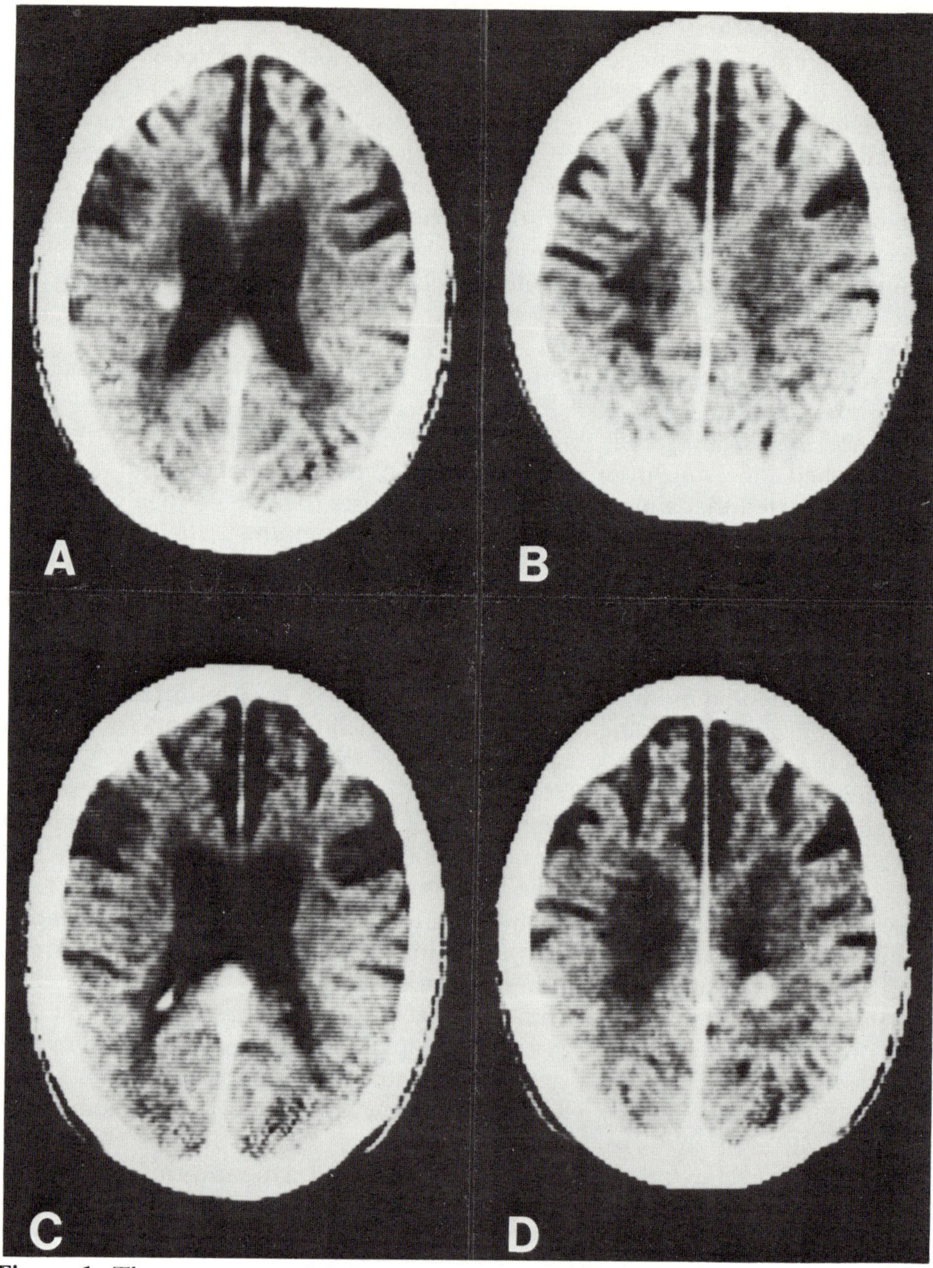

Figure 1. The appearance and disappearance of contrast-ehhancing periventricular lesions on the CT scan of an MS patient over a 32-day period, without treatment. (*a,b*) Sections of the first scan showing an enhancing lesion in the wall of the right lateral ventricle (*a*); (*c, d*) Comparable cuts taken 32 days later. The enhancement seen on the right is no longer evident, but a new enhancing lesion has appeared in the wall of the left lateral ventricle (*d*).

nontheless, it seems likely that CT scanning will play a major role in future treatment trials for MS. Patients in the later stages of the illness, who often have not been suitable for participation in treatment trials in the past because of the difficulty in clinical detection of new lesions, may be able to participate now that this objective form of measurement is available. This may speed the testing of new therapies, and the ability of a therapeutic agent to prevent new lesions visible on CT scanning would be impressive.

Efforts to Influence Natural History

Most therapeutic measures that are aimed at changing the natural history of the disease can be classified into four categories. The first is *general immunosuppression* and includes use of such medications as corticotropin (adrenocorticotropic hormone [ACTH]), synthetic adrenal glucocorticoids, cyclophosphamide, and azathioprine. Plasmapheresis is a procedure that probably also belongs in this category. Second, recent efforts have been made to produce *specific immunosuppression* by giving inoculations with MBP. The third category includes agents intended to produce varying forms of *immune enhancement.* These include levamisole, blood and plasma transfusions, immunoglobulins, interferon, and transfer factor. The fourth category includes *miscellaneous therapies* such as dietary treatment and hyperbaric oxygen.

General Immunosuppression

Immunosuppressive treatment of MS finds its rationale both in the pathologic similarities between MS and allergic encephalomyelitis (EAE) in humans and animals and in the fact that EAE can be modified or prevented by immunosuppressive drugs. EAE in humans previously developed as an infrequent complication of old rabies vaccines that contained nervous tissue. Uchimura and Shiraki (15) have demonstrated the striking pathologic similarities between EAE and acute MS; in both illnesses, lesions tend to occur around large veins and in the walls of cerebral ventricles.

MBP, one of the principal proteins of myelin, is capable of producing in animals an acute perivenous demyelinating disease when combined with Freund's complete adjuvant. In some respects, this disease resembles acute perivenous encephalomyelitis in humans and acute MS. Animals injected intracutaneously with MBP and Freund's complete adjuvant usually become ill about the eleventh day, and there is variable paralysis and mortality, depending on species and other factors.

The pathologic similarities between MS and EAE are more striking in the case of chronic relapsing EAE, which can be induced in similar manner in young strain-13 guinea pigs. In this form of EAE, there is a longer latent period between induction and illness (often eight to 12 weeks), but the animals recover and relapse repeatedly over a long period. Pathologic examination discloses demyelinating lesions of different durations in typical locations—periventricularly, in the brain stem, and in the spinal cord (16,17).

ACTH and Adrenal Corticosteroids. The mechanisms of action of ACTH and the synthetic adrenal glucocorticoids are similar. Both cause lysis of lymphocytes and both have antiedema properties and anti-inflammatory action. Moreover, both ACTH and glucocorticoids improve conduction in demyelinated axons, possibly by increasing the efficiency of the sodium-pump mechanism in demyelinated fibers (18). The sodium-potassium-activated adenosine triphosphatase enzyme system is important in promotion of cation exchange across cell membranes and thus is important in repolarization of axonal membranes (19).

A nationwide trial of ACTH in recent exacerbations of MS 10 years ago that involved 10 university centers in the United States confirmed an earlier, British study that showed ACTH to be of some benefit in the treatment of acute relapses (4,20). The U.S. trial lasted about four years. All patients who entered the study had had an acute period of worsening during the previous eight weeks. Patients were admitted randomly to the ACTH or the placebo group, and the study was double blind. All patients were hospitalized and treated for two weeks and then were observed as outpatients for an additional two weeks. Treatment included low-sodium (800 mg) diet approximately 2,000 calories per day; all patients also received 1.0 g potassium chloride three times a day and 15 ml of a mixture of magnesium and aluminum hydroxides (Maalox) or a similar low-sodium antacid between meals and at bedtime. During the first week, each patient received 40 units of ACTH gel or placebo intramuscularly (IM) every 12 hours. For the next four days, 20 units of ACTH or placebo was given every 12 hours. During the last three hospital days, patients received 20 units of ACTH gel or placebo once a day.

Patients were evaluated by several different methods in this study. One method was recording of changes on standard neurologic examination. Another method used a scoring system to record the patient's own daily impression of the severity of individual symptoms. Still another method used a standardized quantitative neurologic examination performed in blind fashion by specially trained physical therapists. This test measured such aspects as the speed of rapid-succession movements of fingers and toes, and included pallesthesiometry, ergogaphy and other techniques of measurement.

Regardless of the method of evaluation, however, patients who received ACTH therapy fared better than the placebo-treated subjects for the first three weeks of observation. By the fourth week the differences between the groups were less evident. However, whenever a difference was seen between the groups at any time during the study, it was almost always in favor of the ACTH-treated group. The study concluded that ACTH modestly hastened the resolution of acute attacks; the estimated advantage of the hormone over placebo seemed to be in the range of 10–15%.

Because the best controlled studies have been performed with ACTH, this hormone remains the mainstay of therapy for acute exacerbations of MS. Many physicians, however now frequently substitute synthetic glucocorticoids for ACTH; prednisone and prednisolone are the glucocorticoids used most widely but some physicians prescribe more potent compounds, such as betamethasone or dexamethasone, for short-term treatment. Such short courses of therapy commonly include prednisone, 80 mg/day for three days, followed by rapid tapering of dosage over another four to seven days. All such regimens should include antacids and abstinence from aspirin, since the combination of aspirin and potent glucocorticoids predisposes the patient to peptic ulceration of the stomach and duodenum. Although there has been extensive experience with the glucocorticoids used in this manner, it should be remembered that their value has not been established by controlled studies.

Long-term moderate-dosage ACTH or glucocorticoids have been shown to be incapable of preventing exacerbations or progression of MS. For example, Millar and co-workers (21) treated 181 patients with 15–25 units of ACTH gel per day for 18 months, while 169 control subjects received placebo. The amount of ACTH given was sufficient to produce signs of hypercorticism, but the treated and control groups fared similarly with regard to MS. The results of this well-controlled study confirmed those of other studies that indicate that long-term *daily* use of adrenal corticosteroids in doses that can be tolerated without an undue complication rate do not benefit patients with MS (21).

Alexander and co-workers (22) have reported long-term high-dosage ACTH to be beneficial in reducing the relapse rate and slowing progression of MS. However, there were many more ACTH-treated patients in this series, and apparently the ACTH and control groups were not treated and evaluated concurrently. Few would attempt to repeat these trials because of the high (21–26%) rate of complications, which included psychosis, peptic ulcer, septicemia, pathologic fractures, and adrenal exhaustion (23). It seems clear both from these studies and from common clinical experience in other areas that long-term high-dosage daily therapy with ACTH or glucocorticoids is hazardous and is contraindicated except in very exceptional circumstances.

Harter et al. (24) suggested that many of the complications of long-term glucocorticoid therapy could be minimized by giving a single, relatively large dose on alternate days. Such alternate-day regimens are feasible when prednisone or prednisolone is used; they cannot be applied with glucocorticoids such as betamethasone or dexamethasone, however, because of the long duration of action of these compounds (two to four days). At present, alternate-day therapy is widely used in patients with severe MS, primarily in those who relapse promptly at the conclusion of short-term therapy. Only one, small controlled study of this form of treatment is available for guidance. In a double-blind crossover study Kibler et al. (25) compared seven patients given 80 mg prednisone in a single dose every other day with patients given placebo. The study lasted two years; patients received prednisone for 65% of the time and placebo for 35% of the time. Six of the seven exacerbations experienced by six patients occurred with placebo treatment.

Kibler and associates (26) commented on an apparent steroid dependency in this small group: the disease tended to worsen shortly after cessation of prednisone treatment. The authors showed that the worsening was not associated with laboratory evidence of adrenal insufficiency.

We, too, have been impressed by the number of patients seen in daily practice who seem to become steroid dependent: clinical evidence of disease activity often resumes when the alternate-day dose of prednisone is reduced below a certain critical level, usually 35–40mg. Such experience points out the need for a properly controlled study of alternate-day glucocorticoids. Alternate-day therapy with prednisone has been shown to be effective in myasthenia gravis, an illness with a defined immune pathogenesis; however, the fact that myasthenia gravis often responds to this regimen was overlooked by clinicians for almost two decades (26,27).

Intrathecal Methylprednisolone. For a number of years, many neurologists have treated MS with methylprednisolone acetate in a special vehicle (Depo-Medrol) in doses of 40–120 mg per intrathecal injection. Although most have abandoned this form of treatment, it continues to be used in some areas. During the 20 years that this treatment was prescribed extensively, it became apparent that it did not prevent exacerbations and that improvement was only a chance occurrence. Insignificant amounts of steroid reach the cisterna magna or cerebral ventricles; moreover, when the drug is released from its depot vehicle, it is absorbed rapidly into the blood.

The subject of intrathecal Depo-Medrol has been reviewed extensively by Nelson and colleagues (28), who point out that this therapy has been complicated by occasional adhesive arachnoiditis. In other instances, prolonged therapy has been associated with fungal and bacterial infections of the meninges.

Azathioprine and Cyclophosphamide. The fact that ACTH is at least slightly effective in MS has encouraged many investigators to use more potent immunosuppressive drugs. For the most part, however, these attempts have been disappointing.

Azathioprine (Imuran), 2–4.7 mg/kg/day for 15–24 months failed to have any advantage over placebo in two separate studies (29,30). Ellison and Myers (31) have recently reviewed the uncontrolled studies of azathioprine in MS. They note that, in seven such studies, 202 patients were treated for approximately one year: 28 patients improved, 106 were unchanged, and 68 worsened. These figures are strikingly similar to the results reported by Millar and co-workers (21) in 199 placebo-treated subjects observed for 1.5 years: 44 improved, 89 were unchanged, and 66 worsened.

Drachman and associates (32) tried cyclophosphamide (Cytoxan), 4.5 mg/kg IV for 10 days, in six consecutive cases. Given in this manner, the drug failed to prevent worsening in all six patients. In another controlled study, Millac and Miller (33), gave cyclophosphamide at a dosage of 75–100 mg orally for one year; three of their patients improved, two were unchanged, and three worsened at the end of the study period. A number of uncontrolled studies have reported benefit from use of the drug, but in several of these studies the agent was used for only a few weeks; prolonged benefit has been claimed even in the absence of maintenance therapy (31). The reported results make it doubtful that prolonged therapy with cylophosphamide is justified, especially in view of the toxicity of the drug, which can induce sterility, mutations, and cancer (34).

Intensive Nonspecific Immunosuppression. Since the results of single-drug therapy with immunosuppressants in MS have not been impressive, some investigators have elected to treat patients with multiple drugs in a more rigorous manner. Lance et al. (35) have reported on the use of prednisone, azathioprine, and horse antilymphocytic globulin (ALG) in the treatment of 14 patients over one year. Most of the patients were in the early phase of the illness, with average relapse rates before treatment of 1.4 per patient per year. During the year of intensive immunosuppression, relapse rates dropped to 0.4 per patient; moreover, when the regimen was discontinued, the relapse rate increased to 1.2 per patient per year. The treatment program included prednisone, 150 mg/day, tapered to 20 mg/day by the seventh day and continued at this dosage for one year. Azathioprine, 3 mg/kg/day for one year; and normal horse immunoglobulin G, 60 mg/kg on day 1 and 30 mg/kg on day 4. ALG, 500 mg per infusion, was introduced on day 5 with 15 infusions over a three-week period.

Although Lance et al. (35) felt that the risks of treatment were clinically acceptable, it was noted that most patients showed positive results on urine and throat cultures at some time during treatment and required antibiotics. One patient had herpes zoster, and three developed thrush. Two had anaphylactoid reactions and one had serum sickness from ALG. Duodenal ulcer with bleeding developed in one patient, and a vertebral compression fracture occurred in another. Three of the 14 patients experienced significant depression.

Phasmapheresis. The relatively recent demonstration of marked benefit from plasmapheresis in some patients with serious cases of myasthennia gravis has stimulated the use of this method in MS. For many years hthere have been periodic reports of demyelinating activity in the serum of some patients and some reports of antimyelin antibodies (36–38). More recently, antibodies to oligodendrocytes have been reported in MS patients (39).

The possibility of the removal of some of these potentially demyelinating substances from the blood by plasmapheresis certainly deserves consideration. However, it should be remembered that the pathogenetic significance of antibodies in serum of MS patients is not nearly as well documented as it is in that of myasthenia gravis patients. In fact, many studies suggest that antimyelin antibodies, in MS are relatively nonspecific and occur in other neurologic diseases as well, especially in amyotrophic lateral sclerosis (36, 38).

Dau and co-workers (40) have reported on the use of plasmapheresis in conjunction with azathioprine (3 mg/kg/day). Five patients with slowly progressive MS were treated with a series of 20 plasma exchanges performed at one- to two-week intervals; a volume equivalent to the patients' total plasma volume was exchanged each time. Supplemental gamma globulin was given after each session, and the patients received 100 mg prednisone/day for five days after each exchange. The authors reported a modest degree of improvement in areas of recent worsening, usually beginning after the third exchange. However, two temporary exacerbations occurred during the course of the treatments. No conclusions about the place of this form of treatment in MS can be drawn from this report, although the worsening during the course of therapy in two cases is sobering in light of the multiple modes of treatment that were given. Other investigators have used plasmapheresis to treat MS but have not yet reported the results, we await these with interest.

Efforts to Induce Specific Immune Suppression

In both the acute and chronic relapsing forms of EAE, the administration of MBP, either plain or mixed with Freund's *incomplete* adjuvant, is capable of either suppression or modification of EAE (41,42). The effectiveness of MBP used in this manner depends both on dosage and on the time of administration in relation to the time the disease is induced. The usefulness of MBP in prevention or treatment of EAE forms the rationale for attempts at specific immune suppression of MS. One possible theoretical problem with this approach is a lack of convincing evidence that MBP is the offending antigen in MS. Antibodies to MBP cannot be detected in sera of MS patients, even with very sensitive techniques. While lymphocyte transformation in response to MBP does occur in some patients, this response appears to be nonspecific and may be seen both in other neurologic diseases and in healthy subjects (43).

Campbell and colleagues (44) gave 5 mg human MBP 1M to 64 patients in a study that lasted about 18 months. Some patients reported subjective benefit, especially lessened fatigue, but the reported results did not allow definite conclusions. The authors suggested, however, that the effort showed no adverse effects of MBP treatment, and they recommended further efforts at this approach with higher dosages of MBP.

Gonsette et al. (45) gave 35 patients either human or bovine MBP, 5 mg/week; the average duration of therapy was 7.5 months, and all patients were observed for at least two years after the conclusion of treatment. Forty-six percent of patients suffered relapse during MBP therapy, and the treatment was promptly stopped when relapse occurred. The annual relapse rate for the group as a whole during the two years before MBP treatment was 0.75 per patient; during the two years after the conclusion of therapy, the annual relapse rate was 0.7 per patient. On the basis of these results, the investigators properly considered MBP therapy a failure.

More recently, Salk and co-workers (46) have initiated a study of the administration of much larger quantities of porcine MBP to nine patients with MS. Daily doses of MBP ranged from 0.5–3.0 mg/kg subcutaneously. Initially, the investigators had hoped that a brief, two-week course of therapy would effectively immunize the patients; however, one of the first patients treated in this manner worsened several days after MBP treatment was stopped. Since then, treatment has been given on a daily basis and has continued indefinitely; several of the patients now have been treated for at least a year and have received cumulative doses of MBP of more than 40 g (47). Larger doses were employed in this study on the basis of previous experiments with animals, which indicated that the effective suppression of EAE in guinea pigs depends on dosage, timing, and duration of treatment. The details of the results of this treatment regimen in human studies have not yet been reported.

Efforts to Enhance Immune Response

Repeated efforts to isolate infectious agents from the tissue or CSF of MS patients usually have been unsuccessful. Occasional viruses have been isolated, but it is doubtful that these are of etiologic significance, since the isolations usually were not reproducible in other cases. Suspicions that MS might be caused by a latent, defective, or slow virus have led to many attempts to enhance the immune response nonspecifically. Johnson (48) has reviewed in detail the evidence for a viral etiology of MS (49).

Efforts to transmit MS to nonhuman primates with use of brain emulsions or cultured cells from MS plaques usually have not been successful, even after many years of observation (49–51). However, a recent report by Rorke and associates (52) describes a chimpanzee who, three years after inoculation with MS explant cells, developed acute quadriplegia with demyelinating lesions in spinal cord root-entry zones and in proximal dorsal roots; there was a proliferation of Schwann cells in the lesions. The authors did not consider this to be a case of Guillain–Barré polyradiculopathy but did suggest herpesvirus as a possible cause, in view of the location of the lesions. Warren and Koprowski (53) have called attention to evidence that suggests a defective herpes simplex infection as the cause of MS.

Whole-Blood Transfusion

Alexander and colleagues (54) administered 500 ml fresh whole blood to 50 patients at weekly intervals for six weeks: 46% of the patients improved, 12% worsened, the remainder were unchanged. These results, of course, indicate no benefit in a short-term study, since the transfusions did not prevent exacerbations. However, the report indicated one other finding of interest: 14% of the patients had allergic reactions to the transfusions, as compared with only 0.4% of similar reactions in the general hospital population.

Pooled Immunoglobulins

Miller and co-workers (55) gave pooled human gamma globulin, 500 mg IM every two weeks for six months, to nine MS patients. This group fared no better than nine others, who received saline injections on the same schedule.

Transfer Factor

Transfer factor, which basically is a dialysate of disrupted lymphocytes, has been prepared from lymphocytes of non-MS patients whose lymphocytes react strongly with exposure to measles antigen. Several studies have suggested that the pathogenesis of MS may involve a defect in thymus-derived lymphocytes (T cells), especially in the response to myxovirus antigens.

Two major studies have used transfer factor in treatment of MS (56,57). Fog and collaborators (57), in Copenhagen, have recently reported the results of a long-term study of 16 treated patients and 16 untreated controls. There were no clinical differences in the two groups at the end of 13 months, even though tranfer factor increased the reactivity of lymphocytes to measles virus in the treated patients.

Levamisole

Levamisole is an immunomodulator whose mechanism of action is unknown; however, it has been shown to be capable of correcting defective cell-mediated immunity and thus of decreasing excessive production of immunoglobulin (58). Dau and co-workers (59) have reported that five of seven patients worsened during the first 12 weeks of treatment with levamisole. Ellison and Myers (31) have reviewed the uncontrolled studies of levamisole and found that of 32 treated patients, three improved, 19 were unchanged, and 10 worsened in treatment periods of usually less than one year. A double-blind placebo-controlled study by Camenga (60) and Gonsette failed to show a statistically significant difference between placebo-treated subjects and those treated with levamisole. Ellison and Myers (31) believe that levamisole probably is not useful in the treatment of MS, but they suggest that related compounds that are capable of correcting certain immune deficiencies may prove useful in the future.

Interferon

Interferon, a low-molecular-weight acid-resistant protein that is produced by virus-infected cells may protect adjoining cells from viral attack in some patients. The substance can be found in many virus-infected tissues and in serum of patients with clinical viral infections.

Formal reports of the results of interferon treatment have not been published, primarily because the substance is difficult and expensive to prepare. Interferon is not likely to benefit MS patients, since it cannot be found in the typical lesions of MS by sensitive assay methods (61).

Miscellaneous Methods

Low-Fat Diet

Swank (62) suggested that slowing of the circulation in response to ingestion of diets high in fat "sludging" of blood might play a role in the pathogenesis of MS, and he has cited worldwide evidence that MS is more common in the populations that consume excessive amounts of fat. Other investigators have since called attention to a striking exception: the diet of white South Africans typically is very high in saturated fat, but the incidence of MS allegedly is low (63).

Swank (64) also reported the results of a 17-year study of a low-fat diet in a large series of patients. Basically the diet restricts the daily consumption of animal fat to 15 g, plus an additional maximum of 30–50 ml of vegetable oil. Of 146 patients who received the diet, 118 showed good compliance over an average period of 17 years. The rest of the patients had a less rapidly progressive course and a lower death rate than a comparison series of patients described in the literature. Moreover, there was clear indication that adoption of the diet soon after diagnosis yielded the best results.

Swank's experience is difficult to evaluate, however, because the comparison group was not followed concurrently. The decrease reported in the frequency of exacerbations is not necessarily significant, since the patients were used as their own controls; as already noted, exacerbation rates typically are higher in the early years of the illness. In later years, new lesions may be expressed less distinctly or not at all in patients who already have considerable functional deficit.

However, although it is difficult to prove the efficacy of the low-fat diet from these results, there remains a possibility that the diet is at least partially effective in the treatment of MS. Reduced fat in the diet also has been a component of the raw-vegetable-and-fruit diet advocated by Evers (65).

Gluten-free Diet

A great deal of publicity has recently been given to the alleged benefits of a diet that eliminates gluten-containing foods and restricts carbohydrates, coffee, and alcohol. The rationale for this diet was the improvement noted by a single patient who adopted this approach. Liversedge (65) has reported on a two-year study of 37 patients who adhered to this diet: relapses occurred at a rate of about 0.5 per patient per year, and the average Kurtzke disability status score decreased from 4.1 to 4.6 during adherence to the diet. This experience indicates that the diet is incapable of preventing either relapses or worsening.

Dietary Supplements of Linoleic and Linolenic Acids

Sinclair (66) has proposed that a diet deficient in certain long-chain polyunsaturated fatty acids (PUFA) might cause a biochemical defect that results in MS. Adequate dietary intake of linoleic and linolenic acid is essential, since synthesis of other fatty acids can occur if there is an adequate supply of these two 18-carbon-atom compounds. Baker et al. (67) reported a reduced concentration of linoleic acid in the serum of MS patients. While some investigators have confirmed this finding, there are at least four separate reports in which the serum concentration of linoleic acid in MS patients has been found to be similar to that in control subjects (68). It seems unlikely, therefore, that an instability of myelin in MS is caused by a dietary deficiency of linoleic acid.

However, the early studies in this area prompted Millar and colleagues (69) to conduct a controlled trial of linoleate supplement in the diet of MS patients. The treated patients were given 30 ml of an emulsion of sunflower seed oil that contained 8.6 g linoleic acid, twice a day; control subjects received a similar emulsion of olive oil that contained 3.8 g oleic acid. Although the subjects were admitted to the study in a randomized manner, there apparently was some initial dissimilarity between the treated patients and the controls: the latter group contained more patients with short histories of MS.

At the end of two years, the 36 patients on linoleate supplementation had had 41 relapses, whereas the 39 controls had had 62 relapses; moreover, there was an indication that the relapses in the control patients were more severe. The authors commented on the difficulty in interpreting the results because of the dissimilarity.

Paty et al. (70) in western Ontario, attempted to reproduce the results of Millar et al. They used linoleic acid supplementation for 30 months in the diets of 76 MS patients but failed to show any benefit as compared with controls.

The saga of attempts to alter the course of MS with polyunsaturated PUFA such as linoleic and linolenic acid continues, however. It has been suggested recently that their effect in producing some immunosuppression occurs via induction of prostaglandins synthesis and that gamma linolenic acid is more active in this regard. Evening-primrose oil (Naudicelle) contains about 72% linoleic acid and 9% gamma linolenic acid and has been shown to have a beneficial effect on the survival of patients with renal transplantation and in the inhibition of EAE (71,72).

Bates and co-workers (73) have reported the results of a two-year study of various PUFA regimens in patients with early relapsing MS. The 116 patients in this trial were divided into four groups and treated with Naudicelle capsules, oleic acid capsules, a spread containing 23 g linoleic acid daily, and a spread containing 16 g oleic acid daily, respectively. There was no difference in the four groups in frequency of relapse or general deterioration of function. The group that received the high daily dose of linoleic acid had less severe and prolonged relapses; however, this effect was described as marginal, although it was consistent with the findings of Millar et al. The annual exacerbation rates in this study (0.8–0.5 per patient) were characteristic of the early years of MS. One must conclude that the effect of PUFA in MS is unimpressive, although there is some slight evidence in favor of advising patients to supplement their diets with sunflower seed oil.

Hyperbaric Oxygen

The breathing of oxygen under high pressure (OHP) has been used effectively in treatment of gas gangrene, burns, air embolism, and a number of other conditions. Jacobs et al. (74,75) have reported that OHP improves cognitive function in the aged. In these studies, elderly patients breathed oxygen at 2.5 atmospheres absolute (ATA) for 90 minutes twice a day for 15 days; at the end of that period, they demonstrated significant improvement on the Wechsler memory scale, the Bender gestalt memory phase, and other tests of cognitive function as comparison with a control group. OHP at 2 ATA reduces elevated intracranial pressure by arterial vasoconstriction (76).

Recently, OHP has been used sporadically in the treatment of MS. There is no good rationale for this treatment, although it should be recalled that Swank and Nakamura (77) and Roizin et al. (78) have suggested that, in MS, the intravascular aggregation of blood cells after high-fat meals might reduce the amount of oxygen available to the brain.

Neubauer (79) has recently reported improvement in a large number of patients receiving a course of 20 treatments with hyperbaric oxygen, with follow-up treatments every one to three months thereafter. OHP chambers are expensive and the availability of facilities is limited. Until controlled studies confirm benefit from OHP, the method cannot be recommended; the results reported so far are consistent with the natural course of the illness.

Maintenance of Mobility

Exercise Programs

There are few objective data to indicate the effect of vigorous physical exercise on patients with either mild MS or only mild evidence of disease activity. In the absence of such data, many physicians adopt a moderate approach and recommend that strenuous exercise programs be avoided. However, we have been impressed with the fact that many mildly affected patients, especially those who seem to recover fairly completely from each attack, can tolerate vigorous exercise, such as tennis and running, without evidence that exercise predisposes them to relapse. One patient of the authors is convinced that high-dosage steroids for two to three days in combination with a daily set of tennis is the best way for him to abort or shorten incipient relapse (1).

On the other hand, probably most patients (i.e., those with moderate disability) find that prolonged exercise usually accentuates existing symptoms and causes old symptoms to return transiently. In most cases this phenomenon probably results from a slight increase in body temperature produced by the exercise. Conduction block in demyelinated axons occurs at much lower temperatures than in normal axons; thus, many patients find that an increase in body temperature of only a fraction of a degree may be associated with general fatigue and decreased mobility and visual acuity (80). Many such patients are benefited significantly for 30–60 minutes after cool baths or swimming; the dramatic though transient benefits of hypothermia were clearly demonstrated many years ago (81). Thus, for many moderately affected patients, the only vigorous exercise that can be tolerated is swimming.

There is little doubt, however, that mild intermittent exercise, with frequent rest periods, is helpful in maintaining mobility, improving coordination, and lessening spasticity. Gait training under the guidance of a trained physiotherapist or a family member who has received proper instructions is beneficial for many patients.

During acute relapse, especially with more severe attacks, most patients complain of a feeling of overwhelming fatigue and will not cooperate in exercise programs. In such patients, restricted activity is necessary but prolonged bed rest should be avoided.

Motor Weakness

Although exercise programs may compensate for mild motor weakness, they are much less effective when weakness is moderate or severe. Bracing has a place in improving the gait of patients who have significant weakness of dorsiflexors of one or both feet; either a molded polypropylene brace or a short-leg aluminum brace with a 90° stop at the ankle can be used in such instances.

Ataxia

The mildly ataxic patient usually can benefit from gait training—learning to walk with a broadened base. In moderate ataxia, coordination exercises may be tried but they are usually ineffective; a cane, Canadian crutches, or a weighted walker may be necessary to provide adequate stability. A vehicle resembling an ordinary grocery market cart, properly weighted, often allows ataxic patients to be ambulatory in a relatively safe manner.

Spasticity

The early referral of patients to a physical therapist, and the assiduous use of active or passive range-of-motion exercises for weak extremities, will prevent contractures of muscles and tendons. Contractures greatly worsen the symptom of spasticity by increasing the afferent volley from tendon and muscle during attempted movement. Patients with mild spasticity may not require treatment; in many such patients, the spasticity of the quadriceps group serves a supportive function, and drugs that diminish spasticity do so at the expense of buckling of the knees when the patient is erect. Some patients, however, find significant benefit from antispasticity compounds and have moderate to marked improvement in their gait; in most cases, therefore, a trial of drug therapy is indicated.

Three drugs are available for the treatment of spasticity at present: dantrolene sodium (Dantrium), diazepam (Valium), and baclofen (Lioresal). We seldom use dantrolene because it may cause hepatotoxicity and because its mechanism of action is interference with excitation-contraction coupling in muscle. In effect, the drug produces muscle weakness (82). Diazepam is effective in some patients, but for many the dosage needed to relieve spasticity is also unpleasantly sedative.

The most effective agent for the treatment of spasticity is baclofen; this drug apparently acts by interfering with the release of excitatory transmitter from primary afferent nerve terminals (83). The effective dosage is highly individual; some patients respond to low dosages, whereas others find no relief with dosages less than 60–80 mg/day. The manufacturer recommends that the total daily dose not exceed 80 mg. The most common side effect of baclofen is drowsiness, although this effect may not be noted. In any event the drowsiness is almost always less than that which occurs with effective doses of diazepam. Tolerance to the sedative effect of baclofen often develops with continued treatment. Nausea is a relatively rare side effect. The drug has been remarkably free of serious hematologic, hepatic, or renal toxicity.

In general, antispasticity drugs are most effective in the treatment of troublesome clonus or recurrent flexor or extensor spasms. As already noted, however, the drug also may be of benefit in other settings. In addition, they also may lessen spasm of the external urethral sphincter, thus reducing the volume of residual urine in some patients with urinary bladder dysfunction.

A few unfortunate patients have intense spasticity that is refractory to all routine treatments, including drug therapy. When such patients have had complete paraplegia without useful bowel or bladder function for at least two years (usually a reliable indicator of irreversibility), destructive procedures for relief of spasticity may be considered to facilitate nursing care. Local nerve blocks with anesthetic solutions or phenol have been used, but the greatest success is usually obtained with intrathecal injections of phenol (84). Other patients have had good results with a Bischof myelotomy (85, 86). This is a selective longitudinal myelotomy that divides connections between anterior and posterior gray matter in the spinal cord, thus interrupting the reflex arc. It must be emphasized that such destructive procedures usually are not necessary and should be undertaken only when the physician, patient, and family are convinced that remission will not occur.

Treatment of Genitourinary Problems

Sexual dysfunction is distressingly frequent in MS; since the symptom is often concealed, the exact incidence is unknown. However, anonymous questionnaires have revealed that problems exist at some time in as many as 90% of men and 72% of women with MS (87). Dysfunction is often intermittent.

Sexual disability, when it is caused by the disease, almost always is associated with disturbance of urinary bladder function. If the latter does not exist, a psychological cause for the impotence or frigidity is likely; this may be treated by psychiatric or psychological therapy. Failure to achieve erection is the most common symptom of sexual malfunction in men with organic impotence and MS; such patients do not experience nocturnal erections, which is important evidence that the condition is not of psychological origin. When the problem is permanent, a penile prosthesis can be implanted.

Disturbance of bladder function is also extremely common in MS patients

(88,89). The most common symptoms, in order of occurrence, are urgency, frequency, incontinence, hesitancy, and urinary retention. Bradley (90) has found abnormal cystometrograms in virtually all patients referred to a neurourology clinic; detrusor hyperreflexia (spastic detrusor) was present in approximately two-thirds of patients and detrusor hyporeflexia in the remainder. Detrusor hyperreflexia is manifested by frequency, urgency, and a low bladder capacity; although the detrusor is spastic, it is also weak, and accumulation of residual urine is common. Measurement of the volume of residual urine is important in cases of detrusor hyperreflexia and arreflexia. Patients with MS often tolerate residual volumes of up to 200 ml without complication; however, urinary infection from stasis is a constant threat.

Clean, nonsterile self-catherization is now the treatment of choice when residual urine volume is high; this method may also be used on a regular schedule to relieve mild urinary incontinence. However, when incontinence is severe in men it is best treated with a condom disposable catheter ("Texas catheter") draining into a receptacle bag attached to the leg. In women, severe incontinence is a more difficult problem; when the problem is intermittent it is best treated with a plastic indwelling Foley catheter. Permanent incontinence in women can be treated by implantation of an artificial sphincter or by an ileal conduit operation (88,89).

The urgency associated with detrusor hyperreflexia can often be diminished by the use of tincture of belladonna or propantheline bromide (Pro-Banthine); the latter should be used sparingly, since frequent use can increase the volume of residual urine or cause urinary retention. In the case of detrusor arreflexia bethancol (Urecholine), 10–30 mg three or four times a day, may provide relief. As already noted, the use of antispasticity drugs such as baclofen may reduce the volume of residual urine by decreasing the spasticity of the urinary sphincter.

Treatment of Paroxysmal Complications

Convulsive Seizures. Grand mal or focal seizures occur in about 2% of MS patients. They are usually readily treated with ordinary anticonvulsant regimens, such as phenytoin (Dilantin) and phenobarbital.

Trigeminal Neuralgia. Paroxysmal facial pains that are indistinguishable from idiopathic tic douloureux occur in about 5% of MS patients. As in the idiopathic disorder, the problem usually is intermittent, lasting a few weeks at a time. The pain usually responds well to adequate doses of carbamazepine (Tegretol); the usual monitoring of hematologic and hepatic status is indicated when using this drug in MS, even for brief courses. Rare persistent cases of facial pain that do not respond to anticonvulsants can be treated with radiofrequency rhizotomy.

Paroxysmal Dyasthria and Ataxia. A few patients with MS have a peculiar syndrome of paroxysmal dysarthria and ataxia; the symptoms arise suddenly, last a few seconds or a minute or two, and recur frequently during the course of the day (90). The symptom complex apparently represents a rare kind of brain-stem epilepsy, since it usually disappears promptly with adequate doses of phenytoin.

Painful Tonic Spasms. Painful tonic spasms are an unusual symptom peculiar to MS and should not be confused with ordinary spasticity (91). Typically patients experience sudden painful spasms of a tonic nature in a hand and foot on one side of the body; there are no clonic movements, which distinguishes the syndrome from ordinary focal epilepsy, and there is no alteration of consciousness. The spasms are stimulus-sensitive, and usually the provoking stimulus is a change in posture (e.g., rolling over, sitting up). A recent patient of ours had an abnormal electroencephalogram with small sharp waves over the contralateral temporal lobe and paroxysmal bitemporal slowing. The spasms usually respond well to anticonvulsant medication; they commonly are present for a few weeks and then disappear, allowing withdrawal of the medication.

Phychosocial Problems

Effects of MS on the Patient

Few diseases have a more marked psychosocial impact on the patient than MS. Early in the illness, anxiety often results from uncertainty about the diagnosis. In many cases of benign MS, reassurance concerning the nondisabling course is important, and in many instances profound psychological or social problems do not develop. However, patients with progressively disabling disease encounter additional stress. As they become dependent on others, especially when sexual and urinary complications develop, marital problems and discord frequently arise. The divorce rate is distressingly high. A problem that requires study is the effect on children of chronic illness in a parent.

In the later stages of MS, organic mental changes are relatively common, although they often go unrecognized by the patient or family. Frank dementia develops in some patients as a result of multiple cerebral lesions.

Effects of Stress on MS

It is common for patients and physicians to relate the onset of recent worsening of MS to emotional stress. Russell (92), Bramwell (93), McAlpine and Compston (94), and Adams et al (95), have noted instances of this relation. Paulley (96) has even suggested initiation of a controlled trial of dynamically oriented psychotherapy.

Stress, of course, is virtually universal and there are substantial problems in inferring a cause-and-effect relation between stress and relapse. The main difficulty is that there is no simple, reliable means of quantitating psychological stress. There apparently is too much diurnal variation in serum levels of cortisol to use this method as an objective measurement. Moreover, Pratt (97) has found that, although emotional upset preceded the onset of MS in 38% of patients, it preceded the onset of other neurologic conditions in a substantial proportion (26%) of cases as well. Nonetheless, although present data do not prove a causal relation between psychological problems and the worsening of MS, further study on this subject is needed.

Management

We have found that a truthful approach is the most satisfactory way of managing patients with early MS. Patients should receive as much accurate information as possible; in many cases this can be given by the physician, but in other settings a group counselor who is familiar with MS and its vagaries can function effectively. Educational conferences and groups are often organized by local or regional MS societies for the purpose of informing patients, families, and the general public about MS. It is important, however, to direct individual patients and families to the sources of specific information that they need most. Patients with benign MS, for example, may become more anxious upon hearing detailed discussions of wheelchairs and the care of chronic bladder dysfunction. However, the families of patients with advanced disability can benefit from courses in home nursing care. Such courses typically outline the essentials of proper nutrition, skin care, bowel and bladder problems, positioning, range-of-motion exercises, and methods of improving function in the activities of daily living.

Hartings and co-workers (98) have described a program of group counseling as part of a comprehensive care program for MS patients. They emphasize the importance of early *routine* psychological assessment. Patients are then assigned to proper information or therapy groups. Such procedures probably help to prevent many of the psychosocial problems that ordinarily arise under the usual system of crisis assessment of psychological status. Such routine evaluation also allows the patient to avoid the stigma frequently attached to psychological or psychiatric referral.

OTHER DEMYELINATING DISEASES

Most forms of Schilder's disease and neuromyelitis optica probably are variants of MS (99), and the preceding discussion is applicable to such cases (100).

There is no effective treatment for adrenal leukodystrophy, globoid-cell leukodystrophy (Krabbe's disease), metachromatic leukodystrophy, or other, even rarer leukodystrophies.

Acute Disseminated Encephalomyelitis

Acute disseminated encephalomyelitis (ADE) is a perivenous demyelinating disease that usually follows acute viral infections of childhood, such as measles, mumps, varicella, rubella, or, occasionally, a nonspecific viral infection. In most cases the illness is self-limited and the prognosis generally is good; an exception is measles encephalomyelitis, which, fortunately, occurs much less frequently since the advent of measles vaccination. It is difficult to evaluate various forms of treatment in these disorders because the acute illnesses usually subside naturally, often in a sudden and dramatic fashion. However, ADE is considered by many to be an analogue of EAE, and adrenal glucocorticoids are often used in therapy.

Acute Hemorrhagic Leukoencephalopathy

In acute hemorrhagic leukoencephalitis, the most explosive and lethal form of demyelinating disease, massive therapy with dexamethasone or betamethasone is indicated. Although mortality from this disease remains high, a few patients have recovered (101).

REFERENCES

1. Carter S, Sciarra D, Merritt HH: The course of multiple sclerosis as determined by autopsy proven cases. Res Publ Assoc Res Nerv Ment Dis 28:471–511, 1950.
2. Bauer HJ: Problems of symptomatic therapy in multiple sclerosis. Neurology 28:8–20, 1978.
3. Müller R: Disseminated sclerosis. Acta Med Scand [Suppl] 222:1949.
4. Rose AS, Juzma JW, Kurtzke JF, et al: Cooperative study in the evaluation of therapy in multiple sclerosis: ACTH vs. placebo. Final report (part 2). Neurology 20:1, 1970.
5. Kuzma JW, Namerow NS, Tourtellotte WW, et al: An assessment of the reliability of three methods used in evaluating the status of multiple sclerosis. J Chronic Dis 21:803–814, 1969.
6. McPherson TA, Gilpin A, Seland TP: Radioimmunoassay of CSF for encephalitogenic basic protein: a diagnostic test for MS? Can Med Assoc J 107:856–859, 1972.
7. Cohen SR, Herndon RM, McKhann GM: Radioimmunoassay of myelin basic protein in spinal fluid. N Engl J Med 295:1455–1457, 1976.
8. Radue EW, Kendall BD: Iodide and xenon enhancement of computed tomography in MS. Neuroradiology 15:153–158, 1978.
9. Cole M, Ross RJ: Plaque of MS seen on computerized transaxial tomogram. Neurology 27:890–891, 1977.
10. Lane B, Carroll BA, Pedley TA: Computerized cranial tomography in diseases of white matter. Neurology 28:592–597, 1978.
11. Sears ES, Tindall RSA, Zarnow H: Active multiple sclerosis—enhanced computerized tomographic imaging of lesions and effect of corticosteroids. Arch Neurol 35:426–434, 1978.
12. Harding AE, Radue EW, Whiteley AM: Contrast enhanced lesions on computerized tomography in multiple sclerosis. J Neurol Neurosurg Psychiatry 41:758, 1978
13. Aita JF, Bennett DR, Anderson RE, et al: Cranial CT appearance of acute multiple sclerosis. Neurology 28:241–255, 1978.
14. Lebow S, Anderson DC, Mastri A, et al: Acute multiple sclerosis with contrast enhancing plaques. Arch Neurol 35:435–439, 1978.
15. Uchimura I, Shiraki H: A contribution to the classification and the pathogenesis of demyelinating encephalomyelitis. J Neuropathol Exp Neurol 16:139–202, 1957.
16. Wisniewski HM, Keith AB: Chronic relapsing experimental allergic encephalomyelitis: an experimental model for multiple sclerosis. Ann Neurol 1:144–148, 1977.
17. Raine CS, Stone SH: Animal model for multiple sclerosis. NY State J Med 77:1693–1696, 1977.
18. Arnason BGW, Chelmicka-Szorc E: Effect of hydrocortisone on nerve conduction in experimental peripheral nerve segmental demyelination. Neurology 20:390, 1970.
19. Katz AI, Epstein FH: Role of sodium potassium activated adenosine triphosphatase in the reabsorption of sodium by the kidney. J Clin Invest 46:1999,. 1967.
20. Miller H, Newell DJ, Ridley A: Multiple sclerosis. Treatment of acute exacerbations with corticotrophin (ACTH). Lancet 2:1120, 1961a.
21. Millar JHD, Vas CJ, Noronha MJ, et al: Long-term treatment of multiple sclerosis with corticotrophin. Lancet 2:429, 1967.
22. Alexander L, Cass LJ: Present status of ACTH therapy in multiple sclerosis. Ann Intern Med 58:454, 1963.
23. Cass LJ, Alexander L, Enders M: Complications of corticotropin therapy in multiple sclerosis. JAMA 197:173, 1966.
24. Harter JG, Reddy WJ, Thorn GW: Studies on an intermittent corticosteroid dosage regimen. N Engl J Med 269:591–596, 1963.
25. Kibler RF, Paty DW, Re PK, et al: Effect of large doses of adrenocorticoids on the course of EAE and multiple sclerosis. In: *Multiple Sclerosis: Immunology, Virology, and Ultrastructure.* Edited by F Wolgram, GW Ellison, JG Stevens, et al. New York, Academic Press, 1972, pp. 511–538.
26. Johns TR, Crowley WJ, Miller JW, et al: The syndrome of myasthenia and polymyositis with comment on therapy. Ann NY Acad Sci 184:64–71, 1971.
27. Warmolts JR, Engel WK: Benefit from alternate day prednisone in myasthenia gravis. N Engl J Med 286:17–21, 1972.

28. Nelson DA, Vates TS, Thomas RB: Complications from intrathecal steroid therapy in patients with multiple sclerosis. Acta Neurol Scand 49:176–188, 1973.

29. Silberberg D, Lisak R, Zweiman B: Multiple sclerosis unaffected by azathioprine in pilot study. Arch Neurol 28:210–212, 1973.

30. Swinburn WR, Liversedge LA: Long-term treatment of multiple sclerosis with azathioprin. J Neurol Neurosurg Psychiatry 36:124–126, 1973.

31. Ellison GW, Myers LW: A review of systemic non-specific immunosuppressive treatment of multiple sclerosis. Neurology 28:132–139, 1978.

32. Drachman DA, Paterson PY, Schmidt RT, et al: Cyclophosphamide in exacerbations of multiple sclerosis. J Neurol Neurosurg Psychiatry 38:592–597, 1975.

33. Millac P, Miller H: Cyclophophamide in multiple sclerosis. Lancet 1:783, 1969.

34. Gershwin ME, Goetzl EJ, Steinberg AD: Cyclophosphamide: use in clinical practice. Ann Intern Med 80:531–540, 1974.

35. Lance EM, Kremer M, Abbosh J, et al: Intensive immunosuppression in patients with disseminated sclerosis. Clinical response. Clin Exp Immunol 21:1–12, 1975.

36. Hughes D, Field EJ: Myelotoxicity of serum and spinal fluid in multiple sclerosis: a critical assessment. Clin Exp Immunol 2:295, 1967.

37. Lisak RP, Zwiman B, Norman M: Antimyelin antibodies in neurologic diseases: immunoflurescent demonstration. Arch Neurol 32:163–167, 1975.

38. Caspary EA: Humoral factors involved in immune processes in multiple sclerosis and allergic encephalomyelitis. Br Med Bull 33:50–53, 1977.

39. Abramsky O, Lisak RP, Silberberg DH, et al: Antibodies to oligodendroglia in patients with multiple sclerosis. N Engl J Med 297:1207–1211, 1977.

40. Dau PC, Petajan JH, Johnson KP, et al: Plasmapheresis and immunosuppressive drug therapy in multiple sclerosis. Paper presented at meeting of the American Academy of Neurology, Chicago, April 27, 1979.

41. Eylar EH, Jackson JJ, Rothenberg G, et al: Suppression of the immune response: reversal of the disease state with antigen in allergic encephalomyelitis. Nature 236:74–76, 1972.

42. Raine CS, Traugott U, Stone SH: Suppression of chronic allergic encephalomyelitis: relevance to multiple sclerosis. Science 201:445–448, 1978.

43. Hughes RAC, Gray I, Clifford-Jones R, et al: Immune response to myelin basic protein in multiple sclerosis. Proc Soc Med 70:874–876, 1977.

44. Campbell B, Vogel PJ, Fisher E, et al: Myelin basic protein administration in multiple sclerosis. Arch Neurol 29:10–15, 1973.

45. Gonsette RE, Delmotte P, Demonty L: Failure of basic protein therapy for multiple sclerosis. J Neurol 216:27–31, 1977.

46. Salk J, Westall FC, Romine JS, et al: Studies on myelin basic protein administration in multiple sclerosis patients. In: *Proceedings of the International Symposium on Progress in MS Research*, Gottingen, West Germany, September 14–15, 1978. Edited by HJ Bauer. New York, Springer-Verlag (in press).

47. Romine JS, Salt J, Wiederholt WC, et al. Studies on myelin basic protein administration in multiple sclerosis patients. Preliminary report of clinical observations. In: *Proceedings of the International Symposium on Progress in MS Research*, Gottingen, West Germany, September 14–15, 1978. Edited by HJ Bauer. New York, Springer-Verlag (in press).

48. Johnson RT: The possible viral etiology of multiple sclerosis. Adv Neurol 13:1–46, 1975.

49. Hudson NP, Grinker RR: Negative results from transfer of material from human active multiple sclerotic to Macacus rhesus under optimum conditions. Arch Pathol 16:373–376, 1933.

50. Gibbs CJ Jr, Gajdusek DC, Alpers MP: Attempts to transmit subacute and chronic neurological diseases to animals. In: *Pathogenesis and Etiology of Demyelinating Diseases*. New York, S. Karger, 1969, pp. 519–551.

51. Sibley WA, Kalter SS, Lagu a JF: Attempts to transmit multiple sclerosis to newborn and germfree non-human primates: a ten year interim report. In: *Proceedings of the International Symposium on Progress in MS Research*, Gottingen, West Germany, September 14–16, 1978. Edited by HJ Bauer. New York, Springer-Verlag- (in press).

52. Rorke LB, Iwasaki Y, Koprowski H, et al: Acute demyelinating disease in a chimpanzee three years after inoculation of brain cells from a patient with MS. Ann Neurol 5:89–94, 1979.

53. Warren KG, Koprowski H: Can a defective herpes simplex virus cause multiple sclerosis? Perspect Biol Med 22:10–18, 1978.

54. Alexander L, Loman J, Lesses MF, et al: Blood and plasma transfusions in multiple sclerosis. Res Publ Assoc Res Nerv Ment Dis 28:178–200, 1950.

55. Miller HG, Foster JB, Newell DJ, et al: Multiple sclerosis: therapeutic trials of chloroquine, soluble aspirin and gamma globulin. Br Med J 5370:1436–1439, 1963.

56. Zabriskie JB, Utermohlen V, Espinoza LR, et al: Immunologic studies with transfer factor in multiple sclerosis patients. Neurology 25:490, 1975.

57. Fog T, Pederson L, Raun N, et al: Long term transfer factor treatment for multiple sclerosis. Lancet 1:851–853, 1978.

56. Brugmans J, Schuermans V, DeCock W, et al: Restoration of host defense mechanisms by levamisole. Life Sci 13:1499–1504, 1973.

59. Dau PC, Johnson KP, Spitler LE: The effect of levamisole on cellular immunity in multiple sclerosis. Clin Exp Immunol 26:302–309, 1976.

60. Camenga DL: Safety and efficacy of levamisole in multiple sclerosis. Edited by WA den Hartog Jaeger, GW Bruyn and APJ Heijstee. In: *Abstracts of the Eleventh World Congress of Neurology.* International Congress Series No. 427. Amsterdam, Excerpta Medica, 1977, pp. 331–332.

61. Sibley WA, Tourtellotte WW: Interferon assay of multiple sclerosis tissue. Trans Am Neurol Assoc 93:124–126, 1968.

62. Swank RL: Multiple sclerosis: a correlation of its incidence with dietary fat. Am J Med Sci 220:421–425, 1950.

63. Liversedge LA: Treatment and management of multiple sclerosis. Br Med Bull 33:78–83, 1977.

64. Swank RL: Multiple sclerosis: twenty years on the low fat diet. Arch Neurol 23:460–474, 1970.

65. Evers J: *Meine Therapie der Multiplen Sklerose. Monatskurse ärztl.* Fortbildung, 1954–55.

66. Sinclair HM: Deficiency of essential fatty acids and atherosclerosis etc. (letter). Lancet 1:381–383, 1956.

67. Baker RWR, Thompson RHS, Zilkha KJ: Serum fatty acids in multiple sclerosis. J Neurol Neurosurg Psychiatry 27:408–413, 1964.

68. Wolfgram F, Myers L, Ellison G: Serum linoleic acid in multiple sclerosis. Neurology 25:786–788, 1975.

69. Millar JHD, Zilhka KJ, Langman MJS, et al: Double blind trial of linoleate supplementation of the diet in multiple sclerosis. Br Med J 1:765–768, 1973.

70. Paty DW, Cousin HK, Read J, et al: Linoleic acid in multiple sclerosis: failure to show any therapeutic benefit. Acta Neurol Scand 58:53–58, 1978.

71. McHugh MI, Wilkinson R, Elliott RW, et al: Immunosuppression with polyunsaturated fatty acids in renal transplantation. Transplantation 24:263–267, 1977.

72. Mertin J, Stackpoole A: Suppression by essential fatty acids of experimental allergic encephalomyelitis is abolished by indomethacin. Prostaglandins Med 1:276, 1978.

73. Bates D, Fawcett PRW, Shaw DA, et al: Polyunsaturated fatty acids in treatment of acute remitting multiple sclerosis. Br Med J 2:1390–1391, 1978.

74. Jacobs EA, Winter PM, Alvis HJ, et al: Hyperoxygenation effect on cognitive functioning in the aged. In: *Proceedings of the 4th International Congress on Hyperbaric Medicine.* Edited by J Wada and T Iwa. Baltimore, Williams and Wilkins, 1970, pp. 448–451.

75. Jacobs EA, Alvis HJ, Small SM: Persistence of intermittent hyperoxygenation in the elderly. In: *Proceedings of the Fifth International Hyperbaric Congress.* Simon Fraser University, Burnaby, British Columbia, pp. 439–445.

76. Miller JD, Ledingham IM: The effect of hyperbaric oxygen on intracranial pressure in experimental cerebral edema. In: *Proceedings of the 4th International Congress on Hyperbaric Medicine.* Edited by J Wada and T Iwa. Baltimore, Williams and Wilkins, 1970, pp. 453–455.

77. Swank RL, Nakamura H: Convulsions in hamsters after cream meals. Arch Neurol 3:594–600, 1960.
78. Roizin L, Abell RG, Winn J: Preliminary studies of sludged blood in multiple sclerosis. Neurology 3:250–260, 1953.
79. Neubauer RA: Treatment of multiple sclerosis with monoplace hyperbaric oxygen. J Fla Med Assoc 65:101, 1978.
80. Davis FA: Pathophysiology of multiple sclerosis and related clinical implications. Mod Treatment 7:890–902, 1970.
81. Watson CW: Effect of lowering body temperature on the symptoms and signs of multiple sclerosis. N Engl J Med 261:1253, 1959.
82. Ellis KO, Bryant SH: Excitation-contraction uncoupling in skeletal muscle by dantrolene sodium. Naunyn-Schmiedebergs Arch Pharmacol 274:107–109, 1972.
83. Davidoff RA: Pharmacology of spasticity. Neurology 28:46–51, 1978.
84. Cain HD: Subarachnoid phenol block in the treatment of pain and spasticity. Paraplegia 3:152–160, 1966.
85. Bischof W: Zur dorsalen longitudinalen Myelotomia. Abl Neuroshir 28:123–126, 1967.
86. Laitinen L, Singorinas E: Longitudinal myelotomy. J Neurosurg 35:536–540, 1971.
87. Lilius HG, Valtonen EJ, Wikstrom J: Sexual problems in patients suffering from multiple sclerosis. J Chronic Dis 29:643–647, 1976.
88. Tarabuley E: Bladder disturbances in multiple sclerosis and their management. Mod Treatment 7:941–960, 1970.
89. Bradley WE: Urinary bladder dysfunction in multiple sclerosis. Neurology 28:52–58, 1978.
90. Andermann F, Cosgrove JBR, Lloyd-Smith D, et al: Paroxysmal dysarthria and ataxia in multiple sclerosis. Neurology 9:211, 1959.
91. Matthews WB: Tonic seizures in disseminated sclerosis. Brain 81:193, 1958.
92. Russell JSR: In: *A System of Medicine,* vol. 7, Edited by C Allbutt and HD Rollerston. London, Macmillan, 1911, p. 809.
93. Bramwell B: The prognosis in disseminated sclerosis. Edin Med J 18:16, 1917.
94. McAlpine D, Compston N: Some aspects of the natural history of disseminated sclerosis. Q J Med 21:135–167, 1952.
95. Adams DK, Sutherland JM, Fletcher WB: Early clinical manifestations of disseminated sclerosis. Br Med J 2:431, 1950.
96. Paulley JW: Psychotherapy for multiple sclerosis (letter). Lancet 1:1206, 1978.
97. Pratt RTC: An investigation of the psychiatric aspects of disseminated sclerosis. J Neurol Neurosurg Psychiatry 14:326, 1951.
98. Hartings MF, Pavlou MM, Davis FA: Group counseling of MS patients in a program of comprehensive care. J Chronic Dis 29:65–73, 1976.
99. Adams RD: A comparison of the morphology of the human demyelinative diseases and experimental allergic encephalomyelitis. In: *Allergic Encephalomyelitis.* Edited by MW Kies and ED Alvord. Springfield, IL, 1959, pp. Charles C Thomas.
100. Ellison PH, Barron KD: Clinical recovery from Schilder disease. Neurology 29:244–251, 1979.
101. Byers RK: Acute hemorrhagic leukoencephalitis: report of three cases and review of the literature. Pediatrics 56:727–735, 1975.

11

Management of Seizure Disorders

J. Bruni

B.J. Wilder

Epilepsy represents the most common disorder treated by neurologists (1). Proper management of epileptic patients requires an accurate diagnosis. The classification of seizures recommended by the International League Against Epilepsy on the basis of electroencephalographic (EEG) characteristics and clinical features is the most useful (2). The major groups of seizures are: (*1*) generalized, convulsive, and nonconvulsive; (*2*) partial, simple, and complex; and (*3*) unilateral. Partial seizures eventually may become generalized. The progression from a partial to a generalized seizure may occur with such rapidity that the focal onset is not clinically obvious. In generalized seizure disorders, the EEG usually shows generalized, relatively synchronous abnormalities. In partial seizures, EEG examination may reveal focal abnormalities and, in adults, neoplasms, vascular malformations, glial scars or meningocerebral cicatrices, and cystic lesions may be responsible for these findings. It is not uncommon in the pediatric population to see focal abnormalities on EEG, with diffuse cerebral disorders and toxic-metabolic conditions.

Although medical management of epileptic patients is the most important aspect of therapy, it is not the only consideration. Comprehensive management of the patient also requires attention to the social, vocational, and psychologic aspects of the condition. Although certain guidelines can be given for the medical management of epileptic patients, no specific rules or regimens are applicable to each individual patient.

The control of seizures in most epileptic patients is based on regular administration of antiepileptic drugs. Successful medical treatment consists of complete freedom from attacks and no significant disability from drug therapy. None of the antiepileptic drugs available at present is curative. Each successful therapy may be seen as suppressive, with the drug limiting the initiation or spread of

This work was supported by the Medical Research Service of the Veterans Administration Hospital and the Epilepsy Research Foundation of Florida, Inc. Dr. Bruni was sponsored by the Ministry of Health, Ontario, Canada.

cerebral seizure activity. Patients must be educated about the nature of their condition. They should be aware of precipitating or aggravating factors and should understand fully the importance of rigid drug compliance.

Management of epileptic patients is a dynamic process, and drugs may have to be altered at times in an orderly sequence. Proper use of antiepileptic drugs will result in good to excellent seizure control in 70–80% of patients with epilepsy; complete control can be achieved in 60% of patients (3). Treatment is less successful in children with infantile spasms and hypsarrhythmic EEG patterns and in those with frequent myoclonic and akinetic attacks. Adolescents or adults with complex partial seizures or multifocal abnormalities on EEG often present a difficult therapeutic problem, both in seizure control and in behavioral and psychological adjustment. Nocturnal seizures are often difficult to control completely. Medical therapy is most successful in the treatment of idiopathic generalized tonic-clonic, simple absence or petit mal, and simple partial or focal seizures. In each patient, practical goals should be set without producing unacceptable adverse reactions to drugs.

Successful and comprehensive management of epileptic patients depends on familiarity with basic pharmacologic principles and the toxicology of antiepileptic drugs, awareness of the social and behavioral problems of patients, and some knowledge as to whether a given patient will benefit from surgical therapy. The following is an outline that will be followed in this chapter:

- Pharmacokinetic Principles of Medical Therapy
  - Absorption
  - Distribution
  - Biotransformation
  - Excretion
  - Monitoring of antiepileptic drugs
  - Drug interactions
- Pharmacology of Antiepileptic Drugs
- Mechanisms of Action of Anticonvulsant Drugs
- Medical Management of Seizure Disorders
- Toxicity of Antiepileptic Drugs
- Management of Psychosocial Problems and Vocational Rehabilitation
- Neurosurgical Treatment of Epilepsy

PHARMACOKINETIC PRINCIPLES OF MEDICAL THERAPY

The understanding of certain pharmacologic principles as they apply to antiepileptic drugs simplifies anticonvulsant therapy and allows the physician to obtain maximal benefit from all the drugs used. Important concepts of pharmacokinetics include biologic half-life, drug bioavailability, distribution, steady state, therapeutic range, and drug interactions. Pharmacokinetic principles allow the physician to describe the time course of drug concentrations as a function of dose and schedule. These components can serve to individualize antiepileptic drug therapy while they make allowances for differences in absorption, distribution, protein binding, biotransformation, and excretion that may arise from multiple factors.

The recent development of sensitive analytic techniques that permit accurate measurement of drug concentrations in plasma and other biologic fluids has contributed greatly to the efficacy and safety of antiepileptic drugs. Several excellent reviews are available for a more detailed analysis on the pharmacologic aspect of antiepileptic drugs (4–14).

In the following section we present the pharmacokinetic principles that form the basis for the medical management of epileptic patients.

Absorption

Physiologic and pathologic factors that influence the gastrointestinal absorption of antiepileptic drugs include the presence or absence of food, bile salts, gastrointestinal motility, splanchnic blood flow, pH of gastric secretions, solubility in lipids and water, drug formulation, and interaction with other drugs. Most antiepileptic drugs are absorbed by passive diffusion in the un-ionized state. Changes in gastric pH may influence drug absorption by changing the ratio of un-ionized to ionized drug, by influencing drug solubility, or by changing gastric motility. The effects of food on drug absorption vary. Solubility of a compound in lipids determines the drug's transport across biologic membranes, and its solubility in water is important for maintaining the drug in solution. Biliary secretions affect drug dispersion in the intestinal tract and enhance absorption.

The influence of formulation on drug availability can be illustrated by phenytoin. Phenytoin suspension may produce satisfactory plasma levels of drug at average dose ranges in some patients who do not achieve therapeutic plasma levels with capsule formulations. The bioavailability of different brands of phenytoin may also vary, and careful monitoring of plasma levels of drug is required both to prevent toxicity and to achieve a therapeutic effect (15–17).

The concurrent administration of another drug may theoretically influence the bioavailability of the first drug by influencing gastric pH, gastric motility, splanchnic blood flow, or the formation of insoluble complexes.

Intramuscular (IM) administration of phenytoin and diazepam is not recommended because these drugs are absorbed erratically and unpredictably (13,18–21). Phenytoin, because of its insolubility at physiologic pH, forms crystals that are absorbed slowly. If both oral and intravenous (IV) routes are contraindicated, dosage regimens that allow for delayed absorption by IM administration have been proposed (18,22–24). The role of the IM route of drug administration has been reviewed recently (25).

Intravenous administration of a drug is indicated when a therapeutic effect must be achieved quickly. Bioavailability is complete, rapid, and predictable with this route. Controlled IV administration of diazepam and phenytoin is the preferred route in status epilepticus (26–28).

Distribution

The pharmacokinetics of drug distribution may influence the time of onset, peak effect, magnitude, and duration of drug action. Drug distribution depends on blood flow to regional tissue, cardiac output, pH gradients, plasma-protein binding, and the permeability of cell membranes (10). Drug distribution also influences the amount of available drug at receptor sites and the rate of drug metabolism and excretion.

After absorption, antiepileptic drugs are distributed widely to tissue reservoirs and the central nervous system (CNS). The binding of drugs to plasma proteins has a varied effect on distribution and metabolism. The net effect of drug competition for protein receptor sites is complex (10,29). Reduced protein binding of phenytoin is observed in renal failure; this leads to lower total (i.e., unbound plus bound) plasma levels of phenytoin, which may be compensated for by increases in the free (unbound) active portions (10,11,30–33). Hepatic disease may influence the protein binding of phenytoin by changing the physical characteristics of albumin, thus affecting the plasma concentration of the drug (34). The effects of plasma- and tissue-protein binding of drugs are important considerations in drug distribution (35,36).

Biotransformation

Most antiepileptic drugs are metabolized by the cytochrome P-450 system in hepatic microsomes. Metabolism usually changes drugs into more polar and less biologically active compounds. However, some metabolites have significant anticonvulsant activity and may be primarily responsible for the anticonvulsant effect. The hepatic microsomal enzymes are responsible for a variety of reactions, including conjugations and oxidations.

The hepatic microsomal enzymes have a low substrate specificity. Although they are incompletely developed in the newborn, their activity in children is enhanced. Hepatic enzymes are subject to induction or inhibition, and their susceptibility to enzyme induction is determined genetically. The molecular mechanisms of enzyme inhibition and stimulation have been reviewed (37–40).

Theoretically, altered metabolism of an antiepileptic drug is predictable when the effects are not a function of drug concentration and active metabolites are not formed. Increased drug clearance, reduced steady-state drug concentration, and decreased duration of action of an antiepileptic agent result from enhanced drug metabolism. In such situations, the drug half-life and total drug action are decreased. Inhibition of drug metabolism has the opposite effect. Drug interactions that may result from concurrent administration of antiepileptic drugs are discussed in a subsequent section.

Although the liver is the most significant organ for metabolism of antiepileptic drugs, the lungs, kidneys, and gastrointestinal tract also contribute, but to a minor degree.

Excretion

The basic mechanisms of renal excretion of drug are glomerular filtration and tubular secretion. Nonionic back diffusion of drugs also may occur across the renal tubular cells. Glomerular filtration can be influenced by hemodynamic factors and protein binding. Lipid solubility influences passive back diffusion. Fifty to sixty percent of phenobarbital may be eliminated by the kidneys. Alkalinization of the urine leads to enhanced excretion of phenobarbital (41,42), while impaired renal function may lead to decreased excretion of unmetabolized phenobarbital. Excretion of phenytoin metabolites also may be decreased (31,33); however the drug's metabolites are inactive.

Drugs and their metabolites may be partially excreted in bile by passive diffusion or active transport. Lipid-soluble drugs are reabsorbed in the small intestine and thereby complete the enterohepatic circulation. Although the excretion of drugs in breast milk and saliva contribute little to drug elimination, sedation and/or hyperactivity may occur in breast-fed babies of mothers who receive phenobarbital or primidone. Salivary excretion of drugs has led to the development of assays of drug in saliva (43–47). Saliva levels of phenytoin correlate with free levels in plasma and cerebrospinal fluid (CSF). Secretion of phenobarbital in saliva is pH dependent. The lungs are an important route of elimination for paraldehyde.

Monitoring of Antiepileptic Drugs

Monitoring of antiepileptic drugs has become part of the routine management of epileptic patients. Such monitoring has improved medical treatment and has increased the safety of antiepileptic drugs (48–61). Plasma concentrations of antiepileptic drugs are a function of dosage, the fraction of the dose that reaches the circulation, the dosage schedule, and the drug clearance.

The biologic activity of antiepileptic drugs is proportional to the amount of drug that reaches the CNS. This is in dynamic equilibrium with the plasma concentration of drug; thus, the plasma level is a better guide to the drug's effect than is the drug dosage. A correlation also exists between plasma levels of drug and dose-related adverse effects (49,53,62,63).

Determinations of plasma levels of drug are helpful clinically in measuring compliance, preventing dose-related toxic side effects, and achieving a therapeutic range for each patient. Plasma determinations should be performed only when the drug is at steady state. When drug dosage is changed, it is necessary to wait for five elimination half-lives in order for the drug to reach a new steady state. For example, phenytoin has a half-life of 24 hours. Therefore, after a dosage change the drug does not reach a new steady state for five days. This information is important to the prevention of excessively rapid increases in drug dosage. Plasma monitoring of antiepileptic drugs also may be helpful in alerting the physician to the presence of possible drug interactions when the patient is receiving multiple therapies.

Lack of correlation between the administered dose of an antiepileptic drug and its plasma level may be attributable to several factors (4,5,53). These include:

1. Individual differences in absorption, volume of distribution, biotransformation, and excretion of antiepileptic drugs. Genetic factors are important in the regulation of antiepileptic drug metabolism (64).
2. Noncompliance, the most common cause of subtherapeutic plasma levels (65–67).
3. Differences in the nature of drug formulation that result in altered bioavailability (15–17).
4. Presence of gastrointestinal, hepatic, or renal disease that interferes with absorption, metabolism, or excretion of antiepileptic drugs (4,9).

5. Abnormal protein binding such as may occur in hypoproteinemia and in renal and hepatic diseases.
6. Pharmacokinetic drug interactions in which the addition of another drug either inhibits or enhances the absorption, metabolism, or excretion of the first drug (10,68–73).
7. Environmental factors which influence drug metabolism (e.g., exposure to chemicals).
8. Saturation kinetics of some antiepileptic drugs, such as phenytoin (74,75) and dose-dependent elimination of carbamazepine (76). Phenytoin concentration may increase disproportionately with increasing dosage. This is an example of zero-order kinetics, in which drug metabolism (rate of reaction) is independent of drug concentration, since the hepatic microsomal enzymes become saturated. At high doses, small increases in drug dose result in large increases in plasma drug concentration (Fig. 1). In first-order kinetics, drug metabolism and/or elimination depends on drug concentration. Plasma levels increase in linear fashion depending on dosage (Fig. 2). With increasing dosage, clearance of carbamazepine increases but the mechanism is not certain. Fortunately, in low therapeutic ranges of plasma levels of drug, most antiepileptic agents generally are metabolized by first-order kinetics.

The indications for monitoring of antiepileptic drugs derive from the considerations described above. These can be summarized as follows:

1. At initiation of therapy, to determine whether a satisfactory plasma level has been achieved.
2. When drug dosage is changed and a new steady state is achieved.
3. When seizures are uncontrolled, to determine compliance, rapid drug metabolism, or whether the epilepsy is resistant to the drug.
4. During the development of intercurrent illness, such as hypoproteinemia, or gastrointestinal, hepatic, or renal disease.
5. If toxic symptoms or subtle behavioral changes occur that may be drug related.
6. When drug interaction is suspected.
7. During pregnancy, when alterations in absorption and metabolism of antiepileptic drug may necessitate adjustment of dosage (77).
8. When factors are present that modify response to antiepileptic drugs at receptor sites (e.g., electrolyte or acid-base disturbances, anoxia).
9. During prepuberty-puberty, when changes in drug metabolism may necessitate adjustment of dosage.
10. During research trials of antiepileptic drugs.

The technique of choice for measurement of plasma levels of antiepileptic drug is gas-liquid chromatography (GLC). This technique offers a high degree of accuracy and specificity and also allows for simultaneous measurement of several drugs. Phenytoin, primidone, phenobarbital, carbamazepine, valproic acid, and ethosuximide can be measured by GLC (78–82). Previously, less sensitive or more complicated spectrophotometric (83) and colorimetric (84) methods were used.

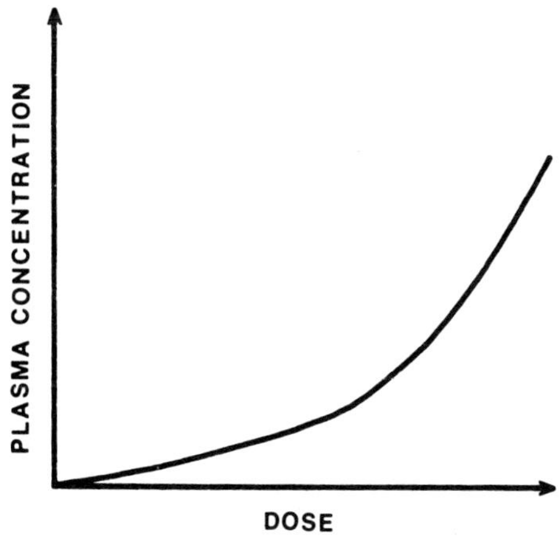

Figure 1. Hypothetical dose-plasma relationship for drugs that exhibit zero-order kinetics (e.g., phenytoin).

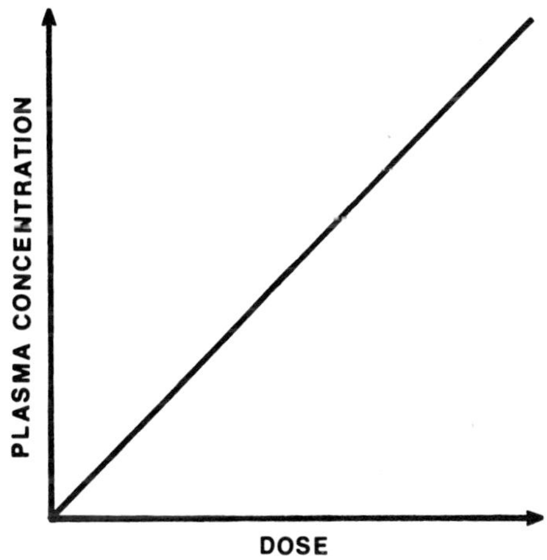

Figure 2. Hypothetical dose-plasma relationship for drugs that exhibit first-order kinetics (e.g., phenobarbital).

At present, radioimmunoassays and enzyme immunoassays are being evaluated for use in measurement of phenytoin, phenobarbital, carbamazepine, primidone, and diazepam (85,86). High-pressure liquid chromatography (87) and gas chromatography–mass spectrometry (88) also are being evaluated but are not readily available for most clinical laboratories.

Drug assays performed by most laboratories measure the total plasma or serum concentration of drug and not only the free (unbound), biologically active drug. This limitation must be recognized, since it is only the free drug that penetrates the CNS to act on receptors. Toxicity also correlates better with concentration of free drug (4,62). This requires special consideration in the presence of hypoproteinemia and hepatic and renal disease. Hepatic disease may lead to a decrease in plasma-protein binding of phenytoin, carbamazepine, and valproic acid, with a subsequent change in drug metabolism.

The concept of a therapeutic range is a statistical one. It represents the range of plasma levels of drug associated with optimal control of seizures in most patients without producing unacceptable toxic effects. Some patients may be controlled with subtherapeutic levels, and their dosages should not be increased in order to raise the plasma level of drug. In some patients, toxic effects may occur with subtherapeutic or low therapeutic levels as a result of differences in patient susceptibility to adverse reactions. If the side effects are unacceptable, either the drug dosage should be reduced or another drug introduced.

The optimal potential of monitoring antiepileptic drugs has yet to be achieved. More significance will be derived from plasma levels when laboratories routinely measure and report concentrations of free drug. The possibility of measuring saliva levels of antiepileptic drugs as an indicator of free drug in plasma is being investigated (43–47).

Drug Interactions

Some general principles of interaction of antiepileptic drugs have been discussed. Interactions are of two types: pharmacodynamic, which occur when one drug directly affects the action of another at the receptor site; and pharmacokinetic, which result from alterations in the absorption, distribution, biotransformation, or elimination of one drug by another. Pharmacodynamic interactions do not change plasma levels of drug; however, they may result in potentiation or antagonism of drug effect. In contrast, pharmacokinetic interactions usually change plasma level of drug. In the following section the major interactions involving the commonly used antiepileptic drug will be presented.

Absorption

Antacids and antihistamines may interfere with absorption of phenytoin. Although phenobarbital may interfere with the absorption of some drugs, such as phenytoin, the effect is minimal. Phenobarbital decreases the absorption of griseofulvin and bishydroxycoumarin (89–91). Phenytoin decreases the absorption of folate, vitamins C and D, and calcium.

Protein Binding

Protein-binding interactions are important considerations with the use of drugs that are highly protein bound. Displacement of anticonvulsant drugs from binding sites makes them more readily available for metabolism. Decreased plasma concentrations of drug may result if the drug-metabolizing enzymes are unsaturated; if enzyme saturation has occurred, high drug concentrations may result. Carbamazepine may decrease total body levels of phenytoin partly as a result of this mechanism. Although concurrent administration of valproic acid with phenytoin results in lower total levels of the latter (72,92–94) this effect appears to be transient (95).

Biotransformation and Excretion

When phenytoin and phenobarbital are administered to experimental animals, the drugs cause an increase in liver size and protein content. The effects of the addition of phenytoin to phenobarbital vary, however (91,96), and this interaction usually is not significant in clinical practice. Phenobarbital is a major metabolite of primidone, and concurrent administration of these drugs results in a significant increase in phenobarbital levels. Data on phenytoin-benzodiazepine interactions conflict (68,97,98). Carbamazepine may lower phenytoin levels by enzyme induction (100) Valproic acid results in elevation of phenobarbital levels (72,93).

Antiepileptic drugs may also interact with drugs used for other medical conditions (73). Interactions between phenytoin and other concurrently administered drugs are shown in Tables 1 and 2.

Drug Potentiation

The concurrent administration of phenobarbital and primidone may produce toxic effects. The sedative effects of phenobarbital and diazepam may potentiate each other.

PHARMACOLOGY OF ANTIEPILEPTIC DRUGS

The important pharmacologic variables of the antiepileptic drugs are presented in Table 3. The following sections complete the pharmacologic data.

Phenytoin and Other Hydantoins

Gastrointestinal absorption of phenytoin is slow and erratic. Peak plasma levels occur 8 to 12 hours after a single dose. Phenytoin is metabolized primarily to 5-hydroxyphenyl-5-phenylhydantoin (HPPH) in the liver and is conjugated and excreted in the urine. Urinary HPPH accounts for approximately 70% of the ingested dose. Small amounts of dihydrodiol and 3-0-methyl catechol metabolites are excreted in the urine (101). Phenytoin metabolism varies among individuals, and measurements of blood levels of the drug should be obtained. The drug is well tolerated by most patients in single daily doses of 4–7 mg/kg. Initiation of therapy can be done by loading the patient orally with a dose of 10–13 mg/kg over a four-hour period (102). The half-life of phenytoin is 10–40 hours.

Failure to achieve a therapeutic range of 10–20 μg/ml with daily doses of 500–600 mg suggests poor compliance, malabsorption, or increased metabolism. Deficiency of hepatic hydroxylating enzymes may result in intoxication with small doses.

Intravenous administration of phenytoin is safe and effective in patients with status epilepticus, although administration should not exceed 50 mg/min. A total dose of 13 mg/kg should be given to produce a maximal response. Intramuscular administration produces moderate pain at the site of injection. Absorption is erratic and slow because of drug crystallization; thus, this mode of administration is not generally recommended. If both oral and IV routes are contraindicated, dosage schedules for IM administration of phenytoin are available (21,23,24).

During pregnancy, decreased plasma levels of phenytoin have been reported despite a constant phenytoin dose; this may lead to an increase in frequency of

Table 1. Drugs That Affect Plasma Phenytoin Concentrations

Increase[a]	*Decrease*
Disulfiram	Carbamazepine
Sulthiame	Ethanol
Isoniazid	Valproic acid
Dicoumarol	Phenobarbital[b]
Phenyramidol	Primidone[b]
Phenobarbital	Salicylates (massive doses)
Primidone	Folic acid
Chloramphenicol	Phenylbutazone
Methylphenidate	Diazepam[b]
Sulfamethiozole	Chlordiazepoxide[b]
Phenylbutazone	Clonazepam[b]
Sulfaphenazone	
Ethosuximide	
Chlorpromazine	
Prochlorperazine	
Propoxyphene	

[a] In decreasing order of probability.

[b] Rare in clinical situations; conflicting data.

Table 2. Drugs Whose Plasma Concentrations are Decreased by Phenytoin

Digitoxin
Bishydroxycoumarin
Metyrapone
Birth Control Pills
Dexamethasone
Doxycycline
Phenylbutazone
Cortisol
25-hydroxycholecalciferol
Thyroxine

seizures (77,103,104). Frequent determinations of plasma level serve as a useful monitor of changing phenytoin requirements.

Mephenytoin is chemically and pharmacologically related to phenytoin. It is metabolized in the liver by demethylation to nirvanol, which is responsible for most of its toxicity. Toxic reactions may be serious, and thus mephenytoin is indicated only rarely.

Ethotoin is a low-potency hydantoin that is used occasionally in the treatment of convulsive seizures.

Carbamazepine

Considerable individual variation exists in the absorption of carbamazepine. Peak plasma levels are generally achieved within six or more hours after admin-

Table 3. Pharmacologic Variables of Antiepileptic Drugs

Drug	*Absorption*	*Peak (hr)*	V_D *(1/kg)*	*t½ (hr)*	*Time to Reach Steady State (days)*	*Protein Binding (%)*	*Major Metabolites*	*Antiepileptic Activity of Metabolite*
Phenytoin	Slow	8–12	0.5–0.8	10–40[a]	7–9	70–95	Hydroxylated phenytoin	
Primidone	Slow-to-moderate	2–4	0.6–0.7	6–18	4–7	0	Phenobarbital, phenylethylmalonamide	+
Phenobarbital	Moderate	4–7	0.7–1.0	50–150	14–21	40–60	Hydroxylated phenobarbital	+
Carbamazepine	Slow-to-moderate	6–24	0.8–1.4	12–35[a]	3–4	70–80	Carbamazepine epoxide	+
Ethosuximide	Rapid	3–7	0.7–0.9	20–60	7–10	0–10	Hydroxylated metabolites	
Valproic Acid	Rapid	1–4	0.15–0.4	8–12	4	90–95	Glucuronide conjugate	?
Trimethadione	Rapid	1–3	0.8	14–16	30[c]	0	Dimethadione	+
Clonazepam	Rapid	1–3	2.4	22–33		47	7-Aminoderivative	
Methsuximide	Rapid	1–4		2–4[b]		0–10	*N*-Desmethylsuximide	+
Diazepam (oral)	Very rapid	0.5–3	1–2	27–48+	4–10	90–96	*N*-Desmethyldiazepam	+
							N-Methyloxazepam	+

Abbreviations: V_D, a measure of the apparent volume of distribution of a drug in the body; peak, time of occurrence of maximal plasma level after dose of a drug; t½, the time required for the drug concentration to decrease by one-half after absorption and distribution.

[a]Half life is dose dependent.

[b]Rapidly metabolized.

[c]Time for active metabolite to reach steady state.

istration. Initiation of therapy should be gradual in order to minimize gastrointestinal side effects, which usually are transient. Administration should be twice a day because the drug's half-life is 12–35 hours (usually 12–14 hours). Daily doses of 7–15 mg/kg generally result in therapeutic plasma levels of 4–10 μg/ml. Carbamazepine is excreted in the urine as carbamazepine epoxide and carbamazepine dihydroxide (105,106). It is not clear whether the metabolites possess anticonvulsant properties in humans.

Barbiturates

Barbiturates with significant anticonvulsant properties include phenobarbital, mephobarbital, and metharbital. Phenobarbital is absorbed completely from the gastrointestinal tract and reaches peak plasma levels after four to seven hours. The half-life ranges from four to seven days. Daily doses of 1–5 mg/kg generally result in therapeutic plasma levels of 20–45 μg/ml. Phenobarbital may be administered in a single bedtime dose. The drug is metabolized predominantly by hepatic parahydroxylation and partially excreted unchanged in the urine (107). Mephobarbital and metharbital have no advantages over phenobarbital and, because of their cost and unpredictable absorption, should not be used as primary antiepileptic drugs.

Primidone

Primidone is absorbed rapidly from the gastrointestinal tract, with peak plasma levels occurring in two to four hours. The drug has a half-life of 6 to 18 hours (108). Daily doses of 10–25 mg/kg produce therapeutic plasma levels of 7–15 μg/ml. Primidone may be started in multiple daily doses of 5 mg/kg and increased in 5 mg/kg increments at weekly intervals. Initiation of therapy with primidone may sometimes necessitate increasing the drug in even smaller increments because of side effects.

Primidone is metabolized in the liver to phenylethylmalonamide and phenobarbital (109). Both metabolites possess anticonvulsant properties, and phenobarbital ultimately accounts for 15–20% of the ingested primidone. After two to three weeks of primidone therapy, therapeutic plasma levels of phenobarbital are reached; these values can be used to monitor the efficacy of the therapy.

Ethosuximide

Ethosuximide is absorbed rapidly, with peak plasma levels occurring in two to four hours. The drug has a half-life of 30–60 hours (110). An initial dose of 250 mg/day is recommended for the first week, with subsequent increases at weekly intervals until control is achieved or until somnolence appears. Doses of 20–30 mg/kg/day generally reach a therapeutic plasma level of 40–100 μg/ml. Urinary excretion of ethosuximide accounts for 13 to 19% of the dose (110); the rest is metabolized by the liver.

Valproic Acid

Valproic acid is absorbed rapidly from the gastrointestinal tract, with peak plasma levels occurring in one to four hours. The recommended initial dose is 15 mg/kg/day, with increases of 5–10 mg/kg/day at weekly intervals until seizures are controlled or side effects prevent further increases. Administration with meals may reduce the initial nausea without decreasing absorption. Valproic acid has a short half-life (8 to 12 hours) and should be administered in three divided daily doses. The effective therapeutic range is 50–100 μg/ml (61). Elimination of valproic acid is rapid; it is metabolized primarily in the liver and is excreted as the glucuronide conjugate. Other metabolites in the urine are 2-propyl-hydroxy-pentanoic acid and 2-propyl-glutaric acid (111). Unmetabolized drug also is present in the urine.

Clonazepam

Clonazepam is absorbed rapidly from the gastrointestinal tract, and peak plasma levels occur in one to three hours. Daily doses of 0.1–0.2 mg/kg/day produce average therapeutic plasma levels of 20–80 ng/ml. The half-life of clonazepam is 22–38 hours. The initial daily dosage for adults should be 0.05 mg/kg. Less than 5% of the administered dose appears unchanged in the urine, and about 30% appears in the urine as unconjugated metabolites; the rest are conjugated metabolites (112).

Diazepam

Orally administered diazepam is absorbed rapidly, with maximal blood levels occurring in 30 minutes to three hours. The total daily dose is 0.15–2 mg/kg/day. Orally administered diazepam has a biphasic decay curve, with a phase I half-life of 2 to 10 hours and a phase II half-life of 27 to 48 or more hours (113). The drug usually is administered in divided doses. The biologic half-life after an IV dose is 30 minutes to 4 hours. When diazepam is administered IV for the treatment of status epilepticus, a total single dose of 0.05–0.15 mg/kg can be administered. If used alone, the dose can be repeated every 30–60 minutes. The total daily IV dose should not exceed 200 mg. Extreme caution should be exercised with the use of IV diazepam in children and the elderly. The principal metabolites of diazepam are *N*-desmethyldiazepam and *N*-methyloxazepam, both of which possess anticonvulsant activity (114).

Trimethadione

Orally administered trimethadione is absorbed rapidly, with peak levels occurring after one to three hours (as observed in animal studies) (115). The total daily dose is 10–25 mg/kg. Although the plasma half-life is 14–16 hours, most of trimethadione is converted to the metabolite dimethadione, which has a half-life of 6 to 12 days. Unmetabolized trimethadione contributes approximately 15% to the drug's anticonvulsant activity, and the remainder is attributed to dimethadione (115). The therapeutic range (as dimethadione) is 600–900 μg/ml.

Therapeutic levels of trimethadione are not well established; however, the drug level reflects drug intake in the previous 12–24 hours. Because dimethadione has a long half-life, its levels reflect trimethadione intake over the previous few weeks.

Other Antiepileptic Drugs

Acetazolamide is used occasionally as adjunctive therapy. It is absorbed rapidly, with peak levels occurring after two to three hours. The dosage range is 5–10 mg/kg/day. Effective blood levels are reported to be 10–14 μg/ml (116). Acetazolamide is excreted unchanged by the kidneys.

Methsuximide is absorbed and metabolized rapidly, with peak concentrations occurring after one to four hours (117). The dosage range is 10–15 mg/kg/day, which produces therapeutic plasma levels of 15–30 μg/ml (as the *N*-desmethyl metabolite). Methsuximide is metabolized to *N*-desmethylsuximide, which probably is responsible for the drug's anticonvulsant properties.

Phenacemide may be effective in the control of complex partial seizures. However, because the drug has serious side effects, its use is rarely justified.

MECHANISMS OF ACTIONS OF ANTICONVULSANT DRUGS (118–120)

The basic mechanisms of action of antiepileptic drugs frequently are obscure. However, certain biochemical and neurophysiologic effects are known, and these are important in prediction of clinical efficacy. It is probable that multiple mechanisms of action account for the efficacy of these agents. Membrane stabilization probably is relevant to some or all of the antiepileptic drugs. Important biochemical effects include changes in cerebral monoamines in cerebral electrolytes, and in oxidative metabolism. Important neurophysiologic effects include elevation of the threshold for seizures, limitation of spread and propagation of seizures, and decrease of both seizures afterdischarge and posttetanic potentiation. Table 4 gives a summary of the mechanisms of action of anticonvulsant drugs.

Phenytoin

Phenytoin suppresses local spread of epileptiform activity without significantly affecting the epileptic focus. The drug does not alter the seizure threshold. Phenytoin exerts a blocking effect on posttetanic potentiation as a result of the stabilization of excitable neuronal membranes. Another action of phenytoin on the suppression of seizure spread may be caused by the facilitation of discharge of Purkinje cells in the cerebellum. Important biochemical effects that probably are important in the actions of phenytoin include increased sodium transport and inhibition of presynaptic calcium uptake, with the possible result of reduced neurotransmitter release. Phenytoin also inhibits accumulation of adenosine 3′:5′-cyclic phosphate (cyclic AMP) and cyclic GMP.

Table 4. Mechanism of Action of Various Anticonvulsant Drugs

	Mechanism of Action	
Drug	*Electrophysiologic*	*Biochemical*
Phenytoin	Decreases PTP, seizure propagation, and excitability of peripheral nerve; increases Purkinje cell discharges.	Increases Na transport and levels of glutamine, serotonin, and GABA; decreases Ca uptake, cAMP, cGMP, glutamic acid, and transmitter release.
Barbiturates	Increase threshold for chemical and electrical stimulation; decrease action potential amplitude, seizure propagation, and excitability of peripheral nerve.	Decrease ACh and ATP synthesis, cerebral energy metabolism, and presynaptic Ca flux.
Primidone	Increases threshold for electrical and chemical stimulation; decreases seizure propagation.	
Carbamazepine	Decreases transmission of anterior ventral nucleus of thalamus; increases threshold for electrical stimulation.	Decreases Na conductance (with high concentrations); inhibits accumulation of cAMP.
Succinimides	Increase threshold against pentylenetetrazol and electroshock seizures.	Decrease potassium permeability.
Valproic Acid	Decreases seizure propagation; increases threshold for bicuculline, picrotoxin, and pentylenetetrazol seizures.	Increases GABA levels and membrane conductance of potassium; decreases levels of succinate and cGMP.
Benzodiazepines	Increase threshold for electroshock and pentylenetetrazol seizures.	Decrease potassium permeability; actions similar to clonazepam and glycine.
Trimethadione	Causes antifacilitation of thalamic circuits; increases threshold for electroshock and pentylenetetrazol seizures.	Decreases potassium permeability; increases intracellular CO_2 accumulation with disruption of cellular metabolism.

Abbreviations: PTP, posttetanic potentiation; cGMP, cyclic GMP; ACh, acetylcholine; ATP, adenosine triphosphate.

Barbiturates

Phenobarbital acts as a general CNS depressant and affects primarily the polysynaptic pathways. Depression of posttetanic potentiation is not an important factor in the action of these drugs. Barbiturates suppress the spread of seizure discharge and increase the convulsive threshold for electrical and chemical stimulation. The drugs also inhibit calcium flux in presynaptic endings and depress metabolism of cerebral energy.

Primidone

The efficacy of primidone as an antiepileptic drug depends on the antiepileptic properties of the parent compound and its metabolites phenobarbital and phenylethylmalonamide. Primidone reduces seizure propagation and increases seizure threshold to electrical and chemical stimulation.

Succinimides

Ethosuximide provides maximal protection against the clonic seizures produced by pentylenetetrazol, whereas phensuximide and methsuximide provide maximal protection against electroshock tonic seizures. Similar to the effect of trimethadione, ethosuximide reduces synaptic transmission during repetitive stimulation without depressing transmission of single impulses.

Carbamazepine

Physiologic studies have shown depression of synaptic transmission in the trigeminal nucleus of the cat. Depression of transmission in the nucleus ventralis anterior of the thalamus also occurs; this may be pertinent because this nucleus has been implicated in the generalization and spread of seizure discharge. High doses of carbamazepine cause some depression of posttetanic potentiation. Carbamazepine inhibits accumulation of cyclic AMP and, in high concentrations, decreases sodium conductance.

Valproic Acid

Electrophysiologically, valproic acid does not influence the epileptic focus. The drug suppresses seizure propagation and increases the threshold to seizures induced by picrotoxin, bicuculline, and pentylenetetrazol. The biochemical effects responsible for the antiepileptic effects of valproic acid may be related to evaluation of brain levels of GABA, decrease of brain levels of cyclic GMP, and/or increased conductance of potassium membrane.

Benzodiazepines

The most striking anticonvulsant effect of diazepam is against pentylenetetrazol-induced seizures. The drug also blocks seizures induced by strychnine, picrotoxin, tetanus toxin, and electroshock. Diazepam blocks seizures after stimulation of the central lateral thalamus. Experimentally, diazepam augments inhibitory discharges of Purkinje cells. In addition, the drug increases presynaptic inhibition, decreases membrane potential, decreases action potentials in presynaptic terminals, and increases postsynaptic inhibition. The concept of benzodiazepine receptors has been advanced recently. The actions of clonazepam are similar in some respects to those of diazepam. Neurochemically, the former mimics the action of glycine, which is a spinal cord inhibitory transmitter.

Trimethadione

Trimethadione increases the threshold against pentylenetetrazol-induced and electroshock seizures and reduces the response to repetitive electrical stimulation. The drug also decreases rhythmic activity in thalamic circuits. Such rhythmic activity may be important in the pathophysiology of absence seizures. Biochemically, trimethadione causes accumulation of carbon dioxide in brain cells and may disrupt cellular metabolic processes by inducing intracellular acidosis.

MEDICAL TREATMENT OF SEIZURE DISORDERS

The goal of medical management of seizure disorders is prevention of recurrent seizures without production of unacceptable toxicity. General principles of therapy for the most common seizure disorders will be outlined, although some minor differences may exist between physicians' preferences regarding first drugs to be used for a particular type of seizure. Table 5 divides the antiepileptic drugs into primary, or major, drugs and secondary drugs and outlines indications for their use. Physicians should be familiar with optimal dosage schedules; metabolic products; absorption, distribution, and elimination characteristics; half-lives; major toxic effects; and drug interactions peculiar to these agents. This knowledge should form the background that the physician will use in managing the epileptic patient. Secondary drugs often are of value in some situations, particularly when primary drugs have resulted in allergic or idiosyncratic reactions; they also can be useful in combination with one or more of the primary drugs.

Except for special circumstances or specific seizure types, therapy should commence with a single drug; after initiation of the drug, the physician should wait for a steady state to occur. The dosage then should be adjusted to achieve seizure control at a level that generally does not exceed the therapeutic range. Unacceptable adverse effects may limit the maximal dosage that a particular patient can tolerate. The therapeutic range and toxicity may vary widely in different persons; thus, therapeutic ranges are presented only as guidelines for treatment. Often, achievement of therapeutic plasma levels is associated with optimal seizure control. However, some patients are not completely or satisfactorily controlled, even though the frequency and severity of seizures are reduced or the character of the seizures is altered. When control is unsatisfactory, another drug should be considered. Certain combinations of drugs potentiate the antiepileptic effects of each individually; however, some combinations may significantly potentiate toxicity.

The major exceptions to initiation of therapy with a single drug are (*1*) patients with both absence and generalized tonic-clonic seizures; (*2*) patients with other, frequent, mixed seizures; and (*3*) patients with frequent or clustered tonic-clonic seizures or partial seizures with secondary generalization.

The section that follows will discuss specific seizure types and the drugs that are more efficacious in treatment.

Table 5. Anticonvulsant Agents That Are Currently Available

Generic Name	*Trade Name*	*Total Daily Dose (per kg body weight)*	*Principal Indications*
Major (Primary) Drugs			
Phenytoin, Diphenylhydantoin (DPH)	Dilantin	4–7 mg	Generalized convulsive seizures (grand mal); simple and complex partial seizures (psychomotor)
Carbamazepine	Tegretol	7–15 mg	Generalized convulsive seizures (grand mal); simple and complex partial seizures
Phenobarbital	Luminal	1–5 mg	Generalized convulsive seizures (grand mal); simple partial seizures (usually in combination with DPH)
Primidone	Mysoline	10–25 mg	Generalized convulsive seizures (grand mal); simple and complex partial seizures (psychomotor)
Ethosuximide	Zarontin	20–30 mg	Absence seizures (petit mal)
Valproic Acid	Depakene	10–60 mg	Absence seizures (petit mal); myoclonus
Secondary Drugs			
Clonazepam	Clonopin	0.1–0.2 mg	Absence seizures (petit mal); myoclonus akinetic attacks; infantile spasms
Trimethadione	Tridione	10–25 mg	Absence seizures (petit mal)
Paramethadione	Paradione	10–25 mg	Absence seizures (petit mal)
Mephenytoin	Mesantoin	7–12 mg	Generalized convulsive seizures (grand mal); simple and complex partial seizures
Ethotoin	Peganone	10–20 mg	Generalized convulsive seizures (grand mal); simple and complex partial seizures

Metharbital	Gemonil	2.5–10 mg	Generalized convulsive seizures (grand mal); simple partial seizures (usually in combination with DPH)
Mephobarbital	Mebaral	2.5–10 mg	Generalized convulsive seizures (grand mal); simple partial seizures (usually in combination with DPH)
Methsuximide	Celontin	10–15 mg	Generalized convulsive seizures (grand mal); simple and complex partial seizures
Phenacemide	Phenurone	25–45 mg	Complex partial seizures (psychomotor)
ACTH		40–60 units/day, total	Infantile spasms
Corticosteroids		5–60 mg/day, total	Infantile spasms
Diazepam	Valium	0.15–2 mg	Myoclonus; absence seizures (petit mal); status epilepticus
Chlordiazepoxide	Librium	1–4 mg	Alcoholic withdrawal seizures
Paraldehyde		0.3–0.7 ml	Alcoholic withdrawal seizures; as an adjunct in status epilepticus
Dextroamphetamine	Dexedrine	0.1–0.3 mg	Tonic seizures; antisoporific to counteract side effects of other drugs
Methylphenidate	Ritalin	0.2–0.6 mg	Tonic seizures; antisoporific to counteract side effects of other drugs

Generalized Major Attacks (Grand Mal) and Simple Partial Seizures (Focal)

Phenytoin, carbamazepine, phenobarbital, and primidone are the most useful drugs for treatment of generalized convulsive seizures (grand mal) and partial (focal) attacks. Phenytoin and phenobarbital in combination act synergistically as anticonvulsants. Similarly, phenytoin and primidone often are useful in combination. The combination of phenobarbital and primidone, however, results in potentiation of sedation and usually is avoided. Since a significant proportion of primidone is converted metabolically to phenobarbital, there usually is little reason for the two to be given concurrently. The four drugs may be used in the following order and combinations: (*1*) phenytoin, (*2*) carbamazepine, (*3*) phenytoin and carbamazepine, (*4*) phenytoin and phenobarbital, (*5*) phenytoin and primidone, (*6*) carbamazepine and phenobarbital, and (*7*) carbamazepine and primidone.

Initial therapy can consist of phenytoin alone or carbamazepine alone. Primidone probably is as potent as phenytoin; however, disagreeable side effects, principally sedation, malaise, and minor personality alterations, are more frequent with primidone. We use the drug as a primary antiepileptic agent infrequently. However, a Veterans Administration cooperative study is under way to assess the role of primidone as a primary antiepileptic agent in treatment of generalized tonic-clonic, complex, and simple partial seizures. No evidence is available to suggest that multiple therapy leads to better seizure control in most cases than monotherapy (121,122). The use of phenobarbital alone is recommended frequently in initial therapy in children because it is safe and inexpensive. Some patients (children more frequently than adults) may be controlled with phenobarbital alone; however, it is usually necessary to add another agent to this regimen. Somnolence frequently is an initial problem, particularly with drug combinations. Small doses of dextroamphetamine, methylphenidate, or methamphetamine may be indicated rarely if somnolence persists. The sedative effects of barbiturates usually subside with continued use of the drug.

Valproic acid may be useful as adjunctive therapy if the regimens described above fail to achieve satisfactory control. Only 30–40% of patients have a satisfactory response to this agent (111,123–125).

Complex Partial Seizures (Psychomotor Attacks)

For patients with complex partial seizures, phenytoin, carbamazepine, and primidone are equally useful. Carbamazepine may be used alone or in combination with either phenytoin or primidone or both. It is one of the major anticonvulsants, especially in this type of seizure disorder. Phenobarbital is used occasionally as a supplemental medication but may at times result in worsening of the disorder as manifested by an increase in the frequency of attacks. Significant control can be achieved in 50 to 70% of patients with these three anticonvulsants, either alone or in combination. If automatisms occur in association with major attacks (grand mal), the attacks usually are alleviated. Rarely, methsuximide has been found to be of benefit, although tolerance to its antiepileptic effect frequently develops. When methsuximide is combined with primidone, oversedation may occur.

Valproic acid occasionally may be helpful in 30–50% of patients (111,123–125) and may be tried as adjunctive therapy if other medical therapies have failed. Acetazolamide also may be a useful adjunct in patients with premenstrual seizures.

Absence Seizures (Petit Mal)

Ethosuximide and valproic acid are first-order agents for the treatment of petit mal seizures; second-order drugs are listed in Table 5. If the patient has concomitant grand mal attacks, treatment should be instituted according to the schedule detailed above. The drug of choice is ethosuximide. Valproic acid is equally effective, but closer monitoring of plasma levels of drug and hepatic and hematologic variables is required. Trimethadione is used only rarely because of its potentially serious side effects. Use of trimethadione may decrease the threshold for major attacks. Failure of these drugs to control this type of seizure is an indication for the use of clonazepam.

Tables 6 and 7 list the major anticonvulsant drugs that are most useful in treatment of generalized tonic-clonic and simple and complex partial and absence seizures. The tables give both generic and trade names and outline the dosages for each. The total daily doses and dosage schedules that we recommend are tabulated also.

Infantile Spasms and Myoclonic Seizures

Infantile spasms are generalized epileptic attacks that are age specific. Infantile spasms usually begin in the first year of life. They may be idiopathic or associated with chromosomal abnormalities, cerebral trauma, tuberous sclerosis, or immunization. The EEG usually is abnormal and is characterized by hypsarrhythmia or, occasionally, polyspike activity and irregular slow waves. Infantile spasms are difficult to treat but may respond to high doses of adrenocorticotropin or corticosteroids. Clonazepam and diazepam are also of benefit sometimes. Infantile spasms have been reviewed recently (127).

Myoclonic seizures in older children and adults may be associated with familial degenerative diseases; the Lennox–Gastaut syndrome is particularly difficult to treat. The Lennox–Gastaut syndrome is an epileptic encephalopathy of childhood that is characterized by akinetic or atonic seizures, myoclonus, and slow spike and wave abnormalities on EEG. Multiple drug therapy is often required for management of these seizure types. Valproic acid appears to be the most promising drug for the treatment of these myoclonic disorders (94,96). Clonazepam and diazepam have been used with limited success. The ketogenic diet or a medium-chain triglyceride diet may be effective in controlling seizures in this syndrome as well as in other seizure types (128). In the ketogenic diet, the daily fat-to-nonfat (carbohydrate-to-protein) ratio is 4:1. The urine should be tested daily for ketones in order to maintain a high ketone saturation in the blood. Supplementary calcium and multivitamins should be given with this diet.

Table 6. Major Drugs Used in the Treatment of Generalized Convulsive (Grand Mal) and Simple and Complex Partial Seizures

Drug or Combination	*Trade Name*	*Formulations*	*Daily Dose*	*Method of Administration*	*Therapeutic Plasma Level*	*Comments*
Phenytoin	Dilantin	Capsules: 50, 100 mg Suspension: 30 mg/5 cc 125 mg/5 cc	4–7 mg/kg	Single daily dose	10–20 μg/ml	
Phenobarbital (alone in children)	Luminal	Tablets: 15, 30, 60, 100 mg	1–5 mg/kg	Single daily dose	20–40 μg/ml	
Primidone	Mysoline	Tablets: 50, 250 mg Suspension: 250 mg/5 cc	10–25 mg/kg	Twice-daily or divided daily doses	7–15 μg/ml	
Carbamazepine	Tegretol	Tablets: 200 mg	7–15 mg/kg	Twice-daily or divided daily doses	4–10 μg/ml	
Phenytoin/primidone			10–25 mg/kg			
Phenytoin/primidone *or* Phenobarbital/ Methsuximide or Valproic Acid			10–15 mg/kg[a]		15–30 μg/ml[b] 50–100 μg/ml[c]	Primidone or phenobarbital may be withdrawn slowly after dosage and plasma levels are stable.
Phenytoin/Primidone *or* Phenobarbital/ Carbamazepine						Phenytoin may be withdrawn slowly over three to four weeks after dosage and plasma levels are stable.

[a]Methsuximide.

[b]*N*-desmethyl metabolite of methsuximide.

[c]Valproic acid.

Table 7. Major Drugs Used in the Treatment of Absence Seizures (Petit Mal)

Drug or Combination	*Trade Name*	*Formulations*	*Daily Dose*	*Method of Administration*[a]	*Therapeutic Plasma Level*	*Comments*
Ethosuximide	Zarontin	Capsules: 250 mg Solution: 250 mg/5 cc	20–30 mg/kg	Twice-daily doses	40–100 μg/ml	
Valproic Acid	Depakene	Capsules: 250 mg Suspension: 250 mg/5 cc	10–60 mg/kg	Three divided daily doses	50–100 μg/ml	
Trimethadione	Tridione	Capsules: 150, 300 mg Solution: 200 mg/5 cc	10–25 mg/kg	Twice-daily doses		
Ethosuximide/Valproic Acid						
Ethosuximide or Valproic Acid-Trimethadione			10–25 mg/kg[c]		600–900 μg/ml[b]	
Ethosuximide		Capsules: 250 mg Syrup: 250 mg/5 cc				Phenytoin or other combinations listed if generalized convulsive or partial seizures coexist.
Clonazepam	Clonopin	Tablets: 0.5, 2 mg	0.1–0.2 mg/kg	Two-three divided daily doses	20–80 ng/ml	Phenytoin or other combinations listed if generalized convulsive or partial seizures coexist.
Acetazolamide	Diamox	Tablets: 250 mg	5–15 mg/kg	Two-three divided daily doses		May be a useful adjunct in both convulsive and absence seizures and can be used with any of the combinations listed.

[a] All drugs may be administered in equally divided doses; however, single or twice-daily doses may be more convenient for the patient.

[b] Dimethadione metabolite of trimethadione.

[c] Trimethadione.

Neonatal Seizures

Neonatal seizures occur in about 0.5–0.8% of infants. The seizures generally occur in the first month of life. Seizure phenomena in newborns differ from those in older children because of immaturity of the CNS in the former. Well-developed, generalized tonic-clonic seizures are rare in newborns. Seizures that occur in premature infants may be difficult to recognize because they may resemble normal reflex responses or random movements.

The etiology of neonatal seizures is unknown in 25% of patients. In the remainder, multiple factors may be responsible. These include metabolic disorders, infections, drug withdrawal, birth trauma and hypoxia, and congenital malformations (129,130).

Treatment of neonatal seizures is directed primarily at the underlying etiologic factors, if possible. Therapy should be instituted quickly to prevent cerebral damage. After an airway is established and oral secretions are removed, an IV line should be introduced. A blood sample should be obtained for determination of concentrations of glucose, sodium, calcium, and magnesium. Examination of the CSF should be performed to rule out CNS infection. The IV administration of 5 ml of 25% glucose should be the first line of approach. If seizures continue, hypoglycemia can be excluded as the cause. Calcium gluconate, 4 mg/kg of a 5% solution, can be administered slowly IV. The EEG should be monitored during administration. If seizures or tetany persist, magnesium sulfate, 20–50 mg/kg in a 2% solution, can be administered IV. Intravenous administration of 50 mg pyridoxine hydrochloride is indicated if the seizures still persist. If seizures continue despite all these measures, phenobarbital, 10–20 mg/kg, should be administered slowly IV. Phenobarbital can be continued orally at a dosage of 5 mg/kg/day in two divided doses. Diazepam and phenytoin generally are not used. Measurements of plasma concentrations of phenobarbital should be used to guide therapy. General measures that require attention are maintenance of adequate hydration, maintenance of body temperature, and prevention of aspiration.

Febrile Seizures

Febrile seizures are defined as seizures that occur in any child with a rectal temperature of 38°C or more in the absence of CNS infection. Febrile seizures occur most often in children between the ages of 6 months and 3 years. However, both the definition and prophylaxis of this condition are controversial (131). In children who have experienced a febrile seizure, it is important to treat the fever and its cause. If the child is still convulsing on examination, the seizure can be terminated with administration of diazepam, 0.1–0.3 mg/kg injected slowly IV. This dose may be repeated in 20 minutes, and larger doses may be necessary. Particular attention should be given to prevention of cardiopulmonary depression. CSF examination should be performed to exclude CNS infection.

Controversy exists as to the effectiveness of prophylaxis with phenobarbital (131–135). Prolonged treatment with phenobarbital is not entirely innocuous, since the drug causes behavioral changes and irritability. The treatment regimen for a particular child must be individualized, and if prophylactic treatment with phenobarbital is chosen, therapeutic plasma levels must be maintained. The greatest chance of recurrence of febrile seizures is in young children; therefore most patients younger than 3 years of age probably should receive treatment. Children older than 3 years who have a brief initial convulsion should not be treated prophylactically. Once prophylaxis is chosen, it should be continued to the age of 4 or 5 years. Recently, recommendations have been made for prophylaxis in any child with any of the following criteria: (*1*) age less than 18 months; (*2*) abnormal EEG seven to 10 days after seizure; (*3*) family history of seizure disorders; (*4*) seizures lasting longer than 15 minutes, occurring more than once in 24 hours, or focal in type; (*5*) presence of a chronic neurologic deficit (136). If the patient cannot tolerate phenobarbital, primidone may be substituted. Any child who has another febrile seizure should receive prophylaxis regardless of the other criteria. Phenytoin is ineffective in children younger than 3 years. However, if phenobarbital and primidone are not well tolerated, phenytoin may be used for prophylaxis in children older than 3 years.

Status Epilepticus

Status epilepticus is a state of continuing or recurring seizures in which recovery between attacks is incomplete. Among the varieties of status epilepticus are prolonged partial seizures, simple and complex epileptic confusional states that may last for hours or even days, petit mal status, and grand mal convulsive status. The last type is by far the most serious and life threatening and, unless it is terminated naturally or therapeutically, results in death (137). Status epilepticus may appear in patients with recurring or chronic seizure disorders as a complication of abrupt withdrawal of anticonvulsant drugs. Furthermore, severe and continuing convulsions are a frequent complication of acute diseases that affect the brain (138). Such diseases include meningitis or encephalitis, toxemia of pregnancy, hypertensive encephalopathy, uremia, an expanding intracranial lesion, and acute electrolyte disturbances such as hyponatremia. Whatever the precipitating cause, the treatment of status epilepticus requires skill and judgment, with a careful balance between the harmful and beneficial effects of the therapy.

As with other conditions that cause coma, strict attention must be directed to maintenance of an adequate airway, tracheobronchial toilet, and hydration. Rapid general and neurologic examinations are required to detect evidence of CNS infection, trauma, increased intracranial pressure, cerebral hemorrhage, or metabolic encephalopathy. Blood samples should be taken for assessment of electrolytes, blood urea nitrogen, glucose, lactic acid, toxicology, and levels of anticonvulsants. Drug treatment is directed toward termination of the seizures, and relatively large dosages frequently are required. As usual, the physician administering anticonvulsant agents IV must be prepared for the possibility of respiratory arrest and the need for ventilatory assistance. In some instances, the assistance of an anesthesiologist who is skilled in the management of patients under sedation should be obtained.

In some instances, the choice of treatment and medication depend on the cause of the status. For example, hyponatremic convulsions respond rapidly to judicious IV administration of hypertonic sodium chloride. The choice of agent also may be limited by its metabolic fate or route of excretion. In patients with renal or hepatic failure, great care must be taken in the administration of large amounts of barbiturates. A bolus of 25–50 ml of 50% glucose should be administered IV early in the course of grand mal status.

In grand mal, petit mal, and simple or complex partial or focal status there are a number of effective ways to terminate the status medically. Different clinicians prefer different regimens on the basis of their familiarity with a particular drug and method of administration.

For the past four years we have used IV phenytoin as the initial drug of choice and have found it to be effective in terminating status in 80% of patients (139). The drug penetrates the CNS rapidly. Intravenous phenytoin has the particular advantages of not producing CNS depression or significantly changing results of the neurologic examination. Furthermore, we have not encountered adverse side effects with this drug. Intravenous diazepam, phenobarbital, and paraldehyde often result in significant sedation, respiratory depression, alteration of neurologic signs, and sometimes hypotension. Such a situation is undesirable if the clinical situation does not permit adequate neurologic examination before cessation of seizure activity, if the patient is elderly, or if the patient has compromised pulmonary function.

Intravenous injection of diazepam may produce immediate cessation of the seizure (140,141); however, unless a major drug is used, seizure activity will resume, and additional IV injections will be required. We prefer a single initial injection of 5–10 mg diazepam coupled with simultaneously administered phenytoin.

When phenytoin is the drug of choice, whether alone or in combination with diazepam, phenobarbital, or paraldehyde, the drug should be given in the full recommended dose of 13 mg/kg. Although we have not observed hypotension or cardiac irregularities with use of phenytoin, caution should be exercised when arrhythmias are present. Electrocardiographic (ECG) monitoring should be done in elderly patients and in patients with known or suspected cardiac disease or conduction abnormalities. The rate of administration should not exceed 50 mg/min. Failure to control or terminate status epilepticus with phenytoin usually occurs when insufficient doses are given.

The depressant side effects of diazepam, phenobarbital, and paraldehyde are neither enhanced nor potentiated by IV phenytoin; however, when combinations of diazepam, phenobarbital, or paraldehyde in therapeutic or even subtherapeutic doses are given, cardiac and respiratory depression can be expected.

If phenobarbital is used in the treatment of status, 5–8 mg/kg can be given slowly and repeated at a dosage of 4 mg/kg every two to six hours. If paraldehyde is selected, the IM, IV, or rectal route may be used. The drug can be given at a dosage of 0.1–0.15 ml/kg, which can be repeated every two to six hours if necessary. The IV route should be used only in emergency situations, and then the drug should be diluted at 1 : 10 ratio of IV solution and administered slowly. When IM paraldehyde is given, nerve trunks should be avoided. If repeated doses are given rectally, mixing the drug with vegetable oil will both prevent irritation and retard absorption.

Rarely, deep anesthesia in addition to phenytoin and phenobarbital may be necessary to control status epilepticus. On several occasions during 15 years of experience, we have used IV lidocaine, which was effective in these severe, refractory cases (142,143). Caution should be exercised with lidocaine because it can cause direct depression of cardiac contractility. The drug can be administered safely at a dosage of 10 mg/kg/hr as long as blood pressure and ECG activity are monitored.

When status epilepticus occurs in an epileptic patient, the inciting cause must be sought. Abrupt drug withdrawal, meningitis, encephalitis, toxemia of pregnancy, hypertensive encephalopathy, uremia, acute electrolyte imbalance, and hypoglycemia are conditions that should be ruled out. In prolonged status epilepticus, respiratory acidosis and metabolic acidosis may occur; if an acid-base disturbance exists, it should be treated.

Table 8 lists the anticonvulsant drugs, dosages, routes and methods of administration, and combinations of drugs that are effective in termination status epilepticus.

Alcohol Withdrawal and Metabolic Seizures

Seizures in the alcoholic patient may have multiple etiologies that require different approaches to treatment. Seizures may be a result of (*1*) an idiopathic seizure disorder, (*2*) acute electrolyte disturbances, hypoglycemia, meningitis, or other toxic-metabolic states, (*3*) trauma, or (*4*) withdrawal. It is important to rule out the other causes before a patient is considered to have alcohol withdrawal seizures.

Alcohol withdrawal seizures, or rum fits, are generalized tonic-clonic seizures that occur during alcohol withdrawal in patients who otherwise have no seizures and have normal EEGs. Withdrawal seizures are most likely to occur between 30 and 48 hours after cessation of drinking. The patient usually experiences one or two attacks (144). Status epilepticus is uncommon in these seizures (145). Forty percent of patients progress to delirium tremens.

Various drugs have been used in the treatment of alcohol withdrawal (146). Paraldehyde is effective in the treatment of seizures, but the drug possesses some undesirable side effects. In most patients the benzodiazepines prevent alcohol withdrawal seizures. If the patient has a history of seizures, the addition of phenytoin in therapeutic doses is indicated. Phenytoin need not be continued beyond the period of withdrawal if the patient does not give a history of seizures that are not related to alcohol. For prevention of withdrawal seizures, all the benzodiazepines probably are equally effective; however, chlordiazepoxide is used most frequently. The dosage may vary from 100–1000 mg/day and may be given orally or IV depending on the severity of the withdrawal reaction. If repeated seizures occur during the withdrawal period, phenytoin may be added to the treatment regimen. If status epilepticus occurs, it should be treated as outlined previously.

The treatment of metabolic seizures should be approached with an aim toward correction of the underlying disturbance (e.g., hypoglycemia, hypocalcemia, hyponatremia, uremia, sepsis). If the patient does not respond adequately, additional anticonvulsant therapy is indicated. Anticonvulsant therapy can be discontinued after the metabolic disturbance is corrected.

Table 8. Drugs Used in the Treatment of Status Epilepticus[a]

Generic (Trade) Name	*Formulations*	*Total Single Dose*	*Method of Administration*	*Comments*
1. Phenytoin (Dilantin)	5- and 2-ml ampoules with 50 mg/ml	13 mg/kg	IV, not to exceed 50 mg/min	
2. Diazepam (Valium)	2- and 10-ml ampoules with 5 mg/ml	0.05–0.15 mg/kg	IV, not to exceed 1–2 mg/min	If used alone, can be repeated every 30 minutes to one hour. Total daily dose should not exceed 100–200 mg. Extreme caution should be exercised when using the drug in children and the elderly. When used in combination with phenytoin, the initial dose rarely needs to be repeated.
3. Phenobarbital (Luminal)		8–15 mg/kg	IV slowly, over 10–15 minutes	Often used after phenytoin; should not be used in combination with diazepam.
4. Paraldehyde		0.1–0.15 ml/kg	IM, IV, or rectally	Most often used in alcoholic withdrawal seizures or after phenytoin. Can be repeated every two to four hours, if necessary. Avoid IV route except in emergency situations.
5. Lidocaine (Xylocaine)	Vials of 1% (10 mg/ml) and 2% (20 mg/ml)	10 mg/kg hr	Calculate rate for IV drip	Monitor blood pressure, pulse, and ECG activity periodically.

[a] The authors use a combination of 1 and 2. These drugs do not potentiate each other except in their anticonvulsant activity. Eighty to ninety percent of patients with status epilepticus respond promptly. The recommended doses of both drugs should not be repeated. Respiration and cardiac activity should be monitored.

Treatment of Single Seizures

Not infrequently, a juvenile or adult patient presents with just a single seizure that has no obvious causes on appropriate investigation. Most often, a single seizure may be caused by severe sleep deprivation, idiosyncratic drug reaction, drug or alcohol withdrawal, isolated posttraumatic seizure, syncopal seizure, or hyperallergic states. Such patients should be observed regularly until it is certain that an underlying structural lesion is not present. The physician also should keep in mind that seizures will subsequently develop in some of these patients. Whether patients with a single seizure should be treated routinely with anticonvulsants depends on many factors. These include whether there is a family history of seizures, the patient's occupation, the patient's willingness to stop driving an automobile temporarily, the availability of close medical supervision, and the patient's appreciation of the situation. This information can be helpful in either predicting the probability of subsequent seizures or recognizing patients who would be at high risk should a second seizure occur.

Termination of Medical Therapy

When an epileptic patient has been treated successfully or is seizure free, the question of withdrawal of medication invariably arises. Most epileptologists are wary of discontinuing medication because there is a high incidence of seizure recurrence when all anticonvulsants are withdrawn. Patients with documented epilepsy who have been seizure free for three to five years have a recurrence rate of 40% after anticonvulsant withdrawal.

We caution patients against withdrawal of medication until they have been seizure free for five years. At that time anticonvulsant drugs may be discontinued sequentially, with termination of the drug presumed least effective initially. A slow decrease in dosage over a period of six to eight weeks follows. If the patient remains seizure free for one month, the second drug is withdrawn in a similar manner, and so on.

Patients should not drive motor vehicles during drug withdrawal. Also, maintenance of close contact with the patient's family is recommended during this period. Stressful situations known to precipitate seizures in epileptic patients are to be avoided.

Therapeutic Failure

Twenty to thirty percent of chronic recurring seizures are refractory to medical therapy. The physician should be constantly alert to the possibility that lack of adequate seizure control may indicate factors other than medical intractability. These factors include:

1. Noncompliance.
2. Inadequate dosage.
3. Improper drug or combination of drugs for the particular seizure disorder.
4. Stressful situations.
5. Progressive neurologic disease.
6. Drug toxicity (rare).

Monitoring of levels of antiepileptic drug is helpful in assessing patient compliance. Toxicity usually is apparent, but psychological or psychotic reactions may occur in the absence of overt signs of drug toxicity. Plasma levels of drug can be extremely useful in assessing these situations. Improper use of drugs or drug combinations can be recognized after reevaluating the initial diagnosis. Reevaluation with more intensive EEG monitoring may be required to distinguish absence seizures from absence-like seizures originating in the temporal lobe. A progressive neurologic disease may be evident only after reevaluation. Physical and emotional stress is frequent cause for exacerbation of seizures. Sleep deprivation, emotional stress, excessive fatigue, alcohol, and irregular and improper dietary habits also may cause recurrence of seizures in a previously controlled patient. History from the patient or an informant may reveal this information and thus allow the physician to counsel the patient effectively.

ANTIEPILEPTIC DRUG TOXICITY

Toxic reactions to antiepileptic drugs can be considered to fall into the following groups: (*1*) acute allergic, dose-related, or idiosyncratic toxic reactions; (*2*) chronic toxicity; (*3*) teratogenic effects; and (*4*) toxic reactions resulting from drug interactions (discussed earlier). The factors that influence drug toxicity include genetic and age-related factors; malnutrition; presence of hepatic, renal, or endocrine disease; and prolonged use of the drug. In our experience, dose-related adverse toxic effects on the CNS that result from either excessive dosage or drug interaction are the most common causes.

Acute Toxicity

Most acute toxic reactions are dose related and usually cause neurologic and gastrointestinal symptoms. Acute allergic reactions are less common and may result in skin rashes or, more rarely, signs or symptoms secondary to hepatic, renal, or hematopoietic involvement. Idiosyncratic reactions are rare but potentially serious.

CNS signs of toxicity result in disturbances in cerebellovestibular, reticulocortical activating, pyramidal, and extrapyramidal systems and in higher cortical integrative function. Generally, the hydantoins induce signs of cerebellovestibular dysfunction (nystagmus, ataxia, incoordination, dysarthria). With more severe toxicity, pyramidal and extrapyramidal disturbances, such as asterixis, dystonic posturing, choreoathetoid movements, and, rarely, myoclonus, may be observed. Epileptic seizures may be exacerbated and, with profound toxicity, stupor and coma may result. Barbiturates generally interfere with the reticulocortical activating system early during therapy, with production of lethargy, somnolence, nystagmus, ataxia and higher cortical dysfunction; stupor and coma also may result. In children and the elderly, irritability may be observed paradoxically. Benzodiazepines may induce early lethargy and somnolence, and carbamazepine may produce ataxia, nystagmus, diplopia, and drowsiness. Nausea may be observed early in the course of therapy; this effect can be alleviated by a gradual increase in dosage.

The succinimides and oxazolidinediones sometimes produce higher cortical dysfunction and/or disturbances of the reticulocortical activating system. Somnolence, lethargy and emotional instability may occur. Trimethadione may produce light blindness (hemeralopia, or defective vision in bright light). Valproic acid may produce transient nausea and vomiting or a fine nonincapacitating tremor. If the patient is receiving other anticonvulsants concurrently, sedation may occur.

Idiosyncratic drug reactions occur in a few susceptible patients. Deficiency of phenytoin parahydroxylation may result in phenytoin intoxication. Barbiturates and phenytoin may induce an acute porphyric crisis. Idiosyncratic reactions are fully discussed in a recent review (147).

Chronic Toxicity

Chronic toxicity may develop insidiously over a prolonged period. The major targets for chronic antiepileptic drug toxicity are (*1*) the nervous system, (*2*) connective tissue and skin, (*3*) hematopoietic system, and (*4*) endocrine and skeletal systems.

Many reports are available on the pathologic changes that can occur in the nervous system after prolonged anticonvulsant therapy; their interpretation, however, is less clear. The relation of phenytoin therapy to cerebellar degeneration has not been proved definitely (148–155). A chronic encephalopathy has been described in association with prolonged phenytoin therapy (156), and a peripheral neuropathy that usually is subclinical also has been described (157–160). The latter is not caused by a deficiency in either vitamin B12 or folate.

Changes in connective tissue and skin that may occur with anticonvulsant therapy include gingival hyperplasia (from phenytoin), Dupuytren's contracture, thickening of subcutaneous tissues, and coarsening of facial features. Valproic acid may cause transient alopecia.

The effects of anticonvulsants on the hematopoietic system include neonatal coagulation defects, immunologic disorders, bone marrow suppression, and folate deficiency. Neonatal coagulation defects have been well documented (161–165). These are caused by a deficiency of vitamin K–dependent clotting factors. It is recommended that a small dose of vitamin K be administered to the mother before delivery or to the infant immediately after delivery. Immunologic disorders include lymphadenopathy resembling lymphoma (166–170) and decreased IgA production (171). Agranulocytosis, pancytopenia, neutropenia, leukopenia, thrombocytopenia, and aplastic anemia occur less frequently with phenytoin, primidone, phenobarbital, and ethosuximide than with other antiepileptic drugs, such as carbamazepine (172). Carbamazepine occasionally may cause transient insignificant leukopenia. Leukopenia of less than 3,000 per mm^3 or a granulocyte count of less than 25% of the total requires a reduction of dosage. Selective erythroid aplasia has been reported to occur with phenytoin (173). Valproic acid has been associated rarely with clinically significant hematologic reactions (111,123,124). Valproic acid also inhibits the secondary phase of platelet aggregation. This effect is not likely to be clinically significant except in patients who receive aspirin or anticoagulants concurrently or who undergo surgery. Folate deficiency may occur in treated epileptic patients, but megaloblastic anemia is rare (174) despite the frequent occurrence of megaloblastosis.

The endocrinologic effects of anticonvulsants include:

1. Osteomalacia (phenytoin, phenobarbital) (175–180).
2. Hyperglycemia (phenytoin) (181).
3. Water and electrolyte disturbances (phenytoin, carbamazepine) (179).
4. Hirsutism, acne, chloasma (phenytoin, phenobarbital).
5. Alopecia (valproic acid) (111,123,124).
6. Abnormalities on thyroid function tests but clinical euthyroidism (phenytoin, valproic acid, carbamazepine) (182–185).
7. Subnormal results on metyrapone and low-dose dexamethasone tests (phenytoin, phenobarbital, carbamazepine) (182).
8. Weight gain (valproic acid) (111,123,124).

Several extensive reviews are available on the toxicology of the antiepileptic drugs (73,147,186–188). Table 9 summarizes the major side effects of these drugs.

Teratogenic Effects

The incidence of congenital malformations in children born to epileptic mothers is higher than in the offspring of nonepileptic mothers. The role played by anticonvulsants in the incidence of congenital malformations is less clear. Data reported between 1964 and 1975 showed that 6% of newborns of drug-treated epileptic mothers had anomalies, while 4.2% of newborns from non-drug-treated epileptic mothers had anomalies (189,190). A higher incidence of anomalies was reported in infants born to mothers who received combined treatment with phenytoin and phenobarbital than with phenytoin or phenobarbital alone (191). Other reports are available that suggest that anticonvulsants have teratogenic effects, with the risk being two to three times higher than in control patients (192–195). Excessive complications during pregnancy and labor in drug-treated mothers also have been observed (196).

Malformations most often associated with anticonvulsant drugs are, in descending order of frequency, cleft lip and palate; cardiac, skeletal and CNS defects; hypospadias, and intestinal atresia. Although there appears to be no single drug that, when taken during pregnancy, has not been associated with malformations, a causal relation is not always easy to prove.

For practical reasons, anticonvulsants should not be discontinued during pregnancy. The risk appears to be minor provided that the patient receives medical care by a physician who anticipates potential problems and takes appropriate action. Careful clinical evaluation and drug monitoring can prevent drug toxicity. New antiepileptic drugs should be avoided in the pregnant patient until further experience is gained with them. Although the mechanisms of antiepileptic drug–induced teratogenesis are uncertain, chromosomal abnormalities, disturbances of mitosis, and folate deficiency may partially be responsible.

Table 9. Toxicity of Various Anticonvulsant Drugs

Acute Toxicity	*Chronic Toxicity*
Gastrointestinal	Dermatologic (skin rashes, acne, chloasma)
Higher Cortical Dysfunction	Connective Tissue (hyperplasia)
Reticulocortical Activating System	Hematopoietic (suppression)
Cerebellovestibular System	Autoimmune (lupus, polyarterities, thyroiditis)
Motor System (pyramidal and extrapyramidal)	Hepatic (hepatocellular damage)
	Renal (nephrotic syndrome)
	Neurologic (encephalopathy, psychosis, personality changes, ataxia)
	Endocrinologic (osteomalacia, hirsutism, hyperglycemia, weight change)
	Lymphatic (lymphadenopathy)
	Teratogenicity

MANAGEMENT OF PSYCHOSOCIAL PROBLEMS AND VOCATIONAL REHABILITATION

The total management of epileptic patients consists of professional medical treatment of seizures, assistance with psychological problems that may be associated with epilepsy, and assistance with vocational rehabilitation. A multiprofessional team approach is required. Management of psychosocial problems improves patients' well-being and helps them to deal with psychological factors that may play a role in triggering seizures.

Most patients with epilepsy have normal personality and intellect; although there is no specific epileptic personality, defects of intellect and personality occur more frequently in epileptic patients than in controls (197). Also, defects in personality or intellect may vary from patient to patient and may be produced by one or more of several factors: (*1*) structural brain disease, (*2*) effects of antiepileptic drugs, (*3*) uncontrolled seizures, (*4*) familial psychological reactions of family members to the illness and (*5*) social isolation (198). There is lack of agreement as to whether patients with complex partial seizures have a higher incidence of psychiatric disturbances than do those with other types of epilepsy (198–204). It also has been suggested that personality and behavioral disorders differ in epilepsy originating in the left or right temporal lobes (203).

The occurrence of psychiatric disorders in epileptic patients is related partly to brain damage, chronicity of the seizure disorder, early age of onset, temporal lobe dysfunction, frightening auras, and restriction of activity (205). Violence is rare during epileptic automatisms (206–208), and the association between epilepsy and criminal behavior is not entirely clear (205). The most common psychiatric disturbances other than personality disorders include depression, anxiety, and psychosis (209).

The psychosocial management of epileptic patients requires proper education of the patient and family concerning epilepsy. The importance of drug compliance should be stressed, the patient's anxieties should be relieved, and all questions should be answered. Children with epilepsy should not be overprotected and should not be allowed to manipulate their environment with their seizures. If overt symptoms of an effective disorder are present, antidepressant drug therapy may be indicated and, if true psychosis is present, piperazine phenothiazines may have to be prescribed. These drugs may rarely cause an increase in seizures but to a lesser degree than the aliphatic and piperidyl phenothiazines. Behavior modification techniques may be of benefit in some patients.

When certain specific problems exist, patients should be referred to the proper agencies that can offer financial assistance, counseling, family planning, and education. Vocational rehabilitation may be able to help patients who otherwise would not gain useful employment. The ability of epileptic patients to drive a motor vehicle alone depends on many factors, and the patient should be seizure free for at least one year before attempting to drive. Factors that should be taken into consideration include:

1. Whether the physician believes the patient is truthful about seizure frequency.
2. Whether the patient is known to be compliant.
3. Whether the patient is under regular medical supervision.
4. Whether the seizures appear to have been prevented by medication.
5. Whether major side effects such as drowsiness, occur.

Patients should obtain specific information from their state department of transportation before applying for a driver's license.

In children with seizures, special educational problems may arise, and some children may require special schooling. Whenever possible the child should be educated in regular classrooms and should be allowed to participate in as many routine activities as possible without being a hazard to himself or herself. The teacher should be aware of the child's medical condition and possible difficulties that may arise concerning language development, emotional maturity, motor development, and behavior. More comprehensive reports are available on this aspect of management (210–220).

SURGICAL THERAPY

A small number of patients with epilepsy can benefit from surgical therapy. Generally, surgical therapy is useful in some cases of partial epilepsy that are unresponsive to optimal medical therapy. Before surgical therapy is considered, certain criteria must be met:

1. A reliable history of seizures and their frequency must be obtained.
2. An adequte trial of anticonvulsants must be conducted.
3. Seizures must be disabling.
4. Unequivocal presence of a seizure focus must be found.
5. There must be a single independent focus that is responsible for the seizures.

6. The focus must be accessible and removable without great risk of neurologic deficit.
7. The patient is potentially capable of leading a useful life if seizures are controlled.
8. A neurosurgical team experienced in this aspect of therapy must be available.

The clinical evaluation of patients requires establishment of the focal nature of the epilepsy. The neurologic history, observation of attacks, neurologic findings on examination, EEG studies, and neuroradiologic examinations are all useful in helping to localize a focal cerebral lesion.

Surgical therapy is usually performed in patients with intractable psychomotor epilepsy. Local cortical excision results either in complete elimination of seizures or in considerable improvement in approximately two-thirds of patients (221–223).

It is important to emphasize to the patient and family that surgery decreases the frequency of seizures but does not cure them. Anticonvulsant therapy usually can be simplified, but most patients will need to continue taking phenytoin or other major antiepileptic drugs that are effective against tonic-clonic seizures.

Other surgical procedures available for the treatment of epilepsy include stereotaxic procedures, cerebral commissurotomy, hemispherectomy, and cerebellar stimulation. These are undertaken in highly selected cases; the efficacy of procedures such as cerebellar stimulation is not clear (224–226). A recent review on the surgical treatment of epilepsy has been published (227).

REFERENCES

1. Masland RL: Commission for the control of epilepsy. Neurology 28:861–862, 1978.
2. Gastaut H: Clinical and electroencephalographical classification of epileptic seizures. Epilepsia 11:102–113, 1970.
3. Schmidt RP, Wilder BJ: *Epilepsy*. New York, FA Davis, 1968.
4. Azarnoff DL: Application of blood level data to clinical trials. Clin Pharmacol Ther 16:183–188, 1973.
5. Vesell ES: Factors causing interindividual variations of drug concentrations in blood. Clin Pharmacol Ther 16:135–148, 1973.
6. Levy G: Pharmacokinetic control and clinical interpretation of steady-state blood levels of drugs. Clin Pharmacol Ther 16:130–134, 1973.
7. Glazko AJ: Antiepileptic drugs: biotransformation, metabolism, and serum half-life. Epilepsia 16:367–391, 1975.
8. Greenblatt DJ, Koch–Weser J: Clinical pharmacokinetics. N Engl J Med 293:702–705, 964–970, 1975.
9. Prescott LF: Pathological and physiological factors affecting drug absorption, distribution, elimination, and response in man. In: *Handbook of Experimental Pharmacology*, vol. 28, part 3. Edited by JR Gillette and JR Mitchell. New York, Springer-Verlag, 1975, pp. 234–257.
10. Shand DG, Mitchell JR, Oates JA. Pharmacokinetic drug interactions. In: *Handbook of Experimental Pharmacology*, vol. 28, part 3. Edited by JR Gillette and JR Mitchell. New York, Springer-Verlag, 1975, pp. 272–314.
11. Hvidberg EF, Dam M: Clinical pharmacokinetics of anticonvulsants. Clin Pharmacokinet 1:101–188, 1976.

12. Gibaldi M, Levy G: Pharmacokinetics in clinical practice. JAMA 235:1864–1867, 1987–1992.

13. Fingl F: Principles of drug absorption, distribution, and metabolism. In: *Antiepileptic Drugs: Quantitative Analysis and Interpretation.* Edited by CE Pippenger, JK Penry and H Kutt. New York, Raven Press, 1978, pp. 221–236.

14. Browne TR: Drug therapy reviews: clinical pharmacology of antiepileptic drugs. Am J Hosp Pharmacol 35:1048–1056, 1978.

15. Arnold K, Gerber N, Levy G: Absorption and dissolution of sodium diphenylhydantoin capsules. Can J Pharmacol Sci 5:89–92, 1978.

16. Pentikainen PJ, Neuvonen PJ, Elfving SM: Bioavailability of four brands of phenytoin tablets. Eur J Clin Pharmacol 9:213–218, 1975.

17. Melikian AP, Straughn GWA, Slynka PL, et al: Bioavailability of 11 phenytoin products. J Pharmacokinet Biopharm 5:133–146, 1977.

18. Dam M, Olesen OV: Intramuscular administration of phenytoin. Neurology 16:288–292, 1966.

19. Kostenbauder HP, Rapp RP, McGovern JP, et al: Bioavailability and single dose pharmacokinetics of intramuscular phenytoin. Clin Pharmacol Ther 18:449–456, 1975.

20. Wilensky AJ, Lowden AJ: Inadequate serum levels after intramuscular administration of diphenylhydantoin. Neurology 23:318–324, 1973.

21. Serrano EE, Wilder BJ: Intramuscular administration of diphenylhydantoin. Arch Neurol 31:276–278, 1974.

22. Wilder BJ, Serrano EE, Ramsay EE, et al: A method of shifting from oral to intramuscular diphenylhydantoin administration. Clin Pharmacol Ther 16:507–513, 1974.

23. Perrier D, Rapp R, Young B, et al: Maintenance of therapeutic plasma levels via intramuscular administration. Ann Intern Med 85:318–321, 1976.

24. Wilder BJ, Ramsay RE: Oral and intramuscular phenytoin. Clin Pharmacol Ther 19:360–364, 1976.

25. Greenblatt DJ, Koch–Weser J: Intramuscular administration of drugs. N Engl J Med 295:542–546, 1976.

26. Lombroso CT: Treatment of status epilepticus with diazepam. Neurology 16:629–634, 1966.

27. Wallis W, Kutt H, McDowell F: Intravenous diphenylhydantoin in treatment of acute repetitive seizures. Neurology 18:513–525, 1968.

28. Wilder BJ, Ramsay RE, Willmore LJ, et al: Efficacy of intravenous phenytoin in the treatment of status epilepticus: kinetics of central nervous system penetration. Ann Neurol 1:511–518, 1977.

29. Koch–Weser J, Sellers EM: Binding of drugs to serum albumin. N Engl J Med 294:311–316, 526–531, 1976.

30. Reidenberg MM, Odar–Cederlof I, von Bahr et al: Protein binding of diphenylhydantoin and desmethylimipramine in plasma from patients with poor renal function. N Engl J Med 285:264–267, 1971.

31. Letteri JM, Mellk LT, Louis S, et al: Diphenylhydantoin metabolism in uremia. N Engl J Med 385:648–652, 1971.

32. Hooper WD, Bochner F, Eadie MJ, et al: Plasma protein binding of diphenylhydantoin: effects of sex hormones, renal and hepatic disease. Clin Pharmacol Ther 15:276–282, 1974.

33. Gugler R, Shoeman DW, Huffman DH, et al: Pharmacokinetics of drugs in patients with the nephrotic syndrome. J Clin Invest 55:1182–1189, 1975.

34. Porter RJ, Layzer RB: Plasma albumin concentration and diphenylhydantoin binding in man. Arch Neurol 32:298–303, 1975.

35. Jusko WJ, Gretch M: Plasma and tissue protein binding of drugs in pharmacokinetics. Drug Metab Rev 5:43–140, 1976.

36. Gillette JR, Pang KS: Theoretic aspects of pharmacokinetic drug interactions. Clin Pharmacol Ther 22:623–639, 1977.

37. Conney AH: Pharmacological implications of microsomal enzyme inductions. Pharmacol Rev 19:317–366, 1967.
38. Kuntzman R: Drugs and enzyme induction. Annu Rev Pharmacol 9:21–36, 1969.
39. Anders MW: Enhancement and inhibition of drug metabolism. Annu Rev Pharmacol 11:37–56, 1971.
40. Richens A, Woodford FP: *Anticonvulsant Drugs and Enzyme Induction.* Amsterdam, Elsevier, 1976.
41. Waddell WJ, Butler TC: The distribution and excretion of phenobarbital. J Clin Invest 36:1217–1226, 1957.
42. Weiner IM, Mudge GH: Renal tubular mechanisms for excretion of organic acids and bases. Am J Med 36:743–762, 1964.
43. Schmidt D, Kupferberg HJ: Diphenylhydantoin, phenobarbital, and primidone in saliva, plasma and cerebrospinal fluid. Epilepsia 16:735–741, 1975.
44. Cook CE, Amerson E, Poole WK, et al: Phenytoin and phenobarbital concentrations in saliva and plasma measured by radioimmunoassay. Clin Pharmacol Ther 18:742–747, 1975.
45. Horning MG, Brown L, Nowlin J, et al: Use of saliva in therapeutic drug monitoring. Clin Chem 23:157–164, 1977.
46. Danhoff N, Breimer DD: Therapeutic drug monitoring in saliva. Clin Pharmacokinet 3:39–57, 1978.
47. Mucklow JC, Bending NR, Kahn GC, et al: Drug concentration in saliva. Clin Pharmacol Ther 24:563–570, 1978.
48. Sherwin AL, Robb JP, Lechter M: Improved control of epilepsy by monitoring plasma ethosuximide. Arch Neurol 28:178–181, 1973.
49. Buchtal F, Svensmark O: Aspects of the pharmacology of penytoin (Dilantin) and phenobarbital relevant to their dosage in the treatment of epilepsy. Epilepsia 1:373–384, 1960.
50. Kutt H: Diphenylhydantoin: relation of plasma levels to clinical control. In: *Antiepileptic Drugs.* Edited by DM Woodbury, JK Penry, and RP Schmidt. New York, Raven Press 1972, pp. 211–218.
51. Buchtal F, Lennox–Buchtal MA: Phenobarbital: relation to serum concentration to control of seizures. In: *Antiepileptic Drugs.* Edited by DM Woodbury, JK Penry, and RP Schmidt. New York, Raven Press, 1972, pp. 335–343.
52. Buchtal F, Lennox–Buchtal MA: Diphenylhydantoin: relation of anticonvulsant effect to concentration in serum. In: *Antiepileptic Drugs.* Edited by DM Woodbury, JK Penry, and RP Schmidt. New York, Raven Press, 1972, pp. 193–209.
53. Kutt H, Penry JK: Usefulness of blood levels of antiepileptic drugs. Arch Neurol 31:283–288, 1974.
54. Kutt H: Pharmacodynamic and pharmacokinetic measurements of antiepileptic drugs. Clin Pharmacol Ther 16:243–249, 1974.
55. Lund L: Anticonvulsant effect of diphenylhydantoin relative to plasma levels. Arch Neurol 31:289–294, 1974.
56. Feldman RG, Pippenger CE: The relation of anticonvulsant drug levels to complete seizure control. J Clin Pharmacol 16:51–59, 1976.
57. Troupin AS, Green JR, Levy RH: Carbamazepine (Tegretol®) as an anticonvulsant. A pilot study. Neurology 24:863–869, 1974.
58. Dam M, Jensen A, Christiansen J: Plasma level and effect of carbamazepine in grand mal and psychomotor epilepsy. Acta Neurol Scand [Suppl] 60:33–38, 1975.
59. Booker HE, Celesia GG: Serum concentrations of diazepam in subjects with epilepsy. Arch Neurol 29:191–194, 1973.
60. Dreifuss FE, Penry JK, Rose SW, et al: Serum clonazepam concentrations in children with absence seizures. Neurology 25:255–258, 1975.
61. Bruni J, Wilder BJ, Willmore LJ, et al: Clinical efficacy of valproic acid in relation to plasma levels. Can J Neurol Sci 5:385–387, 1978.

62. Booker HE, Darcey B: Serum concentrations of free diphenylhydantoin and their relationship to clinical intoxication. Epilepsia 14:177–184, 1973.

63. Booker HE: Primidone: relation of plasma levels to clinical control. In: *Antiepileptic Drugs.* Edited by DM Woodbury, JK Penry, and RP Schmidt. New York, Raven Press, 1972, pp. 373–376.

64. Kutt H: Biochemical and genetic factors regulating Dilantin metabolism in man. Ann NY Acad Sci 179:704–722, 1971.

65. Gibberd FB, Dunne JF, Handley AJ, et al: Supervision of epileptic patients taking phenytoin. Br Med J 1:147–149, 1970.

66. Buchtal F, Svensmark O: Serum concentrations of diphenylhydantoin (phenytoin) and phenobarbital and their relation to therapeutic and toxic effects. Psychiatr Neurol Neurochir 74:117–136, 1971.

67. Blackwell B: Patient compliance. N Engl J Med 289:249–252, 1973.

68. Kutt H: Interactions of antiepileptic drugs. Epilepsia 16:393–402, 1975.

69. Vree TB, Henderson PT, Van Der Kleijn E, et al: Drug interactions at the metabolic level: a reality in drug treatment of epilepsy. In: *Clinical Pharmacology of Antiepileptic Drugs.* Edited by HS Janz, C Gardner–Thorpe, H Meinardi, et al. New York, Springer-Verlag, 1975, pp. 34–42.

70. Richens A: Interactions with antiepileptic drugs. Drugs 13:266–275, 1977.

71. Rawlins MD: General mechanisms of drug interactions. In: *Drug Interactions.* Edited by DJ Grahame–Smith. Baltimore, University Park Press, 1977, pp. 35–44.

72. Wilder BJ, Willmore LJ, Bruni J, et al: Valproic acid: interaction with other anticonvulsant drugs. Neurology 28:892–896, 1978.

73. Bruni J, Wilder BJ: The toxicology of antiepileptic drugs. In: *Handbook of Clinical Neurology.* Edited by PJ Vinken and GW Bruyn. Amsterdam, North Holland. Volume 37, Part 2, pp. 199–222, 1979.

74. Garrettson LK, Jusko WJ: Diphenylhydantoin elimination kinetics in overdosed children. Clin Pharmacol Ther 17:481–491, 1975.

75. Houghton GW, Richens A: Rate of elimination of tracer doses of phenytoin at different steady-state serum phenytoin concentrations in epileptic patients. Br J Clin Pharmacol 1:155–161, 1974.

76. Cotter LM, Eadie MJ, Hooper WD, et al: The pharmacokinetics of carbamazepine. Eur J Clin Pharmacol 12:451–456, 1977.

77. Ramsay RE, Strauss RG, Wilder BJ, et al: Status epilepticus in pregnancy: effect of phenytoin malabsorption on seizure control. Neurology 28:85–89, 1978.

78. Kupferberg HB: Quantitative estimation of diphenylhydantoin, primidone, and phenobarbital in plasma by gas-liquid chromatography. Clin Chim Acta 29:283–288, 1970.

79. Change T, Glazko AJ: Quantitative assay of 5,5-diphenylhydantoin (Dilantin) and 5-(*p*-hydroxyphenyl)-5-phenylhydantoin by gas-liquid chromatography. J Lab Clin Med 75:145–155, 1970.

80. McGee J: Rapid determination of diphenylhydantoin in blood plasma by gas-liquid chromatography. Anal Chem 42:421–422, 1970.

81. Perchalski RJ, Scott KN, Wilder BJ, et al: Rapid simultaneous GLC determination of phenobarbital, primidone, and diphenylhydantoin. J Pharmacol Sci 62:1735–1736, 1973.

82. Kutt H: Carbamazepine: chemistry and methods of determination. In: *Advances in Neurology,* vol. 11. Edited by JK Penry and DD Daly. New York, Raven Press, 1975, pp. 249–261.

83. Svensmark O, Kristensen P: Determination of diphenylhydantoin and phenobarbital in small amounts of serum. J Lab Clin Med 61:501–507, 1963.

84. Dill WA, Kazenko A, Wolf LM, et al: Studies on 5,5-diphenylhydantoin (Dilantin) in animals and man. J Pharmacol Exp Ther 118:270–279, 1956.

85. Wisdom GB: Enzyme immunoassay. Clin Chem 22:1243–1255, 1976.

86. Schottelius DD: Homogeneous immunoassay system (EMIT) for quantitation of antiepileptic drugs in biological fluids. In: *Antiepileptic Drugs: Quantitative Analysis and Interpretation.* Edited by CE Pippenger, JK Penry, and H Kutt. New York, Raven Press, 1978, pp. 95–108.

87. Evans JE: Simultaneous measurement of diphenylhydantoin and phenobarbital in serum by high performance liquid chromatography. Anal Chem 45:2428–2429, 1973.

88. Horning MG, Lertratanangkoon K, Nowlin J, et al: Anticonvulsant drug monitoring by GC-MS-COM techniques. J Chromatogr Sci 12:630–635, 1974.

89. Busfield D, Child KJ, Atkinson RM, et al: An effect of phenobarbitone on blood levels of griseofulvin in man. Lancet 2:1042, 1963.

90. Rigelman S, Rowland M, Epstein WL: Griseofulvin-phenobarbital interactions in man. JAMA 213:426–431, 1970.

91. Cucinell SA: Phenobarbital—interactions with other drugs. In: *Antiepileptic Drugs.* Edited by DM Woodbury, JK Penry and RP Schmidt. New York, Raven Press, 1972, pp. 319–327.

92. Bardy A, Hari R, Lehtovaara R, et al: Valproate may lower serum phenytoin. Lancet 2:1297–1298, 1976.

93. Vakil SD, Critcheley EMR, Philips JC, et al: The effect of sodium valproate (Epilim) on phenytoin and phenobarbital levels. In: *Clinical and Pharmacological Aspects of Sodium Valproate (Epilim) in the Treatment of Epilepsy.* Edited by NJ Legg. Tunbridge Wells, England, MCS Consultants, 1976, pp. 75–77.

94. Patsalos PM, PT Lascelles: Valproate may lower serum phenytoin. Lancet 1:50–51, 1977.

95. Bruni J, Wilder BJ, Willmore LJ, et al: Valproic acid and plasma levels of phenytoin. Neurology (in press) 1979.

96. Buchanan RA, Sholiton LJ: Diphenylhydantoin—interaction with other drugs. In: *Antiepileptic Drugs.* Edited by DM Woodbury, JK Penry, and RP Schmidt. New York, Raven Press, 1972, pp. 181–191.

97. Edwards VE, Eadie MJ: Clonazepam—a clinical study of its effectiveness as an anticonvulsant. Proc Aust Assoc Neurol 10:61–66, 1973.

98. Houghton GW, Richens A: The effect of benzodiazepines and pheneturide on phenytoin metabolism in man. Br. J Clin Pharmacol 1:334–335, 1974.

99. Cereghino JJ, Van Meter JC, Brock JT, et al: Preliminary observations on serum carbamazepine concentrations in epileptic patients. Neurology 23:357–366, 1973.

100. Richens A, Ahmad S: Controlled trial of sodium valproate in severe epilepsy. Br Med J 4:255–256, 1975.

101. Glazko A: Antiepileptic drugs: biotransformation, metabolism and half-life. Epilepsia 16:367–391, 1975.

102. Wilder BJ, Serrano EE, Ramsay RE: Plasma diphenylhydantoin levels after loading and maintenance dose. Clin Pharmacol Ther 14:797–801, 1973.

103. Mirkin BL: Diphenylhydantoin: placental transport, fetal localization, neonatal metabolism and possible teratogenic effect. J Pediatr 78:229–237, 1971.

104. Mygind KI, Dam M, and Christiansen J: Phenytoin and phenobarbital plasma clearance during pregnancy. Acta Neurol Scand 54:160–166, 1974.

105. Frigerio A, Fanelli R, Biandrate J, et al: Mass spectrometric characterization of carbamazepine-10,11-epoxide, a carbamazepine metabolite isolated from human urine. J Pharmacol Sci 61:1144–1147, 1972.

106. Baker KM, Csentenyi J, Frigerio A, et al: 10,11-Dihydro-10,11-dihydroxy-5H-dibenz/b, f/ azepine 5-carboxamide, a metabolite of carbamazepine isolated from human and rat urine. J Med Chem 16:703–705, 1973.

107. Maynert EW: Phenobarbital, mephobarbital and metharbital: biotransformation. In: *Antiepileptic Drugs.* Edited by DM Woodbury, JK Penry, and RP Schmidt. New York, Raven Press, 1972, pp. 311–317.

108. Gallagher BB, Baumel IP: Primidone: absorption, distribution and excretion. In: *Antiepileptic Drugs.* Edited by DM Woodbury, JK Penry, and RP Schmidt. New York, Raven Press, 1972, pp. 357–359.

109. Gallagher BB, Baumel IP: Primidone: biotransformation. In: *Antiepileptic Drugs.* Edited by DM Woodbury, JK Penry, and RP Schmidt. New York, Raven Press, 1972, pp. 361–366.

110. Change T, Dill WA, Glazko AJ: Ethosuximide: absorption, distribution, and excretion. In: *Antiepileptic Drugs.* Edited by DM Woodbury, JK Penry, and RP Schmidt. New York, Raven Press, 1972, pp. 417–423.

111. Bruni J, Wilder BJ: Valproic acid: review of a new antiepileptic drug. Arch Neurol 36:393–398, 1979.

112. Browne TR: Clonazepam. N Engl J Med 299:812–816, 1978.

113. Browne TR, Penry JK: Benzodiazepines in the treatment of epilepsy. Epilepsia 14:277–310, 1973.

114. Mattson RH: Other antiepileptic drugs: the benzodiazepines. In: *Antiepileptic Drugs.* Edited by DM Woodbury, JK Penry and RP Schmidt. New York, Raven Press, 1972, pp. 497–516.

115. Frey H-H, Schulz R: Time course of the demethylation of trimethadione. Acta Pharmacol Toxicol (Copenh) 28:477–483, 1970.

116. Woodbury DM: Sulfonamides and derivatives: acetazolamide. In: *Antiepileptic Drugs.* Edited by DM Woodbury, JK Penry and RP Schmidt. New York, Raven Press, 1972, pp. 465–475.

117. Glazko AJ, Dill WA: Other succinimides: methsuximide and phensuximide. In: *Antiepileptic Drugs.* Edited by DM Woodbury, JK Penry, RP Schmidt. New York, Raven Press, 1972, pp. 455–464.

118. Woodbury DM: Antiepileptic drugs: pharmacology and mechanisms of action. In: *Epilepsy. Proceedings of the Hans Berger Centenary Symposium.* Edited by P Harris and C Mawdsley. Edinburgh, Churchill Livingstone, 1972, pp. 78–95.

119. Reynolds EH: How do anticonvulsants work? Br J Hosp Med 19:505–512, 1978.

120. Wilder BJ, Bruni J: Mechanisms of action of antiepileptic drugs. In *Journal of Clinical Neuropharmacology.* Edited by HL Klawans. New York, Raven Press (in press).

121. Simonsen N, Olsen PZ, Kuhl V, et al: A comparative controlled study between carbamazepine and diphenylhydantoin in psychomotor epilepsy. Epilepsia 17:169–176, 1976.

122. Sharvon SD, Reynolds EH: Unnecessary polypharmacy for epilepsy. Br Med J 2:1635–1637, 1977.

123. Simon D, Penry JK: Sodium di-n-propylacetate (DPA) in the treatment of epilepsy. Epilepsia 16:549–573, 1975.

124. Pinder RM, Brodgen RN, Speight TM, et al: Sodium valproate: a review of its pharmacological properties and therapeutic efficacy in epilepsy. Drugs 13:81–123, 1977.

125. Villarreal HJ, Wilder BJ, Bauman AW, et al: Effect of valproic acid on spike and wave discharges in patients with absence seizures. Neurology 28:886–891, 1978.

126. Jeavons PM, Clark JE, Maheshwari MC: Treatment of generalized epilepsies of childhood and adolescence with sodium valproate (Epilim). Dev Med Child Neurol 19:9–25, 1977.

127. Lacy JR, Penry JK: *Infantile Spasms.* New York, Raven Press, 1976.

128. Livingston S: *Comprehensive Management of Epilepsy in Infancy Childhood, and Adolescence.* Springfield IL, Charles C Thomas, 1972.

129. Lombroso CT: Seizures in the newborn period. In: *Handbook of Clinical Neurology.* Edited by RJ Vinken and GW Bruyn. Amsterdam, North-Holland, 1974, 15:189–218.

130. Volpe JJ: Neonatal seizures. Clin Perinatol 4:43–63, 1977.

131. Lennox–Buchtal MA: A summing up: clinical session. In: *Brain Dysfunction in Infantile Febrile Convulsions.* Edited by MAB Brazier, and F. Coceani. New York, Raven Press, 1976, pp. 327–351.

132. Faero O, Kastrup KW, Neilson EL, et al: Successful prophylaxis of febrile convulsions with phenobarbital. Epilepsia 13:279–285, 1972.

133. Heckmatt JZ, Houston AB, Clow DJ, et al: Failure of phenobarbitone to prevent febrile convulsions. Br Med J 1:559–561, 1976.

134. Wolf SM, Carr A, David DC, et al: The value of phenobarbital in the child who has a single febrile seizure: a controlled prospective study. Pediatrics 59:378–385, 1977.

135. Bower B: The treatment of epilepsy in children. Br J Hosp Med 19:8–19, 1978.

136. Gellis SS: *The Year Book of Pediatrics.* Year Book Medical Pub

137. Oxbury, JM and Whitty CM: Causes and consequences of status epilepticus in adults. Brain 94:733–744, 1971.

138. Aicardi J, Chevrie JJ: Convulsive status epilepticus in infants and children. A study of 239 cases. Epilepsia 11:187–197, 1971.

139. Wilder BJ, Ramsay RE, Willmore LJ, et al: Efficacy of intravenous phenytoin in the treatment of status epilepticus: kinetics of central nervous system penetration. Ann Neurol 18:513–525, 1977.

140. Lombroso CT: Treatment of status epilepticus with diazepam. Neurology 16:629–634, 1966.

141. Duffy FH, Lombroso CT: Treatment of status epilepticus. In: *Clinical Neuropharmacology,* vol. 3. Edited by HL Klawans. New York, Raven Press, 1978, pp. 51–55.

142. Bernhard CG, Bohm E: Local Anesthetics as Anticonvulsants. Uppsala, Almgvsit and Wicksell, 1965.

143. Khalid MS, Schulz H: The treatment and management of emergency status epilepticus. Epilepsia 17:73–76, 1976.

144. Victor M, Brausch J: The role of abstinence in the genesis of alcoholic epilepsy. Epilepsia 8:1–20, 1967.

145. Victor M, Adams RD: The effect of alcohol on the nervous system. Res Publ Assoc Res Nerv Ment Dis 32:526–573, 1953.

146. Sellers EM, Kalant H: Alcohol intoxication and withdrawal. N Engl J Med 294:757–762, 1976.

147. Booker HE: Idiosyncratic reactions to the antiepileptic drugs. Epilepsia 16:171–181, 1975.

148. Hofman WW: Cerebellar lesions after parenteral Dilantin administration. Neurology 8:210–214, 1958.

149. Utterback RA, Ojeman R, Malek J: Parenchymatous cerebellar degeneration with Dilantin intoxication. J Neuropathol Exp Neurol 17:516–519, 1958.

150. Haberland C: Cerebellar degeneration with clinical manifestation in chronic epileptic patients. (Liepz) Psychiatr Clin 143:29–44, 1962.

151. Snider RS, Del Cerro M: Drug-induced dendrite sprouts on Purkinje cells in the adult cerebellum. Exp Neurol 17:466–480, 1967.

152. Dam M: Number of Purkinje cells in patients with grand mal epilepsy treated with diphenylhydantoin. Epilepsia 11:313–320, 1970.

153. Ghatak NR, Santoso RA, McKinney WM: Cerebellar degeneration following long term phenytoin therapy. Neurology 26:818–820, 1976.

154. Rapport RL, Shaw CM: Phenytoin-related cerebellar degeneration without seizures. Ann Neurol 2:437–439, 1977.

155. Salcman M, Defendini R, Correll J, et al: Neuropathological changes in cerebellar biopsies of epileptic patients. Ann Neurol 3:2–9, 1978.

156. Glaser GH: Diphenylhydantoin: toxicity. In: *Antiepileptic Drugs.* Edited by DM Woodbury, JK Penry, and RP Schmidt. New York, Raven Press, 1972, pp. 219–226.

157. Lovelace RA, Horwitz SJ: Peripheral neuropathy in long-term diphenylhydantoin therapy. Arch Neurol 18:69–77, 1968.

158. Birkit-Smith E, Krogh E: Motor nerve conduction velocity during diphenylhydantoin intoxication. Acta Neurol Scand 47:265–271, 1973.

159. Eisen AA, Woods JF, Sherwin AL: Peripheral nerve function in long term therapy with diphenylhydantoin. Neurology 24:411–417, 1974.

160. Dobkin BH: Reversible subacute peripheral neuropathy induced by phenytoin. Arch Neurol 34:189–190, 1977.

161. Solomon GE, Hilgartner MH, Kutt H: Coagulation defects caused by diphenylhydantoin. Neurology 22:1165–1171, 1972.

162. Solomon GE, Hilgartner MH, Kutt H: Phenobarbital-induced coagulation defects in cats. Neurology 24:920–924, 1974.

163. Evans AR, Forrester RM, Discombe C: Neonatal hemorrhage following maternal anticonvulsant therapy. Lancet 1:517–518, 1970.

164. Kohler HG: Hemorrhage in the newborn of epileptic mothers. Lancet 1:267, 1966.

165. Mountain KR, Kirsh J, Gallus AS: Neonatal coagulation defects due to anticonvulsant drug treatment in pregnancy. Lancet 1:265–268, 1970.

166. Bjornberg A, Holst R: Generalized lymphadenopathy as a drug reaction to hydantoin. Acta Neurol Scand 43:399–402, 1967.

167. Charlton MH, Lunsford D: The role of diphenylhydantoin in the causation of malignant lymphoma. Minerva Med 62:43, 1971.

168. Anthony JJ: Malignant lymphoma associated with hydantoin drugs. Arch Neurol 22:450–454, 1970.

169. Sorrell TC, Forbes IJ, Burness FR, et al: Depression of immunologic function in patients treated with phenytoin sodium (sodium diphenylhydantoin). Lancet 2:1233–1235, 1971.

170. Lukes RJ, Tindle BH: Immunoblastic lymphadenopathy: a hyperimmune entity resembling Hodgkin's disease. N Engl J Med 292:1–8, 1975.

171. Salvin BN, Fenton GM, Laundy M, et al: Serum immunoglobulins in epilepsy. J Neurol Sci 23:353–357, 1974.

172. Pisciotta AV: Carbamazepine: hematologic toxicity. In: *Complex Partial Seizures and Their Treatment.* Edited by DD Daly and JK Penry. New York, Raven Press, 1978, pp. 355–368.

173. Yunis AA, Arimura BK, Lutcher CL, et al: Biochemical lesion in Dilantin-induced erythroid aplasia. Blood 30:587–600, 1967.

174. Reynolds EH: Anticonvulsants, folic acid and epilepsy. Lancet 1:1276–1378, 1973.

175. Hahn TJ, Hendin CR, Scharp CR, et al: Effect of chronic anticonvulsant therapy on serum 25-hydroxycholecalciferol levels in adults. N Engl J Med 287:900–904, 1972.

176. Harris M, Jenkins MV, Wills MR: Phenytoin inhibition of parathyroid hormone induced bone resorption in vitro. J Pharmacol 50:405–408, 1974.

177. Borgstedt AD, Bryson MF, Young LW, et al: Long-term administration of antiepileptic drugs and the development of rickets. J Pediatr 81:9–15, 1972.

178. Christiansen CP, Rodbro P, Lund M: Incidence of anticonvulsant osteomalacia and effect of vitamin D: controlled therapeutic trial. Br Med J 4:695–701, 1973.

179. DeLuca K, Masotti RE, Partington MW: Altered calcium metabolism due to anticonvulsant drugs. Dev Med Child Neurol 14:318–321, 1972.

180. Mosekilde L, Melsen F: Anticonvulsant osteomalacia determined by quantitative analysis of bone changes. Population study and possible risk factors. Acta Med Scand 199:349–355, 1976.

181. Levin SR, Booker J Jr, Smith DF, et al: Inhibition of insulin secretion by diphenylhydantoin in the isolated perfused pancreas. J Clin Endocr Metab 30:400–401, 1970.

182. Charib H, Munoz JM: Endocrine manifestations of diphenylhydantoin therapy. Metabolism 23:515–524, 1974.

183. Cantu RC, Schwab RS: Ceruloplasmin rise and protein-bound iodine fall in human serum during diphenylhydantoin (Dilantin) administration. Trans Am Neurol Assoc 91:201–203, 1966.

184. DiSalle E, Pacifici GM, Morselli PL: Studies on plasma binding of carbamazepine. Pharmacol Res Commun 6:193–202, 1974.

185. Fichsel H: Effect of anticonvulsant drugs on thyroid hormones in epileptic children. Epilepsia 19:111–112, 1978.

186. Plaa GL: Acute toxicity of antiepileptic drugs. Epilepsia 16:183–191, 1975.

187. Reynolds EH: Chronic antiepileptic drug toxicity: a review. Epilepsia 16:319–352, 1975.

188. Wilder BJ: Anticonvulsant drug toxicity. In: *Clinical Neuropharmacology,* vol. 3. Edited by HL Klawans. New York, Raven Press, 1978, pp. 57–84.

189. Speidel BD, Meadow SR: Maternal epilepsy and abnormalities of the fetus and newborn. Lancet 2:839–843, 1972.

190. Janz D: Teratogenic risk of antiepileptic drugs. Epilepsia 16:159–169, 1975.

191. Fedrick J: Epilepsy and pregnancy: a report from the Oxford Record Linkage Study. Br Med J 2:442–448, 1973.

192. South T: Teratogenic effect of anticonvulsants. Lancet 2:1154, 1972.

193. Massey KM: Teratogenic effects of diphenylhydantoin sodium. J Oral Ther Pharmacol 2:380–385, 1966.

194. Miller JHD, Nevin NC: Congenital malformations and anticonvulsant drugs. Lancet 1:328, 1973.

195. Annegers JF, Elveback CR, Hauser WA, et al: Do anticonvulsants have a teratogenic effect? Arch Neurol 31:364–373, 1974.

196. Bjerkedal T, Bahna L: The course and outcome of pregnancy in women with epilepsy. Acta Obstet Gynecol Scand 52:245–248, 1973.

197. Rutter M, Graham P, Yule W: *A Neuropsychiatric Study in Childhood.* Lavenham, Suffolk, Lavenham Press, 1970.

198. Guerrant J, Anderson WW, Fischer A, et al. (editors): *Personality in Epilepsy.* Charles C Thomas, Springfield, IL, 1962.

199. Small JG, Milstein V, Stevens JR: Are psychomotor epileptics different? Arch Neurol 7:187–294, 1962.

200. Gudmundsson G: Epilepsy in Iceland. Acta Neurol Scand [Suppl] 25:43, 1966.

201. Blumer D: Temporal lobe epilepsy and its psychiatric significance. In: *Psychiatric Aspects of Neurologic Disease.* Edited by DF Benson, D Blumer. New York, Grune and Stratton, 1975, pp. 171–197.

202. Rodin EA, Katz M, Lennox K: Differences between patients with temporal lobe seizures and those with other forms of epileptic attacks. Epilepsia 17:313–320, 1976.

203. McIntire M, Pritchard PB, Lombroso CT: Left and right temporal lobe epileptics: a controlled investigation of some psychological differences. Epilepsia 18:377–386, 1976.

204. Bear DM: Quantitative analysis of interictal behavior in temporal lobe epilepsy. Arch Neurol 34:454–467, 1977.

205. Scott DF: Psychiatric aspects of epilepsy. Br J Psychiatry 132:417–430, 1978.

206. Knox SJ: Epileptic automatisms and violence. Med Sci Law 8:96–104, 1968.

207. Fenton GW: Epilepsy and automatism. Br J Hosp Med 7:57–64, 1972.

208. Gunn J: Criminal behaviour and mental disorder. Br J Psychiatry 130:317–329, 1977.

209. Rodin EA: Psychiatric disorders associated with epilepsy. Psychiatr Clin North Am 1:101–115, 1978.

210. Taylor DC: Mental state and temporal lobe epilepsy: a correlative account of 100 patients treated surgically. Epilepsia 13:727–765, 1972.

211. Flor-Henry P: Ictal and interictal manifestations of epilepsy. Specific or nonspecific. Epilepsia 13:773–783, 1972.

212. Rodin E: *The Prognosis of Patients with Epilepsy.* Springfield, IL, Charles C Thomas, 1968.

213. Sigal M: Psychiatric aspects of temporal lobe epilepsy. J Nerv Ment Dis 163:348–351, 1976.

214. Holdsworth L, Whitemore K: A study of children with epilepsy attending ordinary school. Dev Med Child Neurol 16:746–750, 1974.

215. Scott DF: Psychiatric aspects of childhood and adolescent epilepsy. Practitioner 218:417–423, 1977.

216. Mostofsky DI: Behaviour therapy for seizure control. In: *Epilepsy. The Eighth International Symposium.* Edited by JK Penry. New York, Raven Press, 1977, pp. 239–243.

217. Hartlage L, Green J, Offutt L: Dependency in epileptic children. Epilepsia 13:27–30, 1972.

218. Baley C: Social prejudice and the adjustment of people with epilepsy. Epilepsia 13:33–45, 1972.

219. Bruens JH: Psychosis in epilepsy. In: *Handbook of Clinical Neurology*. Vol. 15. Edited by PJ Vinken and GW Bruyn. Amsterdam, North-Holland, 1974, pp. 593–610.

220. Fenton GW: Rehabilitation problems in people with epilepsy. Rehabilitation 96:15–21, 1976.

221. Van Buren JM, Ajome-Marsan C, Mutsuga N, et al: Surgery of temporal lobe epilepsy. In: *Advances in Neurology*, vol. 8. Edited by DP Purpura, JK Penry, RD Walter. New York, Raven Press, 1975, pp. 155–195.

222. Rasmussen T: The role of surgery in the treatment of focal epilepsy. Clin Neurosurg 16:288–314, 1969.

223. Falconer MA, Serafetinides EA: A follow-up study of surgery in temporal lobe epilepsy. J Neurol Neurosurg Psychiatry 26:154–165, 1963.

224. Cooper IS, Amin I, Gilman S: The effect of chronic cerebellar stimulation upon epilepsy in man. Trans Am Neurol Assoc 98:192–196, 1973.

225. Grabow JD, Ebersold MJ, Albers JW, et al: Cerebellar stimulation for the control of seizures. Mayo Clin Proc 49:759–774, 1974.

226. Van Buren JM, Wood JH, Oakley J, et al: Preliminary evaluation of cerebellar stimulation by double-blind stimulation and biological criteria in the treatment of epilepsy. J Neurosurg 48:407–416, 1978.

227. Purpura DP, Penry JK, Walter RD (editors): *Advances in Neurology,* vol. 3. New York, Raven Press, 1974.

12
Treatment of Head and Face Pain

Dewey K. Ziegler

Pain is the symptom responsible for most patient visits to health professionals, and the commonest sites of pain are the head and the low back region. When clear-cut diagnostic entities that cause pain (e.g., myocardial infarctions, acute abdomen) are excluded, diagnostic problems of painful conditions in these regions far outnumber other painful conditions. The 1962 classification of head and face pain devised by an ad hoc committee of the National Institute of Neurology Disease and Blindness (Table 1) (1) can still be used as a framework for discussion of treatment (this structure does have problems, which will be discussed later). In this review, face and head pain will be discussed in the order shown in Table 2.

NEURALGIAS

Trigeminal Neuralgia

Trigeminal neuralgia (tic douloureux) is a clinically well-defined syndrome. Pain is abrupt in onset, extremely severe, very brief in duration, (usually lasting less than a minute), and clearly localized to the distribution of the trigeminal nerve (face, anterior part of the scalp, mucous membranes of the nasal and oral cavities, jaw). Pain often is elicited by slight stimulus of touch, pressure to a point in the affected area (trigger point), or by chewing or even speaking.

In true trigeminal neuralgia, neurologic examination shows no abnormalities. If any neurologic deficit pointing to impaired function of the trigeminal nerve (depressed sensation of the face or cornea) is found, the physician must suspect pain that is symptomatic of a fixed lesion in the posterior fossa of the skull. Signs of cerebellar dysfunction or other neurologic signs carry the same meaning. Sharp facial pain occasionally occurs in other brain-stem lesions, such as multiple sclerosis, although never with a true trigger point.

The etiology of tic douloureux, as that of all neuralgias, remains unknown. Loeser et al. (2) postulate that there are probably multiple sites of abruptly altered decreases in axonal diameter along the trigeminal nerve. These sites

Table 1. Classification of Head and Face Pain

Vascular Headache of Migraine Type
Classic migraine
Common migraine
Cluster headache
Hemiplegic and ophthalmoplegic migraine
Lower-half headache
Muscle-Contraction Headache
Combined Headache (vascular and muscle-contraction)
Headache of Nasal Vasomotor Reaction
Headache of Delusional, Conversion, or Hypochondriacal states
Nonmigrainous Vascular Headaches
Traction headache
Headache from Overt Cranial Inflammation
Headache from Disease of Ocular, Aural, Nasal, and Sinus, Dental, or Other Cranial or Neck Structures
Cranial Neuritides
Cranial Neuralgias

SOURCE: The Ad Hoc Committee on Classification of Headache (composed of Drs. Arnole P. Friedman (chairman), Knox H. Finley, John R. Graham, E. Charles Kunkle, Adrian M. Ostfeld, and Harold G. Wolff): Classification of Headache. *Arch Neurol* 6:173–176, 1962. (Permission given from Dr. Arnold Friedman and Publishers of The Journal of the American Medical Association.)

produce "reflection" of the normal nerve impulse with reverberating impulses, resulting in a "repetitive barrage presented to the central terminals in response to a few afferent discharges from the peripheral receptor terminals" (2).

As in all problems, of pain, treatment must be considered under the rubric of immediate alleviation and prophylaxis. The neuralgias present a particular problem in that the brief character of the pain usually precludes immediate treatment; it is questionable whether regular administration of analgesics is of benefit. The use of analgesics will be discussed in more detail later.

The prophylactic treatment of choice for trigeminal neuralgia is carbamazepine. Although dosage must be tailored to the individual, the initial therapy should begin with 100 mg b.i.d. and be increased gradually over a few weeks to the effective dose, which is usually in the range of 600–1200 mg/day. The effect of the medication is often surprisingly abrupt. The patient discovers that the pain ceases at a specific dosage and recurs within a few hours if the dosage is decreased. Medication should be continued for several months before stepped reduction is attempted to determine whether spontaneous remission has occurred.

Minor side effects of carbamazepine at therapeutic levels are not uncommon and include sensations of dizziness, nausea, and, occasionally, drowsiness and confusion. The elderly are particularly susceptible to these central nervous system (CNS) effects, and the increments in dosage should be made with particular caution in these patients. Therapeutic drug levels should be maintained at 3–12μg/L. Sedative effects occur at toxic drug levels and, unlike phenytoin, are more prominent than ataxia.

The major risk with carbamazepine is the rare one of bone marrow suppres-

Table 2. Defined Entities of Face and Head Pain

Neuralgias of the Anterior Part of the Head and Face
Trigeminal neuralgia
Postherpetic neuralgia (cranial nerves V and VII)
Glossopharyngeal neuralgia
Greater occipital nerve neuralgia
Sphenopalatine (vidian) neuralgia
Atypical Facial Pain
Head Pain from Identifiable Lesions
Skull lesions
Intracranial lesions
Eye disease (corneal lesions, refractive error, orbital lesion, glaucoma)
Nasopharyngeal cavity disease (acute or chronic sinusitis, mucous membrane or other lesion)
Mandibular and dental disease (dental infection or disease, temporomandibular joint disease, malocclusion)
Systemic Disease
Hypertension
Temporal (giant-cell) arteritis
Disseminated lupus erythematosus
Cervical Spondylosis
Head Pain of Multiple Cause (migraine and muscle contraction)
Cluster Headache (migrainous neuralgia)

sion; fatal cases of agranulocytosis have occurred. Aplastic anemia occurred in four of 510 patients with trigeminal neuralgia treated with carbamazepine (3). This dreaded side effect has been reported only very rarely recently, and whether it occurs more frequently with multiple-drug regimens remains unknown. Patients taking carbamazepine must have an initial blood count, with the white cell count and differential count repeated at one-month intervals for three months and at three-month intervals as long as the patient is taking the drug. Unfortunately, discontinuance of the drug to eliminate leukopenia does not always reverse the bone marrow suppression. Patients should be informed of this rare complication and instructed to report any suspicious symptoms, such as sore throat, fever, or easy bleeding or bruising.

Rare cases of toxic hepatitis also have occurred with carbamazepine; therefore, screening tests for liver function should be done, with blood counts. The two most useful tests probably are measurements of serum and of glutamic oxaloacetic transaminase alkaline phosphatase. The drug also has antidiuretic activity. It sometimes produces electrolyte disturbances, which usually are asymptomatic, and it can produce water intoxication (4).

Before carbamazepine was in common use, phenytoin was used as prophylaxis against pain of trigeminal neuralgia. The latter was given in daily doses of 300–500 mg to achieve blood levels of 15–20 μgm/l. Its efficacy is much less consistent than that of carbamazepine. Phenytoin may be added to carbamazepine in patients whose condition is resistant to treatment. Although evidence is lacking, a combination of these drugs should provide further prophylaxis of the pain if their combined action is similar to that in seizures. Toxicity is manifested by ataxia, and the patient should be so informed. Occasional patients are allergic to phenytoin and respond with rash and/or fever. In such cases, the drug should be discontinued. There is a wide variety of other side effects, all of which are rare. They include lymphadenopathy, lupus-like syndrome, peripheral neuropathy, choreoathetotic movements. All are almost invariably reversible with discontinuance of the drug.

If it is demonstrated that the pain of trigeminal neuralgia is not prevented adequately by the drug treatments described above, neurosurgery should be recommended. A variety of surgical procedures for relief of this condition are in use. The more conventional procedures are subtemporal operations with partial sensory-root sections close to the ganglion, and a variety of ablative procedures on peripheral branches of the trigeminal nerve. Avulsion of the supraorbital, infraorbital, and inferior dental nerves, and alcohol injection of the supraorbital and infraorbital nerves are currently in use, and percutaneous electrocoagulation of the trigeminal rootlets by needle penetration of foramen ovale has recently been tried. Medullary tractotomy and decompression of the Gasserian ganglion also have been attempted and are now rarely used because pain eventually recurs. Jannetta (5) reported finding the nerve at the root-entry zone to be compressed and distorted by a variety of conditions—chiefly by anomalous position of the cerebellar artery—and reported relief by decompression of the offending vessel. Evaluation of the comparative efficacy and risks of the various procedures is beyond the scope of this review.

Probably the next most common well-defined neuralgia is postherpetic neuralgia. The herpes zoster virus attacks the cells of the sensory-root ganglion at any level of the neuraxis from the spinal cord to the trigeminal ganglion. The infection is signaled by a vesicular cutaneous eruption in the distribution of that nerve root. Typically only one root of the trigeminal ganglion is affected, and the eruption then appears in the appropriate portion of the face. The eruption is accompanied and followed by severe pain in the area of the eruption, and the pain may persist after the blisters disappear and scar. Any slight touch to the area is then exquisitely painful, although normal appreciation of a "sharp" stimulus is diminished. Occasionally, there is wasting of the muscles that are innervated by the segment whose sensory nerve is affected.

If the eruption is in the distribution of the first division of the trigeminal nerve (upper part of the face, eye and forehead) protection of the cornea from scarring is of paramount importance. If a lesion occurs on the cornea, the eye should be protected by a patch, and an ophthalmologist should be consulted. The use of an antiviral ointment five times a day is indicated. The two agents available for this purpose are vidarabine (Vira-A) and idoxuridine (Stoxil). Rarely, ophthalmoplegia and optic neuritis accompany herpes zoster of the first division of the trigeminal nerve.

Although postherpetic neuralgia responds to carbamazepine less consistently than does idiopathic neuralgia, the drug should be tried; phenytoin should be added as described above if there is no response. If drugs are ineffective, various types of counterstimulation of the skin may be beneficial. Mechanical stimulation to the scarred area with a vibrator has been reported effective (6). Relief of pain has been reported also with use of self-administered electrical stimulation to the skin of the affected area. A pulsed stimulus with voltage controlled by the patient is used in 15-minute treatments from two to 14 times a week (7). Repeated anesthesia of the skin with ethyl chloride spray over a period of weeks or months has been reported successful (8).

No type of surgery has been consistently effective for any extended period in patients with postherpetic neuralgia. In particular, sections of the posterior roots have been ineffective. Probably some central pain mechanism is established during the herpetic infection and cannot be destroyed by deafferentation procedures. On the other hand, electrical and mechanical stimulation may work by activating the central analgesic mechanism described in recent years.

Geniculate ganglion neuralgia, a variety of postherpetic neuralgia described by Ramsay-Hunt, occurs in herpes zoster that affects the ganglion of the seventh cranial nerve (9). The eruption is in the tragus, antihelix, and external meatus and, occasionally, on the drum head of the ear. Eruption sometimes appears on the soft palate and the anterior two-thirds of the tongue. Severe facial weakness on the side of the eruption occurs in all patients, usually after a latent period. Fortunately, the pain seems to be limited to the acute period, and postherpetic pain is rare.

Another, rare neuralgic pain, glossopharyngeal neuralgia, is localized to the posterior nasopharynx and oropharynx. It is precipitated by chewing, swallowing, or touching areas of the mucous membranes of the oropharynx. The entity usually is idiopathic but has been described rarely with intracranial vascular anomalies and tumors, multiple sclerosis, and anomalies of the base of the skull, such as Paget's disease. Several cases of cardiac arrest leading to syncope secondary to glossopharyngeal neuralgia have been reported; the syncope can be ameliorated by treatment with atropine and usually is cured by nerve section. Because of the rarity of this condition, experience with treatments has been limited. However, carbamazepine has been reported to give control (10). A variety of surgical procedures also have been utilized for this condition, usually avulsion of the nerve either in the neck or intracranially in the posterior fossa.

A less well-defined condition is greater occipital nerve neuralgia. The greater occipital nerve is formed primarily from the second cervical nerve root and supplies the posterior part of the scalp. Occasionally, a patient complains of severe lancinating posterior head pain, and tenderness is encountered on applying pressure over the inion, where the greater occipital nerve is relatively near the surface. Blocking the nerve at this point with local anesthetic has given temporary relief to some patients, and there have been reports of more prolonged relief by severance of the nerve. Unlike trigeminal neuralgia, however, there are almost never trigger points that produce pain from touch stimuli. Furthermore, the series reported suggest that it is difficult to isolate this syndrome from other types of intermittent posterior head pain, and controlled studies of the pain control have not been done.

Severe pain at the base of the nose that radiates into the orbital area, with signs of vasodilatation in the face, has been ascribed to neuralgia of the sphenopalatine ganglion or vidian nerve and has been called Sluder's neuralgia. This is a poorly defined entity, and its distinction from many forms of severe headache, notably migrainous neuralgia, is difficult if not impossible. The patients described did not have the brief, lancinating pains characteristic of other neuralgias. The diagnostic feature of the condition is said to be relief of pain by anesthesia of the sphenopalatine ganglion. The literature is sparse, however, and the entity is debatable (11).

ATYPICAL FACIAL PAIN

An unfortunate group of patients suffer from a poorly defined condition known as atypical facial neuralgia. Unlike trigeminal neuralgia, pain in this condition is long lasting and often continuous. It often is felt beyond the confines of the distribution of the trigeminal nerve, such as in the upper neck, into and behind the ear, or deep in the head. True trigger points are almost invariably absent. Onset occasionally follows known mandibular, dental, or nasopharyngeal disease; it is always mandatory to rule out lesions in these areas scrupulously.

A large percentage of patients with atypical facial pain have severe psychiatric disease. Depression is extremely common (12), and severe personality disorders with hypochondriacal and paranoid features frequently are present. Intermittent psychosis also has been described (13). The boundary between this condition and what has been called *chronic migrainous neuralgia* or *chronic cluster headache* is not clear. These patients rarely respond to carbamazepine. Some may be helped by tricyclic antidepressants or by tricyclic drugs in combination with substituted phenothiazines, as in the treatment of intractable pain elsewhere in the body. The use of chlorophenesin carbamate has been reported to be of some benefit (14). The psychiatric status of these patients must be watched carefully, and formal psychotherapy may be needed. Of all types of patients with head and face pain studied by Sweet (120), these patients were found to be the most resistant, and only one responded to any kind of nerve or vessel surgery.

HEAD PAIN CAUSED BY IDENTIFIABLE LESIONS

Face and head pain occasionally occur with localized diseases of the skull; in such cases, pain usually is clearly localized to the areas affected. Treatment is directed toward the primary disease. Rarely is intermittent headache characteristic of such disease processes. The same is true of headaches that accompany brain tumors.

Headache is often, but not always, a manifestation of increased intracranial pressure, whether caused by a mass or by the physiologic disturbance known as pseudotumor. There are few data on the frequency of relief of headache following relief of increased intracranial pressure. The pain itself probably is the result of stimuli to intracranial arterial walls and intracranial dura, and a reduction of intracranial pressure could well lead to sudden dilation of intracranial arteries, which in turn produces headache. Pain occurs with the occasional lesions that irritate the fifth or ninth cranial nerves. Some intracranial aneurysms produce this symptom, and severe head pain is part of Tolosa–Hunt syndrome, an intracranial granulomatous condition that causes ophthalmoplegia.

Pain is severe with many corneal lesions but is absent in many other ophthalmic diseases, such as glaucoma. Although "eye strain" probably is a poorly defined vague term in relation to headache, refractive error can lead to feelings of stress associated with the effort of reading, and sustained contraction of the neck and scalp muscles may result in pain. Correction of the refractive error can lead to amelioration of the headache.

Many lesions of the nasopharyngeal cavity produce head pain. Usually the pain is fairly well localized and is persistent rather than intermittent; the lesions can be visualized. Acute sinusitis produces severe aching in the face, but chronic sinusitis is markedly overdiagnosed as a cause for chronic or recurrent headache. Many of these patients probably have headache that is not related to sinus disease. Rarely should patients be given prolonged treatment for reduction of edema in sinus membranes as a treatment for recurrent or chronic headache. Patients can acquire an addiction resulting from ingestion of large amounts of antihistamine decongestant medications.

The pain of dental disease is well known, is almost invariably well localized, and often demands strong analgesia (to be discussed later). Disease of the temporomandibular joints is not a common cause of face pain and occurs occasionally in the course of arthritis. At present, many cases of head pain are ascribed to malocclusion, and extensive orodental repairs are being recommended. However, the connection of headache to this problem often is dubious.

SYSTEMIC DISEASE

Does relief of hypertension relieve the headache associated with that condition? Certainly hypertension is associated with headache to a most inconstant degree, although it does appear that the relation is clearer when diastolic pressure is very high or when pressure has been rising rapidly (15,16). Treatment of hypertension, of course, is of prime importance and often results in relief of headache. Severe headache with hypertension, however, is not an indication for emergency treatment, and *sudden* changes in blood pressure should not be sought merely because hypertension is present. It is inadvisable to prescribe ergotamine, a vasoconstrictor, to hypertensive patients.

The vasculitides are the disease processes associated most specifically with headache. Giant-cell or temporal arteritis is a disease of the elderly that is characterized almost without exception by palpable, usually tender, superficial temporal arteries, headache, and elevated sedimentation rate. A high index of suspicion for this disease should be maintained, since the arterial disease if left untreated, often attacks the retinal arteries and produces blindness. Treatment consists of adrenal steroid compounds. An average regimen is prednisone, 40–50 mg/day for several months. The dosage of prednisone should be lowered gradually several months after all symptoms of disease (headache, fever, tender temporal arteries) have subsided and the sedimentation rate has returned to normal. In one recent series, 26 of 63 patients were able to stop prednisone therapy after two years (17). In order to reduce side effects from steroids, alternate-day drug treatment has been proposed. This regimen, however, has been shown to control the disease much less effectively (18). With this long-term treatment, care must be taken to guard against the side effects of peptic ulceration by use of antacids, to prescribe low-sodium high-potassium diets, and to watch for evidence of confusion, psychosis, or osteoporosis.

Disseminated lupus erythematosus in its early stages is also commonly characterized by severe headache.

CERVICAL SPONDYLOSIS

Chronic intermittent pain caused by arthritic disease of the cervical spine is frequently referred to various parts of the head, characteristically to the midline of the occipital or frontal region. Pain may be caused by any type of lesion of the vertebrae or soft tissues, but chronic pain, particularly in the elderly, is usually the result of osteoarthritic disease. Such pain is commonly reproduced by neck movement or by maintenance of the neck immobile for extended periods, as during sleep. Sustained muscle contraction of paracervical muscles to prevent movement of the arthritic joints frequently occurs and also can produce pain. In addition to analgesics, treatment of this condition includes intermittent heat, massage of paracervical muscles, occasional immobilization of the neck with a soft collar, and muscle relaxants in moderate dosages. For example, diazepam, 5–10 mg, may be helpful, particularly at bedtime. Patients who habitually awaken with headache of this type may benefit from changing head posture when retiring; this can be accomplished, for example, with use of a supporting pillow to provide slight neck flexion.

HEAD PAIN OF MULTIPLE CAUSE, INTERMITTENT HEADACHE, AND MIGRAINE AND MUSCLE CONTRACTION

Among the substantial number of patients who are subject to recurrent headaches, relatively few demonstrate the specific etiologies of eye, ear, nose, throat, cervical spine, intracranial, or systemic disease. In the vast majority, these illnesses are either absent or inconsistently related to headache. Even when disease is known to be present, the degree of pain produced varies. Individual differences in threshold for pain may be one of many variables that determine which patient with cerebral neoplasm, for example, will develop headache. An analogy may be drawn to epilepsy, in which it has been shown that seizures following head trauma occur much more frequently in patients with a family history of seizures than in those without.

For the remaining patients who suffer from intermittent headache of unknown pathology, there seems to be a relatively huge number of variables associated with production of headache. It is this large population whose headache patterns are termed *common migraine, classic migraine, complicated migraine, muscle contraction headache* or *combined headache.* There is a large body of knowledge—biochemical, physiologic, genetic, psychological—about all these conditions, but there are few clues as to the sequence of the data with regard to the genesis of the headache.

In this review, I will take the somewhat unorthodox point of view that, from the standpoint of therapy, the severity of the symptom is more important than the diagnosis, for which the criteria are uncertain and controversial. There is increasing evidence that this categorization of headache syndromes implies knowledge that we do not have. Philips (19) has analyzed the clinical headache phenomena from a random sample of 1488 individuals and found that "there is little evidence for two discrete types of head pain," (i.e., migraine and muscle contraction). For example, approximately one-quarter of both men and women with tension headache had a single vascular symptom, and neither the site nor the time of occurrence sharply differentiated the headache types. Ziegler et al. (20) also found, with principal components factor analysis of headache symptoms, that characteristics of migraine did not cluster in one factor and those of tension in another (20). Bakal and Kaganov (21) found, as did Philips, on comparison of patients with either muscle-contraction or migraine headache, that the location of head pain was not specific to diagnostic groups. These investigators also found higher surface electromyographic (EMG) activity in scalp muscles in patients with migraine than in those with muscle-contraction headache; in fact, many of the latter patients had no more muscle contraction than did the controls. The indistinguishability of neck and scalp muscle contraction in migraine patients from that in patients with tension headache has been reported by other investigators as well, (22,23) who have suggested that the muscle spasm appears to be a consequence rather than the cause of headache.

In the following pages, therefore, the treatment of attack and prophylaxis of headache will be discussed in terms of severe headache and mild to moderate headache. Obviously many severe headaches could be designated as migraine, and many of the mild ones, as muscular-contraction.

TREATMENT OF MILD TO MODERATE HEADACHES OF UNKNOWN CAUSE

Rest and Mechanical Therapy

It is common knowledge that headaches often occur in the setting of excessive pressure, and brief periods of conscious relaxation often can alleviate such headaches significantly. It also is common for headaches to occur after periods of sustained emotional disturbance, with concomitant unrealized and involuntary contraction of neck and scalp muscles. Again, repeated periods of deliberate relaxation may be therapeutic (specific techniques will be discussed later).

With this type of headache, massage of the scalp or the neck muscles and the use of mechanical vibrators is often of striking benefit.

Pharmacologic Therapy

Certainly the standard analgesic that usually is used for mild headache is acetylsalicylic acid (aspirin), in general, 0.6 g every four hours until pain subsides is the optimal dose. There is little evidence to correlate pain relief with salicylate plasma levels of salicylate. Aspirin usually is innocuous, but regular ingestion of the drug may produce epigastric distress, gastrointestinal bleeding, and benign gastric ulcers. Large doses produce tinnitus, sweating, tachycardia, and tachypnea. Extremely toxic doses lead to hyperthermia, hyperventilation in acidosis, coma and death. Evidence for greater or quicker analgesic action with buffered aspirin is not convincing. Aspirin does inhibit platelet aggregation and therefore can prolong bleeding time.

Phenacetin and acetophenidin are used in patients who cannot tolerate salicylates; the usual dosage is 0.3–0.6 g every four hours. Ingestion of large amounts of these drugs causes methemoglobinemia and sulfhemoglobinemia, with cyanosis, dyspnea, and weakness. Phenacetin can also cause hemolytic anemia.

A large variety of mixtures containing aspirin, phenacetin, and caffeine are in common use for mild to moderate headaches. It has not been proved that these compounds are superior to aspirin alone, although many patients are convinced that they are. The danger of psychological dependence on these mixtures, is real and many persons take several of these tablets daily to "prevent" headaches. Such large doses of phenacetin have been cited to cause papillary necrosis of the kidney as well (24,25). The importance of warning patients of these dangers cannot be overemphasized.

Acetaminophen is also in extremely common use and is found in more than 200 formulations marketed for symptomatic relief of pain, cough, and colds in addition to headache. It is absorbed rapidly from the gastrointestinal tract and is metabolized by the liver; the metabolic products are excreted by the kidney. Comparable single doses of aspirin (600 mg.) and acetaminophen (1,000 mg.) studied in the setting of pain resulting from orthopedic surgery or unresectable cancer were reported to have produced statistically indistinguishable degrees of analgesia. Acetaminophen has the advantage of not causing gastric ulceration or prolongation of bleeding time. Large, toxic doses of acetaminophen, however, are hepatotoxic, and suicide attempts with the drug result in severe hepatitis. Myocardial damage, renal tubular necrosis, and hypoglycemia also can result from massive doses of acetaminophen. The onset of symptoms usually is gradual. If discovered early, overdosage with acetaminophen should be treated with activated charcoal to reduce absorption. The drug of choice for severe hepatotoxicity from acetaminophen poisoning is cysteamine (b-mercapto-ethylamine).

Indomethacin should never be used as analgesic for headache.

Psychotropic "Anxiolytic" Drugs

Few aspects of this subject are more difficult to address than the place of psychotropic drugs in the treatment of pain, and of headache in particular. It has come increasingly to the attention of the medical community in recent years, particularly since the studies of Beecher (26), that pain is the result of various amounts of two elements: (*1*) noxious stimuli to the body, and (*2*) emotional response to the stimuli and emotional state of the individual. What is evaluated as pain by the patient will vary markedly when either element is altered. Since it is generally assumed that many mild to moderate headaches are brought on and accompanied by emotional tension, it is reasonable to try to reduce the emotional tension, and therefore the CNS component of pain, with use of a combination of analgesics and sedatives. In common use are preparations containing aspirin, phenacetin, and a barbiturate. Several favorable reports appeared with the introduction of these compounds, (27–29), and there is little doubt that they ameliorate many episodes of headache. The psychotherapeutic effect of patient–doctor interaction, however, is powerful in this clinical problem, and use of placebo has been reported to result in 50% improvement.

One rationale for the use of these combination compounds has been that tension headaches derive from painful tension in neck and scalp muscles. The muscle relaxation that is thought to result from the action of barbiturates would lead to alleviation of pain. As noted earlier, however, recent studies have cast doubt on the consistent association between any particular variety of headache and such muscle contraction. It still is not certain that the muscle contraction causes the headache.

Other lines of evidence, however, indicate that headache, like other pain, is influenced markedly by centrally acting drugs. Diazepam, for instance, is commonly used as a tranquilizer. Although diazepam has had no influence on the threshold for experimentally induced pain or on the sensory discriminative component of pain (30), it has been clearly demonstrated to "affect the emotional–motivational component of the pain experience and thereby to reduce the aversive drive associated with continuing pain" (30–32).

For practical reasons, it is inadvisable to give a patient continuous anxiolytic medication for presumed frequent tension headaches. Strong psychological dependency on the medication results, and insomnia and increased CNS stimulation occasionally result after withdrawal from regularly used large amounts.

Prophylaxis

A variety of possible etiologic factors are encountered in the patients who are subject to episodic headaches, and although large numbers of factors are not encountered in any single case, it is wise to search for as many as possible. In patients who must read for long periods, occasionally unsuspected visual refractive errors are present, and the resultant visual strain may lead to sustained and eventually painful scalp and cervical muscle contractions. Similarly, certain occupations, such as those that necessitate prolonged bending over some apparatus, can lead to the same type of "muscle spasm."

It also seems probable that mild hypoglycemia can produce headache in predisposed persons. Such persons should not miss meals and should avoid excessive intake of carbohydrates. Loss of sleep is a provocative factor in certain individuals. Another possible etiologic factor is a daily regimen almost completely devoid of physical exercise, and regular exercise, such as walking, swimming, or calisthenics, is occasionally strikingly therapeutic. Ingestion of large amounts of coffee has become common in many workplaces, and cessation of the coffee habit has given rise to the entity of caffeine withdrawal headache.

Emotional stress probably is the most important of all environmental influences in the genesis of recurrent mild headache. Resolution of the patient's problems, be they financial, physical, or domestic, is often beyond the capabilities of the physician, but it is the physician's responsibility to at least become sufficiently well acquainted with the patient to form an intelligent judgment as to the degree of such stress and its importance in the symptom complex. For patients with evidence of depression, antidepressant drugs or hospitalization may be indicated, with due regard to the degree of suicidal risk with that individual. Often, regular medical visits with the concerned physician are therapeutic in unknown ways. It is a mistake to assume, however, that emotional stress causes all recurrent headache. Specific therapies designed to reduce various kinds of tension will be discussed later.

TREATMENT OF SEVERE HEADACHES

It was emphasized previously that pain is difficult to quantitate; therefore, it is somewhat artificial to recommend certain drugs for certain degrees of headache severity. The analgesics discussed earlier, of course, are often used in severe headache. Nevertheless, the following drugs should be used for extreme pain only and should be given to patients only occasionally and with strict limitations.

Analgesics

Codeine

Codeine is one of the most powerful oral analgesics. It is effective at doses of 30–65 mg and is even more effective when combined with aspirin. Its potential for addiction is low and causes little respiratory depression; however, it can produce nausea, vomiting, dizziness, and some sedation. Tolerance to the drug does develop.

Propoxyphene

The merits of propoxyphene (Darvon) have been debated widely, and the conclusion of Beaver may here be quoted. It is a

> mild oral analgesic which . . . is of questionable efficacy in doses lower than 65 mg. The drug is approximately ½ to ⅔ as potent as [codeine and] . . . in 32 mg to 65 mg doses is certainly no more and possibly less, effective than the usually used doses of aspirin or APC. [There is] a rational basis for the use of a combination of an antipyretic-analgesic, such as aspirin, with a narcotic-type analgesic, such as codeine or dextropropoxyphene, and several studies would indicate that such significant summation of analgesic effect does indeed occur (33,34).

Propoxyphene alone, then, does have analgesic properties; it also does not produce gastric ulceration or prolonged bleeding time, as does aspirin. Patients frequently abuse propoxyphene, however, and deaths have occurred from its ingestion to produce euphoria or other CNS effects. Overdosage with propoxyphene leads to rapid onset of symptoms that may fluctuate appreciably and lead abruptly to delirium, convulsions, and respiratory and cardiac depression (35). Regular use of large amounts of the drug (600–825 mg/day) can cause a slight but significant abstinence syndrome on withdrawal (36). The napsylate salt of propoxyphene (Darvon-N) has been introduced because it is less soluble and more stable than the hydrochloride and lacks convulsant properties. Therefore, it is considered to pose less danger in case of overdosage.

Pentacozine

Pentacozine is a benzyomorphine derivative that is said to lack potential for addiction. Halpern (36), however, states that addiction to the drug has occurred. Some patients have developed hypertension, tachycardia, nausea, and dizziness. An oral dose of 50 mg seems to be approximately equivalent to 60 mg codeine.

Oxycodone

Oxycodone is a synthetic analgesic that is marketed in a mixture with aspirin, phenacetin, and caffeine. The potency of 10–15 mg of the mixture is said to equal that of 120 mg codeine or 10 mg morphine. It clearly is a powerful analgesic drug with fewer side effects than morphine but with clear danger of addiction. Addiction to oxycodone has been observed with much greater frequency than addiction to codeine (36).

Ergotamine

Introduced as a possible therapeutic agent for migraine in 1926 and in general use for the past 30 years, ergotamine is still something of a puzzle in terms of effectiveness. It has a well-known vasoconstrictive action on the walls of arteries, demonstrated both in animals and humans. In a series of classic experiments, Wolff (118) and collaborators demonstrated that, in some migraine attacks, decreased pulsation of the superior temporal artery occurred before the attack (during phenomena suggestive of cerebral vasoconstriction) and that increased pulsation occurred at the time of, and presumably was partially the cause of, the migrainous pain. Ergotamine decreased the amplitude of these pulsations markedly, and this reduction presumably accounted for relief of the pain.

A mass of clinical literature has supported the use of ergotamine in migraine attacks. In 1936, O'Sullivan (37) conducted an uncontrolled study and found that subcutaneous ergotamine gave relief in 92% of migraine attacks, that oral ergotamine gave relief in 70% of attacks. In 1957, Friedman and Merritt (38) reported that in 1,644 patients with migraine, 80% were relieved with parenteral ergotamine and 50% were relieved with oral ergotamine. In a rare controlled study, Ostfeld (39) found that oral ergotamine, 5 mg, gave significantly greater benefit than placebo in migraine attacks. Selby and Lance reported (40) excellent response in 47% and good response in 34% of 263 patients with diagnosed migraine.

Other, more recent studies, however, have cast doubt on the specificity of ergotamine as therapy for migraine attacks. In a study of 88 women with migraine, Waters (41) reported no significant differences between use of 2–3 mg oral ergotamine and placebo. Hakkarainen et al. (42) reported no significant difference between ergotamine and the analgesic dextropropoxyphene in preventing migraine attacks in a trial of 525 acute attacks, dextropropoxyphene was superior to ergotamine in ameliorating attacks that did occur. Barrie et al. (43) studied the daily use of ergotamine as a prophylactic agent in a group of patients subject to recurrent headache. They found "no suggestion [that] the most classical of migrainous patients respond better, or worse, to ergot derivatives as used here, than the patients with mild bilateral headaches lacking characteristic migrainous features." Yet higher doses of all the ergot derivatives were significantly more effective than lower doses on the basis of reported severity of attacks (43).

Do these discrepant results aid in our judgment of the usefulness of ergotamine? It would seem that they bring into focus three issues: (*1*) the magnitude of the placebo effect, (*2*) the question of dosage of ergotamine, and (*3*) the problem of the susceptible headache syndrome. These specific issues are discussed below.

As to placebo, all controlled studies of therapy for headache have found strikingly high percentages of placebo benefit—from 50 to 75% (39,41,44). It is clear that uncontrolled studies of therapeutic agents for this symptom have little merit.

As to adequate dosage, in his negative report Waters (41) used 2–3 mg oral ergotamine, whereas Ostfeld used 5 mg. As noted above, the early literature cited the clear superiority of parenteral medication in alleviating the problem of drug absorption.

Only within recent years have techniques for measurement of blood levels drugs become available, and few studies have been done in this area. Meier and Schreier (45) found plasma levels of 1 mg/ml one hour after subjects ingested two tablets containing 2 mg ergotamine tartrate, 200 mg caffeine. Orton (46) found no ergotamine in the plasma of three patients at 60 to 75 minutes after ingestion of 2 mg ergotamine for an acute attack, and in only one of 13 patients who habitually took 1–8 mg ergotamine daily. It is not certain, however, that plasma levels of ergotamine completely reflect the biologic activity of the drug. For example, Eadie (47) has demonstrated that, after an initial rise, plasma levels rapidly fell to unmeasurable levels after intravenous (IV) injection of the drug, but that nausea and vomiting still occurred. In 1972, Eadie (47) also demonstrated minimal absorption of ergotamine from the buccal mucosa after patients retained the drug in the mouth. Sutherland et al. (48) confirmed this finding with use of ergotamine solutions. They concluded that probably only about .03 mg of ergotamine (of the 2.0 mg. in a sublingual tablet) might be expected to cross the buccal mucosa in five minutes (48). The conclusion is that therapy by this route results in ineffective plasma levels of drug. Caffeine facilitates gastric absorption of ergotamine, and a combination of the two agents may offer some advantages; caffeine also has some vasoconstrictive effect. Tablets containing caffeine and ergotamine usually contain 2 mg of the latter. A good trial regimen for the treatment of severe headache (migraine) is use of two caffeine–ergotamine tablets when pain reaches a high intensity. Additional tablets can be taken twice at 30-minute intervals, with care not to exceed four tablets in 24 hours or 12 tablets per week.

Nausea and emotional distress frequently are problems, and common ergotamine preparations in both oral and rectal forms contain belladonna alkaloids and a barbiturate, which aid in control of these symptoms. The possible problems from anticholinergic effects and sedation however, must be kept in mind. Unless a reliable patient is certain of the onset of severe headache, ergotamine should not be used before the pain is severe, since this habit may lead to overmedication. As already noted, absorption of the drug from the upper gastrointestinal mucosa is inconsistent; whether it is better from the rectum is unknown, but certainly in cases of severe nausea the suppository can be tried, either of ergotamine alone or with a sedative. Again, this should be taken with the recognition of the need for adequate dosage; 1 unit should be taken at the onset of severe pain and repeated in one-half hour if relief does not occur.

Failure of the effect of the drug by these routes may still mean lack of drug absorption, and trials should be made of the inhalation route. Presumably, the drug passes the pulmonary epithelium readily, but this benefit also raises the possibility of excess ergot effect. In a controlled trial, Crooks et al. (49) found that the therapeutic effect of inhaled ergotamine was significantly superior to placebo and sublingual administration in a controlled trial. In some patients, subcutaneous injection of 0.25–0.5 mg ergotamine tartrate is necessary and predictably therapeutic.

Concerning the usefulness of ergotamine in headache syndromes, despite its use for over 40 years, the specificity of ergotamine in migraine continues to be challenged. Although Lennox et al. (50) noted an absence of therapeutic effect of ergotamine in nonmigrainous headache, it is clear that migraine is far from a homogeneous entity. It is common for mild headaches to have some migrainous features (41,51), and, as noted, Barrie et al. (43) have noted a therapeutic effect of ergotamine in a wide range of headache types. It may well be that response to ergotamine, as Ostfeld postulated, is a better operational definition of a variety of headache than any other.

In summary, ergotamine probably is specific for certain cases of headache. When given parenterally, its effect is clearest; when given orally, large doses must be used. Because of the unknown amount of absorption, evaluation of the drug's effect is extremely difficult. Further studies should be carefully controlled in view of the repeated reports of placebo response in 50% of cases.

Even if ergotamine continues to prove efficacious in migraine, problems remain regarding the mechanism. The drug has alpha-adrenergic blocking properties, and its vasoactive action is amphoteric—that is, it causes vasoconstriction at low vascular resistance and vasodilation at high resistance. It also inhibits reuptake of neuronally liberated noradrenalin into storage sites.

The toxic effects of ergotamine have long been known; its cerebral manifestations were documented in medieval Europe, when massive poisonings occurred from the ingestion of rye contaminated with the fungus *Claviceps purpurea*. Overt ergotism usually produces vasospasm in the extremities, which may be prolonged and lead to gangrene. Ordinarily this results from prolonged use of large doses of ergotamine (more than 20 mg/week) but it has occurred with smaller doses (52–54). Persons with sepsis, preexisting vascular disease, hyperthyroidism, hepatitis, renal disease, or anemia may be abnormally sensitive to the drug (55). If ergotamine must be given to a pregnant woman, it should be given at small dosages.

The early symptoms of vascular insufficiency to the extremities are changes in skin color, pain (particularly on exertion), and weak or nonpalpable pulses. Several studies have documented angiographically the variation in the nature of the vasoconstriction in the arteries (56–60). Discontinuance of the drug and the use of antispasmodics, such as papaverine, usually reverse these early symptoms.

Vasoconstriction from ergotamine, while particularly dangerous in the arteries that supply skeletal muscle, also occurs in coronary arteries and can produce angina (61,62). In addition, ischemic neuropathy, presumably related to vascular obstruction at a site between the femoral and popliteal arteries, has been reported recently (63). Ergotism also has caused spasm of mesenteric and renal arteries (64, 65) and optic nerve papillitis presumably due to retinal ischemia (66).

Ergotism also affects the cerebral vessels and massive poisoning presumably accounted for the delirium, seizures, coma, and dementia in the ancient epidemics reported. It has been speculated that the "hysteria" epidemic that allegedly accounted for the phenomenon of witches in Salem, Massachusetts, was due to ergot intoxication (67). Several angiographic studies have shown vasoconstriction from ergotamine to occur in the carotid arteries, producing both focal neurologic signs and diffuse cerebral dysfunction (confusion) (68,69).

The relation between ingestion of ergot and symptoms of ergotism is sometimes difficult to establish (70). A paradoxic increase in headache has also been reported with excess ergotamine therapy; the mechanism of this effect is unknown (71).

The exact frequency of toxicity from ergotamine treatment also is unknown. Muscular blood flow decreased demonstrably in one series of patients who were taking large doses (72), and arterial blood pressure in the feet frequently was abnormal in another series and rose with discontinuance of the medication (73). In a recent series of 43 patients who were taking large weekly doses of ergotamine, 13 had cardiovascular symptoms and five had signs of peripheral neuropathy (presumably ischemia).

In summary, therapy with ergotamine is not innocuous and must be monitored. The prescribing physician must warn the patient of the symptoms of ergotism, be constantly alert to intercurrent disease, and avoid prescribing continuous ergot medication or excessive doses.

Other Drugs

The sympathomimetic agent isometheptene also has been reported to abort migraine attacks. The drug is available only in combination with acetaminophen and the relaxant-analgesic dichloralphenazine. One double-blind crossover trial found isometheptene to be superior to the ergotamine–caffeine combination in the treatment of headache; the former also caused less nausea and vomiting (74). Another double-blind study found treatment with the compound superior to placebo and the analgesic component of the pill with which it was combined (75).

Antiemetics and Tranquilizers

Nausea and vomiting frequently accompany severe headache. In addition to the discomfort they cause, these gastrointestinal disturbances effectively prevent absorption of drugs given orally. In choosing an antiemetic, preference should be given to an agent that has some tranquilizing properties, since the induction of emotional calm will reduce the patient's need for potent analgesics. Suppositories of some phenothiazines are often helpful and should be given in adequate amounts. For example, prochlorperazine may be given in a 25-mg suppository to an agitated, nauseated headache sufferer and may be repeated if needed in 45 minutes to one hour. If sleep can be induced, the patient often awakens with little or no headache. The antiemetic tranquilizers should be used liberally to obviate the demands of the patients for injectable opiates, which they soon discover are markedly effective but whose dangers are obvious.

Patients who are examined after having suffered severe headache with vomiting for hours or days usually require fluid and electrolyte replacement. After initial blood chemistries have been determined, IV fluids should be started with care to maintain appropriate electrolytes. A useful commonly used solution is 5%

dextrose in half-normal saline. An antiemetic and sedative agent, such as rectal or parenteral prochlorperazine, also must be given. During sedation, care must be taken to protect the patient from aspiration of vomitus; the patient should be kept in the lateral decubitus position.

Prophylaxis

Possibly of more importance than the treatment of the attack of severe headache is the attempt to decrease the frequency and severity of future attacks. Such treatment may be pharmacologic or nonpharmacologic.

Pharmacologic

Over the years, a large assortment of medications has been reported to be of benefit in preventing or alleviating the severity of severe episodic headache (migraine). The choice as to which of these agents will be discussed must be somewhat artibrary. The subsequent paragraphs will review the following: (*1*) beta-adrenergic blocking agents (propranolol); (*2*) serotonin antagonists (methysergide, cypropheptadine); (*3*) blockers of central vasomotor reflexes (clonidine); (*4*) tricyclic antidepressants (amitriptyline); and (*5*) vasodilators (papaverine).

Beta-adrenergic Blocking Agents. The only beta-adrenergic blocking agent approved for use in the United States is propranolol. The drug proved effective in the treatment of angina pectoris, but its mechanism of action is still uncertain. Propranolol also is effective in treatment of any rapid cardiac arrhythmia, symptoms of hypertrophic subaortic stenosis, and hypertension. In the course of antihypertensive therapy, its prophylactic effect against migraine was discovered serendipitously and its use for this purpose is now approved.

Several controlled studies have now confirmed the prophylactic effect of propranolol in many kinds of severe headache. Side effects have been minimal, although bradykinesia and a mild, usually asymptomatic, decrease in blood pressure occurs. There have been no studies contesting its usefulness in migraine.

Whether the prophylactic effect is due solely to the beta-adrenergic blocking action of the drug is unknown. Sjaasted and Stensrud (76) found that D-propranolol, which has only slight beta-blocking properties, also had a significant antimigraine action, although less than that of L-propranolol (Inderal). They suggest that other properties of propranolol may be at work (76).

Several beta-adrenergic blocking agents are available outside the United States, and the effect of one of them, prindolol, has been studied in migraine. Two studies have found it ineffective (76,77), and one found it effective (78). Why propranolol should be more effective than other beta-adrenergic blocking drugs remains an enigma.

The appropriate dosage for propranolol has not been studied systematically. In most studies, 120–160 mg/day has been administered in divided doses, but it has been pointed out that hepatic clearance of the drug "varies twentyfold between patients so that the relationship between oral dosage and plasma concentration is extremely variable. To achieve an effective plasma level the daily oral dose can vary from 40 to 800 mg or more" (79). There have been no studies of either the efficacy of high doses of propranolol in refractory cases or of correlations between plasma concentrations of propranolol and efficacy in treatment of migraines.

Use of propranolol is contraindicated in patients with asthma, severe bradycardia, and cardiac failure. Patients who are taking maintenance dosages of propranolol and receive epinephrine can develop bradycardia and an excessive pressor response. There is also some evidence of excessive vasoconstriction in some patients who take propranolol and who subsequently use ergotamine; therefore, the latter drug should be used with more caution in subjects taking propranolol. Side effects are uncommon. Orthostatic hypotension may occur, and occasional cases of cardiac failure (in the elderly) and mental depression have been reported. If the drug must be discontinued, withdrawal should be accomplished over a two-week period, since abrupt discontinuance of the drug in cardiac patients has resulted in angina and myocardial infarction; patients should be warned about this effect.

The issue of how long patients with severe headache should be maintained on propranolol has been studied infrequently and the same is true of other prophylactic drugs. Certainly patients should be weaned from the drug after several months.

Antiserotonin Agents. Sicuteri (79a) has speculated that serotonin might play a part in migraine because (*1*) ergotamine, the drug with the most specific antimigraine effect, has antiserotonin activity, and (*2*) depletion of body serotonin stores, such as by reserpine or parachlorophenylalanine, may induce pain and, in many persons, headache. On the basis of this evidence, he introduced the antiserotonin agent methysergide as a prophylactic agent against migraine and migrainous neuralgia. It has proved to be consistently effective and has been reported to give good or excellent results in 60–90% of patients in various series (80–81). The usual maintenance dosage is 6–8 mg/day in divided doses; this reduces both the frequency and severity of the headaches.

Unfortunately, side effects are common with methysergide. The less serious but annoying ones are nausea, dizziness, and "dreamy" states, which occur in about 7–25% of patients (82,83). Anthony et al. (78) believe all these side effects can be minimized by beginning treatment with a test dose of 1 mg, then increasing the dosage gradually to the required amount, and, finally, reducing it to the lowest effective level.

However, methysergide also has vasoconstrictive properties, and claudication or angina develops in a few patients. Graham (82) points out the extreme variability of this complication, with occasional patients showing vascular spasm on very small daily doses. He recommends that the drug not be given to persons who have "overt evidence of vascular disease, whether arterial or venous in origin and it should be used with caution and frequent supervision in patients in the older age groups and those with significant hypertension and other states. . . ." (82). Graham also urges reduction in amounts of ergotamine given to patients receiving methysergide.

When methysergide is administered continuously for long periods (more than four months), it can produce retroperitoneal, pleural, or cardiac valvular fibrosis. These complications are extremely rare and are almost invariably reversible with discontinuance of the medication. In order to avoid these complications, however, methysergide should be discontinued gradually after not more than four months of administration, and the patient should be given a "drug holiday." For cluster headache or migrainous neuralgia, for which methysergide is equally effective, the drug should be given only during the several weeks of the cluster itself.

The only other antiserotonin drug available is cyproheptadine. It also has been reported to relieve migraine, although in a smaller percentage of cases than methysergide (78,84,85). The drug also has some antihistaminic activity. Its side effect is drowsiness, but the vasoconstrictor action apparently is lacking.

Blockers of Central Vasomotor Reflexes. Clonidine causes a decrease in blood pressure, probably from depression of CNS centers that control autonomic function. The drug is thought to inhibit the vasomotor center of the medulla oblongata. It lowers peripheral vascular resistance and slows the heart rate by decreasing excitation of the postganglionic sympathetic axon of the cardiac nerves. At present, its major use is as an antihypertensive agent. The drug also has a vasoconstrictive effect on vascular smooth muscle, but the pressure response that reflects this action is brief and is not thought to occur with oral medication (86).

There have been a few studies of its success as a prophylactic agent against migraine in doses of 75–150 μg/day (87,88). One study, however, found its effect no superior to that of carbamazepine, which in turn had been found not to be superior to placebo (78).

Orthostatic hypertension can occur with clonidine. CNS depressants should not be administered concomitantly. Patients should be warned that abrupt discontinuance of clonidine may result in potentially dangerous hypertension.

Tricyclic Antidepressants. The tricyclic compounds used as antidepressants produce two neurotransmitter effects that could have an effect on migraine headaches. The drugs inhibit uptake of norepinephrine into nerve endings to varying degrees, presumably resulting in depletion of norepinephrine, and they inhibit uptake of serotonin by platelets, presumably resulting in depletion of serotonin. Amitriptyline, the amine most studied, has more effect on serotonin than on the norepinephrine system (89).

The usual dosage of amitriptyline has been 75–150 mg/day in divided doses; side effects are common unless the initial dose is low (25 mg) and then is raised gradually. For the first several days, the drug should be given only at times of sleep, and the patient often first notes some lessening of insomnia. The prophylactic effect against headache is reported in approximately 70% of cases.

The common side effects of amitriptyline are due to its anticholinergic actions and its CNS effects. Dryness of the mouth often occurs but is seldom troublesome. Occasionally, weakening of bladder contraction causes some urinary retention, particularly in men with prostatism. An occasional case of decreased potency is encountered. Sedation is the most common side effect; in many patients it is a transient disturbance, in others it is so troublesome as to prohibit use of the drug. Increased appetite with resultant weight gain is a common, often most unpleasant, side effect.

If patients receiving amitriptyline need for any reason to be given parenteral injections of one of the sympathomimetic amines levarterenol, epinephrine, or phenylephrine, these medications should be administered with great caution. Excessive pressor responses and, in the case of epinephrine, cardiac dysrhythmias, have been reported.

Is the prophylactic effect of amitriptyline on migraine related to its antidepressant action? It is of interest that in two studies (75,90), amitriptyline was reported to be of benefit in tension headaches, suggesting that the drug had primarily a psychotherapeutic action. Yet two of the recent studies on migraine have specifically noted the beneficial effect of the drug in patients who were not depressed (44,91).

Vasodilators. On the basis of the theory that vasoconstriction regularly precedes and is responsible for the vasodilation that produces the pain of migraine, vasodilators have been tried in patients with migraine. There have been two brief reports of the use of papaverine as a prophylactic agent in migraine. In an uncontrolled study, eighteen of 20 adults migraine that was refractory to other medications obtained relief with 150 mg papaverine b.i.d. (92). In a controlled study, 80% of children with migraine experienced excellent or good drug effect, as compared with 17% of placebo patients (93).

Nonpharmacologic Prophylaxis

Recent decades have seen the emergence of many varieties of nonpharmacologic prophylactic regimens for headaches. Some of these therapies have been alleged to be specific for tension or muscle-contraction headache, and some for migraine. Other studies have claimed success for chronic intractable headache, without specification of type.

These therapies can be divided into the following categories:

1. Voluntary raising of digital skin temperature. This therapy has been used with and without autogenic phrases (i.e., phrases that suggest relaxation and drowsiness). It has also been used with and without some type of feedback by which the muscle contraction is transformed into a signal that enables the subject to see or hear another signal that indicates success or failure (biofeedback).
2. Voluntary contraction of the superficial temporal artery.
3. Learning to control and enhance EEG alpha activity.
4. Voluntary relaxation of muscles, particularly of the neck and scalp. Such techniques also have been used with and without biofeedback.
5. Hypnosis, often used with hand-temperature biofeedback.
6. Behavioral self-management.

Voluntary Raising of Digital Skin Temperature. Enthusiasm for learning or conditioning therapies probably can be traced to the demonstration by Miller that experimental animals can be taught "control" over a wide variety of visceral functions with use of conditioning techniques (94). Clinical studies demonstrating some conditioning of cardiac functions, blood pressure, and seizure discharges in humans followed (95). In 1973, Sargent, and co-workers (96) reported on 28 patients with migraine or tension headache who were treated with a combination of autogenic phrases (suggesting relaxation and warmth of extremities) and feedback from digital skin temperature that the patient was attempting to raise. Twelve of 15 migraine patients and two of four tension headache patients reported improvement. The investigators found that the "majority" of patients could produce warmth in their hands in one to eight weeks (96). Mitch et al. (97) studied 20 migraine patients with roughly the same regimen as Sargent et al. and reported improvement in 65% of patients in two or more of the following areas: intensity of headache, frequency of headache, duration of headache, and amount of medication required. Blanchard and Young (95) cite two other anecdotal studies that have reported benefit to migraine patients with the same combination of techniques (98,99).

The same percentages of improvement have been reported with the technique of suggesting of increased digital temperature *without* the autogenic phrases. Turin and Johnson (100) claimed that all seven of their subjects learned the peripheral warming quickly and that all subjects showed significant decreases on three indices of migraine activity during warming. Reading and Mohr (101) reported a similar study in six migraine patients; biofeedback was used in the latter study but not in the Turin and Johnson study. Wickramasekera (102) also reported hand-warming alone to be therapeutic, with use of *neither* autogenic phrases nor biofeedback.

The most recent controlled study (103) of the effectiveness of the hand-warming treatment, however, contains surprising information. Migraine patients were *less* able to produce vasodilatation on demand than were control subjects; the results were more striking in the temporal artery than in digital arteries. Biofeedback had no significant advantage over relaxation treatment. The authors also point out that their results (with temporal artery volume) argue against the hypothesis that increased blood volume in the hand results in decreased blood volume in the head—the mechanism by which hand-warming presumably would be effective (103).

Voluntary Contraction of the Superficial Temporal Artery. There clearly has been considerable controversy over the rationale of a treatment for migraine that concentrates on the peripheral circulation. One study (104) has reported results in measurement of "pulse waves from the forehead recorded plethysmograph . . . directly above the temporal artery." Experimental subjects were given visual feedback from pulsation of the forehead skin and were notified that they would be trained to reduce the pulsation. Control patients were given analogous notification with respect to pulsation in the index finger. The experimental group demonstrated highly significant vasoconstriction in the extracranial arteries. In this very interesting study, both groups "seemed equally convinced at the end of training that they would be able to control their headache," but only the experimental group demonstrated a significant decrease in major migraine attacks.

In summary, numerous studies have reported success in patients with migraine using procedures whose common denominator is training patients to alter the caliber of an artery. The problem remains the evaluation of the placebo effect. Turin and Johnson (100) feel that they have overcome this problem by demonstrating that "hand cooling" suggestions led to no improvement in migraine, whereas hand-warming always did. Yet it is quite possible that the emotional implications of warmth are different from those of coolness and that suggestions of increased warmth inevitably carry suggestions of general relaxation.

Learning to Control and Enhance EEG Alpha Activity. It appears that only one report has dealt with the alleviation of headache by enhancement of alpha activity on EEG. The patient studied had severe headache resulting from head injuries and in some instances was allegedly able to prevent pain by going into a "high alpha state" (105).

Voluntary Relaxation of Muscles. Therapy for headache directed at relaxation of scalp and neck muscles derives support from a 1954 study that called attention to contraction of these muscles during tension and anxiety (106). In the 1960s, the Colorado group began to treat tension headaches by playing back surface recording over the allegedly contracted muscles so that patients could see or hear when they were achieving relaxation. In a 1973 report (107), six patients who received true feedback were compared with six who received pseudofeedback. The former group showed a significant reduction in headache and frontalis muscle activity. Correlation between weekly headache activity and of weekly frontalis activity on EMG for the whole period was found to be as high as +.90 for the experimental group. Another, recent, uncontrolled study (108) of 18 patients with "muscle tension headache or neck pain" reported marked decline in the mean "pain index" (an amalgam of frequency, duration, and intensity of headache) with use of EMG feedback. However, follow-up results showed the number of hours of pain to be only slightly fewer than during baseline value, with a decline in intensity.

How important is the specific biofeedback technique, and how specific is it to tension headache? Several studies have reported benefit to headache patients who used instruction in muscle relaxation (109,110) or muscle relaxation with transcendental meditation (111). As noted, Price and Tursky (103), in their study of digital vasodilatation and headache amelioration in response to biofeedback and to tape recorded teaching of relaxation, found that "there was no significant advantage for biofeedback over . . . a relaxation treatment" (103). Hay and Madders (109) reported on another mode of therapy for headache patients that consists of simple relaxation exercises as part of group therapy. Fifty-two percent of patients reported a decrease in frequency and severity of headache. This study was on migraine rather than tension headaches. A recent study (112) of 27 patients compared biofeedback of frontalis muscle activity with verbal instruction in relaxation and found no difference between the two in effectiveness; both were significantly better than a placebo, however, which was presented to the patient as a muscle relaxant.

Hypnosis. Other kinds of psychological treatment of severe headache also have yielded positive results. In a group of patients who were taught self-hypnosis as a prophylactic measure, 10 of 23 achieved complete remission during the last three months of the trial (113). Another interesting study compared biofeedback for hand warming, for EEG alpha enhancement, and training for self-hypnosis in 33 patients with migraine. All treatments showed significant and comparable reduction in occurrence of headaches (114).

Behavioral Self-Management. Mitchell and White (115), in the most recent of a series of papers, have reported a 73% reduction in frequency of migraine attacks in subjects who were taught problem analysis and appropriate control skills in self-management. The stated aim of the training is to minimize both the symptom-oriented approach and the dependence on a therapist; rather, the therapy stresses gaining techniques of self-knowledge, of discovering what is stressful for the individual, and of concentration on altering these patterns. This therapy, of course, assumes that migraine is almost invariably the result of an excessive or disordered response to environmental stress, an assumption that is far from proved.

How can the bewildering results of these nonpharmacologic therapies be summarized? Studies with a negative view of these methods are few, and it appears that relaxation instruction, EMG feedback, conditioning of hand-warming, conditioning of temporal-artery constriction, and behavior modification work. The evidence that distinguishes effectiveness of the techniques in migraine as opposed to muscle-contraction headache is sparse. An interesting study comparing the hypnotizability of migraine patients who were subjected to three treatment regimens—hand-warming, EEG alpha enhancement, and self-hypnosis—is relevant here. All three groups showed significant improvement, and there were no significant differences in improvement among any of the treatment groups. The "high hypnotizable" group, however, showed significantly greater improvement with all treatments than the "low hypnotizable" group. The conclusion was that the "more suggestible subjects are apt to respond favorably to treatment situations where they have high expectations of being helped than are low suggestible subjects, producing what is often referred to as the placebo effect. In short, the particular biofeedback treatments were not necessarily the relevant variables in producing these effects" (114). This statement is reminiscent of the study of vasodilatation by Price and Tursky: "First, and in the short run, digital, vasodilation (and presumably autonomic relaxation) can be produced by any treatment that has face value for a subject" (103).

With the evidence we have at present, we cannot conclude that any one of these training techniques is superior to another. It is clear that the careful attention of a therapist to the patient's problem is common to all and may account for a large part of the therapeutic effect despite attempts at control. On the other hand, a less nihilistic concept is that better division of patient populations can be devised. It is possible that specific profiles of symptoms and personality characteristics in headache-prone persons may be shown to be important factors in the response of patients to one of these therapies and not the others.

CLUSTER HEADACHE

There is controversy as to the relation of the syndrome known as cluster headache, or migrainous neuralgia, to migraine. Certain features seem to identify these patients and their illness—the occurrence predominantly in men, the nocturnal attacks, the brevity and severity of attacks, and the vasodilatation of the nose and sclera. One of the names of the syndrome ("clusters") refers to the tendency for attacks to occur with great frequency in limited periods. A variation of the syndrome that is without the characteristic of temporal clustering has also been described (chronic migrainous neuralgia).

Attacks of cluster headaches at times respond to ergotamine. The same regimen described earlier can be used. Of course, prophylaxis at the onset of a series of clusters should be sought, and methysergide has been effective for this in the dosage described earlier. A recent series (116) reported marked improvement in 53% of 77 patients who received 600–800 mg methysergide/day for cluster headache.

Recently, daily treatment with prednisone has been introduced as prophylactic treatment. One initial dose used was 60 mg/day, with the dose tapered over a period of several weeks (117). Unfortunately, headaches recurred in some patients when the steroid dosage fell below 15 mg/day. Alternate-day steroid treatment also has been reported to be of benefit. Cyproheptadine, an antiserotonin drug, has been tried in some patients, with cessation of cluster (118). The poorly defined chronic cluster headache has been reported to be markedly improved in several patients with use of lithium carbonate, 600 mg/day for seven days, and 900 mg for another 14 days (116).

In 1969 White and Sweet (119) reported results of surgery in patients with intractable cluster headache. Resection of the superficial temporal artery was reported to provide "striking relief" in three of 14 patients. The authors also reviewed the published evidence for benefit from section of the superficial petrosal nerve and reported their results with this procedure. In most patients headache recurred; in three of the original eight, long-lasting improvement was recorded (119). More recently Sweet (120) has reported relief of pain in four of eight patients with migrainous neuralgia with use of controlled thermocoagulation of the trigeminal ganglion and rootlets. It should be emphasized, however, that (*1*) the course of cluster headache is unpredictable, (*2*) there is a low rate of long-lasting improvement with these surgical procedures, and (*3*) the procedures have complications and markedly different rates of success in the hands of different surgeons.

REFERENCES

1. Ad Hoc Committee on Classification of Headache of National Institute of Neurological Diseases and Blindness: Classification of headache. In: *Handbook of Clinical Neurology*, vol. 5. Edited by PJ Vinken and GW Bruyn. Amsterdam, North-Holland, 1968.
2. Loeser JD, Calvin WH, Howe JF: Pathophysiology of trigeminal neuralgia. Clin Neurosurg 24:527–537, 1977.
3. Gaylord JJ, Redpath TH: The side-effects of carbamazepine. Proc R Soc Med 62:615–616, 1969.
4. Rado JP: Water intoxication during carbamazepine treatment. Br Med J 2:479, 1973.
5. Jannetta PJ: Treatment of trigeminal neuralgia by suboccipital and transtentorial cranial operations. Clin Neurosurg 24:538–549, 1976.
6. Russell WR, Espir MLE, Morganstern FS: Treatment of post-herpetic neuralgia. Lancet 1:242, 1957.
7. Nathan PW, Wall PD: Treatment of post-herpetic neuralgia by prolonged electric stimulation. Br Med J 3:645–647, 1974.

8. Taverner D: Alleviation of post-herpetic neuralgia. Lancet 2:671–673, 1960.
9. Boudreau JC, Oravec J, White TD, et al: Geniculate neuralgia and facial nerve sensory systems. Arch Otolaryngol 103:473–481, 1977.
10. Jamshidi A, Masroor MA: Glossopharyngeal neuralgia with cardiac syncope. Arch Intern Med 136:843–845, 1976.
11. Vail HH: Vidian neuralgia. Ann Otol Rhinol Laryngol 41:837–856, 1932.
12. Dalessio DJ: Some reflections on the etiologic role of depression in head pain. Headache 8:28–31, 1968.
13. Delaney JF: Atypical facial pain as a defense against psychosis. Am J Psychiatry 133:1151–1154, 1976.
14. Paulson GW: Atypical facial pain. Oral Surg 43:338–341, 1977.
15. Weiss NS: Relation of high blood pressure to headache, epistaxis, and selected other symptoms. N Engl J Med 287:631–633, 1972.
16. Badran RHA, Weir RJ, McGuiness JB: Hypertension and headache. Scott Med J 15:48–51, 1970.
17. Sorensen PS, Lorenzen I: Giant-cell arteritis, temporal arteritis and polymyalgia rheumatica: a retrospective study of 63 patients. Acta Med Scand 201:207–213, 1977.
18. Hunder GG, Sheps SG, Allen GL, et al: Daily and alternate-day corticosteroid regimens in treatment of giant cell arteritis: comparison in a prospective study. Ann Intern Med 82:613–615, 1975.
19. Philips C: Headache in general practice. Headache 16:322–329, 1977.
20. Ziegler DK, Hassanein R, Hassanein K: Headache syndromes suggested by factor analysis of symptom variables in a headache prone population. J Chronic Dis 25:353–363, 1972.
21. Bakal DA, Kaganov JA: Muscle contraction and migraine headache: a psychophysiologic comparison. Headache 17:208–215, 1977.
22. Pozniak-Patewicz E: 'Cephalgic' spasm of head and neck muscles. Headache 15:261–266, 1976.
23. Magora F, Magora A, Abramsky O, et al: An electromyographic investigation of the neck muscles in headache. Electromyogr Clin Neurophysiol 14:453–462, 1974.
24. Hutchinson HE, Jackson JM, Cassidy P: Phenacetin-induced haemolitic anaemia. Lancet 2:1022–1024, 1962.
25. Walton SB, Smith IB: Fatal nephritis in chronic phenacetin poisoning. Am J Med 28:127–134, 1960.
26. Beecher HK: Anxiety and pain. JAMA 209:1080, 1969.
27. Collins IS: 'Fiorinal' in the treatment of tension headache and other painful states associated with nervous tension. Med J Aust 2:448, 1968.
28. Sproule BC: 'Fiorinal' in the treatment of tension headache and other painful states associated with nervous tension. Med J Aust 1:739–740, 1968.
29. Monckton G: Drugs for headache of migrainous, vascular or muscular origin. Can Med Assoc J 91:175–176, 1964.
30. Hall GM, Whitwam JG, Morgan M: Effect of diazepam on experimentally induced pain thresholds. Br J Anaesth 46:50–53, 1974.
31. Chapman CR, Feather BW: Effects of diazepam on human pain tolerance and pain sensitivity. Psychosom Med 35:330–340, 1973.
32. Chapman CR: Some pitfalls in the psychophysical assessment of drug effects: another look at the effects of diazepam on pain thresholds. Br J Anaesth 47:640, 1975.
33. Beaver WT: Mild analgesics. I. A review of their clinical pharmacology. Am J Med Sci 250:577–604, 1965.
34. Beaver WT: Mild analgesics. II. A review of their clinical pharmacology. Am J Med Sci 251:576–599, 1966.
35. Carson DJL, Carson ED: Dextropropoxyphene poisoning. Br Med J 2:105–106, 1976.

36. Halpern LM: Analgesic drugs in the management of pain. Arch Surg 112:861–869, 1977.
37. O'Sullivan ME: Termination of one thousand attacks of migraine with ergotamine tartrate. JAMA 107:1208, 1936.
38. Friedman AP, Merritt HH: Treatment of headache. JAMA 163:1111, 1957.
39. Ostfeld AM: A study of migraine pharmacotherapy. Am J Med Sci 241:192–198, 1961.
40. Selby G, Lance JW: Observations on 500 cases of migraine and allied vascular headache. J Neurol Neurosurg Psychiatry 23:23–32, 1960.
41. Waters WE: Controlled clinical trial of ergotamine tartrate. Br Med J 2:325–327, 1970.
42. Hakkarainen H, Gustafsson B, Stockman O: A comparative trial of ergotamine tartrate, acetyl salicyclic acid and a dextropropoxyphene compound in acute migraine attacks. Headache 18:35–39, 1978.
43. Barrie MA, Fox WR, Weatherall M, et al: Analysis of symptoms of patients with headaches and their response to treatment with ergot derivatives. Q J Med 37:319–336, 1968.
44. Couch JR, Ziegler DK, Hassanein RS: Evaluation of amitriptyline in migraine prophylaxis. Trans Am Neurol Assoc 99:33–37, 1974.
45. Meier J, Schreier E: Human plasma levels of some anti-migraine drugs. Headache 16:96–104, 1976.
46. Orton D: Ergotamine tartrate levels using radioimmunoassay. In: *Current Concepts in Migraine Research.* Edited by R Green. New York, Raven Press, 1978, pp. 79–84.
47. Eadie MJ: The use of ergotamine in migraine. Med J Aust 2(suppl):26–29, 1972.
48. Sutherland JM, Hooper WD, Eadie MJ, et al: Buccal absorption or ergotamine. J Neurol Neurosurg Psychiatry 37:1116–1120, 1974.
49. Crooks J, Stephen SA, Brass W: Clinical trial of inhaled ergotamine tartrate in migraine. Br Med J 1:221–224, 1964.
50. Lennox WG, von Storch TJC, Solomon P: The effect of ergotamine tartrate on non-migrainous headaches. Am J Med Sci 192:57–61, 1936.
51. Ziegler DK: Tension headache. Med Clin North Am 62:495–505, 1978.
52. Enge I, Silvertssen E: Ergotism due to therapeutic doses of ergotamine. Am Heart J 70:665, 1965.
53. Diamant-Berger F, Pasticier A, Haas C, et al: Artériospasme généralisé sévère après dose thérapeutique minime d'ergotamine. Sem Hop Paris 48:3395–3399, 1972.
54. Cameron EA, French EB: St. Anthony's fire rekindled: gangrene due to therapeutic doses of ergotamine. Br Med J 2:28, 1960.
55. Katz AI, Massry SG: Arteriospasm after ergotamine tartrate in infectious hepatitis. Arch Intern Med 118:62–64, 1966.
56. Bagby RJ, Cooper RD: Angiography in ergotism. Report of two cases and review of the literature. AJR 116:179–186, 1972.
57. Yater WM, Cahill JA: Bilateral gangrene of feet due to ergotamine tartrate used for pruritis of jaundice. JAMA 106:1625–1631, 1936.
58. Pader E: Leriche syndrome in a patient with prolonged and continuous use of ergot derivatives. Vasc Dis 4:380–388, 1967.
59. Iuel J, Mune O: Peripheral arterial insufficiency in ergotism. Vasc Dis 4:159–166, 1967.
60. Tator CH, Heimbecker RO: Unilateral arm ischemia due to ergotamine tartrate. Can Med Assoc J 95:1319–1321, 1966.
61. Fagerberg S, Jorulf H, Sandberg CG: Ergotism, arteriospastic disease and recovery, studied angiographically. Acta Med Scand 182:769–772, 1967.
62. Wendkos MH: The anti-anginal effect of rapidly acting nitrates in subjects with ergot-induced angina. Am J Med Sci 253:39–43, 1967.
63. Perkin GD: Ischaemic lateral popliteal nerve palsy due to ergot intoxication. J Neurol Neurosurg Psychiatry 37:1389–1391, 1974.
64. Holmes G, Martin E, Tuba S: Mesenteric vascular occlusion in pregnancy: suspected ergot poisoning. Med J Aust 2:1009–1011, 1969.

65. Fedotin MS, Hartman C: Ergotamine poisoning producing renal artery spasm. N Engl J Med 283:518–520, 1970.

66. Gupta DR, Strobos RJ: Bilateral papillitis associated with Cafergot therapy. Neurology 22:793–797, 1972.

67. Caporael LR: Ergotism: the satan loosed in Salem? Convulsive ergotism may have been a physiological basis for the Salem witchcraft crisis in 1692. Science 192:21–26, 1976.

68. Brohult J, Forsberg O, Hellstrom R: Multiple arterial thrombosis after oral contraceptives and ergotamine. Acta Med Scand 181:453–456, 1967.

69. Richter AM, Banker VP: Carotid ergotism. Radiology 106:339–340, 1973.

70. Senter HJ, Lieberman AN, Pinto R: Cerebral manifestations of ergotism. Report of a case and review of the literature. Stroke 7:88–92, 1976.

71. Wainscott G, Volans G, Wilkinson M: Ergotamine-induced headaches. Br Med J 2:724, 1974.

72. Leinonen H, Hokkanen E, Waltimo O: Ergotism and muscular blood flow measured by the ^{133}Xe-clearance method (abstract). In: *Headache-76*. Joint Meeting of the Italian Headache and the Scandinavian Migraine Societies, Florence, June 2–3, 1976. Book of Abstracts (as referred to in article by Hokkanen, E., Waltimo, O., and Kallanranta, T.: Toxic Effects of Ergotamine Used for Migraine, Headache, 18:95–98, 1978, Reference #11). Pp. 19–20.

73. Dige-Petersen H, Lassen NA, Noer I, Tønnesen KH: Subclinical ergotism. Lancet 2:65–66, 1977.

74. Yuill GM, Swinburn WR, Liversedge LA: A double-blind crossover trial of isometheptene mucate compound and ergotamine in migraine. Br J Clin Pract 26:76–79, 1972.

75. Diamond S, Baltes BJ: Chronic tension headache treated with amitriptyline—a double-blind study. Headache 11:110–116, 1971.

76. Sjaasted O, Stensrud P: Clinical trial of a beta-receptor blocking agent (LB-46) in migraine prophylaxis. Acta Neurol Scand 48:124–128, 1972.

77. Ekbom K, Lundberg PO: Clinical trial of LB-46: an adrenergic beta-receptor blocking agent in migraine prophylaxis. Headache 12:15–17, 1972.

78. Anthony M, Lance JW, Somerville B: A comparative trial of prindolol, clonidine and carbamazepine in the interval therapy of migraine. Med J Aust 1:1343–1346, 1972.

79. Ahlquist R: Appraisal and reappraisal of cardiac therapy: present state of alpha and beta adrenergic drugs. III. Beta blocking agents. Am Heart J 93:117–120, 1977.

79a. Sicuteri F: Vasoneuractive substances and their implication in vascular pain. Res Clin Stud Headache 1:6–45, 1967.

80. Pedersen E, Moller CE: Methysergide in migraine prophylaxis. Clin Pharmacol Ther 7:520–526, 1966.

81. Shekelle RB, Ostfeld AM: Methysergide in the migraine syndrome. Clin Pharmacol Ther 5:201–204, 1964.

82. Graham JR: Methysergide for prevention of headache: experience in five hundred patients over three years. N Engl J Med 270:67–72, 1964.

83. Rooke ED, Rushton JG, Peters GA: Vasodilating headache: a suggested classification and results of prophylactic treatment with UML 491 (methysergide). Proc Mayo Clin 37:433–443, 1962.

84. Miller J, Fishman A: A serotonin antagonist in the treatment of allergic and allied disorders. Ann Allergy 19:164–171, 1961.

85. Curran DA, Lance JW: Clinical trial of methysergide and other preparations in the management of migraine. J Neurol Neurosurg Psychiatry 27:463–469, 1964.

86. Putnam P: Clonidine (Catapres): a new antihypertensive agent. Heart and Lung 5:457–460, 1976.

87. Shafar J, Tallett ER: Evaluation of clonidine in prophylaxis of migraine. Lancet 1:403–407, 1972.

88. Heathfield KWG, Raiman JD: The long-term management of migraine with clonidine. Practitioner 208:644, 1972.

89. Bopp B, Biel JH: Minireview: anti-depressant drugs. Life Sci 14:415–423, 1974.

90. Lance JW, Curran DA: Treatment of chronic tension headache. Lancet 1:1236–1239, 1964.

91. Gomersall JD, Stuart A: Amitriptyline in migraine prophylaxis: changes in pattern of attacks during a controlled clinical trial. J Neurol Neurosurg Psychiatry 36:684–690, 1973.

92. Poser CM: Papaverine in prophylactic treatment of migraine. Lancet 1:1290, 1974.

93. Sillanpaa M, Koponen M: Papaverine in the prophylaxis of migraine and other vascular headache in children. Acta Paediatr Scand 67:209–212, 1978.

94. Miller NE: Learning of visceral and glandular responses. Science 163:434–445, 1969.

95. Blanchard EB, Young LD: Self-control of cardiac functioning: a promise as yet unfulfilled. Psychol Bull 79:145–163, 1973.

96. Sargent JD, Walters ED, Green EE: Psychosomatic self-regulation of migraine headaches. In: *Seminars in Psychiatry*, vol. 5. Edited by L Birk. New York, Grune and Stratton, 1973, pp. 415–428.

97. Mitch PS, McGrady A, Iannone A: Autogenic feedback training in migraine: a treatment report. Headache 16:267–270, 1976.

98. Peper E: Biofeedback training: holistic and transpersonal frontiers. In: *Mind/Body Integration. Essential Readings in Biofeedback.* Edited by E Peper, S Ancoli, M Quinn. New York, Plenum Co., 1979, chap. 10, pp. 151–162.

99. Weinstock SA: A tentative procedure for the control of pain: Migraine and tension headaches. In: *Biofeedback and Self-Control 1972.* Edited by D Shapiro, TX Barber, LV DiCara, et al. Chicago, Aldine, 1972. Pp. 510–512.

100. Turin A, Johnson WG: Biofeedback therapy for migraine headaches. Arch Gen Psychiatry 33:517–519, 1976.

101. Reading C, Mohr PD: Biofeedback control of migraine: a pilot study. Br J Soc Clin Psychol 15:429–433, 1976.

102. Wickramasekera I: Temperature feedback for the control of migraine. J Behav Ther Exper Psychiat. 4:343–345, 1973.

103. Price KP, Tursky B: Vascular reactivity of migraineurs and non-migraineurs: a comparison of responses to self-control procedures. Headache 16:210–217, 1976.

104. Friar LR, Beatty J: Migraine: management by trained control of vasoconstriction. J Consult Clin Psychol 44:46–53, 1976.

105. Gannon L, Sternbach RA: Alpha enhancement as a treatment for pain: a case study. J Behav Ther & Exper Psychiat 2:209–213, 1971.

106. Sainsbury P, Gibson JF: Symptoms of anxiety and tension and accompanying physiological changes in the muscular system. J Neurol Neurosurg Psychiatry 17:216–224, 1954.

107. Budzynski TH, Stoyva JM, Adler CS, et al: EMG biofeedback and tension headache: a controlled outcome study. Psychosom Med 35:484–496, 1973.

108. Peck CL, Kraft GH: Electromyographic biofeedback for pain related to muscle tension: a study of tension headache, back and jaw pain. Arch Surg 112:889–895, 1977.

109. Hay KM, Madders J: Migraine treated by relaxation therapy. J R Coll Gen Pract 21:664–669, 1971.

110. Lutker ER: Treatment of migraine headaches by conditioned relaxation: a case study. Behav Ther 2:592–593, 1971.

111. Warner G, Lance JW: Relaxation therapy in migraine and chronic tension headache. Med J Aust 4:298–301, 1975.

112. Cox DJ, Freundlich A, Meyer RG: Differential effectiveness of electromyographic feedback, verbal relaxation instructions and medication placebo with tension headaches. J Consult Clin Psychol 43:892–898, 1975.

113. Anderson JAD, Basker MA, Dalton R: Migraine and hypnotherapy. Int J Clin Exp Hypn 23:48–58, 1975.

114. Andreychuk T, Skriver C: Hypnosis and biofeedback in the treatment of migraine headache. Int J Clin Exp Hypn 23:172–183, 1975.

115. Mitchell KR, White RG: Behavioral self-management: an application to the problem of migraine headaches. Behav Ther 8: 213–222, 1977.

116. Kudrow L: Comparative results of prednisone, methysergide and lithium therapy in cluster headache. In: *Current Concepts in Migraine Research.* Edited by R Green. New York, Raven Press, 1978, pp. 159–163.

117. Couch JR, Ziegler DK: Prednisone therapy for cluster headache. Headache 18:219–221, 1978.

118. Wolff HG: *Wolff's Headache and Other Head Pain.* Revised by DJ Dalessio. New York, Oxford University Press, 1972, pp. 348–353.

119. White JC, Sweet WH: *Pain and the Neurosurgeon: A Forty Year Experience.* Springfield, IL, Charles C Thomas, 1969, pp. 359–372.

120. Sweet WH: Controlled thermocoagulation of trigeminal ganglion and rootlets for differential destruction of pain fibers: facial pain other than trigeminal neuralgia. Clin Neurosurg 23:96–102, 1976.

13
Management of Back and Neck Pain

Charles Jablecki

There are many serious causes of back and neck pain, including primary and metastatic tumors to the vertebral spine, intraspinal tumors of nervous or leptomeningeal origin, and septic or aseptic inflammation of the leptomeninges, bone, or soft supporting tissues. More commonly, however, back and neck pain are related to stress or trauma to the muscles, ligaments, bones, intervertebral disks, and spinal nerve roots (1). The purpose of this chapter is to outline an approach to the management of acute and chronic back and neck pain that results from these causes.

ACUTE BACK AND NECK PAIN

Muscle Strain or Ligament Sprain

The sudden onset of back or neck pain may reflect muscle strain or ligament sprain after a hyperflexion-hyperextension injury of the neck, sudden extension of the back after prolonged lumbar flexion, or a sudden twisting movement of the neck or back. The pain is localized to the back or neck without radiation into the extremities, and there are no paresthesias, weakness, or reduction of deep-tendon reflexes to suggest spinal nerve or root damage. The spine movements may be quite limited by pain and paravertebral muscle spasm, and the muscles and bones may be tender to palpation. Plain radiographs, which should include anterior-posterior, lateral, and oblique views, are normal, with no evidence of fracture or displacement.

The principles of therapy are similar to those for treatment of muscle strain or ligament sprain in an extremity. First, the patient should be given bed rest to reduce movement of the painful area. If the pain is in the neck, sandbags should be positioned to limit neck and head motion. If the pain is in the thoracic or lumbosacral region, the patient should assume a comfortable reclining position. While in many cases the patient chooses the modified Trendelenburg position, with the back slightly elevated and the knees slightly flexed, some patients may find that lying in the lateral decubitus position is more comfortable. Generally, it is best to permit the patient to use the bathroom, since this is less stressful than attempting to use a bedpan.

Second, steps should be taken to reduce inflammation and promote healing. For the first two days after the onset of the pain, moist cold should be applied directly to the painful area. A moist towel containing crushed ice should be applied for a period of 10–20 minutes four to five times a day while the patient is awake. If local signs of damage (muscle spasm, percussion tenderness, limitation of spine movement by pain), persist for more than two days, then moist heat (hot towels) should be applied in a similar fashion. If the patient insists on remaining ambulatory because the symptoms are mild, relative immobilization of the neck may be achieved by using a soft cervical collar or dry towel folded lengthwise and wrapped around the neck. Relative immobilization of the lumbosacral spine may be obtained by using a corset. In both cases, the patient should be advised to lie down during the day as frequently as possible and to use moist cold or heat as noted above.

Third, patients at bed rest should be provided with adequate analgesics. Aspirin or acetaminophen, 650 mg, should be given every three to four hours and supplemented with codeine, 30–60 mg, or Percodan (oxycodone with aspirin, phenacetin, and caffeine) as needed while the patient is awake. Overuse of analgesics should be avoided both if the patient insists on remaining ambulatory and at night to permit the patient to detect pain and make reflex movements should they unconsciously assume a position that aggravates the injury.

Finally, after the initial discomfort has largely subsided, the patient may start a program of graded exercises to assist in strengthening extensor and flexor muscles of the spine and to increase the range of motion. This recommendation is analogous to the range-of-motion exercises encouraged in patients with inflammatory disorders of other joints to prevent fibrosis and subsequent painful limitation of motion. If the patient does not respond to the approach outlined above, the diagnosis of soft-tissue injury may be erroneous. On the other hand, the physician should be certain that the patient has in fact followed the course of therapy as outlined. The need for compliance should be emphasized to the patient at the initiation of treatment.

Soft-Disk Protrusion

An intervertebral disk protrusion should be suspected in patients who complain of sudden onset of neck or back pain with radicular signs or symptoms. Patients may complain of local neck or back pain that radiates into the shoulder, buttock, or limb and may be accompanied by paresthesias in a dermatome distribution. Both the pain and paresthesias usually worsen with a cough, sneeze, or spine movement. Soft-disk protrusion with consequent irritation of spinal roots may occur in the same stressful situations that cause muscle strain or ligament sprain. It often is possible to identify the affected root from the patient's description of the distribution of the paresthesias plus documentation of muscle weakness and changes in deep-tendon reflexes (Tables 1 and 2). Table 3 outlines a series of maneuvers that change the size of the neural foramen or stretch spinal nerve roots to duplicate, intensify, or relieve radicular pain (2–4). In performing these tests, the physician should be certain that the character and distribution of the pain coincide with the patient's complaints. Plain radiographs of the spine are either normal or show a narrowed disk space that corresponds to the presumed level of disk protrusion. Recently, it has been shown that computerized tomography of the spine can provide direct documentation of disk protrusion without the need for the invasive technique of myelography (5). Myelography, electromyography, (EMG) and nerve-conduction studies usually are not required in the initial phases of management unless the clinical diagnosis of radiculopathy is uncertain.

Patients with suspected cervical, thoracic, or lumbosacral disk protrusions should be treated with bed rest, moist cold followed by moist heat, and analgesics, as outlined for muscle and ligament injuries. In addition, after signs of local tissue damage resolve, a trial of gentle cervical traction for suspected cervical disk protrusion may be tried. In my experience, the best results of cervical traction are seen when response to the foramen compression test intensifies and gentle manual cervical traction gives transient relief of the radicular pain. It is essential that the initial cervical traction be performed under the direction of a qualified physiotherapist so that the optimal force (usually 10–20 pounds) and the direction of the force (usually but not necessarily vertical) can be determined. Cervical traction should be applied five to 10 minutes, three to four times a day. When the patient is not undergoing traction, neck movements should be limited with sandbags or a soft cervical collar if at bed rest or with a collar if ambulatory. Traction does not appear to play a role in the management of thoracic or lumbosacral disk protrusion other than to enforce bed rest. Since the position of pelvic traction may not be the most comfortable position for bed rest, pelvic traction is not recommended, since it may aggravate lumbosacral disk protrusion. Patients with lumbosacral disk protrusion should use crutches or a walker for support when arising to use the bathroom.

There may be some value in the use of systemic corticosteroids in the treatment of lumbosacral disk protrusion. If treatment with bed rest and moist cold followed by moist heat for 10 days does not result in significant improvement, a seven-day course of corticosteroids may produce prompt resolution of symptoms (6). Dexamethasone may be given intramuscularly in divided doses according to the following schedule: first day, 64 mg; second day, 32 mg; third day, 24 mg; fourth day, 12 mg; fifth through seventh day, 8 mg/day.

Williams (7) popularized the use of exercise during the period of bed rest to treat lumbosacral radiculopathies, and his flexion exercises bear his name. His recommendations were based on the assumption that these patients have exaggerated lordosis and that all disk protrusions are due to hyperextension injuries of the lumbosacral spine related to weak flexor muscles. The aim of his exercises is development of the muscles that are responsible for flexion of the lumbosacral spine and stretching of structures that are responsible for extension. However, lumbosacral radiculopathies may, in fact, worsen acutely with these maneuvers and therefore they are not recommended. Also, I believe that patients who derive some benefit from these flexion maneuvers are more likely to have low back pain caused by extensor muscle spasm and not by lumnosacral disk protrusion.

McKenzie (8) has described the more likely mechanism of lumbosacral disk

Table 1. Distribution of Symptoms and Signs of Cervical Root Damage

Root	*Pain*	*Paresthesias*	*Muscle Weakness*	*Depression of Stretch Reflexes*
C-5	Neck, shoulder, lateral arm just distal to elbow	Shoulder	Deltoid, infraspinatus	Biceps, brachioradialis
C-6	Neck, shoulder, scapula, posterolateral arm, radial aspect of forearm	Thumb and index finger	Biceps, brachioradialis, wrist extensors	Biceps, brachioradialis
C-7	Neck, shoulder, scapula, posterolateral arm, dorsal or volar surface of forearm	Middle and index fingers	Triceps	Triceps
C-8	Neck, shoulder, scapula, posteromedial arm, ulnar aspect, forearm	Little and ring fingers	All intrinsic hand muscles	Triceps or none

Table 2. Distribution of Symptoms and Signs of Lumbosacral Root Damage

Root	*Pain*	*Paresthesias*	*Muscle Weakness*	*Depression of Stretch Reflexes*
L-4	Posterolateral hip, anterior thigh	Anterior thigh, across patella, anterolateral aspect of leg	Quadriceps	Quadriceps
L-5	Posterolateral thigh, leg, across dorsum of foot	Lateral calf, dorsum of foot	Tibialis anterior, extensor hallucis longus, posterior tibial, gastrocnemius, gluteus medius	Internal hamstring
S-1	Posterior thigh, leg, into heel	Posterior calf, lateral and plantar aspects of foot	Intrinsic foot muscles, hamstrings, gastrocnemius, gluteus maximus	Gastrocnemius, external hamstring

Table 3. Tests for Radicular Pain

Test	*Description*
Cervical Foramen Compression Test	Narrowing of the cervical foramen is achieved by compression of the vertex of the head while the neck is hyperextended, laterally flexed, and rotated. Results are considered positive if the vertex pressure produces or aggravates the radicular pain.
Manual Cervical Traction Test	Widening of the cervical neural foramen is achieved by manual traction. With the patient sitting, and the head slightly bent, the examiner faces the patient and pulls up on the head with hands turned up and cradling the chin and occiput on each side. Results are considered positive if the radicular pain is relieved transiently by the maneuver. If results are positive, it is likely that cervical traction will be of benefit in the management of the patient's symptoms.
Chin–Chest Maneuver	Causes the spinal cord to ascend into the spinal canal. Ascension of the cord places the spinal-nerve roots under tension, particularly the thoracic and lumbosacral roots. If a nerve root is tethered close to its neural foramen, radicular pain will be induced by the maneuver. The test is best performed with the patient supine and relaxed. The examiner passively flexes the neck so that the chin rests on the chest. Results are considered positive if the maneuver produces or aggravates radicular pain in the thoracic or lumbosacral distribution.
Straight-Leg-Raising Test	Places the fifth lumbar and first sacral roots and the sciatic nerve under tension. The test is best performed with the patient supine and relaxed, with the head supported by a pillow. With the knee extended, the leg is raised passively by the examiner's hand under the calf. In order to eliminate hamstring tightness, the leg is slightly rotated internally and adducted as it is raised. The examiner makes note of the angle of elevation that causes the pain. Results are considered positive if the maneuver produces pain in the back or leg at an angle of less than 70°. In order to eliminate the possibility that the pain produced during the test is related to pathology of the hip or knee joint, the hip

Table 3. Tests for Radicular Pain

Test	*Description*
	and knee should be flexed and the hip rotated externally, a maneuver that moves both joints without stretching the sciatic nerve.
Femoral-Nerve Stretch Test	Places the second, third, and fourth lumbar roots and the femoral nerve under tension. The test is best performed with the patient resting in the prone position. The leg is flexed at the knee and slowly hyperextended at the hip. The examiner notes the distribution of the pain that is induced and the elevation of the knee when the pain occurs. Results are positive if the maneuver produces or aggravates the patient's radicular pain.

protrusion. He suggested that lumbar flexion probably predisposes the patient to lumbosacral disk protrusion by forcing the viscous nucleus of the disk posteriorly as the anterior interdisk space narrows. Posterolateral protrusion through a weakened annular ligament occurs during extension of the spine after prolonged flexion. In patients prone to recurrent lumbosacral disk protrusions, McKenzie noted that it frequently was possible to reproduce the radicular symptoms during an asymptomatic period by having the patients stoop forward (lumbar flexion) for a short time (20 minutes). In addition, it was possible to abolish the pain by gradually restoring lumbar extension. These observations provide the basis for a spinal-extension exercise that can be used to prevent lumbosacral disk protrusion during periods of overuse:

1. Eliminate flexion posture and decrease the frequency of flexion movements during daily activities, including sitting, standing, and lifting.
2. Improve the range of spine-extension movements with the "press up" exercise. To do a press-up, the subject first assumes a prone position. With the hands positioned on the floor next to the shoulders, the subject extends the arms to push the top half of the body up, while the pelvis and legs remain in contact with the floor. The exercise should be done 10 times during each session and repeated four to five times a day.

Theoretically, the exercises permit resolution of nuclear disk distortion with movement of the viscous nucleus anteriorly as the anterior interspace is widened with extension. Direct measurements of intervertebral disk pressures in cadavers and in vivo by Nachemson (9) support McKenzie's theory. Thus, the role of bed rest and the effectiveness of exercises in the treatment of lumbosacral radiculopathies caused by protruded disks may change as our understanding of the mechanics of disk protrusion increases. Currently guidelines are evolving to permit the selection of the best combination of rest and specific exercises to provide optimal nonoperative therapy on an individual basis. Until these guidelines are established, however, it is recommended that neither flexion nor extension exercises be used during acute episodes and that the mainstay of therapy remain bed rest with relative immobilization, moist cold followed by moist heat, and analgesics. With the help of a physiotherapist, a program of exercises may be chosen for use during asymptomatic periods so as to reduce the possibility of recurrent painful episodes.

When symptoms have been present for two to three weeks, EMG is often valuable in confirming the presence of the site of motor-nerve damage, especially if this is combined with needle examination of the paraspinal muscles, which both increases the diagnostic yield of the test and helps to exclude a plexus lesion (Table 4). Nerve-conduction studies, particularly of the median and ulnar nerve, may detect median neuropathy of the wrist or ulnar neuropathy in the cubital tunnel that is masquerading as cervical radiculopathy.

Resolution of soft-disk protrusion with relief of root irritation is manifested by a reduction in the severity and frequency of pain and paresthesias and by increased strength and reduced reflexes. If the patient shows signs of improvement over a week, it is reasonable to continue with the program. However, myelography and cerebrospinal fluid (CSF) examination and surgery should be considered in the following situations:

1. Development of signs or symptoms suggestive of myelopathy or compression of the cauda equina (spastic paresis, bladder or bowel incontinence, transverse sensory level).
2. Progression of radicular weakness over a period of days.
3. Persistence or worsening of radicular pain over a period of weeks.

Myelography before surgical exploration is an important step for several reasons. First, while it frequently is possible to identify the site of cervical disk protrusion on the basis of neurologic signs and symptoms (10), it is not possible to do so reliably in the lumbosacral area. This is because, although the nerve roots exit almost laterally in the cervical area, they travel longitudinally some distance in the lumbosacral area before they exit. Therefore, in the lumbosacral area, a disk protrusion may at L-5 to S-1 (and frequently does) cause neurologic signs and symptoms in the distribution of the first sacral root, even though this nerve root exits below the disk by the full height of a vertebral body. Second, intraspinal lesions other than disk protrusion, such as primary neoplasms of nerve or leptomeningeal origin and arteriovenous malformations, may be responsible for radicular signs and symptoms. It is important to identify the cause of the root damage as well as its location as accurately as possible before surgical exploration so that the appropriate surgical approach can be planned. Finally, CSF removed at the time of myelography should be cultured and analyzed for cells, protein, and glucose. Cytologic studies for malignant cells permit identification of meningeal carcinomatosis as the cause of radicular symptoms. A mild pleocytosis in association with a normal total protein concentration and elevated gamma globulin fraction, as seen in multiple sclerosis, may place an otherwise normal myelographic study in perspective. Lumbar puncture alone is not recommended before myelography and surgery in patients with suspected

Table 4. Incidence of EMG Abnormalities in Radiculopathies

Muscles	*Cervical*	*Lumbosacral*
Paraspinal only	4%	22%
Limb only	38%	22%
Limb and Paraspinal	19%	33%
None	39%	23%

SOURCE: Erik Strieb, Cleveland Clinic, (Cleveland, Ohio) 1979 (unpublished data).

disk protrusion because incomplete or complete block of CSF flow, if present, may worsen the neurologic condition after removal of the fluid.

If myelographic studies confirm the presence of a root lesion caused by soft-disk protrusion, surgical therapy should consist of laminectomy and foramenotomy, with removal of the protruded soft-disk fragment and the remaining disk material to prevent recurrence. The protruded lumbosacral disk should be approached posteriorly. A posterior or posterolateral approach may be used to remove a protruded thoracic disk. In the cervical area, if there are one or even two documented soft-disk protrusions, an anterior approach is recommended over a posterior approach because the former permits direct access to fragments of the disk that may compress the root or cord. If stabilization is needed, it is simpler to obtain a bony fusion from the anterior approach. In addition, the anterior approach allows much less trauma to the extensor neck muscles necessary for postoperative stabilization of the neck, resulting in a more rapid recovery.

The practice of injection of intervertebral disks with the proteolytic enzyme chymopapain has been uncertain in the United States since 1975, when the Food and Drug Administration declared a moratorium on the use of the drug for this purpose (11). Not only is there risk (about 1%) of allergic reaction to the enzyme (including anaphylaxis), but a double-blind cooperative study in the United States failed to show significant benefit from treatment with chymopapain enzyme as compared with treatment with the vehicle in which the enzyme is supplied (12).

CHRONIC BACK AND NECK PAIN

Back and neck pain may be classified as chronic if the patient suffers from recurrent episodes or continous pain over months to years. This pain usually is not caused by muscle strain, ligament sprain, or soft-disk protrusion; therefore, it is not likely to respond to therapy that is directed at these lesions. As with acute back and neck pain, chronic pain may be related to a variety of inflammatory, neoplastic, and congenital malformations (13). This section will address two conditions (spondylosis and spondylolisthesis) that can be diagnosed radiographically and a condition (facet-joint dysfunction) that can be diagnosed on the basis of history and clinical examination.

Spondylolysis

Spondylolysis (14) results from fracture of an intact vertebral neural arch, usually at L-5, that occurs shortly after birth. The fracture may remain asymptomatic, or local pain and tenderness may develop that worsen with weight bearing, movement, and lifting, subside with rest and recumbency. Radicular symptoms related to irritation of the lumbosacral root also may occur. On physical examination of the lumbosacral spine, the physician may document a step-like deformity between the vertebrae if slippage of the superior vertebral body forward has occurred (spondylolisthesis). Plain radiographs are diagnostic, and the oblique films are particularly valuable in documenting the defect of the pars interarticularis if slippage forward has not occurred yet.

During acute exacerbations of pain, the patient should follow the program outlined earlier for treatment of acute back pain (with or without radicular symptoms), since the exacerbation may be due to a superimposed soft-disk protrusion, muscle sprain, or ligament strain. If the radicular symptoms subside with this program, the patient frequently can minimize local pain both by wearing a corset to limit back motions while standing and by performing exercises to strengthen the paraspinal extensor muscles in order to compensate for spinal instability. Myelography and surgery should be considered if the patient has radicular signs and symptoms that fail to improve with nonoperative measures (as described for suspected soft-disk protrusions). Surgery should be considered if the patient has local pain that causes significant disability despite faithful adherence to a program of strengthening the extensor muscles and use of a corset for support. In both cases, myelography is recommended before surgery to determine whether there is concomitant disk protrusion that needs treatment concurrently with the spondylolisthesis. The operation of choice is posterior exploration with removal of the mobile fragment and decompression of the nerve root, followed by fusion of the sliding vertebral bodies.

Spondylosis

Soft-disk protrusions are a common cause of nerve root compression in middle age. Later in life, spondylotic changes are a more common cause of back or neck pain (1). Sondylosis results from a combination of degenerative and proliferative bone changes. These changes may compress spinal nerve roots or the spinal cord and cauda equina by narrowing the neural foramen or the spinal canal, respectively (15). Symptoms and signs, therefore, may be related to nerve root or spinal cord compression, or both. In addition, there usually is limitation of spine movement at the affected level. Narrowing of the spine in the lumbar area has been associated with the syndrome of pseudoclaudication, with weakness, paresthesias, and pain in the lower extremities on prolonged standing or walking (16). Plain radiographs of the affected spinal segment document the degenerative and proliferative changes and EMG may detect evidence of chronic root damage of motor nerves in muscles that are innervated by the damaged spinal cord segments.

The natural history of spondylosis is unpredictable (17). The condition may stablilize, show slight improvement, or progress rapidly. If progression occurs, particularly if signs of myelopathy develop, consideration should be given to surgical therapy. Again, myelography is recommended before surgery to document the extradural defects of spondylosis at multiple levels and to exclude an intradural lesion or superimposed soft-disk protrusion. Because the disease process has already fused the vertebral bodies, complete laminectomy and foramenotomy at multiple levels may be performed without fear of causing spinal instability. The patient should be informed before surgery that transient worsening of symptoms is common postoperatively and that the deficit that existed preoperatively may not improve. The principle reason for surgery is prevention of further progression. Nonoperative therapy of spondylosis usually is disappointing. Cervical traction often makes symptoms worse. A cervical collar and lumbosacral corset may be tried, but they often are of little value unless there is a superimposed soft-tissue injury. Occasionally, exercise under the guidance of a physiotherapist to improve the range of motion of joints helps.

Facet-Joint Dysfunction

There are two types of facet-joint dysfunction that affect the cervical and lumbosacral vertebrae (18). The first is painful hypomobility related to arthritic changes. The pain usually is localized to the low back or neck area and is exacerbated by movements that take place at the facet, such as tilting of the head or shoulders to the opposite side or rotation forward of the opposite shoulder or cheek. The pain is relieved quickly by rest. Radiographs of the affected joint show hyperostosis, and the EMG is normal. Initially, symptoms can be treated with immobilization, moist cold followed by moist heat, and analgesics, as in suspected muscle strains or ligament sprains. Subsequently, a program under the direction of a physiotherapist aimed at improvement of the range of motion of the affected facet with passive movements should be undertaken to prevent recurrent episodes.

Hypermobility of the facet joint also may be a cause of recurrent back or neck pain. Hypermobility may be a consequence of either lax ligaments or diffuse neuromuscular disease, such as muscular dystrophy or amyotrophic lateral sclerosis, in which there is weakness of the supporting paraspinal muscles. Typically, the patient complains of local back or neck pain with prolonged use, as in standing. Physical examination demonstrates a greater-than-normal range of motion of the affected facet, with pain at the extremes of motion. Radiographs of the affected hypermobile joint usually are normal, as is the EMG. Therapy should begin with fitting of a corset or soft collar to provide additional lumbosacral or cervical support. In addition, exercises to strengthen the extensor muscles are helpful, particularly if the underlying neuromuscular disease stabilizes.

SUMMARY

The more common causes of acute back and neck pain reflect the effect of mechanical stress on muscles, ligaments, intervertebral disks, and vertebral bones. The principles of therapy that are valuable in the treatment of soft-tissue injuries in the extremities can be applied to the care of spinal injuries. If these measures fail, there are surgical alternatives. Nonoperative measures usually are successful if the diagnosis is correct and if the patient complies with therapy. Chronic back pain may also be due to the effects of repeated stress on vertebral joints and bones, and the degenerative changes can be documented on radiographic examination. In these cases, therapy should be directed at support of weak structures and improvement of mobility of arthritic joints. If nonoperative therapy fails, surgical decompression of narrowing of the neural foramen or of the spinal canal frequently is necessary to relieve symptoms and to prevent progression of the condition.

REFERENCES

1. Kelsy JL: Epidemology of radiculopathies. In: *Advances in Neurology.* Edited by BS Schoenberg. New York, Raven Press, 1978, 18:385–398.
2. Spurling RG, Scoville WB: Lateral rupture of the cervical intervertebral discs. Surg Gynecol Obstet 78:350–358, 1944.
3. Mayo Clinic Staff: Clinical Examinations in Neurology. Philadelphia, WB Saunders, 1976.
4. Edgar MA, Park, WM: Induced pain patterns on passive straight-leg raising in lower lumber disk protrusion. J Bone Joint Surg 56B:658–667, 1974.
5. Meyer Ga, Haughton VM, Williams AL: Diagnosis of herniated lumbar disk with computerized tomography. N Engl J Med 301:1166, 1979.
6. Green LM: Dexamethasone in the management of symptoms due to herniated lumbar disk. J Neurol Neurosurg Psychiatry 38:1211–1217, 1975.
7. Williams PC: Examination and conservative treatment for disk lesions of the lower spine. Clin Orthop 5:28–39, 1955.
8. McKenzie RA: Prophylaxis in recurrent low back pain. NZ Med J 89:22–23, 1979.
9. Nachemson A: The load on lumbar disks in different positions of the body. Clin Orthop 45:107–122, 1966.
10. Yoss RE, Corbin KB, MacCarty CS, et al.: Significance of symptoms and signs in localization of involved root in cervical disk protrusion. Neurology 7:674–683, 1958.
11. Simpson P: Chymopapain: a case study in federal drug regulation. JAMA 240:195–219, 1978.
12. Schwetschenau PR, Ramirez A, Johnston J, et al.: Double-blind evaluation of interdiscal chymopapain for herniated lumbar disk. J Neurosurg 45:622–627, 1976.
13. Fearnside MR, Adams BT; Tumours of the cauda equina. J Neurol Neurosurg Psychiatry 41:24–31, 1978.
14. Adkins EWO: Spondylolisthesis. J Bone Joint Surg 37B:48–62, 1955.
15. Wilkinson M: The morbid anatomy of cervical spondylosis and myelopathy. Brain 83:589–610, 1960.
16. Blau JN, Logue V: The natural history of intermittent claudication of the cauda equina. Brain 101:211–222, 1978.
17. Pallis C, Jones AM, Spillane JD: Cervical spondylosis. Brain 77:274–289, 1954.
18. Mooney V, Robertson J: The facet syndrome. Clin Ortho 115:144–156, 1976.

Index